Carpal Instability

Jeffrey Yao, MD

Editor

Carpal Instability

The Comprehensive Case-Based Approach

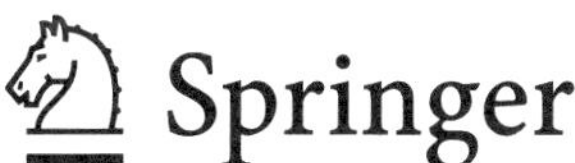
Springer

Editor
Jeffrey Yao, MD
Professor
Hand and Upper Limb Surgery
Department of Orthopedic Surgery
Stanford University
Stanford, CA, USA

ISBN 978-3-031-55871-9   ISBN 978-3-031-55869-6   (eBook)
https://doi.org/10.1007/978-3-031-55869-6

This Springer imprint is published by the registered company Springer Nature Switzerland AG
The registered company address is: Gewerbestrasse 11, 6330 Cham, Switzerland

If disposing of this product, please recycle the paper.

Acknowledgements

As we embarked upon this Comprehensive Casebook on Carpal Instability, I sought to draw on the massive collective international wisdom to assemble the most complete compilation of chapters dedicated to the topic of Carpal Instability. Thanks to our outstanding contributors I believe we have been successful in our quest.

I would like to thank all of our authors who put in countless hours of volunteer effort to share with all of us their expertise in each and every aspect of Carpal Instability. These chapters embody the mastery of the most distinguished experts from around the globe. For this, I and our readership are grateful.

I would also like to acknowledge and thank the incredibly organized and dedicated Springer publishing staff for shepherding us through the process of envisioning the work to its completion.

Last, I would be amiss without thanking my wonderful wife Jennifer and daughters Madeline and Isabella for their continued support of my academic pursuits and being forever understanding and supportive of my unceasing mission to educate.

I hope you enjoy this Casebook!

Jeffrey Yao, MD

Contents

Contributors

Joshua M. Abzug Department of Orthopaedics, University of Maryland School of Medicine, Baltimore, MD, USA

Marcio Aurelio Aita Centro Universitário FMABC (ABC Medical School) ABC Hand Center, Santo André, SP, Brazil

Ahlam Arnaout International Wrist Centers-Clinique du Poignet, Bizet Clinic, Paris, France

Vicente Carratalá Baixauli Hand Surgery Unit, Quironsalud Hospital Valencia, Valencia, Spain

M. Burnier Institut Main-Membre Supérieur, Villeurbanne, France

Matthew B. Burn Hand, Wrist, Elbow & Nerve Surgery, OrthoArkansas, Little Rock, AR, USA

Jack C. Casey Department of Orthopaedics, Alpert Medical School of Brown University & Medical University of South Carolina, Providence & Charleston, RI & SC, USA

Spencer B. Chambers BioSkills and Biomechanics Laboratory, Department of Orthopaedic Surgery, Emory University, Atlanta, GA, USA

Department of Plastic and Reconstructive Surgery, St. Joseph's Hand and Upper Limb Clinic, Western University, London, ON, Canada

Zheng Xu Cheng Wakefield Orthopaedic Clinic, and Centre of Orthopaedic and Trauma Research, University of Adelaide, Adelaide, SA, Australia

Devin W. Collins Florida Orthopedic Institute, Temple Terrace, FL, USA

Fernando Corella Orthopedic and Trauma Department, Hospital Universitario Infanta Leonor, Madrid, Spain

Orthopedic and Trauma Department, Hospital Universitario Quironsalud Madrid, Madrid, Spain

Surgery Department, School of Medicine, Universidad Complutense de Madrid, Madrid, Spain

Greg Couzens Queensland University of Technology: Brisbane Hand and Upper Limb Research Institute, Brisbane, QLD, Australia

Brisbane Hand and Upper Limb Research Institute, Queensland University of Technology, Brisbane, QLD, Australia

Leah R. F. Demetri, MD Department of Orthopedic Surgery, Brigham and Women's Hospital, Boston, MA, USA

Lauren E. Dittman Mayo Clinic, Rochester, MN, USA

Mireia Esplugas Institut Kaplan, Barcelona, Spain

Diego L. Fernandez University of Bern, Bern, Switzerland

Nathaniel Fogel, MD Department of Orthopaedic Surgery, Duke University, Durham, NC, USA

Margaret Woon Man Fok Department of Orthopaedics and Traumatology, Queen Mary Hospital, The University of Hong Kong, Pok Fu Lam, Hong Kong Special Adminstractive Region

John R. Fowler Department of Orthopedics, University of Pittsburgh Medical Center, Pittsburgh, PA, USA

James Tyler Frix Atrium Health Orthopedic Surgery, Charlotte, NC, USA

Marc García-Elías Institut Kaplan, Barcelona, Spain

Francisco Lucas García Hand Surgery Unit, Quironsalud Hospital Valencia, Valencia, Spain

Michael J. Garcia Florida Orthopedic Institute, Temple Terrace, FL, USA

R. Glenn Gaston OrthoCarolina Hand and Upper Extremity Department, Atrium Health Department of Orthopedic Surgery, Charlotte, NC, USA

Charles A. Goldfarb Department of Orthopaedic Surgery, Washington University, St. Louis, MO, USA

Warren C. Hammert Division of Hand Surgery, Department of Orthopaedic Surgery, Duke University Medical Center, Durham, NC, USA

Alex Han Department of Orthopedics & Sports Medicine, Houston Methodist Hospital, Houston, TX, USA

G. Herzberg Clinique Parc & Val Ouest, Lyon, France

Pak-Cheong Ho Department of Orthopaedic and Traumatology, Prince of Wales Hospital, Hong Kong SAR, China

Jerry I. Huang Department of Orthopaedics and Sports Medicine, University of Washington Medical Center, Seattle, WA, USA

Parker Johnsen Cooper University, Camden, NJ, USA

Sanjeev Kakar Department of Orthopedic Surgery, Mayo Clinic, Rochester, MN, USA

Robin N. Kamal Department of Orthopaedic Surgery, Stanford University, Redwood City, CA, USA

Arin E. Kim Montefiore Medical Center, Bronx, NY, USA

Hannah C. Langdell Division of Plastic, Reconstructive, Maxillofacial and Oral Surgery, Department of Surgery, Duke University Medical Center, Durham, NC, USA

Rafal Laredo Orthopedic and Trauma Department, Hospital Universitario Quironsalud Madrid, Madrid, Spain

Orthopedic and Trauma Department, Hospital Universitario Quironsalud Toledo, Toledo, Spain

Ricardo Larrainzar-Garijo, MD Orthopedic and Trauma Department, Hospital Universitario Infanta Leonor, Madrid, Spain

Surgery Department, School of Medicine, Universidad Complutense de Madrid, Madrid, Spain

Steve K. Lee Hospital for Special Surgery, New York, NY, USA

Steven J. Lee Hand and Upper Extremity, Lenox Hill Hospital, New York, NY, USA

Lenox Hill Hospital, New York, NY, USA

Bo Liu Department of Hand Surgery, Beijing Ji Shui Tan Hospital, Capital Medical University and the 4th Clinical College of Peking University, Beijing, China

Alex Lluch Institut Kaplan, Barcelona, Spain

Hand and Wrist Unit, Hospital Vall d'Hebron, Barcelona, Spain

Hayman Lui School of Medicine and Dentistry, Griffith University, Gold Coast, QLD, Australia

Department of Orthopedic Surgery, Mayo Clinic, Rochester, MN, USA

Justin Luis Lenox Hill Hospital, New York, NY, USA

Christophe Mathoulin International Wrist Centers-Clinique du Poignet, El Tarter, Andorra

Jane C. Messina UOC First Orthopaedic Clinic, University of Milan, ASST Gaetano Pini-CTO Orthopaedic Institute, Piazza Cardinal Ferrari 1, Milan, Italy

Steven L. Moran Division of Plastic Surgery, Department of Orthopedics, Mayo Clinic, Rochester, MN, USA

Michelle M. Nguyen Palo Alto VA Medical Center, Palo Alto, CA, USA

Stanford University Medical Center, Stanford, CA, USA

Maureen O'Shaughnessy University of Kentucky, Lexington, KY, USA

Montserrat Ocampos Orthopedic and Trauma Department, Hospital Universitario Infanta Leonor, Madrid, Spain

Orthopedic and Trauma Department, Hospital Universitario Quironsalud Madrid, Madrid, Spain

Kelsey L. Overman Department of Orthopaedic Surgery, Washington University, St. Louis, MO, USA

Anne Owen Department of Orthopedic Surgery, Stanford University Medical Center, Redwood City, CA, USA

H. B. Parikh Department of Orthopaedics, Cedars-Sinai Medical Center, Los Angeles, CA, USA

Pietro S. Randelli UOC First Orthopaedic Clinic, University of Milan, ASST Gaetano Pini-CTO Orthopaedic Institute, Piazza Cardinal Ferrari 1, Milan, Italy

Laboratory of Applied Biomechanics, Department of Biomedical Sciences for Health, University of Milan, Milan, Italy

Research Center for Adult and Pediatric Rheumatic Diseases (RECAP-RD), Department of Biomedical Sciences for Health, University of Milan, Milan, Italy

Shruti Raut Wrightington Hospital, Wigan, UK

Mark Rekant Philadelphia Hand to Shoulder Center, Philadelphia, PA, USA

Department of Orthopaedic Surgery, Thomas Jefferson University, Philadelphia, PA, USA

Marc J. Richard, MD Department of Orthopaedic Surgery, Duke University, Durham, NC, USA

Marco Rizzo Mayo Clinic, Rochester, MN, USA

Melvin P. Rosenwasser Department of Orthopedic Surgery, Columbia University Medical Center, New York, NY, USA

Mark Ross Department of Orthopaedic Surgery, University of Queensland: Brisbane Hand and Upper Limb Research Institute, Brisbane, QLD, Australia

Brisbane Hand and Upper Limb Research Institute, University of Queensland, Brisbane, QLD, Australia

Gustavo Mantovani Ruggiero Hospital Beneficencia Portuguesa de São Paulo, São Paulo Hand Center, Sao Paulo, SP, Brazil

Universita Degli Studi di Milano, Milano, MI, Italy

William Runge Hospital for Special Surgery, New York, NY, USA

Michael Sandow Wakefield Orthopaedic Clinic, and Centre of Orthopaedic and Trauma Research, University of Adelaide, Adelaide, SA, Australia

C. Schaeffer Emory University Hospital, Atlanta, GA, USA

Christine V. Schaeffer Division of Upper Extremity Surgery, Department of Orthopaedic Surgery, Emory University, Atlanta, GA, USA

Ana Scott-Tennent Hospital Arnau de Vilanova, Lleida, Spain

Lauren M. Shapiro Department of Orthopaedic Surgery, University of California, San Francisco, San Francisco, CA, USA

Christian M. Shigley Department of Orthopaedics and Sports Medicine, University of Washington Medical Center, Seattle, WA, USA

Alexander Y. Shin Mayo Clinic, Rochester, MN, USA

S. S. Shin Department of Orthopaedics, Cedars-Sinai Medical Center, Los Angeles, CA, USA

Kathryn J. Stevens Stanford University Medical Center, Stanford, CA, USA

Nina Suh BioSkills and Biomechanics Laboratory, Department of Orthopaedic Surgery, Emory University, Atlanta, GA, USA

José Tabuenca Orthopedic and Trauma Department, Hospital Universitario Quironsalud Madrid, Madrid, Spain

Sumedh C. Talwalkar Wrightington Hospital, Wigan, UK

Sami Tuffaha Johns Hopkins University School of Medicine, Baltimore, MD, USA

Pedro Bronenberg Victorica Instituto de Ortopedia y Traumatología "Carlos E. Ottolenghi," Potosí 4215 (C1199ACK), Buenos Aires, Argentina

Valeria Vismara UOC First Orthopaedic Clinic, University of Milan, ASST Gaetano Pini-CTO Orthopaedic Institute, Piazza Cardinal Ferrari 1, Milan, Italy

Eric R. Wagner Department of Orthopaedic Surgery, Emory University, Upper Extremity Center, Atlanta, GA, USA

Arnold-Peter C. Weiss Department of Orthopaedics, Alpert Medical School of Brown University & Medical University of South Carolina, Providence & Charleston, RI & SC, USA

Scott Wolfe Hospital for Special Surgery, New York, NY, USA

Feiran Wu Birmingham Hand Centre, Queen Elizabeth Hospital, University Hospitals Birmingham, Birmingham, UK

Jeffrey Yao, MD Department of Orthopedic Surgery, Stanford University, Stanford, CA, USA

Jason J. Yoo Department of Orthopaedics, University of Maryland School of Medicine, Baltimore, MD, USA

Nicole A. Zelenski Division of Upper Extremity Surgery, Department of Orthopaedic Surgery, Emory University, Atlanta, GA, USA

Chapter 1
Carpal Bone Anatomy

Spencer B. Chambers and Nina Suh

Introduction

The wrist is a complex joint comprising numerous osseous, tendinous, and ligamentous structures connecting the hand to the forearm. Intrinsic stability in the wrist is facilitated by its delicate inter-bone relationships as each carpal bone is uniquely shaped with various articulations, mobility constraints, and soft tissue attachments. As a construct, this allows for a variety of wrist positions while maximizing gripping stability and power.

Osteology

The wrist comprises eight bones organized into a proximal and distal row (Fig. 1.1) [1]. From the radial to ulnar side, the proximal row comprises the scaphoid, lunate, triquetrum, and pisiform. The distal row comprises the trapezium, trapezoid, capitate, and hamate. The scaphoid is unique in its configuration because it bridges both rows and coordinates movement between them [2]. Each bone comprises a cancellous core, cortical shell, and cartilage surface.

S. B. Chambers · N. Suh (✉)
BioSkills and Biomechanics Laboratory, Department of Orthopaedic Surgery, Emory University, Atlanta, GA, USA
e-mail: nina.suh@emory.edu

J. Yao (ed.), *Carpal Instability*, https://doi.org/10.1007/978-3-031-55869-6_1

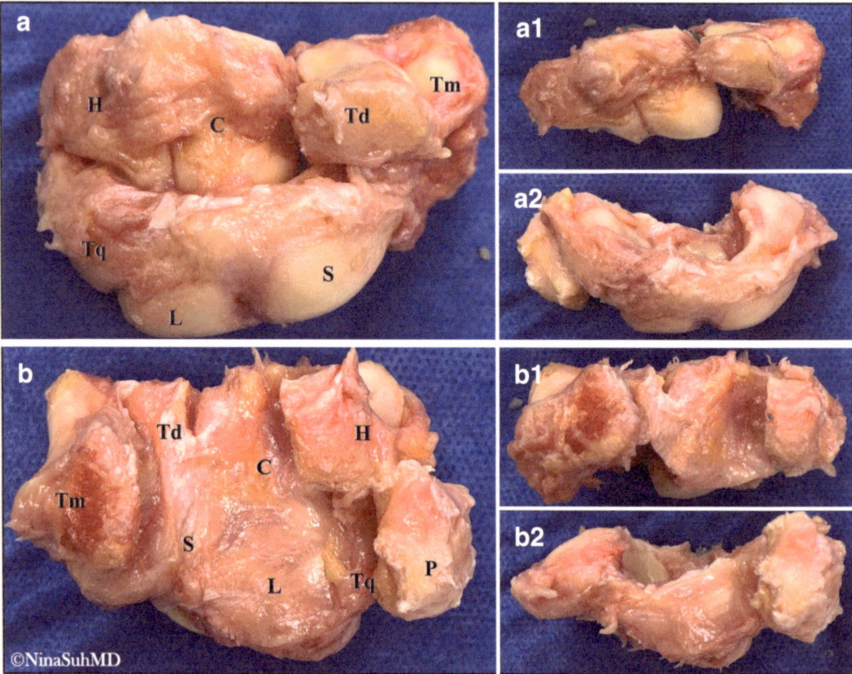

Fig. 1.1 Carpal Anatomy. The carpus is organized into distal and proximal carpal rows with complex topology. (**a**) Dorsal View of Carpus. (**a1**) Dorsal View of Distal Carpal Row. (**a2**) Dorsal View of Proximal Carpal Row. (**b**) Volar View of Carpus. (**b1**) Volar View of Distal Carpal Row. (**b2**) Volar View of Proximal Carpal Row

Scaphoid

The scaphoid is the second largest of the carpal bones and is at the radial side of the carpus (Fig. 1.2). Its name is derived from its boat-like shape (skaphos "boat" Latin), with the superior surface being convex and the inferior surface concave. Over 80% of its surface is covered with cartilage to facilitate articulations with four neighboring carpal bones (trapezium, trapezoid, capitate, and lunate) [3]. There are two primary locations for attachments of ligaments on the scaphoid: (i) the scaphoid tubercle lies on the proximal volar surface which is a rounded projection oriented volarly and serves as the attachment for the transverse carpal ligament, and (ii) a small ridge on the inferior aspect runs the length of the bone and serves as the attachments for the radial collateral ligament. These areas are also of importance because they receive vascular supply to nourish the scaphoid with over 80% of the vascularity entering the distal dorsal ridge from the radial artery. These source vessels then supply the proximal aspect of the scaphoid in a retrograde fashion [4]. The remainder of the vascularity is supplied through the distal tuberosity via volar branches of the radial artery [4].

Fig. 1.2 The Scaphoid. A boat-shaped bone with curvature in two planes articulating with the trapezium, trapezoid, capitate, and lunate. (**a**) The capitate articulation is along the concave ulnar aspect of the bone. (**b**) The proximal radial articulation and distal trapezial articulation are both convex and divided by the dorsal mid-ridge (*) where most of the vascular supply enters the scaphoid

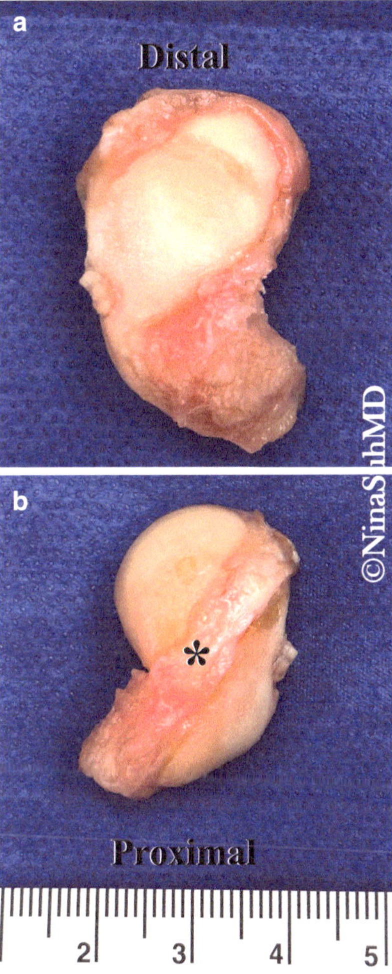

Lunate

The lunate resides in the central aspect of the proximal row and is a wedge or moon-shaped bone (luna "moon" Latin) (Fig. 1.3). Two common morphological variations have been described: Type I has a total of four articulations; proximally with the radius at the radiolunate fossa, radially with the proximal scaphoid pole, ulnarly with the triquetrum, and at the distal central aspect with the capitate. Type II also has an articulation at the distal-ulnar aspect with the hamate. The volar and dorsal aspects of the lunate are non-articulating surfaces and serve as the site of attachments of numerous soft tissue structures including the short and long radiolunate ligaments and are a site of vascular ingrowth. The lunate has a dual blood supply with a dominant source via the dorsal transverse carpal arch. A minor contribution

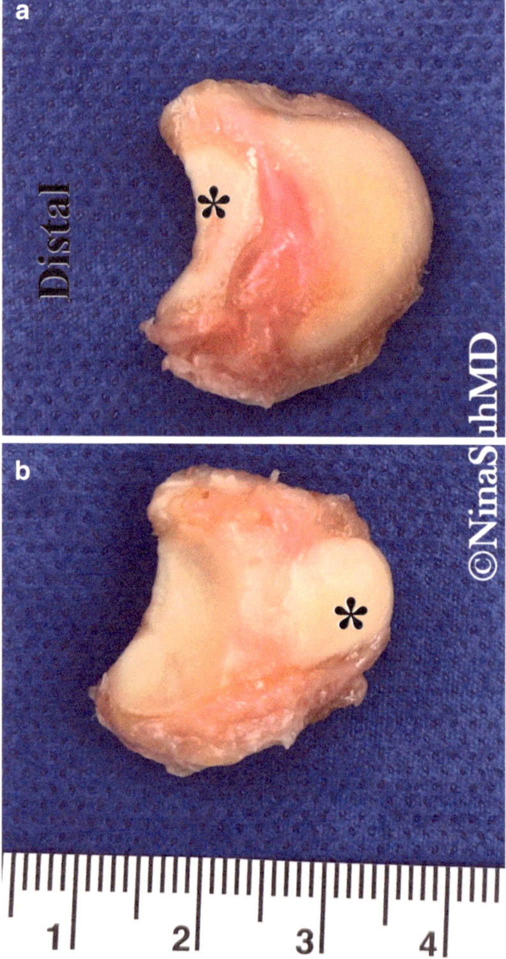

Fig. 1.3 **The Lunate.** A moon-shaped bone with a broad radial articulation in addition to articulations with the scaphoid, lunate, capitate, and in some cases the hamate. (**a**) The convex radiocarpal articulation is noted in addition to the scapholunate articulation (∗). (**b**) The lunocapitate joint is convex forming a tight osseus relationship with the proximal pole of the capitate. The triquetral articulation is broader in comparison to the scapholunate counterpart

also arises from the anterior interosseus artery [5]. The intraosseous blood supply is variable with the majority of lunates having robust anastomoses that can be categorized as "I", "Y", or "X" patterns. However, 20% of lunates receive only a few volar perforators with less robust collateralization [6].

Triquetrum

The triquetrum is the most ulnar carpal bone within the proximal row and is pyramidal shaped (Fig. 1.4). It articulates with the hamate distally, the lunate radially, and the pisiform volarly. Although it is in close approximation with the ulna it does not articulate directly, but rather is related through the triangular

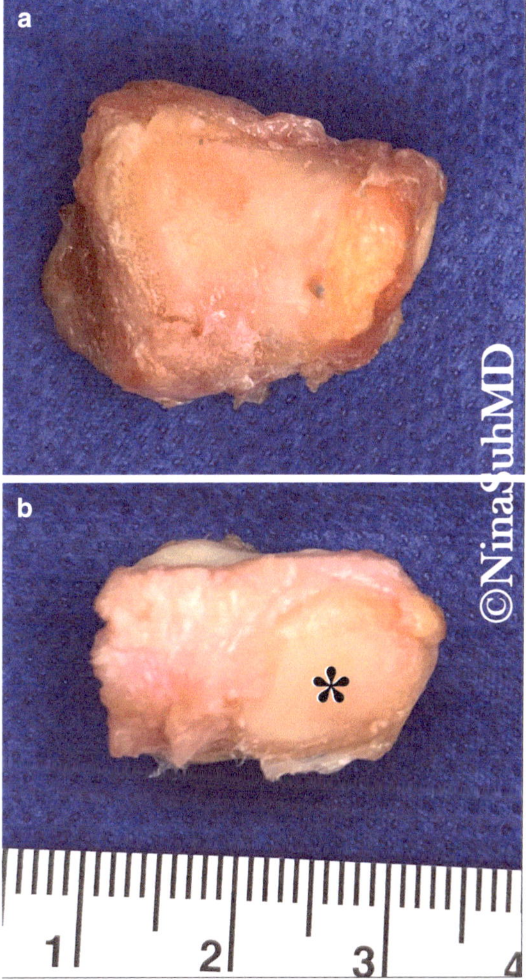

Fig. 1.4 The Triquetrum. A pyramidal-shaped bone that articulates with the pisiform, lunate, and hamate. (**a**) The hamate articulation is broad allowing mobility between these carpal bones. (**b**) Proximally, the convexity mirrors that of the ulnocarpal joint and volarly the pisiform facet is present (∗)

fibrocartilage complex (TFCC). The vascularity to the triquetrum is rich with source vessels from the volar and dorsal branches of the radiocarpal arch arising from the ulnar artery [5].

Pisiform

The pisiform is a sesamoid bone residing over the triquetrum and resides within the substance of the flexor carpi ulnaris tendon (FCU) proximal to its insertion in the base of the fifth metacarpal, in addition to acting as a portion of Guyon's canal (Fig. 1.5). It articulates with the triquetrum but does not contribute to carpal

Fig. 1.5 The Pisiform. A pea-shaped bone articulating with the triquetrum. (**a**) The deep surface of the pisiform is articular allowing a broad joint with the triquetrum (∗). (**b**) Superficially, the pisiform is roughened allowing for an insertion of the flexor carpi ulnaris

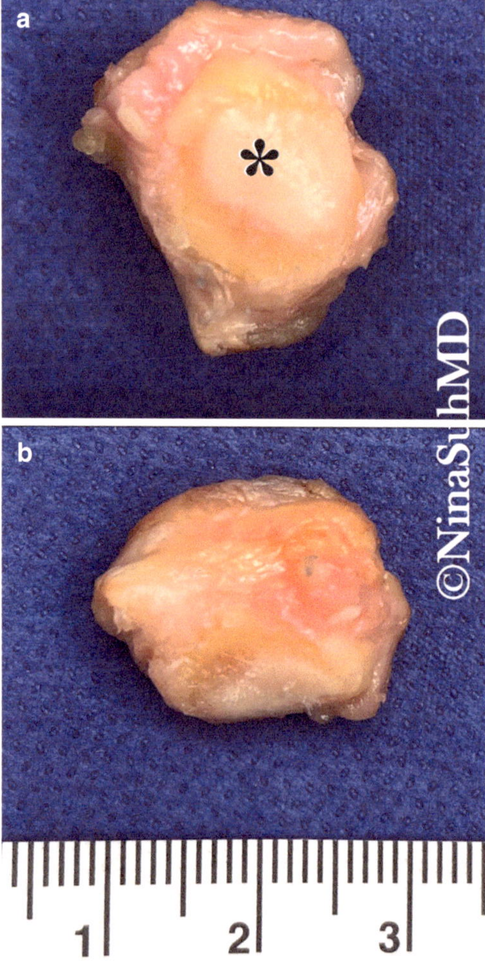

kinematics. The pisiform receives robust vascularity proximally and distally from branches of the ulnar artery, with a rich anastomotic network encompassing the bone [6].

Trapezium

The trapezium is the most radial bone in the distal carpal row and resides at the base of the thumb (Fig. 1.6). It has a biconcave shape with the integration of two saddle joints in orthogonal topology (ginglymoid type hinge joint). This allows for a wide

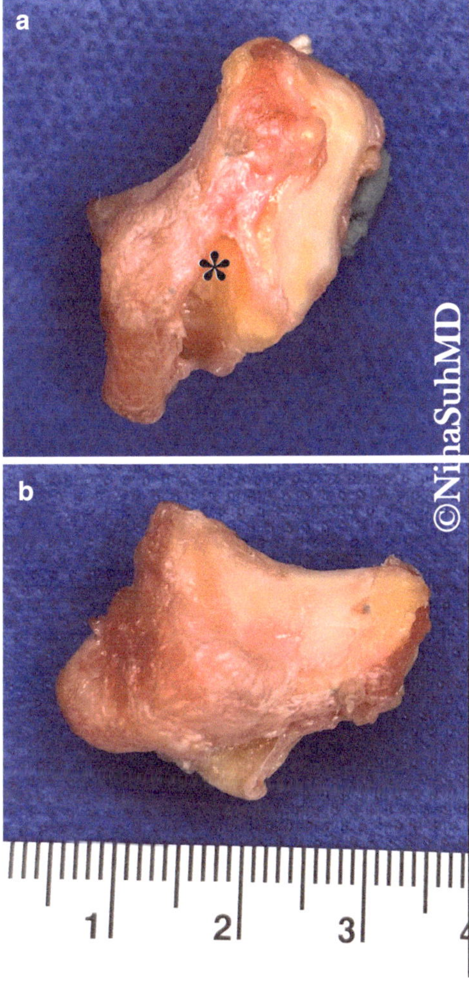

Fig. 1.6 The Trapezium. A biconcave saddle-shaped bone articulating with the first metacarpal, second metacarpal, trapezium, and scaphoid. (**a**) The trapezial joint is supported primarily by ligaments permitting large varieties of motion at the first carpal metacarpal joint. The flexor carpi radialis is intimately associated with the trapezium as it traverses a fibro-osseus tunnel (*). (**b**) The metacarpal articulation forms a ginglymoid joint facilitating flexion and extension in addition to mild abduction and addiction

range of motion of the first metacarpal and the thumb. The volar, dorsal, and radial aspect of the trapezium do not articulate with other bones. These rough areas allow for the insertion of numerous stabilizing tendons and ligaments. At the ulnar distal aspect, the trapezium attaches to the second metacarpal, but little motion occurs at this joint. The ulnar aspect of this bone articulates with the trapezoid, and proximally with the scaphoid. The trapezium is dorsal to the distal pole of the scaphoid, so with radial deviation as the scaphoid impacts into the more dorsal trapezium it forces the scaphoid (and the rest of the intact proximal carpal row) into flexion. The three non-articular surfaces of the trapezium serve as locations of vascular inflow from the radial carpal arch laterally and dorsally, with dominant supply being dorsal [5].

Trapezoid

The trapezoid is the second smallest carpal bone and resides adjacent to the trapezium (Fig. 1.7). It has a wedge-like shape and five faces of articulation. On the radial aspect, the trapezoid articulates with the trapezium. Proximally, there is an articulation with the scaphoid and ulnarly with the capitate. Distally, there are two primary variations. The trapezoid always articulates with the second metacarpal, but in a minority of cases there is also a small distal-ulnar facet that also articulates with the third metacarpal. The trapezoid serves as a bridge between the distal carpal row and the metacarpals but is the least mobile carpal bone, contributing to the stable central aspect of this joint. The dominant blood supply enters via the non-articular dorsal surface of the trapezoid with numerous small perforators [5, 6].

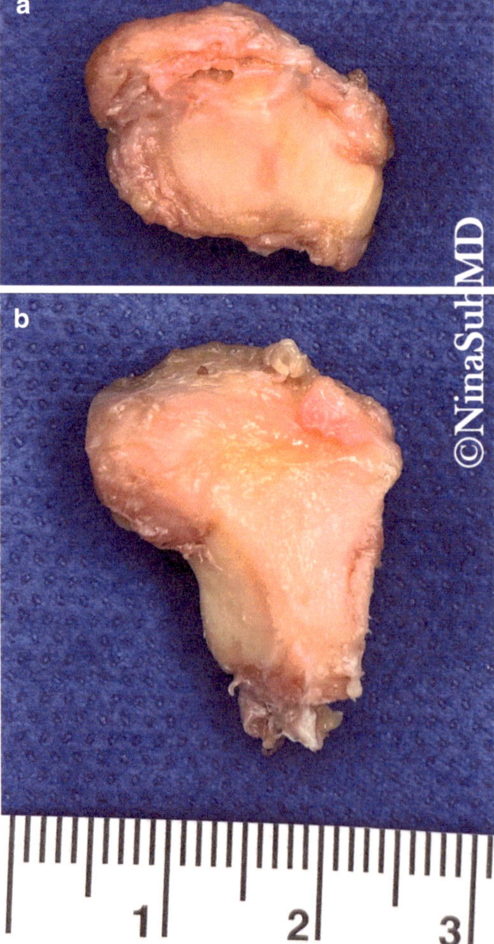

Fig. 1.7 The Trapezoid. A variably shaped carpal bone articulating with the trapezium, second metacarpal, scaphoid, capitate, and in some cases the third metacarpal. (**a**) Distally, the trapezoid forms the second and in some cases a portion of the third carpal metacarpal joint. These are stable joints allowing little motion. (**b**) Proximally, the trapezoid is intimately associated with the trapezium and scaphoid

Capitate

The capitate is the largest carpal bone and is located centrally in the distal carpal row (Fig. 1.8). It comprises the basis of the transverse carpal arch forming a rigid central column of the hand and wrist. Distally, it articulates with the third and fourth metacarpal. There is minimal motion at this joint and functionally the capitate acts as an extension of the base of the third metacarpal. On the radial aspect of the capitate lies the scapho-capitate joint. On the ulnar aspect, the capitate articulates with the hamate. Proximally, the capitate sits within the lesser convexity of the lunate, which allows for flexion and extension at the midcarpal joint. The capitate receives vascular inflow near its neck on the volar and dorsal surfaces [5]. These vessels have considerable connections creating a rich network that supplies the proximal aspect of the capitate in a retrograde fashion [6].

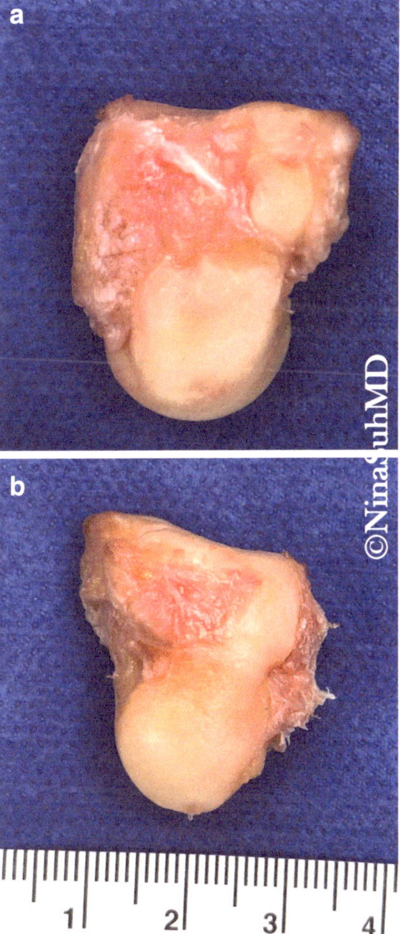

Fig. 1.8 The Capitate. The largest carpal bone articulates with all other carpal bones except the pisiform, in addition to the third metacarpal. In some cases, there are additional articulations with the second and fourth metacarpal. (**a**) Ulnarly, the capitate is a flat through its articulation with the hamate, and proximally is convex to allow flexion and extension with the lunate. (**b**) Radially, the proximal pole of the capitate is spherically allowing complex motion with the scaphoid. Distally, the flat dorsum serves as an insertion site to the extensor radialis brevis (the tendon also inserts on the base of the third metacarpal)

Hamate

The hamate is the most ulnar carpal bone in the distal row and is wedge shaped with an osseous projection volarly (hamulus, "little hook," Latin) that forms a radial portion of Guyon's canal (Fig. 1.9). Distally, the hamate articulates with the fourth and fifth metacarpal, radially with the capitate, and proximally with the triquetrum. The helicoid articulation of the proximal hamate engages the triquetrum during ulnar deviation and forces the triquetrum (and the entire proximal row when intact) into extension. In comparison to the radial sided carpometacarpal joints, there is significant mobility at the ulnar carpometacarpal joint allowing for abduction and positioning of the small finger and power gripping. The body of the hamate receives blood supply over the roughened dorsal surface from perforators of the dorsal carpal arch. Volarly, radiocarpal arch branches perforate the base at the level of the hook to supply this region of the bone [6].

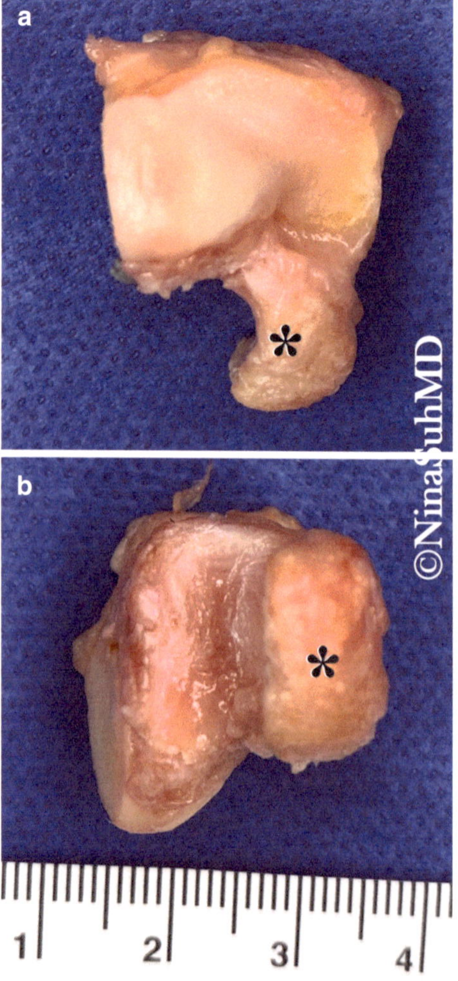

Fig. 1.9 The Hamate. The ulnar-most bone of the distal row that articulates with the capitate, triquetrum, fifth metacarpal, and in some cases the lunate. (**a**) The distal articulation is broad and flat permitting mobility at the carpometacarpal joint. The hook of the hamate (∗) is a curved volar projection that forms a portion of Guyon's canal. (**b**) Radially, the hamate has a flat articulation with the capitate and proximally, a shallow convexity with the triquetrum. The hook is a prominent volar projection (∗)

Soft Tissue Anatomy

There are numerous soft tissues that are important for maintaining joint congruency. Although any crossing tendinous structure may be considered a dynamic stabilizer, these supply secondary support to the static ligaments, and for the purpose of this work only principal tendinous structures will be discussed. Ligaments are categorized as (i) intrinsic: originating and inserting within the carpus, or (ii) extrinsic: originating on the distal radius and/or ulna and inserting onto the carpus.

Extrinsic Carpal Ligaments

There are significant variations in the topology and number of extrinsic carpal ligaments, but each structure can be categorized into three main groups: palmar radiocarpal, palmar ulnocarpal, dorsal radiocarpal (DRC) Additionally, the dorsal intercarpal (DIC) ligament, functions synergistically with the DRC as an extrinsic stabilizer despite originating and inserting within the carpus. The only ligament on the dorsal-ulnar aspect of the wrist is the TFCC. These soft tissue structures form a confluence with the wrist capsule and are best visualized intra-articularly.

Palmar Radiocarpal

The four ligaments in this group are the radioscaphoid ligament (RSL), radioscaphocapitate ligament (RSCL), the long radiolunate ligament (LRLL), and short radiolunate ligament (SRLL). The RSL, RSCL, and LRLL originate from the lateral aspect of the distal radius and are superficial. These ligaments take an oblique course ulnarly and distally to insert on the scaphoid, capitate, and lunate, respectively. The SRLL is a deeper structure and originates from the medial aspect of the radius and travels to the lunate directly.

The RSCL is a particularly important to scaphoid stability and serves as a fulcrum for the scaphoid to rotate. The interval between the RSCL and the LRLL, known as the space of Poirier, is an area of weakness within this complex that the lunate may dislocate through in the setting of significant force.

Palmar Ulnocarpal

Most variation in extrinsic wrist ligaments is found in the ulnar stabilizers, but typically there are three ligaments that can be organized into deep and superficial structures. The ulnar collateral ligament (UCL) is a superficial structure arising from the base of the ulnar styloid. Deeper to this ligament arising from the TFCC are the ulnar triquetral ligament (UTL) and ulnar lunate ligament (ULL). The UCL forms a distal inverted "V", or arcuate ligament in conjunction with the RSCL, whereas the three collective structures (UCL, UTL, ULL) are known as the ulnar carpal ligamentous complex and form a proximal inverted "V" with the LRLL and SRLL.

Dorsal Radiocarpal

There is a single extrinsic radiocarpal ligament on the dorsal aspect of the wrist known as the dorsal radiotriquetral ligament (DRTL) with various thickenings (Fig. 1.10). This is a broad ligament with numerous attachments onto the triquetrum and lunate with some variations including the scaphoid.

Midcarpal Ligaments

There are fewer interosseous ligaments in the midcarpal joint which allows for significant motion. There is only a single dorsal ligament, the dorsal intercarpal ligament (Fig. 1.10), that connects the lunate to the distal scaphoid, trapezium, and trapezoid. In conjunction with the DRC, this ligament forms a lateral V shape and is a critical stabilizer of the proximal carpal row [7]. Volarly, there are many short, strong ligaments that make various connections between the proximal and distal carpal rows. Of these, the most important in the maintenance of scaphoid position are the scaphoid capitate ligament (SCL) and the dorsolateral scaphoid-trapezium-trapezoid ligament (STTL).

Fig. 1.10 Dorsal Wrist Extrinsic Ligaments: There is variability on dorsal wrist ligaments but consistently one large structure arising from the radius and traversing ulnarly is present (dorsal radial triquetral ligament (DRTL)). Withing this structure the dorsal intercarpal ligament (DIC), dorsal radiocarpal ligament (DRC), and dorsal radial ulnar ligament (DRU) are noted

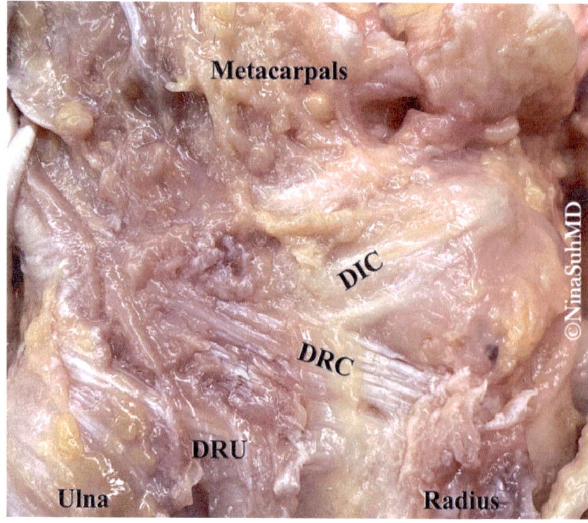

Triangular Fibrocartilage Complex

This ligamentous complex is composed of six main structures: dorsal radioulnar ligaments, volar radioulnar ligaments, a central articular disc, meniscal homolog, ulnar collateral ligament, extensor carpus ulnaris subsheath, and the origin of the UTL and ULL. The primary role of the TFCC is to preserve stability between the radius and ulna, with secondary relationships stabilizing the ulnocarpal joint. The periphery is well vascularized but centrally is relatively avascular, resulting in poor healing of injuries to the articular disc. Foveal tears may lead to instability in the distal radial ulnar joint that in turn cause secondary carpal pathology.

Intrinsic Carpal Ligaments

The intrinsic carpal ligaments constrain motion and ensure intercarpal rotational forces are balanced. This is thought to be most critical in the proximal row where connections between the lunate and the neighboring triquetrum and scaphoid preserve rotatory alignment. The distal carpal bones tend to have more constrained osseus relationships and tighter ligamentous structures, limiting relative motion and creating more stable joints.

Scapholunate Ligament

The Scapholunate Intercarpal Ligament (SLIL) is a C-shaped structure that transfers a flexion moment from the scaphoid to the lunate. It is divisible into three subregions, with the thickest portion being dorsal, measuring 2–3 mm [8]. This component is particularly important in maintaining carpal stability as it ensures the lunate does not enter a dorsal posture which may lead to secondary instabilities such as dorsal intercalated segment instability. In addition to this direct connection, the SLIL also provides stability secondarily through connections to the wrist capsule.

Lunotriquetral Ligament

The lunotriquetral intrinsic ligament (LTIL) is shorter and stronger in comparison to the SLIL, owing to a closer relationship in the motion of the lunate and triquetrum (Fig. 1.11). The LTIL is also subdivided into three regions, but in contrast to the SLIL, the volar LTIL is the thickest [9]. This portion of the ligament transmits the extension moment of the triquetrum to the lunate, balancing the flexion imparted by the scaphoid. The dorsal and proximal components of the LTIL are progressively thinner in comparison, but the still play a principal role in rotational constraint of the lunate [9].

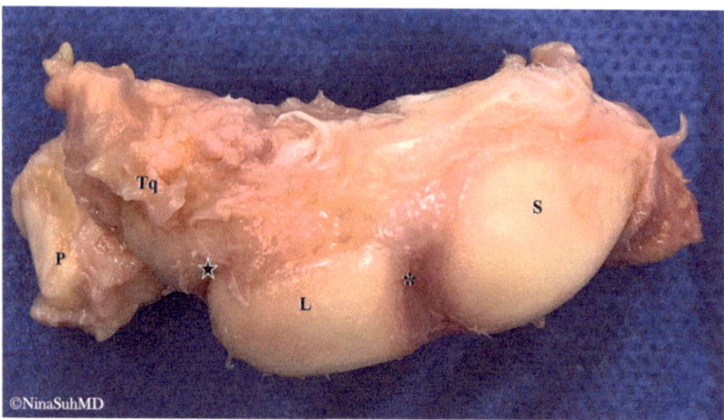

Fig. 1.11 Intrinsic Intercarpal Ligaments of the Proximal Row. The scapholunate intercarpal ligament (SLIL) (*) is a complex C-shaped structure coordinating motion between the scaphoid (S) and lunate (L) that is thickest dorsally. The lunotriquetral intercarpal ligament (LTIL) (black star) resides on the other side of the lunate and is thickened volarly. The LTIL introduces an extending moment to the lunate, and the SLIL provides an antagonistic flexion moment, keeping the lunate balanced in coordination with the distal row. *Tq* Triquetrum, *P* Pisiform

Tendons

On the volar aspect of the wrist, the extrinsic finger flexors (flexor digitorum superficialis, flexor digitorum profundus, flexor pollicus longus) cross the carpus through the carpal tunnel. The carpal tunnel is formed by the transverse carpal ligament (TCL) superficially, the joint capsule deeply, the hook of the hamate ulnarly and the trapezium radially. The flexor carpi radialis is intimately associated with the trapezium (Fig. 1.6) before inserting onto the base of the second metacarpal. The FCU encapsulates the pisiform (Fig. 1.5) prior to inserting into the base of the fifth metacarpal. Dorsally, the extensor tendons cross broadly over the carpus before inserting more distally at the metacarpals or phalanges.

Nerves

Volarly, the median nerve enters the wrist with the extrinsic flexor tendons through the carpal tunnel. The ulnar nerve enters via Guyon's canal which is formed by the pisiform and hook of hamate (Figs. 1.5 and 1.9). Prior to entering Guyon's canal, the ulnar nerve gives off a cutaneous branch which travels dorsally crossing the ulnocarpal joint before becoming cutaneous. The superficial radial nerve also terminates in the dorsal radial sensory branch which crosses in wrist at the radial aspect of the wrist before becoming cutaneous over the thumb, first webspace, index, and dorsum of the hand. In addition to these cutaneous and mixed motor nerves, the wrist joint receives direct innervation from the terminal portions of the anterior interosseus nerve (AIN) and posterior interosseous nerve (PIN).

Blood Vessels

The carpus is supplied via rich intercarpal arches joining the radial and ulnar artery. The ulnar artery crosses the wrist with the ulnar nerve through Guyon's canal before forming the superficial arch. The radial artery has a more torturous path, traversing from volar to dorsal and crossing over the proximal aspect of the scaphotrapezial joint. It then pierces the soft tissues between the first and second metacarpal entering the volar hand and forming the deep arch. In most cases, there is a rich anastomotic network between these two arches, allowing redundant flow.

References

1. Wolfe SW, Pederson WC, Kozin SH. Green's operative hand surgery. 6th ed (Green DP, ed.). Elsevier; 2011.
2. Hirt B, Seyhan H, Wagner M. Hand and wrist anatomy and biomechanics: a comprehensive guide; 2016. https://doi.org/10.1007/s00590-017-1991-z.
3. Sendher R, Ladd AL. The scaphoid. Orthop Clin North Am. 2013;44(1):107–20. https://doi.org/10.1016/j.ocl.2012.09.003.
4. Gelberman RH, Menon J. The vascularity of the scaphoid bone. J Hand Surg Am. 1980;5(5):508–13. https://doi.org/10.1016/S0363-5023(80)80087-6.
5. Gelberman RH, Panagis JS, Taleisnik J, Baumgaertner M. The arterial anatomy of the human carpus. Part I: the extraosseous vascularity. J Hand Surg Am. 1983;8(4):367–75. https://doi.org/10.1016/S0363-5023(83)80194-4.
6. Panagis JS, Gelberman RH, Talcisnik J, Baumgaertner M. The arterial anatomy of the human carpus. Part II: the intraosseous vascularity. J Hand Surg Am. 1983;8(4).375–82. https://doi.org/10.1016/S0363-5023(83)80195-6.
7. Mitsuyasu H, Patterson RM, Shah MA, Buford WL, Iwamoto Y, Viegas SF. The role the dorsal Intercarpal ligament in dynamic and static Scapholunate instability. J Hand Surg Am. 2004;29(2):279–88. https://doi.org/10.1016/j.jhsa.2003.11.004.
8. Berger RA, Imeada T, Berglund L, An KN. Constraint and material properties of the subregions of the scapholunate interosseous ligament. J Hand Surg Am. 1999;24(5):953–62. https://doi.org/10.1053/jhsu.1999.0953.
9. Ritt MJPF, Bishop AT, Berger RA, Linscheid RL, Berglund LJ, An KN. Lunotriquetral ligament properties: a comparison of three anatomic subregions. J Hand Surg Am. 1998;23(3):425–31. https://doi.org/10.1016/S0363-5023(05)80460-5.

Chapter 2
Carpal Instability: Physical Examination Tips and Tricks

Anne Owen and Jeffrey Yao

Carpal Instability: Physical Examination

The proximal row of the carpus provides 60% of wrist motion, allowing for flexion, extension, ulnar and radial deviation [1]. In comparison, the midcarpal row provides 40% of the motion [1]. Allowing for stability and range of motion between bones of the proximal row are the scapholunate interosseous ligament (SLIL) and lunotriquetral interosseous ligament (LTIL) [2]. The SLIL is one of the most important ligaments stabilizing the carpus [1]. It has three anatomic regions: dorsal, volar and proximal [2]. The dorsal component of the SLIL ligament is the strongest. It provides stability against distraction, torsion, and translation [3]. The volar portion provides stability against rotational forces [3]. Disruption of the SLIL ligament and subsequent secondary stabilizers results in a dorsal intercalated segment instability (DISI) pattern of the wrist.

Similarly, the LTIL has three different regions: dorsal, membranous, and volar. In contrast, however, the strongest region of the LTIL is the volar portion [2]. The dorsal LTIL assists in rotational stability [3]. Disruption of the LTIL results in a volar intercalated segment instability (VISI) pattern of the wrist.

With any physical examination, it is important to start with a detailed history and obtaining subjective data from the patient. Discussion should address any previous trauma to the symptomatic wrist, what activities that cause pain, and any deficits in strength and range of motion. If there is an acute SLIL injury, the patient may describe

A. Owen (✉)
Department of Orthopedic Surgery, Stanford University Medical Center,
Redwood City, CA, USA
e-mail: aowen@stanfordmed.org

J. Yao
Department of Orthopedic Surgery, Stanford University, Stanford, CA, USA
e-mail: jyao@stanford.edu

J. Yao (ed.), *Carpal Instability*, https://doi.org/10.1007/978-3-031-55869-6_2

persistent wrist pain, decreased grip strength, and occasionally popping and clicking associated with pain during axial loading activities, particularly with an extended wrist [3]. In the chronic phases of an SLIL injury, the patient may complain of decreased ROM and pain with wrist extension and axial loading [3]. Regarding LTIL injuries, the patient may complain of ulnar-sided wrist pain and decreased grip strength [3].

The physical exam begins with direct observation of the patient's bilateral wrists resting on the exam table. Observe any visible edema/effusion about the dorsum of the wrist. Dorsal wrist effusion at the location of the scapholunate region may indicate a scapholunate dissociation/tear, the beginnings of an SLAC wrist, a dorsal wrist ganglion, or tenosynovitis as seen in patients with rheumatoid arthritis. Evaluate the patient's bilateral wrist extension, flexion, supination, pronation, ulnar and radial deviation to determine any deficits in range of motion (ROM) compared to the contralateral uninjured extremity. During these maneuvers, pain may be elicited with extension and radial deviation [3] or ulnar deviation and flexion [4, 5]. It is also important to determine if the patient has any deficits in sensory and motor functions, particularly in the median nerve distribution. An acute perilunate injury my cause acute carpal tunnel or contusion of the median nerve in up to 25% of cases [1].

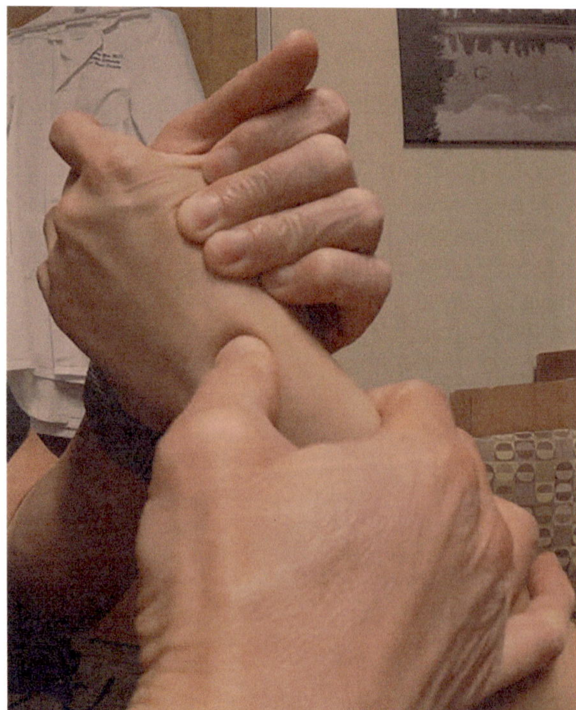

Fig. 2.1 Scapholunate interval

Fig. 2.2 Volar
scapholunate interval

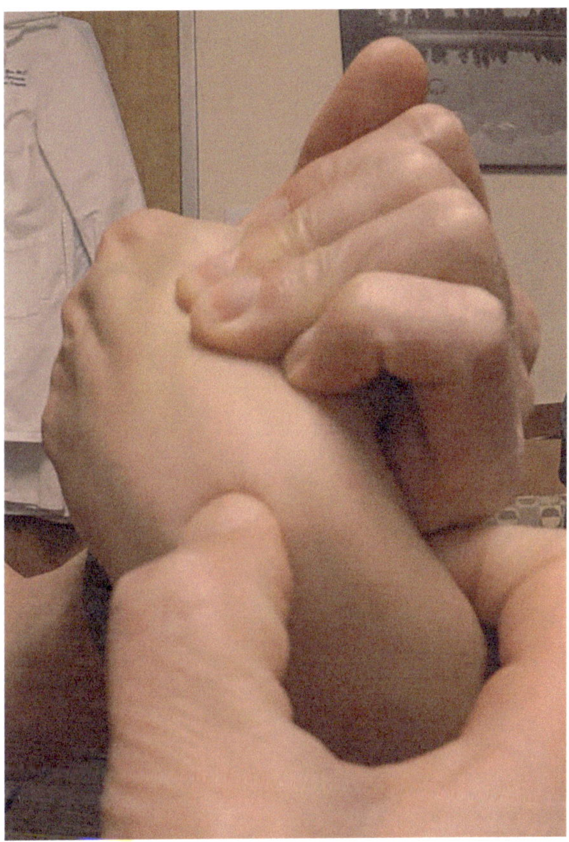

Examination of SLIL

The scapholunate interval is located approximately 1 cm distal to lister's tubercle [6]. Evaluate the dorsal SLIL by applying deep pressure at the scapholunate interval dorsally while the patient's wrist is in neutral (Fig. 2.1). Tenderness in this region may indicate a dorsal scapholunate injury, ganglion cyst, or dorsal wrist impingement syndrome [7]. To evaluate the volar SLIL, flex the wrist slightly and apply deep pressure on scapholunate interval dorsally. If pain is elicited with this maneuver, it may indicate a membranous and/or volar scapholunate injury (Fig. 2.2).

The scapholunate ballottement or scaphoid shear test is suggestive of an SLIL injury. It is performed by stabilizing the scaphoid with one hand, while the other hand stabilizes the lunate. The scaphoid is then shifted from volar to dorsal in relation to the lunate. If this causes pain or has increased ROM compared to contralateral wrist, this is considered a positive scapholunate ballottement [7] (Fig. 2.3).

The Watson shift test, when positive, may indicate a dorsal intercalary instability (DISI) of the carpus [8], or be positive as a result of asymptomatic ligamentous laxity [7]. With one hand, place the thumb on the scaphoid tubercle while the patient's

Fig. 2.3 Scapholunate
ballottement

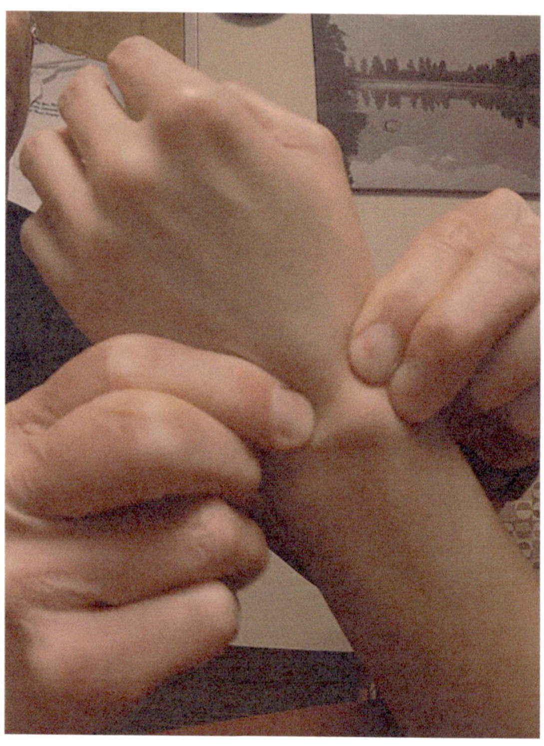

Fig. 2.4 Watson shift
radial deviation

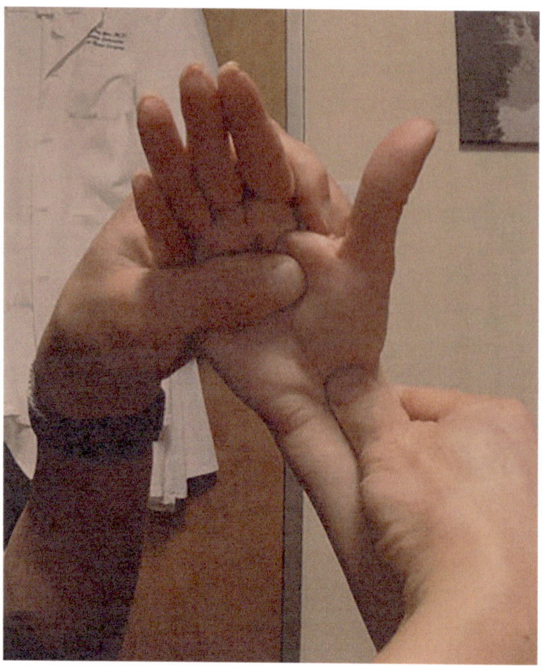

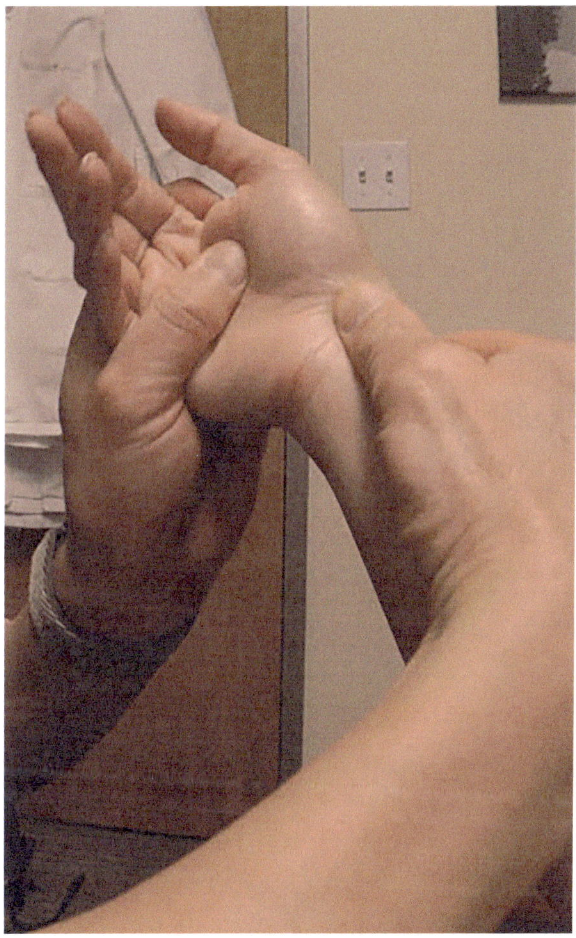

Fig. 2.5 Watson shift ulnar deviation

wrist is in neutral position. Flex the wrist slightly and apply pressure on the scaphoid tubercle volarly while he patient's wrist is manipulated from radial to ulnar deviation [8] (Figs. 2.4 and 2.5). If the SLIL is torn, the proximal pole of the scaphoid translates over the dorsal lip of the radius [7]. Relief of this pressure creates a palpable clunk, as the scaphoid returns to its place within the scaphoid fossa [7]. A palpable clunk is considered a positive Watson shift test. This test should always be performed on both wrists, as a positive test (typically painless) may also be present in the patient with generalized ligamentous laxity.

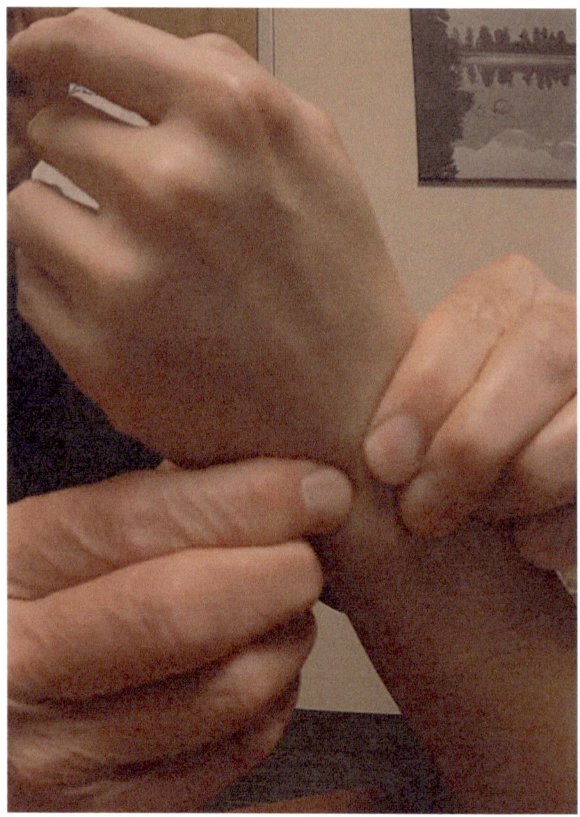

Fig. 2.6 LT Ballottement

Examination of LTIL

The lunotriquetral (LT) interval is located ulnar to the lunate, in line with the fourth ray [4, 7]. Tenderness to palpation about the LTIL dorsally may suggest an LT injury. Other etiologies of ulnar-sided wrist pain such as injuries to the triangular fibrocartilage complex (TFCC), extensor carpi ulnaris (ECU) tendon, ulnar extrinsic ligament injuries, and pisotriquetral pathology must also be considered and ruled out.

The LT ballottement test is performed by stabilizing the lunate and rocking the triquetrum back and forth from volar to dorsal (Fig. 2.6). A positive test elicits pain, clicking, and/or laxity [7].

The LT Shuck Test is performed by stabilizing the dorsal lunate with one hand. The contralateral thumb will apply pressure on the pisotriquetral joint volarly,

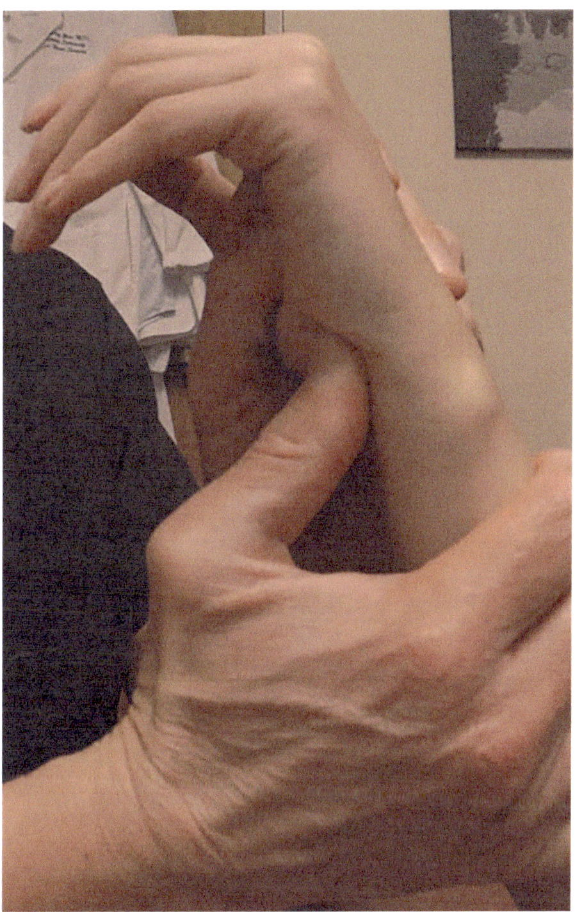

Fig. 2.7 Pisiform boost

creating a shear force at the LT interval. The wrist will be brought to ulnar and radial deviation. A painful clunk is elicited and signifies an LT ligament injury or generalized laxity [5, 7].

The pisiform boost test is performed by placing the thumb on the pisiform volarly, while placing a dorsal load to stress the LTIL ligament indirectly by pushing the triquetrum dorsally (Fig. 2.7). Pain with this test may indicate an LTIL injury but may also be indicative of the presence of pisotriquetral arthritis [7, 9].

Midcarpal Instability Examination

Ligamentous laxity of the wrist, or tears of the dorsal triquetral hamate ligament and/or volar arcuate ligament may lead to midcarpal instability [7]. To test for midcarpal instability, one may perform the midcarpal shift test. The midcarpal shift test

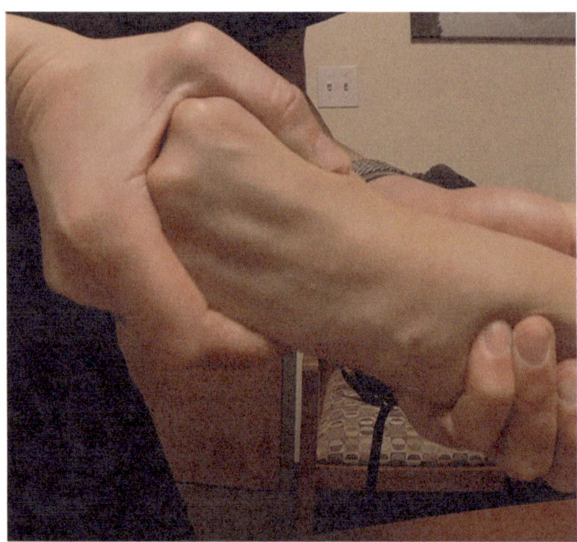

Fig. 2.8 Midcarpal shift load

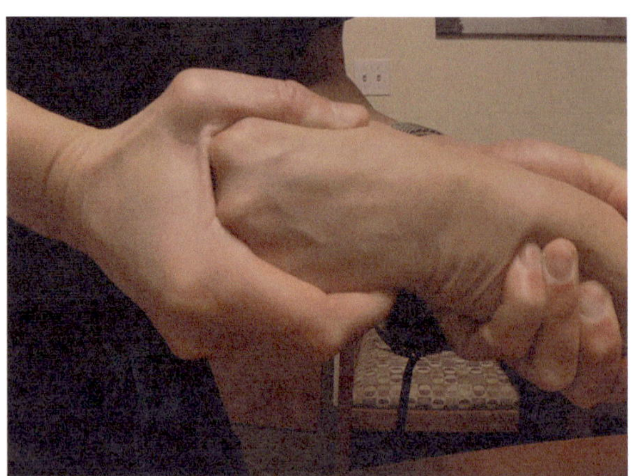

Fig. 2.9 Midcarpal shift ulnar deviation

is performed by putting pressure on the dorsal capitate and loading volarly while ulnarly deviating the wrist simultaneously (Figs. 2.8 and 2.9). A painful clunk is a positive midcarpal shift test [7]. This occurs when the proximal carpal row shifts from flexion to extension and the capitate forces the lunate into extension, and the helicoid articulation of the hamate causes the triquetrum to extend with ulnar deviation of the wrist [7]. Similar to the Watson's shift test, this test should always be done on both wrists, as a positive test may also indicate that the patient may have generalized ligamentous laxity.

Summary

Diagnosis of wrist pathologies can be daunting due to the many underlying bony and soft tissue structures confined in a small anatomic space. When diagnosing carpal instability, it is important to examine the contralateral, uninjured side to rule out any generalized ligamentous laxity.

Good knowledge of the wrist anatomy, biomechanics, and pathologies, as well as an overall understanding of the patient's history, symptomatology, and review of imaging can guide the examiner's decision-making process regarding what exam maneuvers are appropriate to make a sound clinical diagnosis.

References

1. Thomas T, Rayan M, Budoff GM, Baratz JE. Principles of hand surgery and therapy. 2nd ed. Philadelphia: Saunders Elsevier; 2010.
2. Berger RA. The gross and histologic anatomy of the scapholunate interosseous ligament. J Hand Surg. 1996;21(2):170–8.
3. Beeker RW, Rehman U. Carpal ligament instability. Treasure Island (FL): StatPearls Publishing; 2022.
4. Ambrose L, Posner M. Lunate-triquetral and midcarpal instability. Hand Clin. 1992;8(4):653–8.
5. Shin AY, Battaglia MM, Bishop MA. Lunotriquetral instability: diagnosis and treatment. J Am Acad Orthop Surg. 2000;8(3):170–9.
6. Reavey PL, Hammert WC. Examination of the wrist. Plast Reconstr Surg. 2021;147:284e–94e. American Society of Plastic Surgeons.
7. Yao J, Skirven T, Osterman AL, Culp RW. Clinical assessment of the wrist. In: Cooney III WP, editor. The wrist: diagnosis and operative treatment. Lippincott Williams & Wilkins; 2010. p. 119–50.
8. Watson H, Ashmead D 4th, Makhlouf M. Examination of the scaphoid. J Hand Surg Am. 1988;13(5):657–60.
9. Reagan DS, Linscheid RL, Dobyns JH. Lunotriquetral Sprains. J Hand Surg Am. 1984;9(4):502–14.

Chapter 3
Imaging of Carpal Instability

Michelle M. Nguyen and Kathryn J. Stevens

Introduction

Carpal instability refers to symptomatic dysfunction, where the wrist is unable to bear physiologic loads, and exhibits abnormal kinematics during its arc of motion [1]. The Mayo classification divides carpal instability into four patterns [2–8]. The carpal instability dissociative (CID) pattern refers to intracarpal instability occurring in the same carpal row. Carpal instability non-dissociative (CIND) pattern relates to instability at the radiocarpal and/or midcarpal joints. Carpal instability complex (CIC) comprises a combination of CID and CIND. Carpal instability adaptive (CIA) refers to carpal instability occurring secondary to an abnormality extrinsic to the wrist, occurring either in the distal radius and/or distal ulna. The degree of carpal instability is related to the severity of ligamentous and/or osseous injury [3]. Dynamic and static forms of carpal instability are well recognized, particularly with respect to scapholunate and lunotriquetral dissociation [8–10].

Imaging plays an important role in the diagnosis of carpal instability and can identify primary ligamentous and osseous injuries, as well as malalignment of the wrist and associated arthropathy [11]. Imaging modalities of the wrist include radiography, cineradiography, ultrasonography (US), magnetic resonance imaging (MRI), MR arthrography (MRA), and computed tomography (CT). Cineradiography and US allow for dynamic imaging of the wrist, although there are modality specific

M. M. Nguyen
Palo Alto VA Medical Center, Palo Alto, CA, USA

Stanford University Medical Center, Stanford, CA, USA

K. J. Stevens (✉)
Stanford University Medical Center, Stanford, CA, USA
e-mail: kate.stevens@stanford.edu

J. Yao (ed.), *Carpal Instability*, https://doi.org/10.1007/978-3-031-55869-6_3

limitations. In this chapter, we will discuss the diagnostic capability of each imaging modality for carpal instability and review the pertinent imaging findings for the different types of carpal instability.

Radiography

Conventional radiographs are the first line of imaging for patients with wrist pain and instability. Correct positioning of the wrist is vital to evaluate wrist alignment [12]. For the posteroanterior (PA) view, the wrist and forearm are in neutral position with the shoulder in 90° of abduction and the elbow in 90° of flexion [12–16]. On a neutral PA view, the extensor carpi ulnaris tendon groove should be profiled at the radial base of the ulnar styloid [17, 18] (Fig. 3.1). The Gilula arcs outline the radio-carpal and midcarpal joints and should not demonstrate any discontinuity [19] (Fig. 3.1). The joint spaces between the individual carpal bones should be ≤2 mm [20, 21].

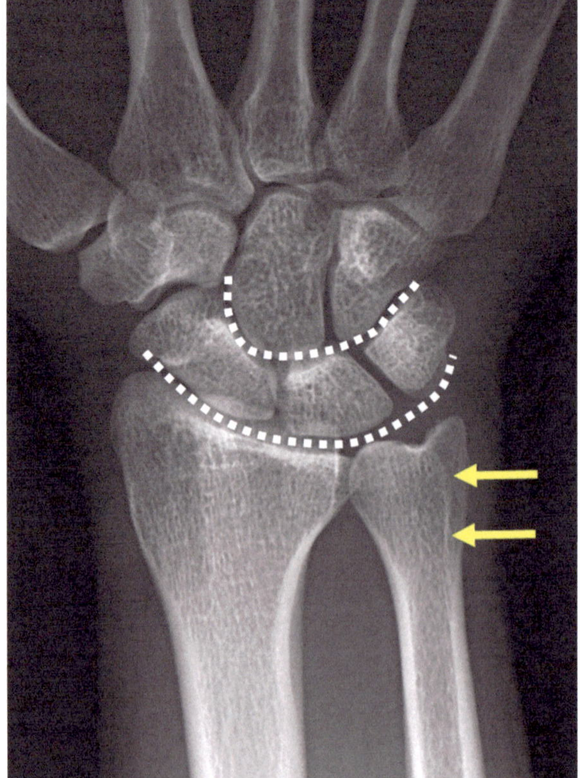

Fig. 3.1 Normal PA radiograph of the wrist. Gilula's arcs are parallel and not disrupted (white dashed lines). The groove for the extensor carpi ulnaris is visible (yellow arrows)

On the lateral view of the wrist, the shoulder is adducted, the elbow is flexed at 90°, and the distal forearm and hand should be resting on the ulnar side [12]. On a correctly positioned lateral view, the pisiform should be located between the volar cortices of the scaphoid and capitate [22] (Fig. 3.2). The longitudinal axis should pass through the radius, lunate, capitate and third metacarpal. The scapholunate angle measured between the scaphoid and lunate axes normally ranges between 30 and 60° [13] (Fig. 3.3a), the capitolunate angle measured between the capitate and lunate axes normally ranges between 0 and 30° [13] (Fig. 3.3b), and the radiolunate angle measured between the radial and lunate axes normally ranges between −15 and +15° [14] (Fig. 3.3c).

Supplemental stress radiographs may be useful in cases of suspected carpal instability with normal appearing PA and lateral radiographs [8]. A "clenched fist" view or modified clenched pencil view may be performed to demonstrate scapholunate dissociation [8, 23]. PA radiographs in ulnar and radial deviation can

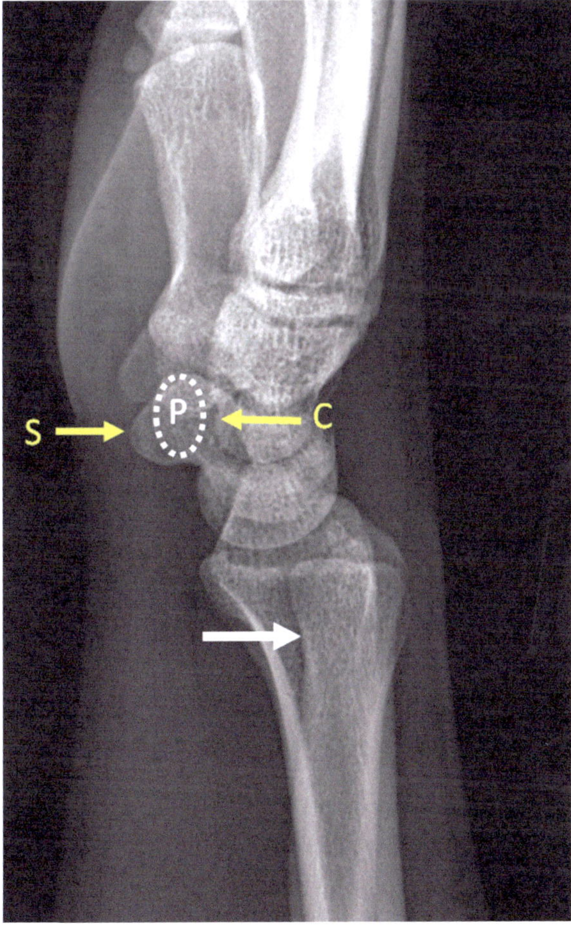

Fig. 3.2 Normal lateral radiograph of the wrist. The pisiform (P, dashed line) is located between the volar cortices (yellow arrows) of the scaphoid (S) and capitate (C). The distal ulna (arrow) overlaps with the radius

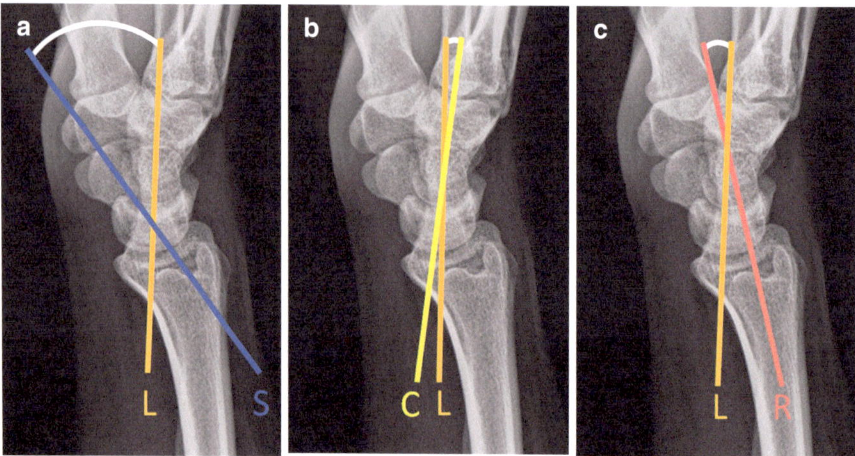

Fig. 3.3 Carpal angles that can be measured on lateral radiographs. (**a**) Normal scapholunate (SL) angle is 30°–60°. (**b**) Normal capitolunate (CL) angle 0°–30°. (**c**) Normal radiolunate (RL) angle −15° to +15°

demonstrate the dynamic relationship of the carpal bones. The distances between the carpal bones are normally equal throughout the carpus and should remain unchanged between radial or ulnar deviation [8, 13].

Cineradiography

Cineradiography uses fluoroscopy to create real-time video images and enables dynamic evaluation of motion induced clicking or snapping of the wrist [24, 25]. Posteroanterior imaging is acquired in the neutral position and in radial and ulnar deviation. Lateral imaging is acquired in the neutral position and in flexion and extension [24, 25]. Patient-induced maneuvers leading to snapping can also be evaluated during the study [26]. However, this modality is limited by low resolution, poor soft tissue contrast and overlapping anatomy [7].

Ultrasonography (US)

US is a useful dynamic imaging modality to evaluate scapholunate instability, but its utility in other types of instability is limited [7]. The normal dorsal scapholunate interosseous ligament (SLIL) is smooth, homogeneous, and echogenic in signal [27] (Fig. 3.4). The sensitivity for diagnosing tears of the dorsal band of the SLIL ranges from 46% to 100%, with specificities of 92%–100% [27–29]. Sensitivity and specificity for evaluating tears of the lunotriquetral ligament are lower and more

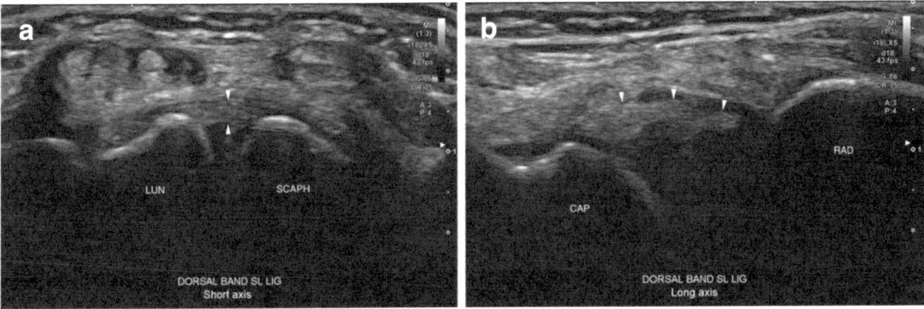

Fig. 3.4 Ultrasound of the normal dorsal band of the scapholunate ligament. (**a**) Short- and (**b**) long-axis ultrasound images obtained over the dorsal aspect of the scapholunate joint with the wrist in a position of moderate volar flexion demonstrate a normal intact dorsal band scapholunate ligament (arrowheads) (*SCAPH* Scaphoid, *LUN* Lunate). The long-axis image has been obtained in the plane of scapholunate joint space which is appreciated as the hypoechoic interval between the capitate (CAP) and radius (RAD). Note the normal fibrillar echotexture of the ligament shown on this short-axis image obtained using a high-frequency (18 MHz) transducer. Image courtesy of John Read, Macquarie University, Sydney, Australia

inconsistent compared to evaluation of the SLIL which may be attributed to the small size of the lunotriquetral ligament and limited ultrasound visualization of the volar and proximal bands [29, 30]. US is also highly dependent on the experience and skills of the operator [27–29]. In addition, a false-negative US may occur with a scarred and chronically torn scapholunate ligament [27]. Quantitative measurements of the scapholunate interval during dynamic maneuvers may be difficult to reproduce due to irregular bony contours of the wrist leading to instability of the US probe [27]. Due to these limitations, US is more commonly used as an adjunct to other imaging modalities [7, 27].

Magnetic Resonance Imaging (MRI) and Magnetic Resonance Arthrography (MRA)

MRI allows for direct visualization of the intrinsic and extrinsic carpal ligaments, as well as the osseous structures and articular cartilage (Fig. 3.5). Both MRI and MRA demonstrate high diagnostic accuracy for detecting intrinsic ligament tears [31–39], with better detection on MRA than conventional MRI [31]. Compared to the traditional 1.5 Tesla (1.5 T) MRI system, imaging on a 3 Tesla (3 T) MRI provides faster scan times, higher signal-to-noise ratio, and higher spatial and temporal resolution [36, 40]. As a result, most hospitals and imaging centers upgrading their equipment usually replace lower strength MRI scanners with 3 T MRI scanners. 3 T MRI is more sensitive than 1.5 T MRI in the detection of interosseous ligament tears with sensitivities ranging from 65% to 89% for scapholunate ligament tears and 60% to 82% for lunotriquetral ligament tears [11, 31, 34, 35]. Three-dimensional (3D) isotropic sequences are now available on most MRI scanners, where the voxels of data

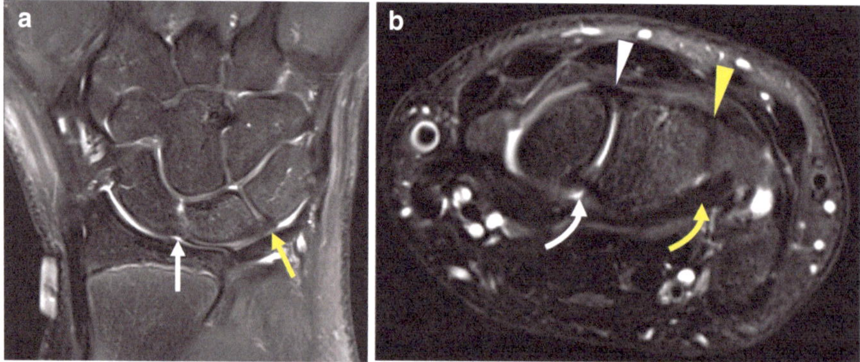

Fig. 3.5 MRI of normal scapholunate and lunotriquetral ligaments. (**a**) Coronal fat-suppressed proton density-weighted image shows intact central fibers of the scapholunate (arrow) and lunotriquetral ligaments (yellow arrow). (**b**) Axial fat-suppressed T2-weighted image shows intact dorsal fibers (arrowhead) and volar fibers (curved arrow) of the scapholunate ligament, and intact dorsal fibers (yellow arrowhead) and volar fibers (yellow curved arrow) of the lunotriquetral ligament

generated by the 3D acquisition measure the same in each direction, allowing images to be reformatted with equal resolution in any direction, and can be acquired with very thin sections of less than 1 mm. A 3D T2-weighted isotropic sequence acquired on a 3 T MRI has been shown to have a high diagnostic accuracy of 91% in detection of partial and complete ligament tears with a sensitivity and specificity for scapholunate ligament tears of 87% and 90%, respectively, and a sensitivity and specificity for lunotriquetral ligament tears of 63% and 97%, respectively [41]. In some institutions, 3 T MRI has replaced MRA of the wrist and is considered the imaging modality of choice when available [40]. Dynamic MRI of the wrist during active motion has been used to demonstrate carpal instability, subluxation/dislocation of the extensor carpi ulnaris tendon with dynamic rotation of the wrist, but is not currently used in clinical practice [42–44].

Computed Tomography (CT) and CT Arthrography (CTA)

Non-contrast CT may help identify occult fractures of the carpal bones, is helpful in evaluating the degree of arthritis in late-stage carpal instability and can aid preoperative planning [13]. Non-contrast CT has little utility in the evaluation of the carpal ligaments. However, CT arthrography is an excellent technique for evaluating the intrinsic carpal ligaments well, as well as any associated injuries to the articular cartilage and or triangular fibrocartilage complex [32, 33]. CTA has high diagnostic accuracy in detecting scapholunate and lunotriquetral ligament tears and is superior to MRI and MRA done on a 1.5 T scanner, especially for partial tears that do not require surgical intervention [32, 33]. CT arthrography may also be appropriate for patients who have metallic hardware in place, where susceptibility artifact from the metal may obscure the ligaments, or in patients with other contraindications to MRI such as intracranial aneurysm clips, cochlear implants, intraocular metallic foreign bodies, pacemakers, implantable cardioverter defibrillators or drug infusion pumps.

Imaging Examples of Carpal Instability

Carpal Instability Dissociative (CID): Scapholunate and Lunotriquetral

Carpal instability dissociative involves derangement within or between bones in the same carpal row. *Scapholunate instability* is the most common type of CID involving the proximal carpal row [45, 46]. In the pre-dynamic stage, the SLIL is partially torn involving the proximal or volar fibers which can diagnosed on MRI or MRA [7] (Fig. 3.6). Conventional and stress radiographs are often normal [7]. In the dynamic stage, the SLIL is partially or completely torn with involvement of the dorsal band, but the secondary stabilizers are intact [7, 26]. The secondary stabilizers of the SLIL are the scaphotrapeziotrapezoid ligament (STTL), radioscaphocapitate ligament (RSCL), and flexor carpi radialis (FCR) tendon on the palmar side, and the dorsal radiocarpal ligament (DRCL) and dorsal intercarpal ligament (DICL) on the dorsal side [26]. Stress PA radiographs or cineradiography may demonstrate scapholunate diastasis while conventional static radiographs are normal [26, 46] (Fig. 3.7). MRI or MRA may demonstrate the SLIL tear with intact secondary ligamentous stabilizers. US may show tearing of the dorsal SLIL on static imaging (Fig. 3.8), as well as instability on dynamic imaging (Fig. 3.9). In the static stage, the secondary stabilizers are torn leading to scapholunate dissociation [46, 47]. PA radiographs demonstrate a widened scapholunate interosseous interval greater than 2–4 mm (Terry Thomas or David Letterman sign) and a scaphoid ring sign due to rotary subluxation of the foreshortened scaphoid [13] (Fig. 3.10). Lateral radiographs may show

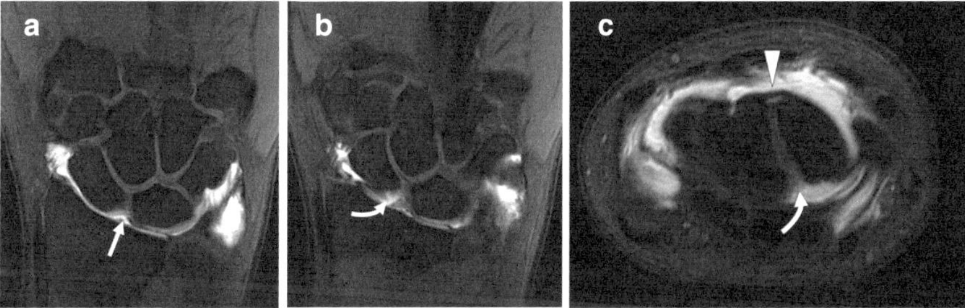

Fig. 3.6 A 28-year-old female with left wrist injury. (**a, b**) Coronal fat saturated T1-weighted MR arthrographic images demonstrate tearing of the proximal (arrow) and volar fibers (curved arrow) of the scapholunate ligament. (**c**) Axial fat saturated T1-weighted MR arthrographic image demonstrates tearing of the volar fibers (curved arrow). The dorsal fibers of the scapholunate ligament remain intact (arrowhead)

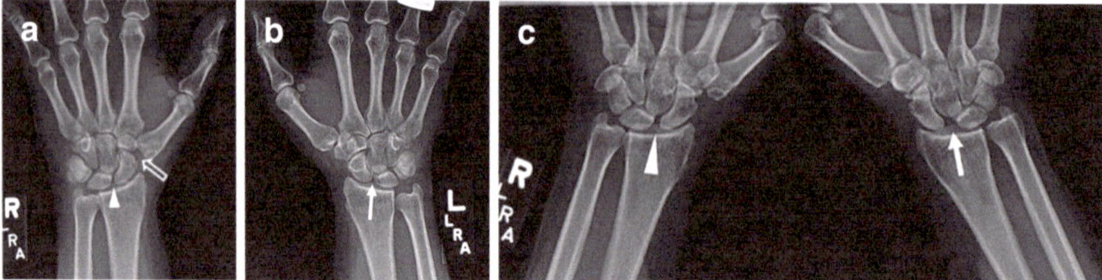

Fig. 3.7 A 51-year-old female with bilateral wrist pain. (**a**) PA radiograph of the right wrist shows a normal scapholunate interval (arrowhead). The patient has had prior trapezial resection (open arrow) for osteoarthritis of their first carpometacarpal joint. (**b**) PA radiograph of the left wrist shows possible mild widening of the scapholunate interval (arrow). (**c**) The pencil grip view (stress view) of both wrists demonstrates marked widening of the scapholunate interval on the left (arrow) and mild widening on the right (arrowhead), compatible with underlying scapholunate ligament injuries bilaterally

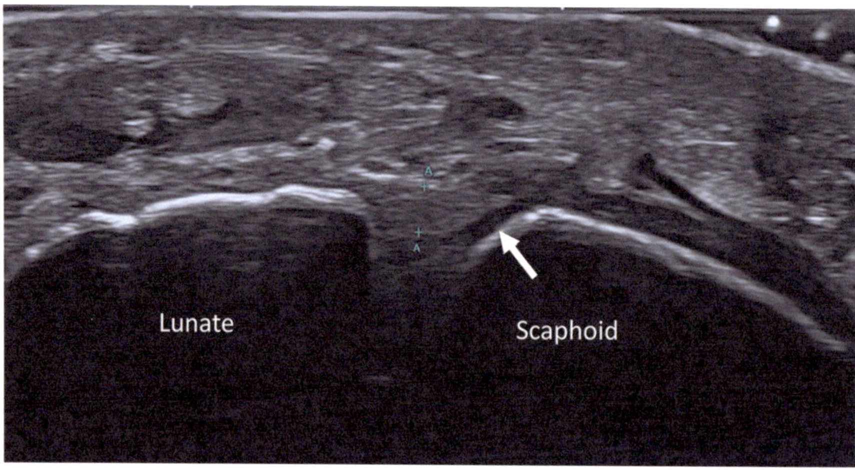

Fig. 3.8 Transverse ultrasound image of the wrist demonstrates a focal tear at the scaphoid attachment of the scapholunate ligament (arrow). It is important to confirm on real-time examination that any apparent defect in fiber continuity is not a scan artifact. This requires the exclusion of anisotropy by appropriate transducer angulation and demonstration of the defect in both transverse and longitudinal imaging planes. Image courtesy of John Read, Macquarie University, Sydney, Australia

dorsiflexion of the lunate and an increased scapholunate angle >60° in dorsal intercalated segmental instability (DISI) [13] (Fig. 3.10). Tears of the SLIL and secondary stabilizers are best diagnosed on MRI or MRA (Figs. 3.10 and 3.11). The late stage of scapholunate instability can lead to osteoarthritis and scapholunate advanced collapse (SLAC), characterized by severe radioscaphoid joint space narrowing and progressive proximal migration of the capitate bone that is interposed between the scaphoid and lunate bones [8] (Fig. 3.12). Nonunion scaphoid fracture

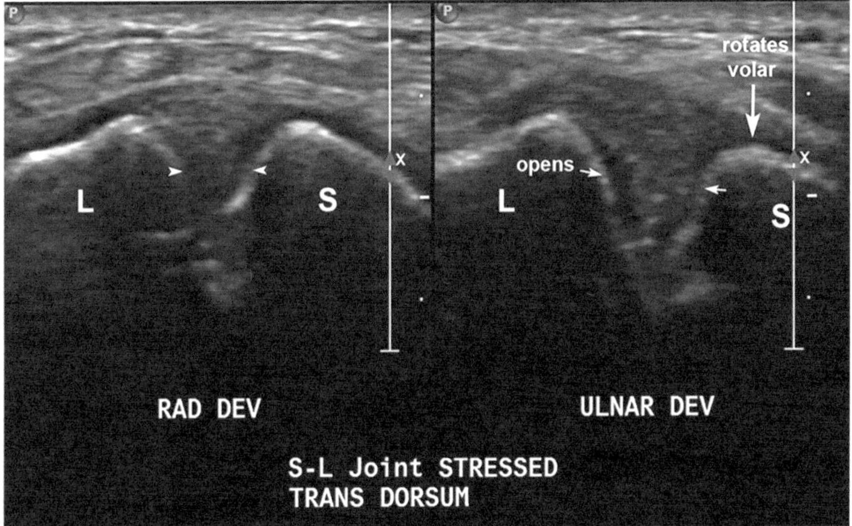

Fig. 3.9 Scapholunate instability. Transverse ultrasound images obtained over the dorsal aspect of scapholunate joint with the wrist placed in positions of active applied end-range radial (RAD DEV) and ulnar deviation (ULNAR DEV) stress demonstrate joint space widening and sagittal plane rotation of the distal pole of the scaphoid in a volar direction relative to the adjacent lunate on the ulnar deviation image. These findings should be interpreted in a clinical context and subjectively compared with the contralateral side to confirm an asymmetrically increased range of motion and exclude innate ligamentous laxity. Image courtesy of John Read, Macquarie University, Sydney, Australia

may also lead to CID, with similar stages of osteoarthritis and collapse of the carpus as seen in scaphoid non-union advanced collapse (SNAC) [8] (Figs. 3.13 and 3.14).

Lunotriquetral (LT) instability can result from tearing of the lunotriquetral interosseous ligament (LTIL) and is often associated with abnormalities of the triangular fibrocartilage complex [26, 48, 49]. Similar to scapholunate instability, LT instability is also classified into pre-dynamic, dynamic and static stages [10, 26]. In the dynamic stage, the LTIL is completely torn whereas in the static stage, the secondary ligamentous stabilizers are torn as well as the LTIL [26]. The main secondary stabilizers of the LTIL are the long radiolunate ligament (LRLL), ulnotriquetral ligament (UTL) and dorsal radiocarpal ligament (DRCL) [26]. In the static stage, PA radiographs demonstrate disruption of Gilula's arcs, proximal migration of the triquetrum and/or LT overlap [8]. Radiographs rarely demonstrate LT widening even in the late stages [8]. In volar intercalated segmental instability (VISI), the lunate may demonstrate a triangular shape on the PA view. On the lateral view, the lunate is flexed and tilted volarly, the proximal capitate is translated volarly, the capitolunate angle is increased (>30°), and the SL angle is decreased (<30°) [8, 11, 13] (Fig. 3.15). Evaluation of the LTIL (particularly the volar and proximal bands) on ultrasound is limited [28, 30]. The LTIL is also difficult to visualize on MRI due to its small size and the oblique course of its volar band [26]. Diagnostic accuracy

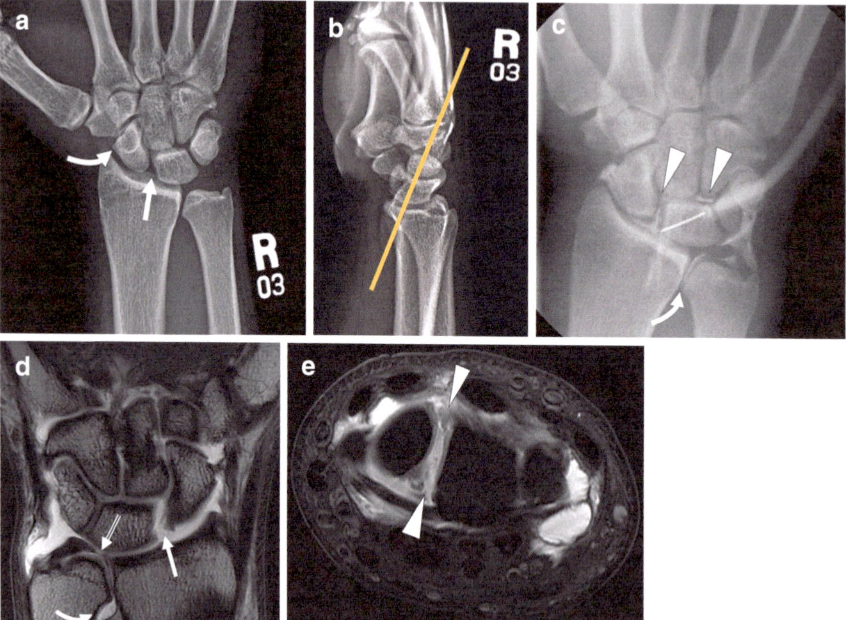

Fig. 3.10 A 22-year-old male with right wrist injury. (**a**) PA radiograph demonstrates mild widening of the scapholunate interval proximally (arrow). A ring-shaped density is present in the distal scaphoid (curved arrow) due to rotatory subluxation from flexion of the scaphoid. (**b**) Lateral radiograph demonstrates dorsal angulation of the lunate (orange line). The scapholunate angle was measured at 82°. (**c**) Wrist arthrogram demonstrates a needle in the scapholunate interval. Injected iodinated contrast is seen extending through the scapholunate interval to the midcarpal joint (arrowheads), indicative of a tear. Contrast is also seen extending into the distal radioulnar joint, compatible with a tear of the triangular fibrocartilage (curved arrow). (**d**) Coronal T1 and (**e**) axial fat-suppressed T1-weighted MR arthrographic images demonstrate a complete full-thickness tear of the scapholunate ligament with disruption of the proximal fibers (arrow), as well as the dorsal and volar fibers (arrowheads). There is also a small tear in the triangular fibrocartilage (short double line arrow) with gadolinium in the distal radioulnar joint (curved arrow)

is improved when arthrography is performed in conjunction with MRI or CT [31–33, 36] (Figs. 3.16 and 3.17). High-resolution 3 T MRI and the inclusion of thin 3D isotropic images which allow images to be reconstructed in any imaging plane may improve the detection of LTIL tears [41] (Fig. 3.18).

Carpal Instability Non-Dissociative (CIND): Radiocarpal and Midcarpal

CIND refers to instability between the carpal rows and is characterized by kinematic dysfunction of the proximal carpal row related to abnormal extrinsic ligaments of the wrist [11, 50]. CIND can occur at the radiocarpal joint, midcarpal joint

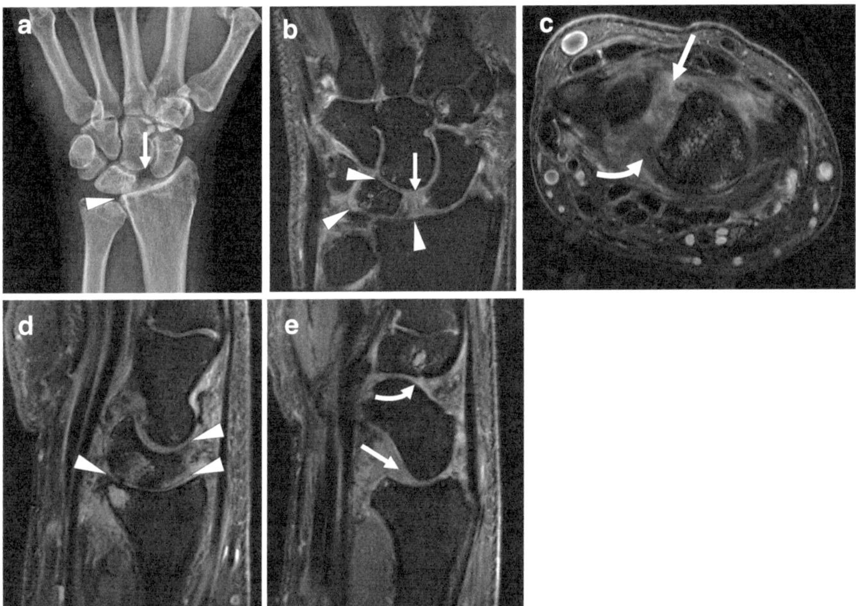

Fig. 3.11 A 65-year-old male with right. (**a**) PA radiograph demonstrates prominent widening of the scapholunate interval (arrow), with narrowing of the radiolunate joint space and subchondral cystic change along the distal radius (arrowheads). Note the ulnar translocation of the lunate and triquetrum. (**b**) Coronal fat saturated T2-weighted image demonstrates tearing of the membranous component of the scapholunate ligament with scapholunate dissociation (arrow), and chondral irregularity and subchondral cystic change along the distal radius, proximal lunate, and proximal capitate (arrowheads). (**c**) Axial fat saturated proton density-weighted image shows complete disruption of the dorsal (arrow) and volar components (curved arrow) of the scapholunate ligament. (**d**) Sagittal fat saturated T2-weighted image demonstrates dorsal tilt of the lunate with chondral thinning and subchondral cystic change along the distal radius, lunate and proximal capitate (arrowheads), compatible with dorsal intercalated segmental instability and a developing SLAC wrist. (**e**) Sagittal fat saturated T2-weighted image demonstrates dorsal translation of the scaphoid relative to the scaphoid fossa of the distal radius (arrow), which can indicate a more severe injury. Chondral irregularity and subchondral cystic change is seen in the trapezoid (curved arrow)

or a combination of both joints, and can be further subdivided by the direction of instability [11, 50, 51]. Imaging is useful to exclude intrinsic ligament tears, evaluate integrity of the extrinsic ligaments and to demonstrate the location and cause of the dynamic "clunk" that can be elicited on clinical examination [11, 51].

Radiocarpal CIND relates to insufficiency or disruption of the obliquely orientated extrinsic radiocarpal ligaments, allowing the proximal row to translocate in an ulnar, volar, dorsal, or radial direction relative to the articular surface of the distal radius [6, 50]. The most common type of radiocarpal instability is ulnar translocation has two distinct patterns. In type I ulnar translocation, the extrinsic radiocarpal ligaments comprising the radioscaphoid (RS), radioscaphocapitate (RSCL), and long radiolunate (LRLL) ligaments are torn which lead to ulnar shifting of the entire

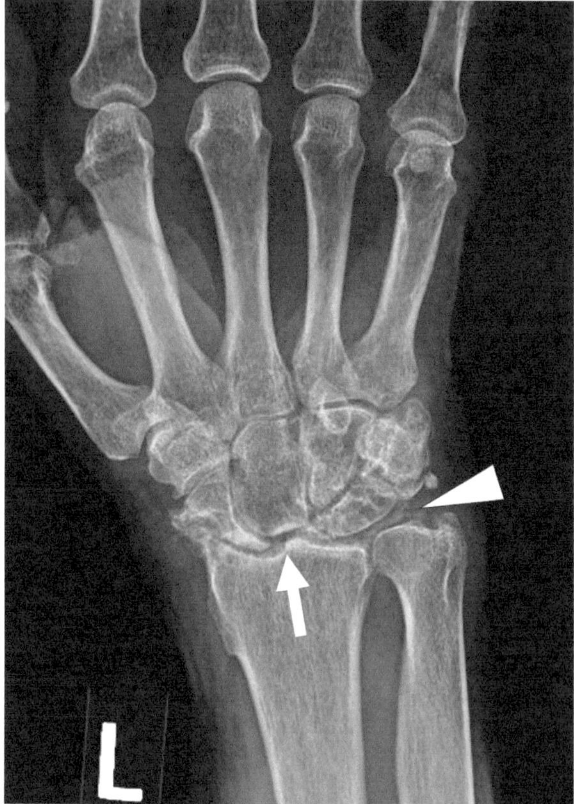

Fig. 3.12 A 72-year-old male with calcium pyrophosphate deposition (CPPD) and severe scapholunate advanced collapse (SLAC) of the left wrist. PA radiograph demonstrates widening of the scapholunate interval with proximal migration of the capitate (arrow). There is severe joint space narrowing in the radiocarpal and midcarpal joints. Chondrocalcinosis is seen in the triangular fibrocartilage (arrowhead)

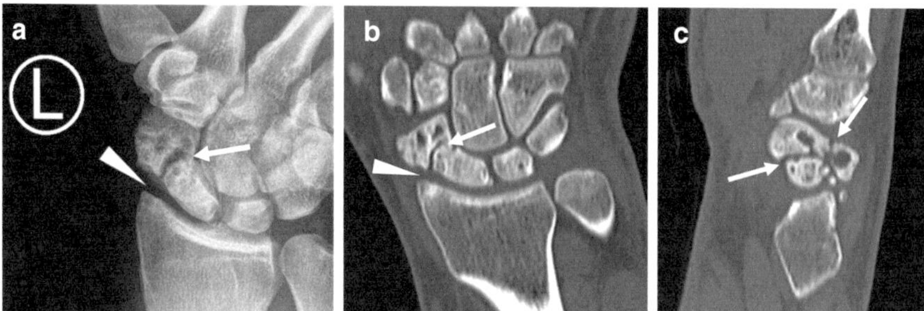

Fig. 3.13 A 29-year-old male with left wrist pain. (**a**) Coned radiograph of the scaphoid demonstrate an ununited fracture of the scaphoid waist (arrows), with adjacent sclerosis and cystic change. There is mild joint space narrowing between the scaphoid and radial styloid with associated subchondral sclerosis and cystic change (arrowhead), compatible with stage 1 scaphoid nonunion advanced collapse (SNAC). (**b**) Coronal and (**c**) sagittal CT reformats again demonstrate the ununited scaphoid fracture with fragmentation of the distal pole (arrows), and mild degenerative changes between the scaphoid and radial styloid (arrowhead)

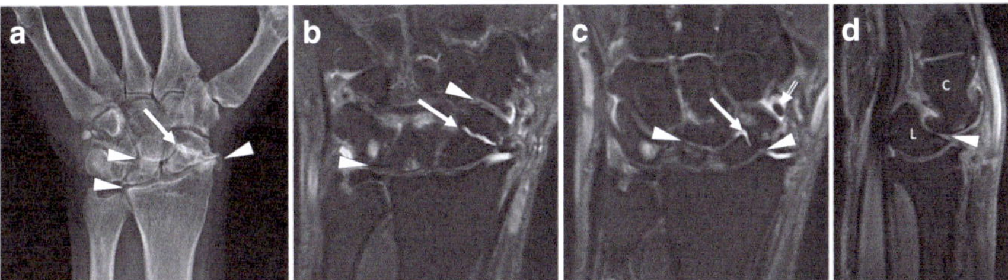

Fig. 3.14 A 58-year-old male with right wrist pain. (**a**) PA radiograph demonstrates scaphoid fracture (arrow) with severe degenerative changes in the radiocarpal and midcarpal joints (arrowheads). (**b**, **c**) Coronal fat-suppressed proton density-weighted images demonstrate a fluid-filled ununited scaphoid waist fracture (arrow) with degenerative changes in the radiocarpal and midcarpal joints (arrowheads). A joint body (short double line arrow) is seen in the joint recess along the distal scaphoid. (**d**) Sagittal fat-suppressed T2-weighted image demonstrates marked dorsal angulation of the lunate (L) with dorsal subluxation of the capitate (C) and marked associated degenerative changes (arrowhead)

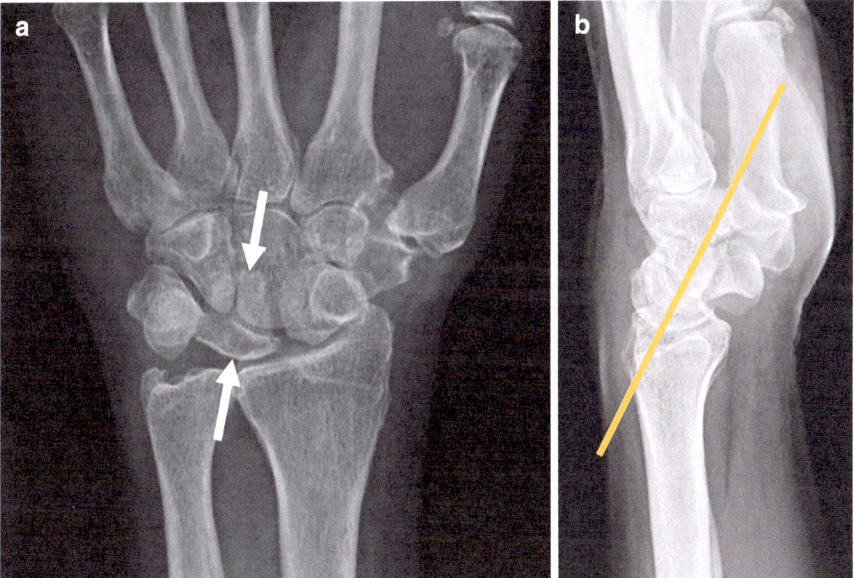

Fig. 3.15 Lunotriquetral instability. (**a**) PA radiograph demonstrates disruption of Gilula's arcs in the mid carpal joints and a triangular lunate (arrows). (**b**) Lateral radiograph demonstrates VISI with volar tilting of the flexed lunate (orange line) and a decreased scapholunate angle (not shown)

carpus [11, 50] (Fig. 3.19). On PA radiographs, there is radioscaphoid widening of >2 mm and decreased radiolunate contact of <50% [8, 50]. In type II ulnar translocation, the SLIL and LRLL are torn leading to ulnar shift of the lunotriquetral block while the scaphoid remains in place (Fig. 3.11), another manifestation of scapholunate dissociation [50]. The second most common type of radiocarpal CIND is radial deviation, followed by frank radiocarpal dislocation [52] (Fig. 3.20).

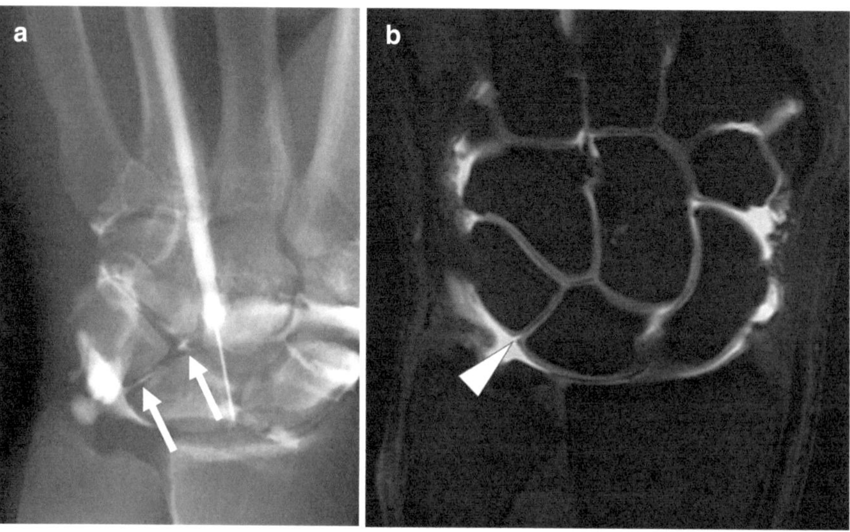

Fig. 3.16 An 18-year-old tennis player with wrist pain. (**a**) Arthrographic image demonstrates a needle in the dorsal radioscaphoid joint. Injected iodinated contrast is seen in the lunotriquetral interval extending to the midcarpal joints indicating a lunotriquetral tear (arrows). (**b**) Coronal fat-suppressed T1-weighted MR arthrographic image demonstrates contrast outlining the tear in the membranous lunotriquetral ligament (arrowhead)

Fig. 3.17 CT arthrogram in a patient with a lunotriquetral ligament tear. Iodinated contrast was injected into the radiocarpal joint and is seen tracking through the lunotriquetral interval (arrowhead) to enter the midcarpal joints, compatible with an underlying tear. Image courtesy of Philip Wong, MD, Emory University, Department of Diagnostic Radiology and Imaging Sciences

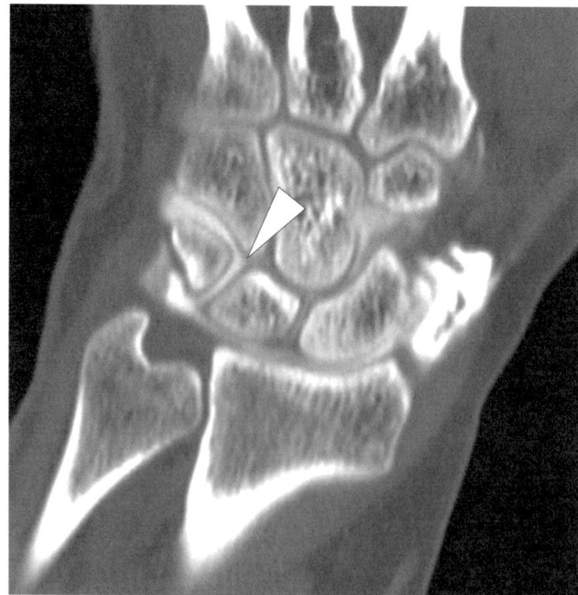

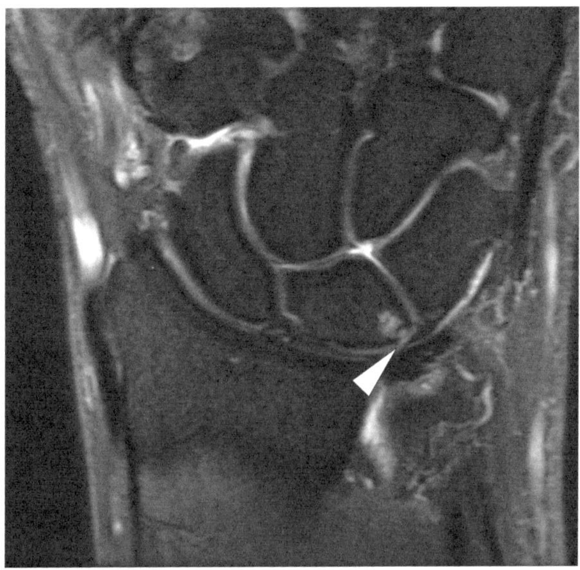

Fig. 3.18 A 54-year-old male with left wrist pain. Coronal fat-suppressed proton density-weighted MR image demonstrates focal detachment of the proximal lunotriquetral ligament from the lunate attachment with adjacent microavulsive cystic change (arrowhead)

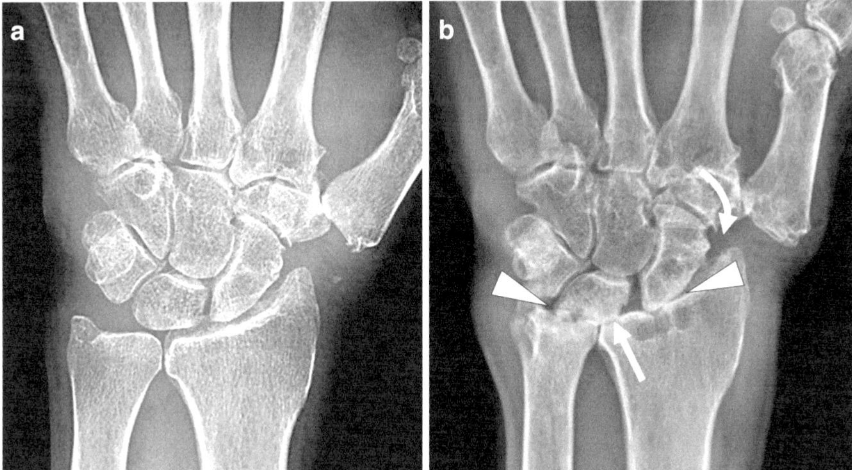

Fig. 3.19 A 43-year-old female with rheumatoid arthritis and radiocarpal instability. PA radiographs at baseline (**a**) and 2 years later (**b**) demonstrate progressive ulnar translocation of the carpus. There is decreased radiolunate contact of less than 50% (arrow). The radial styloid-scaphoid interspace is widened (curved arrow) while the radial-proximal scaphoid, radiolunate and ulnolunate joint spaces are significantly narrowed with the development of erosions and cysts in the carpus, distal radius, and ulna (arrowheads)

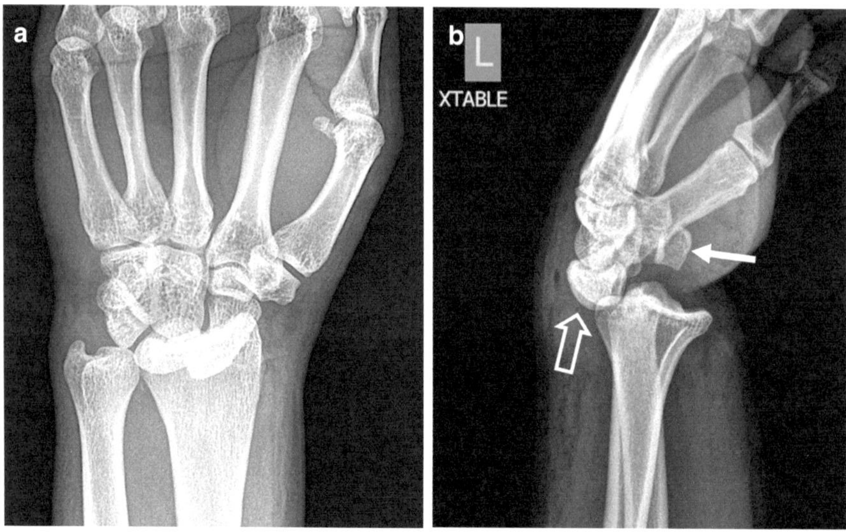

Fig. 3.20 A 25-year-old male with crush injury of left wrist. (**a**) PA radiograph demonstrates the proximal carpal bones overlapping the distal radius. (**b**) Lateral radiograph demonstrates dislocation of the radiocarpal joint with dorsal displacement of the carpus (open arrow) and prominent overlying soft tissue swelling. There is also dislocation of the pisiform bone (arrow)

Midcarpal instability (MCI) is frequently associated with snapping or clunking of the wrist due to symptomatic laxity of the carpal ligaments [51, 53]. MCI is classified into intrinsic and extrinsic categories [54]. The intrinsic category can be further subdivided into palmar, dorsal, or combined MCI instability [53, 54]. Radiographs of MCI may be normal [53]. Depending on the direction and severity of the MCI, radiographs or MRI may demonstrate malalignment between the proximal and distal carpal row, and a VISI or DISI deformity (Fig. 3.21) [8, 53, 54]. Cineradiography can be used to evaluate the dynamic instability of the midcarpal joint and elicit any dynamic clunk as the wrist moves from radial to ulnar deviation [53]. MRI is the preferred imaging modality to evaluate the integrity of the intrinsic and extrinsic carpal ligaments [55].

Carpal Instability Complex (CIC)

Complex carpal instability includes features of both CID and CIND injuries. Most of these complex instabilities are secondary to perilunate injuries [8]. Perilunate instability progresses from a radial to ulnar direction with sequential ligamentous injuries that are classified into four Mayfield stages [4]. Stage I involves SLIL

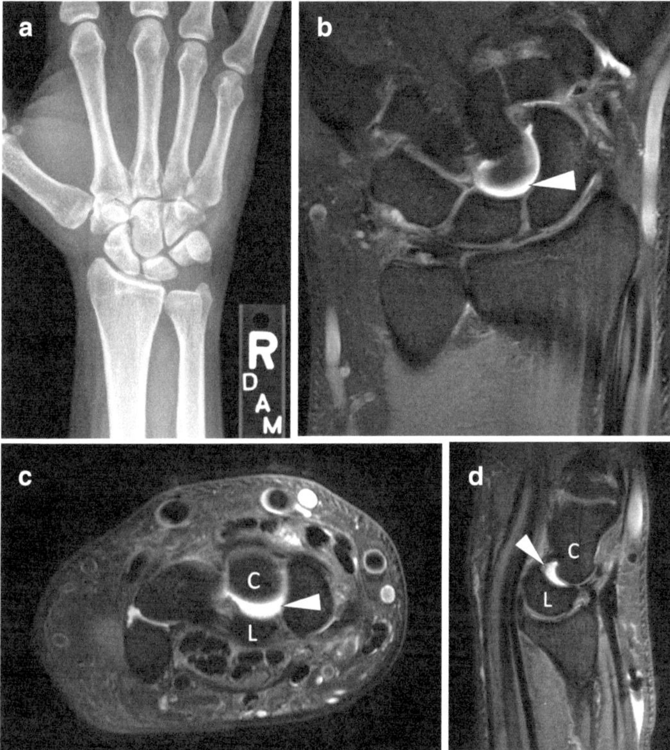

Fig. 3.21 A 47-year-old male with dorsal type non-dissociative midcarpal instability. (**a**) PA radiograph of the wrist is normal. (**b**) Coronal fat-suppressed proton density-weighted image shows abnormal fluid in the midcarpal joint (arrowhead). (**c**) Axial fat-suppressed proton density-weighted image demonstrates increased intraosseous space between the lunate (L) and capitate (C) bones (arrowhead). (**d**) Sagittal fat-suppressed proton density-weighted image shows asymmetric widening of the lunocapitate joint space (arrowhead), dorsal tilt of the lunate, and posterior subluxation of the capitate

disruption leading to scapholunate dissociation. In stage II, there is lunocapitate disruption leading to dislocation of the capitate, commonly dorsally. In stage III, the LTIL is disrupted. In the final stage IV, the lunate is dislocated volarly and the capitate is aligned with the radius [8, 4] (Fig. 3.22). Mayfield classified perilunate injuries into lesser arc and greater arc patterns [4]. Lesser arc injuries are purely ligamentous along the articular surfaces of the lunate [53]. Greater arc injuries occur when there are superimposed fractures of the bones surrounding the lunate as seen in perilunate-fracture dislocations [8, 4] (Fig. 3.23). Radiographs are the first line of imaging to diagnose these injuries [8]. CT can be useful in complex injuries to detect fractures, and MRI can assess the integrity of articular cartilage and carpal ligaments [11].

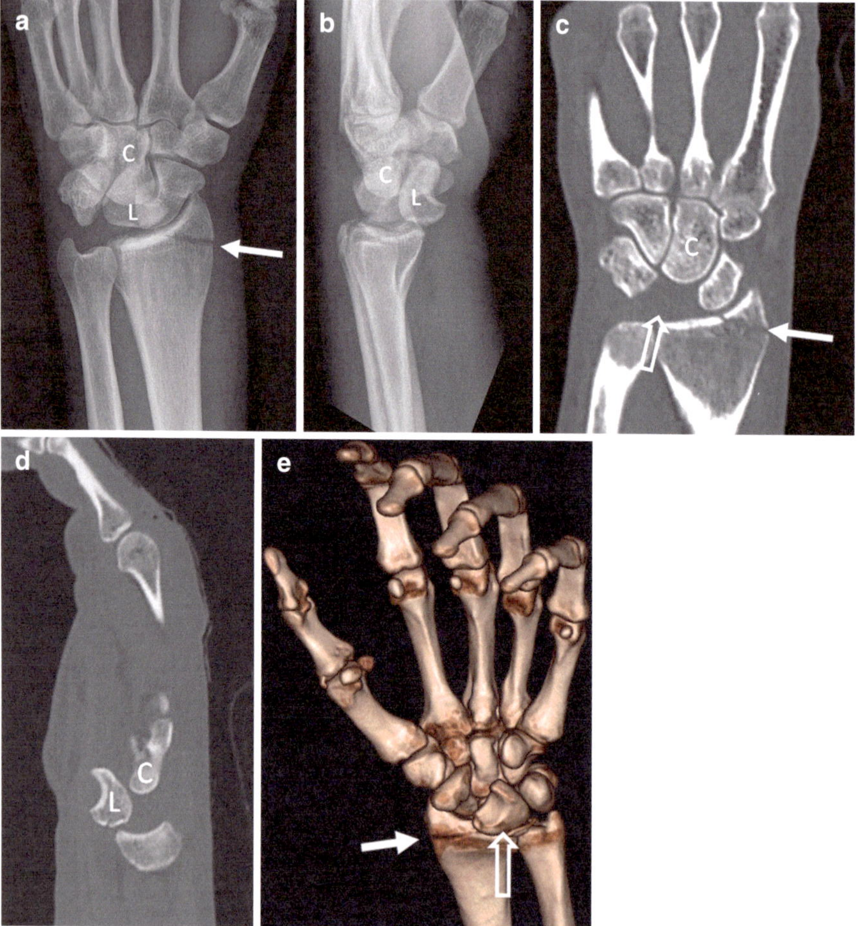

Fig. 3.22 A 33-year-old male with left wrist injury. (**a**) PA radiograph demonstrates a mildly displaced fracture through the radial styloid (arrowhead). The lunate (L) appears triangular in morphology and overlaps the capitate (C), with disruption of the first and second Gilula arcs. (**b**) Lateral wrist radiograph shows volar dislocation of the lunate (L) with respect to the capitate (C). (**c**) Coronal CT reformat shows the radial styloid fracture (arrow) and absence of the lunate in the proximal carpal row (open arrow). (**d**) Sagittal CT reformat confirms volar dislocation of the lunate (L). (**e**) 3D reformatted CT image nicely depicts the dislocated lunate along the volar wrist (open arrow) and radial styloid fracture

Carpal Instability Adaptive (CIA)

Adaptive carpal instability is similar to radiocarpal instability CIND except the cause is related to distal radial or ulnar abnormalities. Malunited distal radial fractures, Madelung's deformity (Fig. 3.24), or excessive resection of the radial styloid process or ulnar head are causes of CIA [8]. Imaging is performed to assess

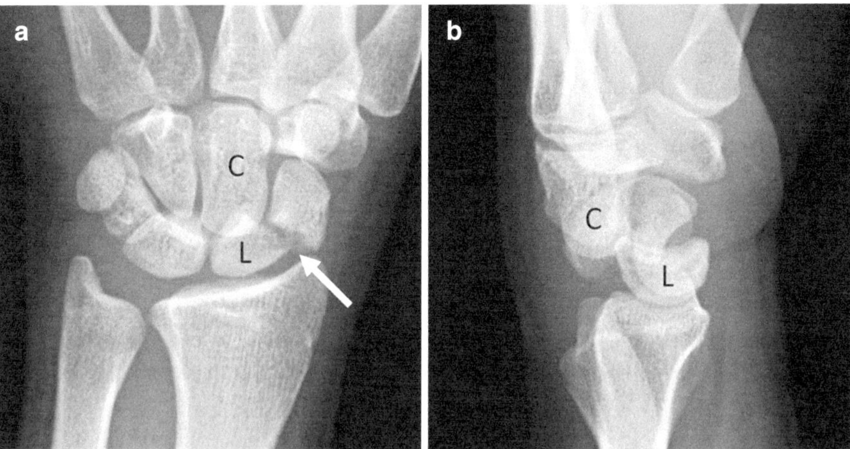

Fig. 3.23 24-year-old male with transcaphoid perilunate dislocation. (**a**) PA radiograph demonstrates a displaced scaphoid waist fracture (arrow) and disruption of the radiocarpal and midcarpal Gilula arcs. (**b**) Lateral radiograph shows that the lunate (L) is in normal alignment with the distal radius, but there is dorsal dislocation of the scaphoid-distal carpal row complex (C) relative to the lunate

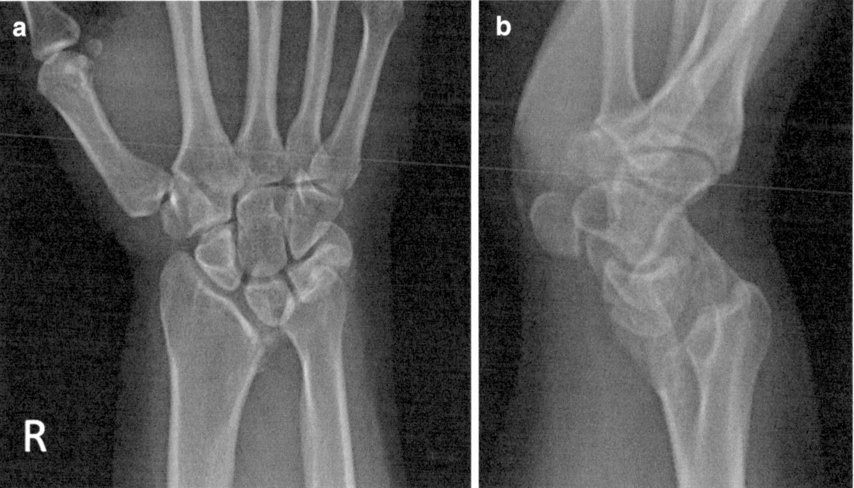

Fig. 3.24 Madelung deformity of the right forearm. (**a**) PA radiograph shows markedly increased radial inclination angle and foreshortening of the ulnar aspect of the distal radius. (**b**) Lateral radiograph demonstrates marked dorsal subluxation of the distal ulna

abnormal anatomy outside the carpus that can lead to adaptive instability [11]. Radiographs and CT can demonstrate these osseous abnormalities well. MRI, MRA, or CTA can be performed to evaluate soft tissue injuries [11].

In summary, imaging plays an important role in the diagnosis of carpal instability and can help guide management. Radiography is the first line of imaging although dynamic types of carpal instability may be normal on conventional radiographs. Cineradiography can capture the clicking of the wrist during dynamic imaging. Ultrasound can be used to diagnose dorsal tears of the scapholunate ligament but is more often used as an adjunct to other imaging modalities. CT arthrography has a high accuracy in the detection of scapholunate and lunotriquetral ligament tears and may be better at detecting partial tears than MRI or MRA performed on lower strength MRI scanners. CT arthrography is the most suitable technique if the patient has metallic hardware in place or contraindications to an MRI scan. Both MRI and MR arthrography have high accuracy in the detection of interosseous ligament tears. However, the high-resolution images produced on 3 T MRI scanners have decreased the use of MR arthrography and CT arthrography in many institutions.

References

1. Garcia-Elias M, Berger RA, Horii E, Kauer J, et al. Definition of carpal instability. The anatomy and Biomechanics Committee of the International Federation of Societies for Surgery of the Hand. J Hand Surg Am. 1999;24(4):866–7.
2. Cooney WP, Dobyns JH, Linscheid RL. Arthroscopy of the wrist: anatomy and classification of carpal instability. Arthroscopy. 1990;6(2):133–40.
3. Wolfe SW, Garcia-Elias M, Kitay A. Carpal instability nondissociative. J Am Acad Orthop Surg. 2012;20:575–85.
4. Mayfield JK, Johnson RP, Kilcoyne RK. Carpal dislocations: pathomechanics and progressive perilunar instability. J Hand Surg Am. 1980;5(3):226–41.
5. Carlsen BT, Shin AY. Wrist instability. Scand J Surg. 2008;97:324–32.
6. Khan M, Lim WY, Resnick D (2012) Carpal instability. In: MRI web clinic Radsource. http://radsource.us/carpal-instability/. Accessed 22 May 2023.
7. Flores DV, Umpire DF, Gómez C, Saad T, Cerezal L, Pathria M. Carpal instability: anatomy, kinematics, imaging, and classification. Radiographics. 2021;41:E155–6.
8. Kani KK, Mulcahy H, Chew FS. Understanding carpal instability: a radiographic perspective. Skeletal Radiol. 2016;45(8):1031–43.
9. Kitay A, Wolfe SW. Scapholunate instability: current concepts in diagnosis and management. J Hand Surg Am. 2012;37:2175–96.
10. Shin AY, Battaglia MJ, Bishop AT. Lunotriquetral instability: diagnosis and treatment. J Am Acad Orthop Surg. 2000;8:170–9.
11. Ramamurthy NK, Chojnowski AJ, Toms AP. Imaging of carpal instability. J Hand Surg Eur Vol. 2016;41E(1):22–34.
12. Beltran H, Greenspan A. Upper limb III: distal forearm, wrist, and hand. In: Greenspan A, editor. Orthopedic imaging: a practical approach. 6th ed. Philadelphia, PA: Lippincott; 2015.
13. Loredo RA, Sorge DG, Garcia G. Radiographic evaluation of the wrist: a vanishing art. Semin Roentgenol. 2005;40(3):248–89.

14. Schmitt R, Prommersberger K. Carpal morphometry and function. In: Schmitt R, Lanz U, editors. Diagnostic imaging of the hand. 1st ed. Thieme; 2008.
15. Mann FA, Wilson AJ, Gilula LA. Radiographic evaluation of the wrist: what does the hand surgeon want to know? Radiology. 1992;184(1):15–24.
16. Sartoris D, Resnick D. Plain film radiography: routine and specialized techniques and projections. In: Resnick D, editor. Diagnosis of bone and joint disorders, vol. 1. 4th ed. Philadelphia, PA: Saunders; 2002.
17. Jedlinski A, Kauer JMG, Jonsson K. X-ray evaluation of the true neutral position of the wrist: the groove for extensor carpi ulnaris as a landmark. J Hand Surg Am. 1995;20:511–2.
18. Levis CM, Yang Z, Gilula LA. Validation of the extensor carpi ulnaris groove as a predictor for the recognition of standard posteroanterior radiographs of the wrist. J Hand Surg Am. 2002;27(2):252–7.
19. Gilula LA. Carpal injuries: analytic approach and case exercises. AJR Am J Roentgenol. 1979;133:503–17.
20. Toms AP, Chojnowski A, Cahir JG. Midcarpal instability: a radiological perspective. Skeletal Radiol. 2011;40(5):533–41.
21. Kindynis P, Resnick D, Kang HS, et al. Demonstration of the scapholunate space with radiography. Radiology. 1990;175:278–80.
22. Yang Z, Mann FA, Gilula LA, Haerr C, Larsen F. Scaphopisocapitate alignment: criterion to establish a neutral lateral view of the wrist. Radiology. 1997;205:865–9.
23. Lawand A, Foulkes GD. The "clenched pencil" view: a modified clenched fist scapholunate stress view. J Hand Surg Am. 2003;28:414–20.
24. Protas JM, Jackson WT. Evaluating carpal instabilities with fluoroscopy. AJR Am J Roentgenol. 1980;135(01):137–40.
25. Pliefke J, Stengel D, Rademacher G, Mutze S, Ekkernkamp A, Eisenschenk A. Diagnostic accuracy of plain radiographs and cineradiography in diagnosing traumatic scapholunate dissociation. Skeletal Radiol. 2008;37(02):139–45.
26. Hesse N, Schmitt R, Luitjens J, Grunz JP, Haas-Lützenberger EM. Carpal Instability: II. Imaging. Semin Musculoskelet Radiol. 2021;25(2):304–10.
27. Dao KD, Solomon DJ, Shin AY, Puckett ML. The efficacy of ultrasound in the evaluation of dynamic scapholunate ligamentous instability. J Bone Joint Surg Am. 2004;86(7):1473–8.
28. Taljanovic MS, Sheppard JE, Jones MD, Switlick DN, Hunter TB, Rogers LF. Sonography and sonoarthrography of the scapholunate and lunotriquetral ligaments and triangular fibrocartilage disk: initial experience and correlation with arthrography and magnetic resonance arthrography. J Ultrasound Med. 2008;27(2):179–91.
29. Finlay K, Lee R, Friedman L. Ultrasound of intrinsic wrist ligament and triangular fibrocartilage injuries. Skeletal Radiol. 2004;33(2):85–90.
30. Boutry N, Lapegue F, Masi L, Claret A, Demondion X, Cotton A. Ultrasonographic evaluation of normal extrinsic and intrinsic carpal ligaments: preliminary experience. Skeletal Radiol. 2005;34(9):513–21.
31. Lee RK, Ng AW, Tong CS, et al. Intrinsic ligament and triangular fibrocartilage complex tears of the wrist: comparison of MDCT arthrography, conventional 3-T MRI, and MR arthrography. Skeletal Radiol. 2013;42(9):1277–85.
32. Moser T, Dosch JC, Moussaoui A, Dietemann JL. Wrist ligament tears: evaluation of MRI and combined MDCT and MR arthrography. Am J Roentgenol. 2007;188:1278–86.
33. Schmid MR, Schertler T, Pfirrmann CW, et al. Interosseous ligament tears of the wrist: comparison of multi-detector row CT arthrography and MR imaging. Radiology. 2005;237(3):1008–13.
34. Hafezi-Nejad N, Carrino JA, Eng J, et al. Scapholunate interosseous ligament tears: diagnostic performance of 1.5 T, 3 T MRI, and MR arthrography-a systematic review and meta-analysis. Acad Radiol. 2016;23(9):1091–103.
35. Andersson JK, Andernord D, Karlsson J, Fridén J. Efficacy of magnetic resonance imaging and clinical tests in diagnostics of wrist ligament injuries: a systematic review. Arthroscopy. 2015;31(10):2014–e2.

36. Lee YH, Choi YR, Kim S, Song HT, Suh JS. Intrinsic ligament and triangular fibrocartilage complex (TFCC) tears of the wrist: comparison of isovolumetric 3D-THRIVE sequence MR arthrography and conventional MR image at 3 T. Magn Reson Imaging. 2013;31(2):221–6.
37. Magee T. Comparison of 3-T MRI and arthroscopy of intrinsic wrist ligament and TFCC tears. Am J Roentgenol. 2009;192(1):80–5.
38. Zanetti M, Bräm J, Hodler J. Triangular fibrocartilage and intercarpal ligaments of the wrist: does MR arthrography improve standard MRI? J Magn Reson Imaging. 1997;7(3):590–4.
39. Dietrich TJ, Toms AP, Cerezal L, et al. Interdisciplinary consensus statements on imaging of scapholunate joint instability. Eur Radiol. 2021;31(12):9446–58.
40. Chhabra A, Soldatos T, Thawait GK, Del Grande F, Thakkar RS, Means KR Jr, Carrino JA. Current perspectives on the advantages of 3-T MR imaging of the wrist. Radiographics. 2012;32(3):879–96.
41. Eladawi S, Balamoody S, Amerasekera S, Choudhary S. 3T MRI of wrist ligaments and TFCC using true plane oblique 3D T2 dual Echo steady state (DESS)—a study of diagnostic accuracy. Br J Radiol. 2022;95(1129):20210019.
42. Henrichon SS, Foster BH, Shaw C, Bayne CO, Szabo RM, Chaudhari AJ, Boutin RD. Dynamic MRI of the wrist in less than 20 seconds: normal midcarpal motion and reader reliability. Skeletal Radiol. 2020;49(2):241–8.
43. Shaw CB, Foster BH, Borgese M, Boutin RD, Bateni C, Boonsri P, Bayne CO, Szabo RM, Nayak KS, Chaudhari AJ. Real-time three-dimensional MRI for the assessment of dynamic carpal instability. PLoS One. 2019;14(9):e0222704.
44. Kaiser P, Kellermann F, Arora R, Henninger B, Rudisch A. Diagnosing extensor carpi ulnaris tendon dislocation with dynamic rotation MRI of the wrist. Clin Imaging. 2018;51:323–6.
45. Larsen CF, Amadio PC, Gilula LA, Hodge JC. Analysis of carpal instability: I. Description of the scheme. J Hand Surg Am. 1995;20(05):757–64.
46. Watson HK, Weinzweig J, Zeppieri J. The natural progression of scaphoid instability. Hand Clin. 1997;13(1):39–49.
47. Mitsuyasu H, Patterson RM, Shah MA, Buford WL, Iwamoto Y, Viegas SF. The role of the dorsal intercarpal ligament in dynamic and static scapholunate instability. J Hand Surg Am. 2004;29(02):279–88.
48. Horii E, Garcia-Elias M, An KN, et al. A kinematic study of lunotriquetral dissociations. J Hand Surg Am. 1991;16(02):355–62.
49. Palmer AK. Triangular fibrocartilage complex lesions: a classification. J Hand Surg Am. 1989;14(04):594–606.
50. Schmitt R, Hesse N, Goehtz F, Prommersberger KJ, de Jonge M, Grunz JP. Carpal Instability: I. Pathoanatomy. Semin Musculoskelet Radiol. 2021;25(2):191–202.
51. Zelenski NA, Shin AY. Management of nondissociative instability of the wrist. J Hand Surg Am. 2020;45(2):131–9.
52. De Villeneuve Bargemon JB, Soudé G, Levadoux M, Viaud-Ambrosino S, Peras M, Camuzard O. Radiocarpal fracture-dislocation: review of the literature, new classification and decision algorithm. Orthop Traumatol Surg Res May. 2023;109(3):103547.
53. Rabinovich RV, Rahman OF, Nasra MH, Polatsch DB, Beldner S. Midcarpal instability. J Am Acad Orthop Surg. 2023;31:834. https://doi.org/10.5435/JAAOS-D-22-00777.
54. Niacaris T, Ming BW, Lichtman DM. Midcarpal instability: a comprehensive review and update. Hand Clin. 2015;31(3):487–93.
55. Ringler MD, Murthy NS. MR imaging of wrist ligaments. Magn Reson Imaging Clin N Am. 2015;23(3):367–91.

Chapter 4
Classification of Intercarpal Ligament Injuries

Jane C. Messina, Valeria Vismara, and Pietro S. Randelli

Introduction

Intercarpal ligament injuries can be caused by acute sprains, trauma of the wrist or micro-trauma, due to repetitive heavy working activities or intensive sports activities. They may be associated to predisposing congenital factors (as ulnar plus). The ligaments mainly involved are scapho-lunate (SL) and luno-triquetral (LT) ligaments. The importance of these lesions is due to symptoms complained by patients especially under load (pain, reduction of grip strength, reduction of wrist motion), and to the potential progression of them leading to carpal instability and degenerative arthritis of the wrist at later stages.

Supplementary Information The online version contains supplementary material available at https://doi.org/10.1007/978-3-031-55869-6_4.

J. C. Messina (✉) · V. Vismara
UOC First Orthopaedic Clinic, University of Milan, ASST Gaetano Pini-CTO Orthopaedic Institute, Piazza Cardinal Ferrari 1, Milan, Italy
e-mail: janechristiane.messina@asst-pinicto.it

P. S. Randelli
UOC First Orthopaedic Clinic, University of Milan, ASST Gaetano Pini-CTO Orthopaedic Institute, Piazza Cardinal Ferrari 1, Milan, Italy

Laboratory of Applied Biomechanics, Department of Biomedical Sciences for Health, University of Milan, Milan, Italy

Research Center for Adult and Pediatric Rheumatic Diseases (RECAP-RD), Department of Biomedical Sciences for Health, University of Milan, Milan, Italy
e-mail: pietro.randelli@unimi.it

J. Yao (ed.), *Carpal Instability*, https://doi.org/10.1007/978-3-031-55869-6_4

Scapho-Lunate Arthroscopic Classification

Scapho-lunate interosseous ligament (SLIOL) injuries are a spectrum of lesions involving the scapho-lunate (SL) ligament and several extrinsic ligaments, this involvement progresses with time and with the use of the wrist, especially due to overload, repetitive traumas or microtraumas, manual work or intensive sports activities and may lead at a later stage to degenerative arthritis and SLAC wrist [1–4].

The mechanism of trauma has been described by Mayfield in 1984 and is related to a trauma that starts from the radial side of the wrist, with the wrist in extension, ulnar deviation, and intercarpal supination [5]. The volar portion of SLIOL is involved first and then the radio-capitate (RC) ligament, radio-triquetral (RT) ligament, and dorso-radiocarpal (DRC) ligament. After the injury to SL ligament (stage I), there is a palmar flexion of the lunate (stage II), a luno-triquetral dissociation (stage III), and then the lunocapitate dislocation (stage IV) [5].

It has been ascertained since many years that the correct staging of these lesions is mandatory before planning a surgical repair [3]. In fact, from the studies of Garcia Elias, there are some parameters that have been proposed in order to define a staging system that can be a guide to treatment. These parameters are integrity of the dorsal part of SL ligament, potential of healing of the ligaments (the repairability of SL ligament remnant), state of secondary stabilisers, reducibility of carpal malalignment, cartilage damage, and ulnar translocation. With these parameters, he has established a staging system and indications to treatment [2, 3].

In order to do the correct staging, we need to have an accurate history of the patient, activities of the patient (work or occupations, sports, and hobbies), X-ray examination, MRI scan and in the recently arthroscopic examination which has given a lot of additional information about intrinsic and extrinsic ligament and cartilage lesions. The developing of arthroscopic examination of the wrist and classification has been able to integrate the information based on Garcia Elias staging system. At the end of the diagnostic process, the surgeon will have a complete picture of the clinical case with the needs and expectations of the patient and will be able to do a correct surgical choice.

The first identification of intrinsic ligament injuries by arthroscopy in the absence of X-rays abnormalities was done by Dautel in 1993 [6]. The arthroscopic classification has been developing during the years and several authors have contributed to define it [6–10]. The Geissler Classification has been widely used for many years [9] and was described in acute SL injuries associated to distal radius fractures. Nevertheless, several anatomical studies have been performed during the past years that clearly show the involvement of extrinsic ligaments and the different resistance strength of the different portions of SLIOL (1–4, 10–12). In fact, the dorsal portion of SLIOL is stronger than the volar and proximal portions and then it is the most important to be repaired [12]. Moreover, we see in the clinical practice that partial ligament injuries are symptomatic and the patient requires treatment.

In the recent years, the classification has evolved by the work of EWAS group, which has developed a thorough classification for acute and chronic injuries, defining partial injuries involving the different portion of SL injuries and involvement of extrinsic ligaments and thus improving the arthroscopic classification [10]. This was based on a study done on cadaver specimen done under fluoroscopic and arthroscopic evaluation, sectioning the different portions of scapho-lunate interosseous ligament and extrinsic ligaments in order to correlate arthroscopic findings to anatomo-pathological damage of intrinsic and extrinsic ligaments in each arthroscopic stage of scapho-lunate injuries [10, 11].

The EWAS classification can be found in Table 4.1 [10, 11].

The wrist is examined from the radiocarpal joint first, standard portals 3–4 and 6R are used and then from midcarpal joint using MCR and MC portals.

In the radiocarpal joint, the normal scapho-lunate ligament is almost invisible and the "baby-buttock" sign (Figs. 4.1 and 4.2) indicates intact intrinsic ligaments, while the protrusion of SL ligament indicates that the ligament is damaged (Fig. 4.3).

The examination of midcarpal joint is more important as it allows the exact staging. The scope is positioned in UMC portal while the probe is positioned in RMC portal. A dynamic laxity test is performed twisting a 2 mm probe in the scapho-lunate joint. The probe is positioned between the scaphoid and the lunate within the SL joint and is twisted in the different portions of the ligament itself. The test should be performed in the anterior portion first, then in the central portion and finally in the posterior portion of SL joint. In this way, it is possible to diagnose which portion of the ligament is damaged and if the extrinsic ligament attachments are still in place or are detached (Table 4.1). Afterwards, the scope is moved to RMC portal and new testing of SL ligament is performed to check the previous evaluation.

The anatomical-arthroscopic and fluoroscopic study revealed the following findings (Table 4.1) [10].

Stage I:

In radiocarpal joint (RC) and midcarpal joint (MC), there is a slight haemorrhage of the SL ligament but no interruption of it. These are usually acute injuries only.

Stage II:

Radiocarpal joint: Slight interruption and minimal protrusion of membranous portion of SL joint (Fig. 4.4a, b).

Midcarpal joint: The tip of the probe can pass through the SL space, but the probe cannot be twisted and there is no widening of the SL space (Video 4.1) (Fig. 4.5a, b).

Stage I and II are stable injuries (that can be treated with simple immobilisation).

Stage IIIA:

In the radiocarpal joint, the Testut ligament can appear thickened and haemorrhagic (pseudo-thickening of Testut ligament). This is not a real thickening, but an indirect sign of involvement of the volar portion of SL ligament and the volar attachment of extrinsic ligaments around SL joint (such as the RSC and the LRL ligaments that may be damaged), which are volar to the Testut ligament and give it this appearance (Video 4.2) (Fig. 4.6a, b).

In the midcarpal joint, testing the laxity with a probe, there is a widening of SL space in its anterior portion (Fig. 4.7). In these cases of anterior widening, a damage

Table 4.1 EWAS Arthroscopic Classification of Scapho-lunate injuries [10, 11]. *DIC* Dorsal intercarpal ligament, *LRL* Long radio-lunate ligament, *RSC* Radio-scapho-capitate ligament, *SRL* Short radio-lunate ligament, *DRC* Dorso radiocarpal ligament

EWAS SL staging A: Acute/C: Chronic Ligaments involved	Arthroscopic findings RC: radio-carpal MC: midcarpal	X-rays
I A only	RC: attenuation of SL ligament, haemorrhage MC: attenuation of SL ligament, haemorrhage. No passage of the probe through SL joint	Stable Not visible at X-rays
II A/C **Tear of central** **membranous portion of SL**	RC: attenuation of SL ligament MC: tip of probe or the whole probe can go through SL space (central part). **Dynamic SL testing neg (no widening of SL space)**	Stable Not visible at X-rays
IIIA A/C **Tear of anterior portion of** **SL**	RC: pseudo-thickening of Testut ligament, possible protrusion of SL MC: anterior SL widening at dynamic instability test, possible involvement of extrinsic volar ligaments (LRL, RSC) **Dynamic Anterior widening of SL space**	Pre-dynamic Not visible at X-rays
IIIB A/C **Tear of dorsal portion of SL**	RC: protrusion of SL ligament MC: partial posterior SL widening at dynamic instability test. Possible injury to DCSS, possible involvement of DIC **Dynamic posterior widening of SL space**	Pre-dynamic Not visible at X-rays
IIIC A/C **Complete SL tear + DIC/** **LRL, RSC**	RC: protrusion of SL ligament, possible step-off, dynamic gap MC: complete SL widening at dynamic instability test, possible step off, involvement of extrinsic ligaments **Dynamic complete widening of SL space (reducible)**	Pre-dynamic Not visible at X-rays
IV A/C **Complete SL tear, DIC,** **DRC, LRL, RSC**	RC: marked protrusion of SL ligament with gap, incongruency SL MC: gap and **passage of the arthroscope** from midcarpal to radiocarpal joint through SL joint, SL diassociation, step off	Dynamic Visible at dynamic X-rays
V C **Complete SL** **tear + multiple extrinsic** **ligament injuries** **(DIC, DRC, LRL, RSL,** **SRL, STT)**	RC: marked protrusion of SL ligament with gap, step off, incongruency of SL, '**drive through sign'** MC: gap and **passage of the arthroscope** through SL joint, SL diassociation, **Radiological signs of instability**, rotatory subluxation of scaphoid	Static Visible at standard X-rays

to the anterior portion of SL ligament, but also a tear of the extrinsic volar ligaments as LRL, RSC ligaments may be present [10], but not always clearly seen by dorsal portals. Sometimes, it is necessary to perform a volar radial portal in the radiocarpal joint.

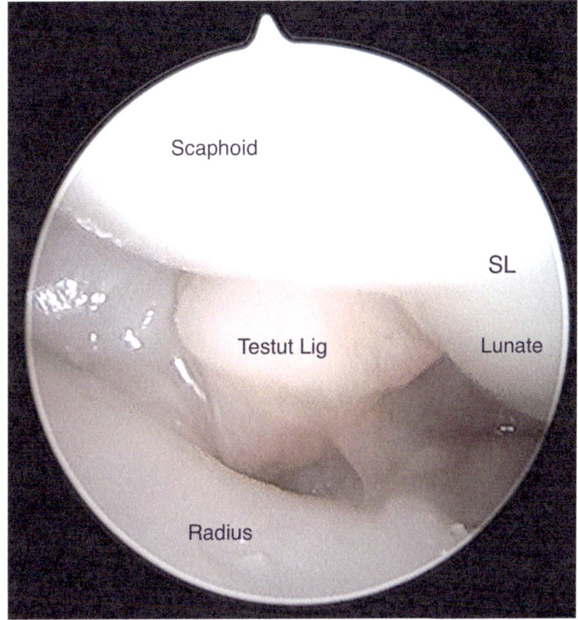

Fig. 4.1 From the radiocarpal joint, we can observe the normal aspect of scapho-lunate (SL) ligament which is invisible between the scaphoid (S) and lunate (L) with the typical aspect of "baby buttock"

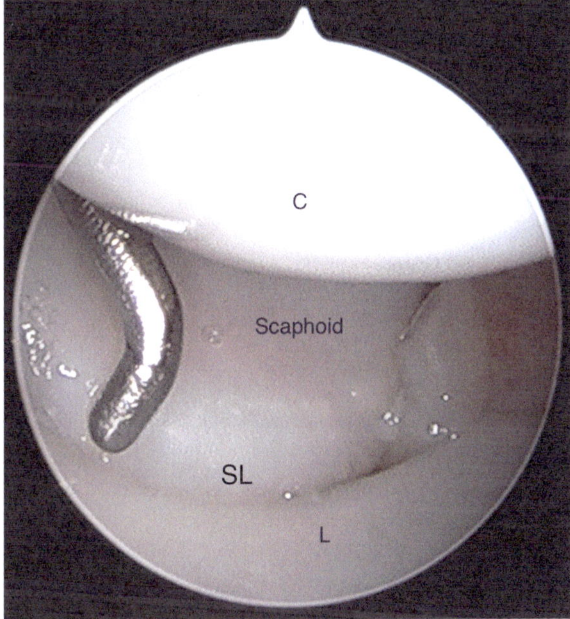

Fig. 4.2 From the midcarpal joint, normal aspect of SL ligament

Fig. 4.3 From the
radio-carpal joint we can
see the protrusion of torn
SL ligament in stage
IIIB. In more advanced
stages the protrusion of the
SL ligament increases

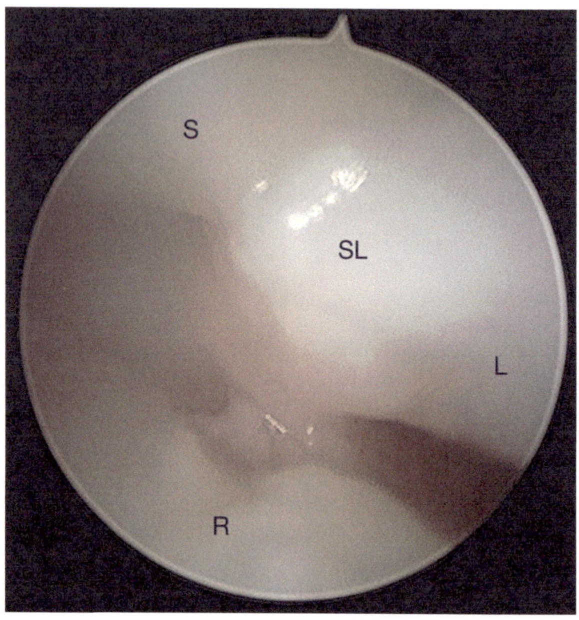

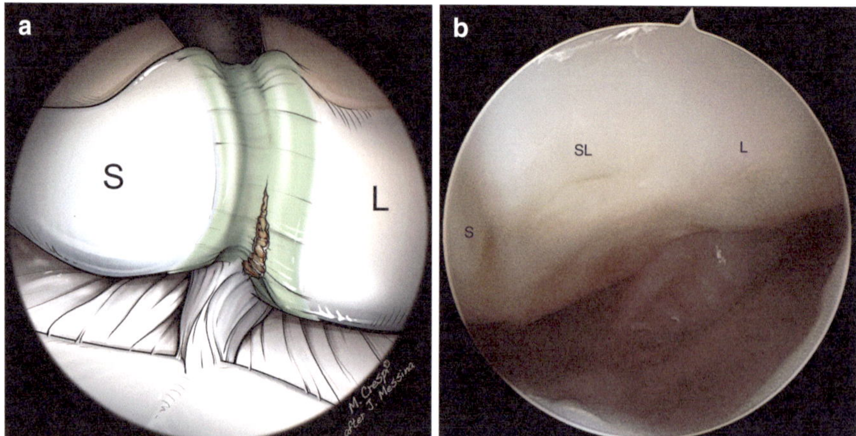

Fig. 4.4 Stage II: (**a** and **b**) From radiocarpal joint, slight protrusion of SL ligament

Stage IIIB:

In the radiocarpal joint, there is a protrusion of SL ligament which increases with the stage and severity if injury (Fig. 4.3).

In the midcarpal joint, there is a widening of the posterior portion of the SL joint. This dorsal widening means a damage of the posterior portion of the SL ligament and the extrinsic ligaments such as the DIC ligament (Video 4.3) (Fig. 4.8a, b).

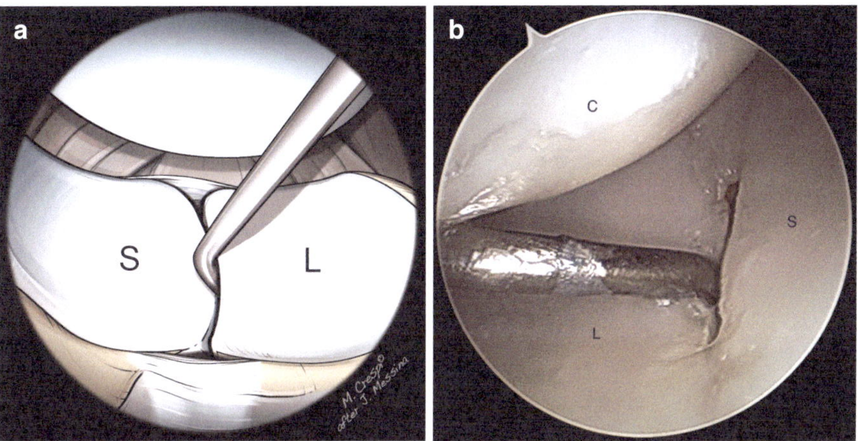

Fig. 4.5 Stage II: (**a** and **b**) From midcarpal joint, the tip of the probe can go through SL joint but there is no widening of SL space

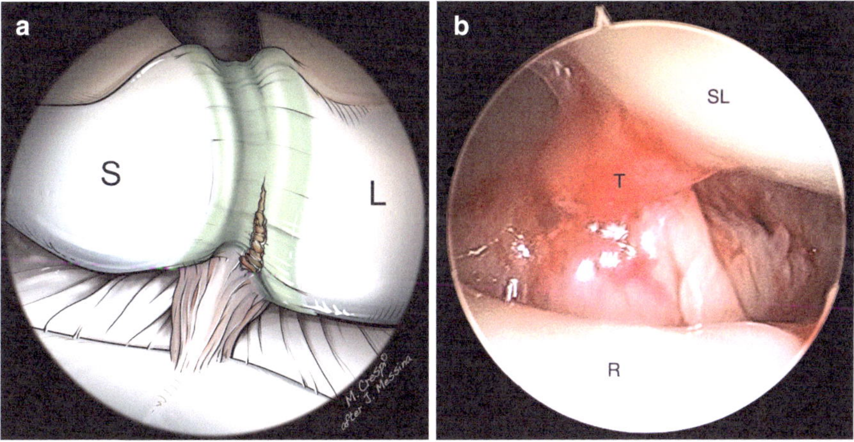

Fig. 4.6 Stage IIIA: (**a** and **b**) in the radiocarpal joint the Tesut ligament (T) appears thickened (pseudo-hypertrophy of Testut), this is an indirect sign of involvement volar portion of SLIOL and of RSC and LRL ligaments, that are anterior to it and may be damaged

A detachment of dorsal scapho-lunate septum (DCSS) can also be present isolated or associated to SL dorsal partial lesion, at this stage. The DCSS is visualised in the radiocarpal joint with the scope in 6R portal and turning it dorsally posteriorly to SL ligament [13] (Fig. 4.9).

Stage IIIC:

In the radiocarpal joint, there is a protrusion of SL ligament which increases with the stage. There can be initial incongruency of SL.

Fig. 4.7 Stage IIIA: in the midcarpal joint there is an anterior widening of SL space twisting the probe

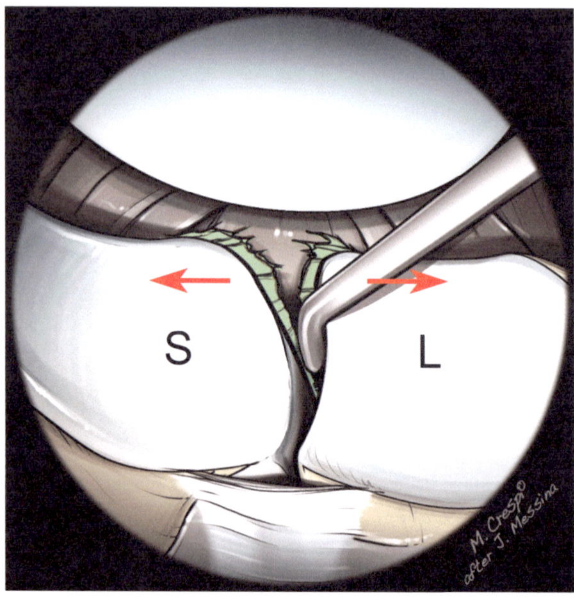

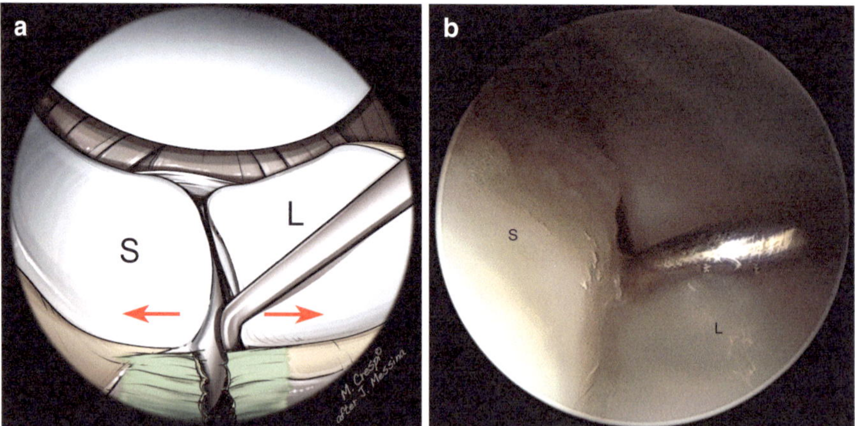

Fig. 4.8 Stage IIIB: (**a** and **b**) in the midcarpal joint there is a widening of the posterior portion of SL ligament

In the midcarpal joint, the tear of SLIOL ligament is complete, and the scaphoid and lunate can be pulled apart by twisting the probe. There can be incongruency of SL space and initial step off. As there is a widening of the whole space with the probe, the damage of SLIOL is complete (either anterior, proximal, and posterior). When the probe is removed, in stage III C, the SL interval closes spontaneously. The volar ligaments such as LRL, RSC ligament, and the DIC are partially torn (Video 4.4) (Fig. 4.10a–b).

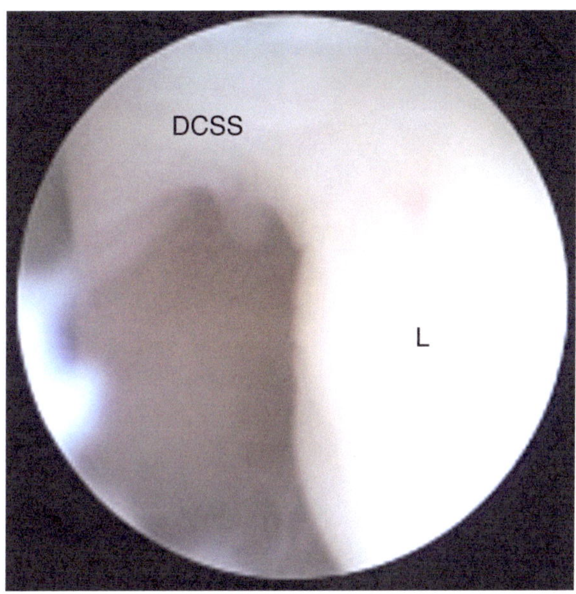

Fig. 4.9 The dorsal scapho-lunate septum (DCSS). It can be damaged in stage IIIB

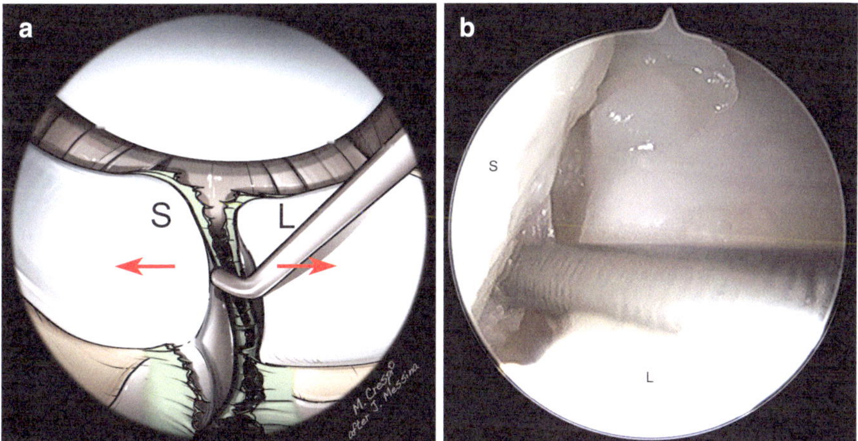

Fig. 4.10 Stage IIIC: (**a** and **b**) from the midcarpal joint we can see the complete widening of the whole SL space twisting the probe, but this is reducible removing the probe. In (**b**) we can also see the step off between scaphoid and lunate

Stage IV:

In the radiocarpal joint, there is a gross protrusion of SL ligament with a gap, step off, incongruency of the joint (Fig. 4.11).

In the midcarpal joint, we can find the widening of the two bones that are disassociated; the SL space is widened, and the arthroscope can go from the midcarpal to the radiocarpal joint. In this stage, there are still no radiological abnormalities on

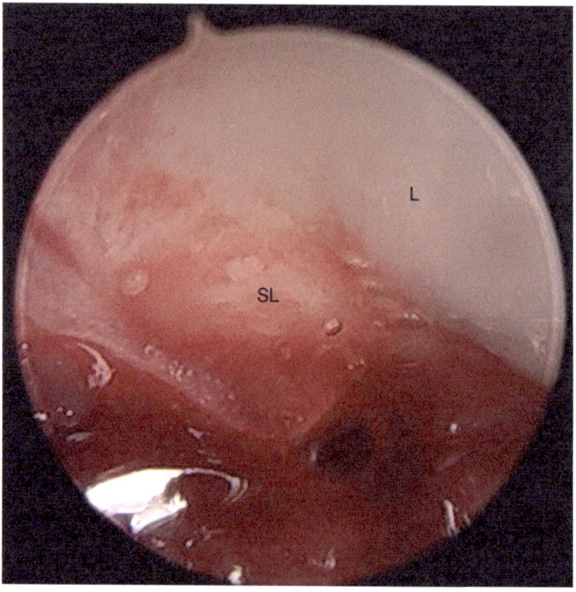

Fig. 4.11 Stage IV: protrusion of SL ligament. From radiocarpal joint a gap is present but not reducible

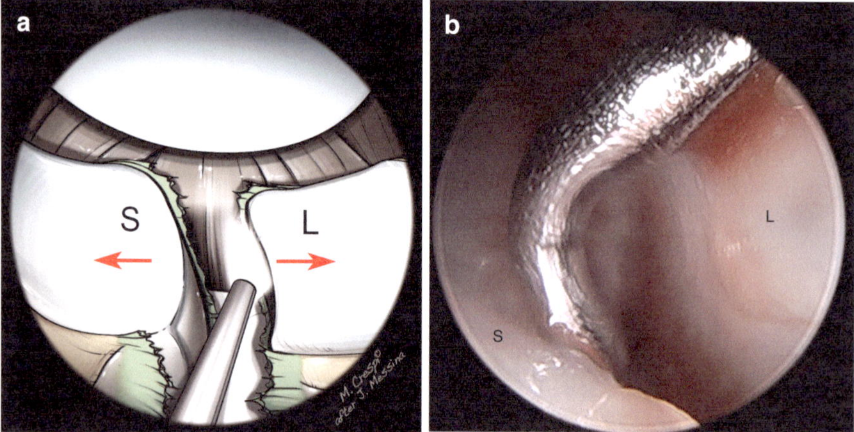

Fig. 4.12 Stage IV: (**a** and **b**). In the midcarpal joint there is a non reducible gap between the scaphoid and lunate, The arthroscope can pass from the midcarpal joint to radiocarpal joint

standard X-rays, but on dynamic X-rays a widening is present. Nevertheless, several extrinsic ligaments are involved, such as the DIC, the LRL, and the RSC ligaments [10] (Video 4.5) (Fig. 4.12a, b).

Stage V:

From 3 to 4 portal the camera enters directly in the SL joint ("drive-through sign") which means that it passes directly in the SL space because there is a wider gap (static scapho-lunate injury). At this stage, there are radiological abnormalities

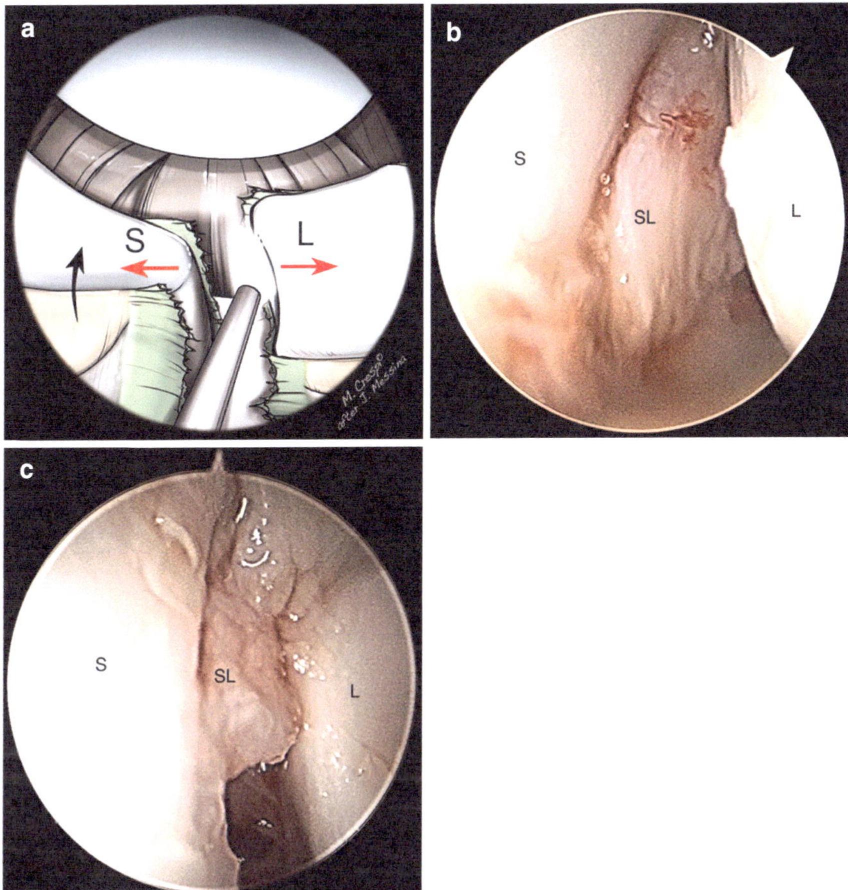

Fig. 4.13 Stage V: (**a** and **b**) from 3–4 portal the arthroscope enters directly in the SL joint ('drive-through' sign), presence of wide gap, increased incongruency of SL and step off which is clearly visible in MC joint (**c**)

(SL gap, DISI deformity etc.) and more extensive involvement of extrinsic ligaments (DIC, DRC, STT, LRL, RSC, SRL) (Video 4.6) (Fig. 4.13a–c). In radiocarpal joint, there can be a gross protrusion of SLIOL (Fig. 4.14).

Advanced stages are commonly found in old chronic injuries, as these injuries evolved in several subsequent steps during the years. However, they can also be present in acute and high energy traumas, like perilunate injuries, high energy distal radius fractures associated to SL ligament injuries, etc.

Arthroscopy allows also the evaluation and staging of cartilage damage and direct extrinsic ligament damage. Cartilage damage can be classified according to ICRS Classification [14] while extrinsic ligament lesions can be evaluated with a specific testing with a probe [15].

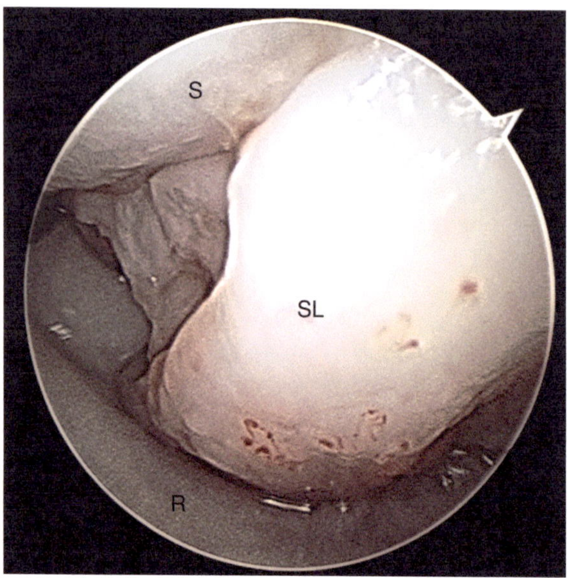

Fig. 4.14 Stage V: gross protrusion of SL ligament in radiocarpal joint (that increases with the stage)

Arthroscopic Luno-Triquetral Classification

The classification used for SL injuries is usually used for the LT tears as well as there are many similarities between the intrinsic ligaments. Nevertheless, there are some small differences in the pathological cases and ligaments involved as anatomy is different at LT joint.

First of all, the volar portion of LT ligament is very strong and isolated volar lesions are rare, they are more frequent in high energy traumas as perilunate dislocations. These are more severe than the volar tears of SL injuries as the volar portion of LT ligament is more resistant than the volar portion of SL ligament (where the dorsal portion of more important) [12]. Among partial tears, the dorsal LT are more frequent and less severe than the volar tears but are nevertheless symptomatic and easy to identify and repair under arthroscopy.

As we know from Mayfield studies, wrist traumas mostly affect the radial side of the wrist as they usually occur with the wrist in extension, ulnar deviation, and intercarpal supination. In fact, in these traumas the LT ligament is involved only at stage III of a perilunate injury [5]. However, there is also another mechanism of trauma that has been described, which is an ulnar-sided trauma in extension, pronation, and radial deviation that can cause LT injuries (reverse perilunate injury). It starts from the ulnar side of the wrist and involves the luno-triquetral ligament first and then progresses to the radial side of the wrist [16–20]. Finally, a certain amount of chronic injuries to LT ligament are caused by ulnocarpal abutment or repetitive minor trauma in an ulnar plus setting; in these cases, the most important thing to consider is restoring the correct length of the ulna, (shortening corrective osteotomy, or wafer procedure), and then repair the LT ligament [21].

Table 4.2 Arthroscopic Classification of lunotriquetral injuries (LT). *DIC* Dorsal intercarpal ligament, *UL* Ulno-lunate ligament, *UT* Ulno-triquetral ligament, *DRC* Dorso radiocarpal ligament, *DIC* Dorso intercarpal ligament, *SRL* Short radio-lunate ligament, *TC* Triquetrocapitate ligament

LT Staging A: Acute/C: Chronic Ligaments involved	Arthroscopic findings RC: radio-carpal MC: midcarpal
I A only	RC: attenuation of LT ligament, haemorrhage MC: attenuation of LT ligament, haemorrhage. No passage of the probe through LT joint
II A/C **Tear of central membranous** **portion**	RC: attenuation of SL ligament MC: tip of probe or the whole probe can go through LT space (central part). **Dynamic LT testing neg (no widening of LT space)**
IIIA A/C **Tear of anterior portion** + volar extrinsic ligaments	RC: hypermobility and LT malalignment MC: anterior LT widening at dynamic instability test. Possible involvement of extrinsic volar ligaments (UL UT, SRL, TC) **Dynamic Anterior widening of LT space**
IIIB A/C **Tear of dorsal portion** + dorsal extrinsic ligaments	RC: hypermobility of LT joint, protrusion LT lig MC: partial posterior LT widening at dynamic instability test. Possible injury to DRC and/or DIC **Dynamic posterior widening of LT space (Fig. 4.15)**
IIIC A/C **Complete LT tear** + involvement of dorsal / volar extrinsic ligaments	RC: Hypermobility and malalignment, dynamic gap, protrusion of LT ligament MC: complete LT widening at dynamic instability test, possible step off, involvement of extrinsic lig volar or dorsal **Dynamic complete widening of LT space-reducible**
IV A/C **Complete** Involvement of multiple extrinsic ligaments	RC: same as IIIC with possible step off MC: non reducible gap **Passage of the arthroscope** from midcarpal to radiocarpal joint through LT joint, LT diassociation if SL involved: possible Floating lunate. Rocking chair sign may be slightly pos if SL involved
V A/C **Complete LT tear** + multiple extrinsic ligament injuries + Radiological Signs	RC: gap, step off, incongruency of LT, MC: gap and **passage of the arthroscope** from midcarpal to radiocarpal joint through LT joint, LT diassociation. Rocking chair sign positive if SL involved **Radiological signs of instability (gap, VISI, Gilula's line altered)**

As mentioned before, the arthroscopic classifications used for SL ligament injuries have been commonly used also for LT injuries, but a specific arthroscopic LT classification, that we have been recently developing, can be found in Table 4.2 (Fig. 4.15).

To classify luno-triquetral injuries, it is important to know that the lunate can have one single concave articular surface (Viegas type I), in the majority of cases, or there could be a crest in the lunate that separates an articular fossa for the capitate and a smaller fossa for the hamate with a biconcave shape (Viegas type II) [22]. If the crest is too close to the LT joint, it could be mistaken as a step off.

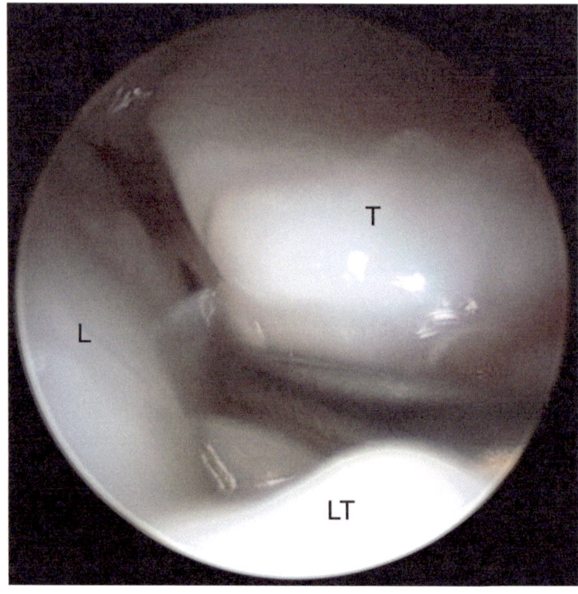

Fig. 4.15 Lunotriquetral (LT) injury stage IIIB. In the midcarpal joint there is a widening of the posterior portion of LT ligament with a detachment of dorsal capsule and DRC ligament

Another factor to take into account is that for testing LT joint, while the camera is in MCR portal, the probe enters from MCU portal this is located more ulnar to LT space, so the probe enters obliquely though the UMC portal, which makes it more difficult to explore the gap (Fig. 4.15).

To evaluate the volar portion of LT ligament, the arthroscope is introduced through the UMC portal and is turned palmar to visualise it, but removal of synovium is needed to have a clear view.

In case of doubts about the laxity of the LT joint from MC joint, it is useful to explore the LT ligament from the radiocarpal joint through the 6R portal. In stages IV and V, the lunate will be completely detached from the triquetrum, and there will be a wide injury of the membranous portion that allow a direct visualisation of the LT joint and articular surfaces.

There can also be combined SL and LT injuries as described by Mayfield, especially in old perilunate injuries or perilunate injuries non-dislocated (PLIND injuries) [23–25]. In those cases, the rocking chair sign is positive as the lunate is completely separated from the scaphoid and the lunate [25].

Discussion

We know from many years that SL are a spectrum of pathologies of different complexity increasing with time in each patient according to the amount of use of wrist, manual activities, overload, sports activities, and subsequent traumas. The arthroscopic evaluation has the aim to classify the lesions and identify anatomo-pathological damage and thus allowing the surgeon to fix specific injuries choosing the more adapted tissue-specific repair technique to repair them [1–5].

Within Garcia Elias staging system, early stages, can be studied under arthroscopy and the arthroscopic classification allows to distinguish the different partial tears of SL ligament in the different portions of SLIOL, and allows a more sophisticated diagnosis of the lesions even at later stages [10].

From our anatomic-fluoroscopic study we have demonstrated that extrinsic ligament injuries are present also in partial injuries, already in the early stages from stage IIIA and then in all more advanced stages [10]. This is important in order to understand that, first of all, there are no isolated injuries of SLIOL but most of them are associated to extrinsic ligament injuries. Secondly, because of that, partial injuries are potential more severe than what we thought. Another important concept is that the repair technique that we use even in partial injuries should thus include extrinsic ligaments repair as well as SLIOL. In fact, the repair of SLIOL alone does not seem too sufficient to repair the damage which involves also the extrinsic ligaments from early stages.

While the stages I and II can heal with simple immobilisation, in stage IIIA we can use arthroscopic capsulodesis techniques of volar repair, recently developed; in stage IIIB, arthroscopic or open techniques of dorsal capsulodesis repair; in stage IIIC, arthroscopic or open techniques of dorsal capsulodesis repair alone or with associate a volar repair. In stages IV and V, reconstruction of SL ligament and extrinsic ligaments with a tendon graft are preferred by the majority of authors [2, 3, 26–31]. The techniques of repair will be developed in the following chapters of this book.

Another point to discuss is the identification of acute of chronic lesions, which is not always easy. Arthroscopy is of great help in this, as it shows directly and in detail the intra-articular clinical state of ligaments with magnification. It is important to evaluate the presence of haemorrhage which indicates an acute trauma and evaluate also the quality of the tissues. If tissues are white and frail, this indicated a chronic injury. The history of the patient is important too, for instance, a recent high energy trauma with a fracture of distal radius or perilunate injury will have frequently acute ligament injuries [8, 9]. A history of numerous previous sprains or traumas, manual work or intensive sports activities indicates, with a high probability, a chronic injury or sometimes there can be a recent minor trauma in the contest of a chronic ligament injury of the wrist. Chronic injuries are important to identify as the treatment will change. In fact, a chronic trauma, will not be treated in acute but a reconstructive procedure with a tendon graft will be planned later.

Another aspect to take into account is that the more the lesion is advanced, the more we will find extensive involvement of extrinsic ligament injuries and cartilage damage and thus the repair and restoration the normal anatomy will be difficult, thus we will have to do a salvage procedure [2, 3, 26, 27]. In fact, in static SL injuries (Stage V) the results of the techniques of reconstruction show a significant amount of recurrence of gap with incomplete correction of DISI, even if stability seems anyways improved [2, 3, 26, 27].

The development of arthroscopic techniques allows us today to repair SL injuries to an early stage with simple procedures and avoiding the progression of the disease and more complex surgeries later on [28–31].

The early identification of these injuries is important in order to treat them early and avoid the progression of the disease and the involvement of several additional extrinsic ligament injuries which are then very difficult to repair in a context of rotatory subluxation of scaphoid.

References

1. Linsheid RL, Dobyns JH, Beabout JW, Bryan RS. Traumatic instability of the wrist. Diagnosis, classification and pathomechanics. J Bone Joint Surg. 1972;54A:1612–32.
2. Garcia Elias M, Lluch A. Wrist instabilities, misalignment and dislocations. In: Wolfe S, Hotchkiss R, Pederson W, Kozin S, Cohen M, editors. Green's operative hand surgery. 7th ed. Philadelphia: Elsevier; 2017; Ch 13. p. 418–78.
3. Garcia-Elias M, Lluch AL, Stanley JK. Three-ligament tenodesis for the treatment of scapholunate dissociation: indications and surgical technique. J Hand Surg. 2006;31(1):125–34.
4. Watson HK, Ballet FL. The SLAC wrist: scapholunate advanced collapse pattern of degenerative arthritis. J Hand Surg Am. 1984;9(3):358–65.
5. Mayfield JK. Wrist ligamentous anatomy and pathogenesis of carpal instability. Orthop Clin N Am. 1984;15(2):209–16.
6. Dautel G, Goudot B, Merle M. Arthroscopic diagnosis of scapho-lunate instability in the absence of X-ray abnormalities. J Hand Surg (Br Eur Vol). 1993;18(2)
7. Dreant N, Dautel G. Development of an arthroscopic severity score for scapholunate instability. Chir Main. 2003;22(2):90.
8. Lindau T, Arner M, Hagberg L. Intraarticular lesions in distal fractures of the radius in young adults: a descriptive arthroscopic study in 50 patients. J Hand Surg Eur Vol. 1997;22(5)
9. Geissler WB. Arthroscopically assisted reduction of intra-articular fractures of the distal radius. Hand Clin. 1995;11(1):19.
10. Messina JC, Van Overstraeten L, Mathoulin CL, Luchetti R, Fairplay T. The EWAS classification of scapholunate tears: an anatomical arthroscopic study. J Wrist Surg. 2013;1(212):105–9.
11. Corella F, Messina JC, Ocampos M, Randelli P. Arthroscopic examination of the wrist. In: Corella F, Heras Palau C, Luchetti R, editors. Carpal ligament injuries and instability. Stuttgart, Germany: Thieme; 2023; chap 7. p. 59–79.
12. Berger RA. The anatomy of the ligaments of the wrist and distal radioulnar joints. Clin Orthop Relat Res. 2001;383(383):32–40.
13. Van Overstraeten L, Camus E, Wahegaonkar A, et al. Anatomical description of the dorsal Capsulo-Scapholunate septum (DCSS)—arthroscopic staging of Scapholunate instability after DCSS sectioning. J Wrist Surg. 2013;02(03):284.
14. Mainil-Varlet P, Aigner T, et al. Histological assessment of cartilage repair: a report by the histology endpoint committee of the international cartilage repair society (ICRS). J Bone Joint Surg Am. 2002;85-A(Suppl 2):45–57.
15. Van Overstraeten L, Camus EJ. A systematic method of arthroscopic testing of extrinsic carpal ligaments: implication in carpal stability. Tech Hand Up Extrem Surg. 2013;17(4):202–6.
16. Reagan DS, Linscheid RL, Dobyns JH. Lunotriquetral sprains. J Hand Surg Am. 1984;9(4):502–14.
17. Shin AY, Battaglia MJ, Bishop AT. Lunotriquetral instability: diagnosis and treatment. J Am Acad Orthop Surg. 2000;8(3):170–9.
18. Nagao S, Patterson RM, Buford WL, Andersen CR, Shah MA, Viegas SF. Three-dimensional description of ligamentous attachments around the lunate. J Hand Surg Am. 2005;30(4):685–92.

19. Garcia-Elias M. Soft-tissue anatomy and relationships about the distal ulna. Hand Clin. 1998;14(2):165–76.
20. Viegas SF. Ulnar-sided wrist pain and instability. Instr Course Lect. 1998;47:215–8.
21. Palmer AK. Triangular fibrocartilage complex lesions: a classification. J Hand Surg Am. 1989;14(4):594–606.
22. Viegas SF, Wagner K, Patterson R, Peterson P. Medial (hamate) facet of the lunate. J Hand Surg Am. 1990;15(4):564–71.
23. Badia A, Khanchandani P. The floating lunate: arthroscopic treatment of simultaneous complete tears of the scapholunate and lunotriquetral ligaments. Hand. 2009;4(3):250–5.
24. Herzberg G. Perilunate Injuries, Not Dislocated (PLIND). J Wrist Surg. 2013;02(04):337–45.
25. Corella F, del Cerro M, Ocampos M, Larrainzar-Garijo R. The "Rocking Chair Sign" for floating lunate. J Hand Surg Am. 2015;40(11):2318–9.
26. Corella F, Del Cerro M, Ocampos M, et al. Arthroscopic ligamentoplasty of the dorsal and volar portions of scapho-lunate ligament. J Hand Surg Am. 2013;38(12):2466–77.
27. Ho PC, Wong C, Tse WL. Arthroscopic assisted combined dorsal and volar scapholunate ligament reconstruction with tendon graft for chronic SL instability. J Wrist Surg. 2015;04(04):252–63.
28. Luchetti R, Papini Zorli I, Atzei A, Fairplay T. Dorsal intercarpal ligament capsulodesis for predynamic and dynamic scapholunate instability. J Hand Surg. 2010;35E(1):32–7.
29. Mathoulin CL, Dauphin N, Wahegaonkar AL. Arthroscopic dorsal capsulo-ligamentous repair in chronic scapholunate ligament tears. Hand Clin. 2011;27:563–72.
30. Del Pinal F, Studer A, Thams C, Glasberg A. An all inside technique for arthroscopic suturing of the volar scapholunate ligament. J Hand Surg. 2011;36A:2044–6.
31. Lui H, Kakar S. Arthroscopic assisted volar scapholunate capsulodesis: a new technique. J Hand Surg Am. 2022;47(11):1124.e-1–124.e6.

Chapter 5
Kinematics of the Scapholunate Ligament

Pedro Bronenberg Victorica and Robin N. Kamal

Case Presentation

A 32-year-old right-handed dominant male presented to the clinic with 2 years of evolution of dorsal- and radial-sided left wrist pain. He does not remember a specific traumatic event before his wrist pain began though he is an avid mountain biker with multiple prior falls. His pain at rest was 0/10, and his activity was not limited when the wrist was in a neutral position. Nevertheless, pain during extension or when loaded was restrictive when activities were performed.

Physical Assessment

Physical examination revealed tenderness at the dorsal scapholunate interval and radioscaphoid joint. He had pain during the Watson shift test without obvious scaphoid subluxation. In addition, he had mild pain with radial and ulnar deviation and loading. The patient was able to make a full fist and extend all digits and denied any numbness or tingling.

P. Bronenberg Victorica
Instituto de Ortopedia y Traumatología "Carlos E. Ottolenghi," Potosí 4215 (C1199ACK), Buenos Aires, Argentina
e-mail: pedro.bronenberg@hospitalitaliano.org.ar

R. N. Kamal (✉)
Department of Orthopaedic Surgery, Stanford University, Redwood City, CA, USA
e-mail: rnkamal@stanford.edu

J. Yao (ed.), *Carpal Instability*, https://doi.org/10.1007/978-3-031-55869-6_5

Diagnostic Studies

Standard radiographs showed changes consistent with an SLAC wrist. The postero-anterior projection (Fig. 5.1a) revealed subtle scapholunate interval widening without a clear positive ring sign. In addition, mild radial styloid breaking and images consistent with chronic fractures of the distal scaphoid pole and lunate, and STT arthritis are seen. In the lateral projection, a DISI deformity with a scapholunate angle of 74° is observed, with lunate extension being the main cause (Fig. 5.1b). Stress views (Fig. 5.2) were performed, showing increased widening of the scapholunate interval in comparison to the uninjured wrist.

Magnetic resonance imaging (MRI) revealed changes in the radial aspect of the lunate, distal scaphoid pole, and radial styloid process consistent with remote trauma including moderate triscaphe degenerative changes and radioscaphoid chondral thinning. Lastly, chronic high-grade tearing involving all components of the scapholunate ligament and widened scapholunate interval measuring 5.6 mm was identified (Fig. 5.3).

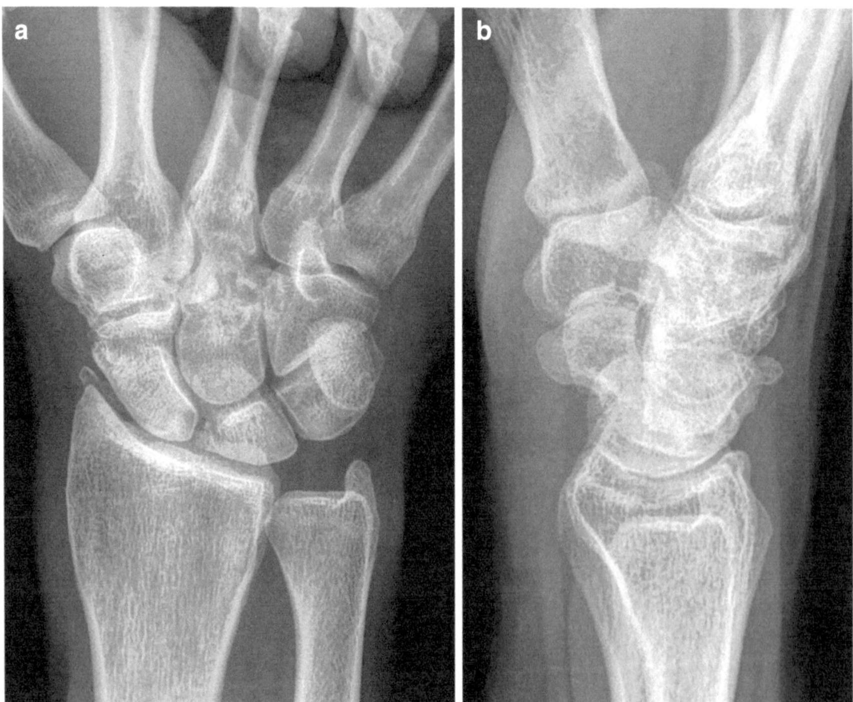

Fig. 5.1 Preoperative posteroanterior (**a**) and lateral (**b**) radiographs. A subtle widening of the scapholunate space and mild radial styloid breaking is observed. The ring sign is not clearly seen as there is no significant flexion of the scaphoid. In the lateral view, a DISI deformity is identified with a scapholunate angle of 74° mainly as a consequence of lunate extension

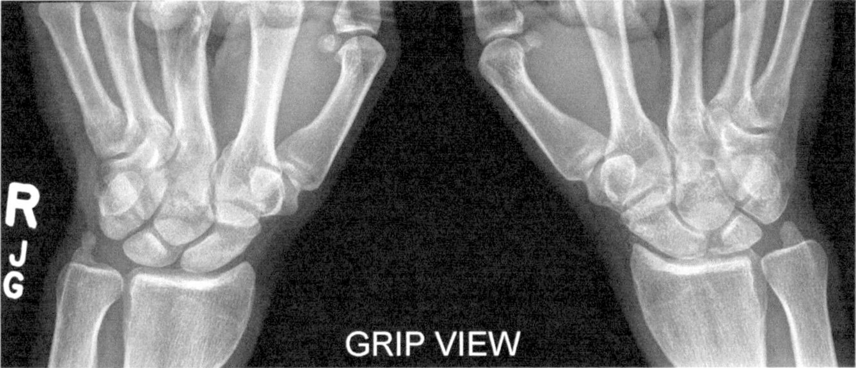

Fig. 5.2 Stress radiographs. Pencil grip view shows a low-grade widening of the left scapholunate interval

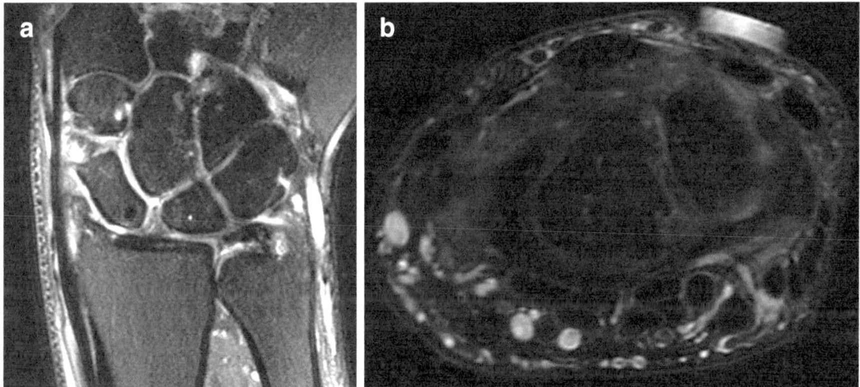

Fig. 5.3 MRI coronal (**a**) and axial (**b**) planes. Images compatibles with chronic high-grade tear involving all components of the scapholunate ligament and widening of 5.6 mm of the scapholunate interval

Diagnosis

Stage I Scapholunate Advanced Collapse (SLAC) and STT arthrosis.

Management Options

Surgical treatment indicated in the presence of a symptomatic SLAC wrist depends essentially on the radiological stage of the patient. In stage I, in which degenerative changes occur only between the scaphoid and radial styloid, radial styloidectomy and scapholunate reconstruction are possible if the scaphoid is still reducible. This corrects the alignment of the carpus, stabilizes the scapholunate joint, and consequently restores the correct distribution of loads across the carpus. It also eliminates symptomatic impingement between the radial styloid and scaphoid.

The range of options for the treatment of scapholunate ligament injuries is very broad, ranging from non-surgical treatment with specific rehabilitation to multiple ligament reconstruction techniques. The latter is a consequence of an incomplete understanding of the kinematics of the carpus, which has led to the development of different techniques that seek to mimic scapholunate kinematics. Generally, treatment of scapholunate ligament injuries depends on the time since the initial trauma, possibility of repairing the SL ligament, whether the carpus is reducible, and the presence of degenerative involvement in the adjacent articular surfaces. In advanced stages, the biomechanical alteration produced by scapholunate ligament injury generates irreversible changes in the adjacent articular surfaces due to loading imbalance through the carpus. Consequently, in advanced stages, only salvage treatments are considered.

Management Chosen for This Case with Rationale

For the treatment of this patient, we completed a 360° scapholunate ligament reconstruction with a tendon graft and internal brace and excision of approximately 4 mm of the radial styloid [1] (Fig. 5.4). When performing this procedure, or any carpal surgical approach, it is important to consider the secondary stabilizers of the SL joint, especially the dorsal intercarpal ligament (DIC). Therefore, we completed a ligament-sparing capsulotomy during the dorsal approach to spare fibers of the DIC (working through windows between capsulotomies within the DIC and dorsal radiocarpal ligament (DRC), opposed to the traditional radially based fiber-splitting capsulotomy.

The 360-reconstruction technique was selected based on its close alignment with the normal anatomy and biomechanical characteristics of the scapholunate ligament. This C-shaped ligament has dorsal, volar, and proximal components. While its most biomechanical important component is the dorsal, with a capacity to resist forces of up to 300 N, its volar component is also capable of resisting forces of up to 120 N. Although it is not as strong as the dorsal component, it can help resist scapholunate rotation. Multiple reconstruction techniques seek to restore solely the dorsal component of the SL ligament, which, although it is the most important, repairing it alone may lead to abnormal kinematics. The 360 procedure is a technique that reconstructs both the volar and dorsal ligaments, similar to techniques reported by Henry and Ho et al. [2, 3].

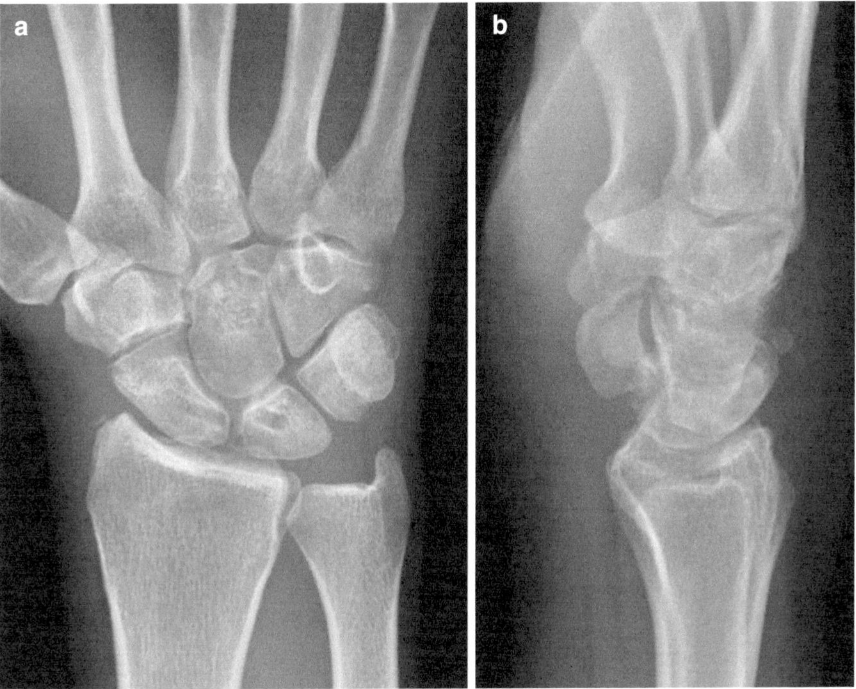

Fig. 5.4 Postoperative posteroanterior (**a**) and lateral (**b**) radiographs at 1-year follow-up. The location of the bone tunnels for the passage of the palmaris longus graft, the radial styloidectomy, and the correction of the scapholunate diastasis and scapholunate angle (45°) are visualized

Clinical Course and Outcome

After the surgery, the patient was immobilized with a short-arm cast for the first 2 weeks. Afterwards, a fabricated dart thrower motion (DTM) (Fig. 5.5) orthosis was designed, and the patient was instructed to remain in the orthosis at all times other than hand hygiene and wound care for the next 2 weeks. Using the DTM orthosis, only the mid-range active range of motion in the DTM plane was allowed. Moreover, under supervision, the patient could remove the orthosis for digital and thumb active range of motion (ROM) and wrist active DTM. The next 2 weeks, the patient continued with active ROM of the wrist in the DTM plane, focusing only on proprioceptive training and progressing to greater end-range motion as tolerated. From week 6 to 10, the patient transitioned to a volar wrist orthosis for sleeping, lifting, and high-risk activities (Fig. 5.6a). He was allowed to begin active ROM in all planes and advance to PROM, light strengthening of grip, pinch, and wrist stabilizers, as tolerated. Light-weight bearing during wrist extension was allowed if the pain was well controlled. After week 10, orthotic use was discontinued, increasing strengthening and sensorimotor training, and progressing to prior level of function as tolerated (Fig. 5.6b).

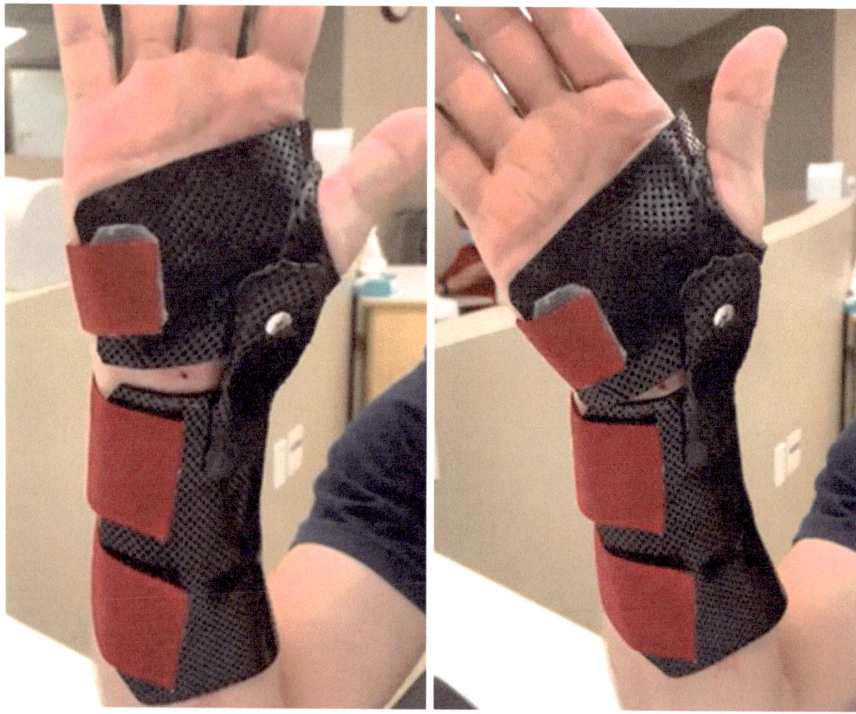

Fig. 5.5 Fabricated dart throwers motion orthosis allows mid-range active range of motion in the DTM plane

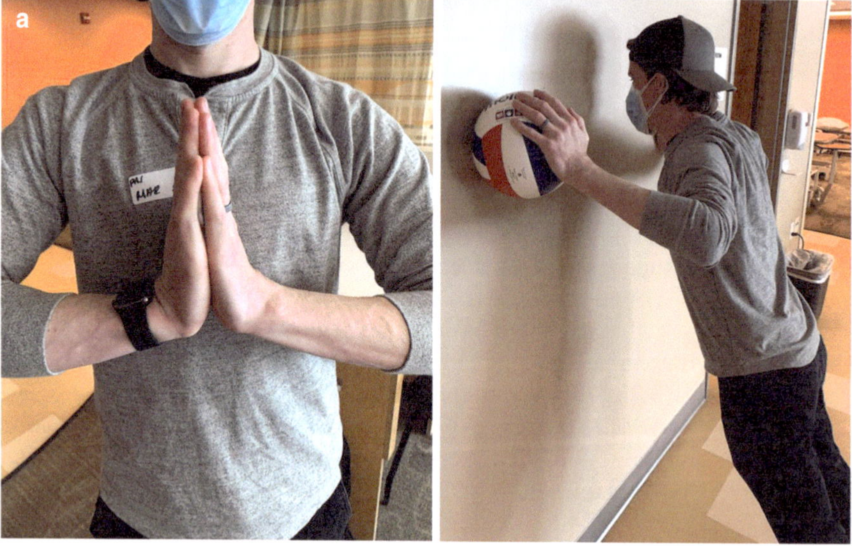

Fig. 5.6 After week 6, patient is allowed to begin active ROM in all planes and advance to PROM (**a**) and after week 10 strengthening, sensorimotor training, and progressing to prior level of function is allowed as tolerated (**b**)

At 1-year follow-up, the patient was pain free. He returned to his normal job and was able to return to mountain biking without any limitations.

Bulleted Clinical Pearls/Pitfalls [3–5, with Figures]

- Scapholunate instability places pathological loads mainly on the radioscaphoid and capitolunate joints, leading to predictable arthritic changes, known as scapholunate advanced collapse.
- When reconstructive surgery is performed, it is as important to attempt to replicate the normal anatomy of the scapholunate ligament when possible, as well as to respect the secondary stabilizers during the surgical approach.
- Ligament-sparing dorsal capsulotomy allows for adequate carpal visualization without detaching the secondary stabilizers of the SL ligament.
- Reconstructive techniques that allow for faster rehabilitation and preclude the need for k-wires are preferred.

Literature Review and Discussion

A thorough understanding of carpal kinematics is essential for understanding the kinematics of the scapholunate ligament. Carpal kinematics describes how carpal alignment changes during wrist movements, whereas carpal kinetics describes how carpal alignment is altered under load [4]. Even today, multiple theories aim to explain these phenomena; however, carpal kinematics continues to be studied. The stability of the carpus is fundamentally determined by the complex interaction between the carpus and the adjacent bones, intrinsic and extrinsic ligaments of the wrist, and forces that pass through the wrist. In addition, other factors, such as clinical laxity or bone morphology, also have a direct influence on carpal stability, although their magnitude is not yet fully understood.

Carpal bones are unique as they have limited tendon insertions, so their mobility is conditioned by their relationship with the base of the metacarpals and with the articular surfaces of the radius and ulna. As previously stated, carpal bone morphology can directly influence kinematic patterns. The clinical and biomechanical effects of morphological changes on the scaphoid and scapholunate joints are uncertain [5]; however, the morphological variations of the lunate are those that would most likely influence scapholunate kinematics. Viegas classifies lunates as type one or two if they articulate only with the capitate, or if they also present a medial facet that articulates with the hamate, respectively [6]. Type II wrists present more scaphoid flexion with radial deviation and relative restriction of midcarpal motion during flexion [7, 8]. This relative stiffness may play a role in the development of dorsal intercalated segment instability (DISI) deformity in the setting of SL tears although this continues to be debated by conflicting reports [9, 10]. Theoretically, the lunohamate joint plays a protective role in providing additional restriction to lunate extension in the absence of an intact scaphoid [9]. This protective property was also evidenced by the lower tendency of Type II lunate wrists to generate DISI in patients with scapholunate dissociation in one report [11].

The relationship between the lunate and the scaphoid during normal wrist movements presents a distinctive characteristic. The axes of rotation of the scapholunate joint during flexion-extension and radioulnar deviation movements vary significantly between patients and positions [12]. This concept contrasts with the hypothesis of the existence of a single axis of motion passing through the center of the scaphoid and lunate articular surfaces and would suggest reconstructions using this approach will not recreate normal kinematics.

Another factor that influences the kinematics of the scaphoid and the entire proximal carpal row is joint laxity, which is another parameter that should be considered when evaluating a patient [13]. There is a linear relationship between scaphoid rotation and the degree of joint laxity. During radioulnar deviation of the wrist in most lax joints, the scaphoid rotates mainly along the sagittal plane of flexion and extension, with slight lateral deviation. Conversely, in patients with less laxity, the scaphoid rotates primarily along the frontal plane of the radioulnar deviation with negligible flexion-extension [14].

The intricate ligament system formed by extrinsic and intrinsic ligaments contributes to the harmonious movement of the carpal bones under load. Extrinsic ligaments originate in a bone outside the carpus and insert into the carpus, whereas intrinsic ligaments have both insertions in the carpal bones [15] (Fig. 5.7a, b) [4]. The scapholunate (SL) and lunotriquetral (LT) ligaments play a central role in the

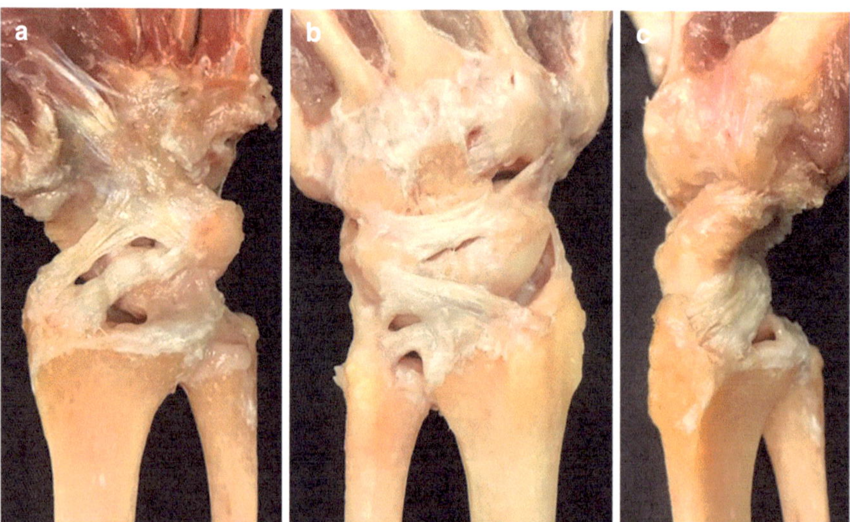

Fig. 5.7 Palmar (**a**), dorsal (**b**), and oblique (**c**) views demonstrating interosseous wrist ligaments and radiocarpal ligaments. Images kindly shared by Ezequiel Ernesto Zaidenberg MD. All Rights Reserved

kinematics of the proximal row of the carpus, with the SL ligament being considered the primary stabilizer of the scapholunate joint [16]. The scapho-trapezoid ligament, which inserts on the distal pole of the scaphoid and trapezium and trapezoid, functions as a secondary stabilizer of the SL joint by restricting scaphoid flexion [17].

Within the extrinsic ligaments, the radioscaphocapitate ligament (RSC), long radiolunate ligament (LRL), short radiolunate ligament (SRL), dorsal intercarpal ligament (DIC), and dorsal radiocarpal ligament (DRC) play an important role as secondary stabilizers of the scapholunate joint [18]. The RSC ligament is the most radial of the volar radiocarpal ligaments, originating proximally at the radial styloid and the volar and radial regions of the scaphoid fossa, and distally at the distal pole of the scaphoid and capitate. This ligament acts as a sling, preventing excessive flexion and pronation of the scaphoid and also prevents ulnar translation of the carpus [19, 20] (Fig. 5.7c). Located ulnar to it, the LRL and SRL limit ulnar translation of the carpus and lunate extension during maximum wrist extension [19, 21]. Finally, the ulnolunate and ulnotriquetral ligaments participate in the stabilization of the lunotriquetral and ulnocarpal joints, thereby influencing the scapholunate joint [22]. The dorsal radiocarpal ligament (DRC) and dorsal intercarpal ligament (DIC) are the most important dorsal ligaments. The DRC originates from the dorsal lip of the distal radius, ulnar to Lister's tubercle, and runs towards the dorsal tubercle of the triquetrum. As it passes over the lunate, it has fibers that insert into the lunate and lunotriquetral ligaments. The DIC originates from the triquetrum and runs towards the scaphoid and trapezium. Like the DRC, it also passes over the lunate and has insertions on it [23]. The DIC ligament elongates with ulnar deviation, whereas the DRC ligament elongates with radial deviation, thereby limiting motion at the extremes of ulnar and radial deviations, respectively [24]. In addition, through their insertions in the scaphoid and lunate, they act as secondary stabilizers of the scapholunate joint, with a marked role in preventing the development of instability when they are functional [25].

Scapholunate ligament injuries are the most common cause of wrist instability [22, 26]. The scapholunate interosseous ligament is divided into three components: dorsal, proximal, and palmar. The dorsal component is thick and is composed of short and transversely oriented collagen fibers. This is the thickest component and provides the greatest biomechanical stability to the scapholunate joint. The proximal component is primarily composed of fibrocartilage, and the palmar region is thin and composed of obliquely oriented collagen fibers [27].

Scapholunate instability places pathological loads mainly on the radioscaphoid and capitolunate joints, leading to predictable arthritic changes known as scapholunate advanced collapse (SLAC) [28]. Previously, it was considered that because the scapholunate ligament is the primary stabilizer of the scapholunate joint, its compromise was sufficient to produce instability [29]. However, more recent studies have shown that injury to the scapholunate ligament in the absence of injury to secondary stabilizers does not necessarily result in scapholunate instability [25, 30]. Even with complete SL ligament injury, the DIC and dorsal capsular attachments to the scaphoid work together to counteract rotatory subluxation of the scaphoid [31].

Similarly, these secondary stabilizers play a major role in stabilizing the lunate and triquetrum during lunotriquetral ligament injury. Isolated injury to this ligament will not produce clinical or radiographic static instability; however, it will result with an aggregate injury to the DRC ligament [32]. The contribution of secondary stabilizers to the stability of the scapholunate joint supports the development of surgical techniques aimed at preserving them during an open dorsal approach to the wrist and highlights the usefulness of repairing/reconstructing them in the event of injury.

Knowledge and understanding of these features have improved our understanding of carpal kinetics. The carpus, radius, and metacarpals were described as a 3-joint link. The strong transverse distal intercarpal ligaments limit the mobility of the distal carpal row; therefore, it is considered a unit along with the base of the metacarpals. Consequently, all the movements are at the level of the proximal carpal row. The kinetic theories have been evolving since Gilford and colleagues noted the function of the scaphoid connecting the radius with the distal carpal row, to Garcia and Elias and collaborators, who suggest that there are opposing forces at each end of the first row of the carpus that neutralize each other [33]. In this kinetic theory, the scaphoid is loaded into flexion by the trapezium and trapezoid, whereas on the other ulnar wrist, the triquetrum is loaded into extension by the hamate. The interosseous ligaments (SL and LT) transfer these loads to the lunate, keeping it in a neutral position, and injury to either affects the kinetics of the first row of the carpus. Thus, injury to the SL causes flexion of the scaphoid and extension of the lunate. In contrast, injury to the LT generates flexion of the lunate and extension of the triquetrum. These abnormal carpal positions lead to abnormal load distribution across the carpus and development of early degenerative involvement.

Even today, with the most advanced imaging techniques and multiple cadaveric and clinical studies performed, the complexity of carpal kinematics is not fully understood. This lack of a complete understanding may explain why there is no reconstructive technique that accurately reproduces the carpal kinematics and is therefore considered the gold standard. However, knowing the factors that influence the biomechanics of the carpus informs the evolution of improved surgical techniques to recreate normal anatomy.

References

1. Kakar S, Greene RM. Scapholunate ligament internal brace 360-degree Tenodesis (SLITT) procedure. J Wrist Surg. 2018;7:336–40. https://doi.org/10.1055/s-0038-1625954.
2. Henry M. Reconstruction of both volar and dorsal limbs of the scapholunate interosseous ligament. J Hand Surg. 2013;38:1625–34. https://doi.org/10.1016/j.jhsa.2013.05.026.
3. Ho P-C, Wong CW-Y, Tse W-L. Arthroscopic-assisted combined dorsal and volar scapholunate ligament reconstruction with tendon graft for chronic SL instability. J Wrist Surg. 2015;4:252–63. https://doi.org/10.1055/s-0035-1565927.
4. Kamal RN, Starr A, Akelman E. Carpal kinematics and kinetics. J Hand Surg. 2016;41:1011–8. https://doi.org/10.1016/j.jhsa.2016.07.105.

5. Schimmerl-Metz SM, Metz VM, Totterman SM, et al. Radiologic measurement of the scapholunate joint: implications of biologic variation in scapholunate joint morphology. J Hand Surg. 1999;24:1237–44. https://doi.org/10.1053/jhsu.1999.1237.

6. Viegas SF. The lunatohamate articulation of the midcarpal joint. Arthrosc J Arthrosc Relat Surg Off Publ Arthrosc Assoc N Am Int Arthrosc Assoc. 1990;6:5–10. https://doi.org/10.1016/0749-8063(90)90089-v.

7. Bain GI, Clitherow HDS, Millar S, et al. The effect of lunate morphology on the 3-dimensional kinematics of the carpus. J Hand Surg. 2015;40:81–89.e1. https://doi.org/10.1016/j.jhsa.2014.09.019.

8. Galley I, Bain GI, McLean JM. Influence of lunate type on scaphoid kinematics. J Hand Surg. 2007;32:842–7. https://doi.org/10.1016/j.jhsa.2007.03.012.

9. Haase SC, Berger RA, Shin AY. Association between lunate morphology and carpal collapse patterns in scaphoid nonunions. J Hand Surg. 2007;32:1009–12. https://doi.org/10.1016/j.jhsa.2007.06.005.

10. Pang EQ, Douglass N, Kamal RN. Association of lunate morphology with carpal instability in scapholunate ligament injury. Hand N Y N. 2018;13:418–22. https://doi.org/10.1177/1558944717709073.

11. Rhee PC, Moran SL, Shin AY. Association between lunate morphology and carpal collapse in cases of scapholunate dissociation. J Hand Surg. 2009;34:1633–9. https://doi.org/10.1016/j.jhsa.2009.06.017.

12. Best GM, Mack ZE, Pichora DR, et al. Differences in the rotation axes of the scapholunate joint during flexion-extension and radial-ulnar deviation motions. J Hand Surg. 2019;44:772–8. https://doi.org/10.1016/j.jhsa.2019.05.001.

13. Best GM, Zec ML, Pichora DR, et al. Does wrist laxity influence three-dimensional carpal bone motion? J Biomech Eng. 2018;140 https://doi.org/10.1115/1.4038897.

14. Garcia-Elias M, Ribe M, Rodriguez J, et al. Influence of joint laxity on scaphoid kinematics. J Hand Surg Edinb Scotl. 1995;20:379–82. https://doi.org/10.1016/s0266-7681(05)80097-x.

15. Taleisnik J. The ligaments of the wrist. J Hand Surg. 1976;1:110–8. https://doi.org/10.1016/S0363-5023(76)80004-4.

16. Short WH, Werner FW, Green JK, Masaoka S. Biomechanical evaluation of the ligamentous stabilizers of the scaphoid and lunate: part II. J Hand Surg. 2005;30:24–34. https://doi.org/10.1016/j.jhsa.2004.09.015.

17. Short WH, Werner FW, Green JK, Masaoka S. Biomechanical evaluation of ligamentous stabilizers of the scaphoid and lunate. J Hand Surg. 2002;27:991–1002. https://doi.org/10.1053/jhsu.2002.35878.

18. Rajan PV, Day CS. Scapholunate interosseous ligament anatomy and biomechanics. J Hand Surg. 2015;40:1692–702. https://doi.org/10.1016/j.jhsa.2015.03.032.

19. Berger RA. The anatomy of the ligaments of the wrist and distal radioulnar joints. Clin Orthop. 2001;383:32–40. https://doi.org/10.1097/00003086-200102000-00006.

20. Siegel DB, Gelberman RH. Radial styloidectomy: an anatomical study with special reference to radiocarpal intracapsular ligamentous morphology. J Hand Surg. 1991;16:40–4. https://doi.org/10.1016/S0363-5023(10)80010-3.

21. Rainbow MJ, Kamal RN, Moore DC, et al. Subject-specific carpal ligament elongation in extreme positions, grip, and the dart thrower's motion. J Biomech Eng. 2015;137:1,110,061–11,100,610. https://doi.org/10.1115/1.4031580.

22. Kitay A, Wolfe SW. Scapholunate instability: current concepts in diagnosis and management. J Hand Surg. 2012;37:2175–96. https://doi.org/10.1016/j.jhsa.2012.07.035.

23. Viegas SF, Yamaguchi S, Boyd NL, Patterson RM. The dorsal ligaments of the wrist: anatomy, mechanical properties, and function. J Hand Surg. 1999;24:456–68. https://doi.org/10.1053/jhsu.1999.0456.

24. Rainbow MJ, Crisco JJ, Moore DC, et al. Elongation of the dorsal carpal ligaments: a computational study of in vivo carpal kinematics. J Hand Surg. 2012;37:1393–9. https://doi.org/10.1016/j.jhsa.2012.04.025.

25. Mitsuyasu H, Patterson RM, Shah MA, et al. The role of the dorsal intercarpal ligament in dynamic and static scapholunate instability. J Hand Surg. 2004;29:279–88. https://doi.org/10.1016/j.jhsa.2003.11.004.
26. Linscheid RL, Dobyns JH, Beabout JW, Bryan RS. Traumatic instability of the wrist. Diagnosis, classification, and pathomechanics. J Bone Joint Surg Am. 1972;54:1612–32.
27. Berger RA. The gross and histologic anatomy of the scapholunate interosseous ligament. J Hand Surg. 1996;21:170–8. https://doi.org/10.1016/S0363-5023(96)80096-7.
28. Trehan SK, Lee SK, Wolfe SW. Scapholunate advanced collapse: nomenclature and differential diagnosis. J Hand Surg. 2015;40:2085–9. https://doi.org/10.1016/j.jhsa.2015.06.110.
29. Short WH, Werner FW, Fortino MD, et al. A dynamic biomechanical study of scapholunate ligament sectioning. J Hand Surg. 1995;20:986–99. https://doi.org/10.1016/S0363-5023(05)80147-9.
30. Short WH, Werner FW, Green JK, et al. Biomechanical evaluation of the ligamentous stabilizers of the scaphoid and lunate: part III. J Hand Surg. 2007;32:297–309. https://doi.org/10.1016/j.jhsa.2006.10.024.
31. Elsaidi GA, Ruch DS, Kuzma GR, Smith BP. Dorsal wrist ligament insertions stabilize the scapholunate interval: cadaver study. Clin Orthop. 2004:152–7. https://doi.org/10.1097/01.blo.0000136836.78049.45.
32. Viegas SF, Patterson RM, Peterson PD, et al. Ulnar-sided perilunate instability: an anatomic and biomechanic study. J Hand Surg. 1990;15:268–78. https://doi.org/10.1016/0363-5023(90)90107-3.
33. Kamal RN, Chehata A, Rainbow MJ, et al. The effect of the dorsal intercarpal ligament on lunate extension after distal scaphoid excision. J Hand Surg. 2012;37:2240–5. https://doi.org/10.1016/j.jhsa.2012.07.029.

Suggested Reading

Kamal RN, Starr A, Akelman E. Carpal kinematics and kinetics. J Hand Surg. 2016;41(10):1011–8.
Berger RA. The anatomy of the ligaments of the wrist and distal radioulnar joints. Clin Orthop. 2001;383:32–40.
Trehan SK, Lee SK, Wolfe SW. Scapholunate advanced collapse: nomenclature and differential diagnosis. J Hand Surg. 2015;40(10):2085–9.

Chapter 6
A Case of Scapholunate Instability Treated by Arthroscopic Dorsal Capsuloligamentous Repair (ADCLR)

Ahlam Arnaout ⓘ and Christophe Mathoulin

Case Presentation

A professional tennis player presented for post-traumatic right wrist pain.

We noted a history of a fall on the right wrist in hyperextension 6 months earlier. The patient described disabling pain, particularly during tennis (holding the racket with his clenched fist), during wrist hyperextension and strength movements (push-ups, getting up from a sofa) and when carrying heavy loads. The pain was located at the dorsal aspect of the wrist.

He also described subjective strength loss and painful "clunks" in certain wrist tilt movements.

The GP ordered plain X-rays which were considered "normal." He was referred for specialist advice.

Supplementary Information The online version contains supplementary material available at https://doi.org/10.1007/978-3-031-55869-6_6.

A. Arnaout (✉)
International Wrist Centers-Clinique du Poignet, Bizet Clinic, Paris, France

C. Mathoulin
International Wrist Centers-Clinique du Poignet, El Tarter, Andorra

Diagnosis

Physical Assessment

The pain was reproduced by palpation of the dorsal scapholunate (SL) joint. The Watson test was positive and painful so as the scaphoid shift test [1, 2]. The lunotriquetral (LT) assessment (Reagan's ballottement test and deep palpation of LT space) was negative.

Pain score was rated at 5 in daily activities and 8 during sports on the VAS scale.

The range of motion (ROM) and grip strength were significantly decreased in comparison with the contralateral unaffected wrist.

– Flexion was 30° versus 70° on the opposite side.
– Extension was 50° versus 85° on the opposite side.
– Radial deviation was 15° versus 25° on the opposite side.
– Ulnar deviation was 20° versus 35° on the opposite side.
– Pronation and supination were normal.
– Grip strength was 30 kg versus 65 kg on the opposite non-dominant side.

Imaging Assessment

– Bilateral and comparative plain X-rays (antero-posterior and lateral) and dynamic views (ulnar deviation, radial deviation, clenched fist) were ordered. The clenched fist view showed a dynamic opening of the SL space greater than 3 mm (Fig. 6.1).
– Arthro CT-scan showed a large scapholunate ligament tear (Fig. 6.2).

The Confirmed Diagnosis was Made Intraoperatively by Arthroscopic Assessment

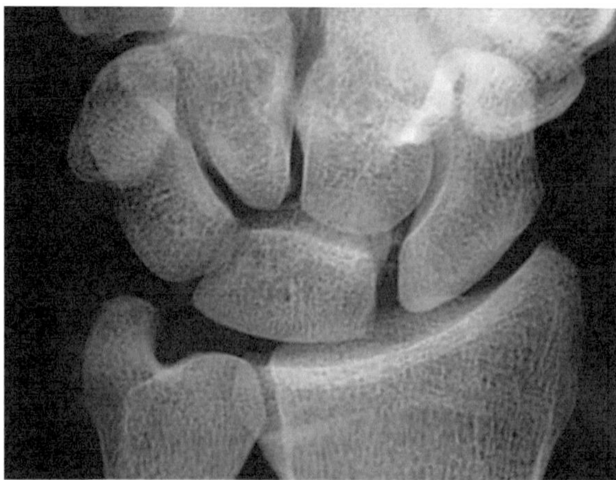

Fig. 6.1 Preoperative clenched fist view: dynamic opening of SL space

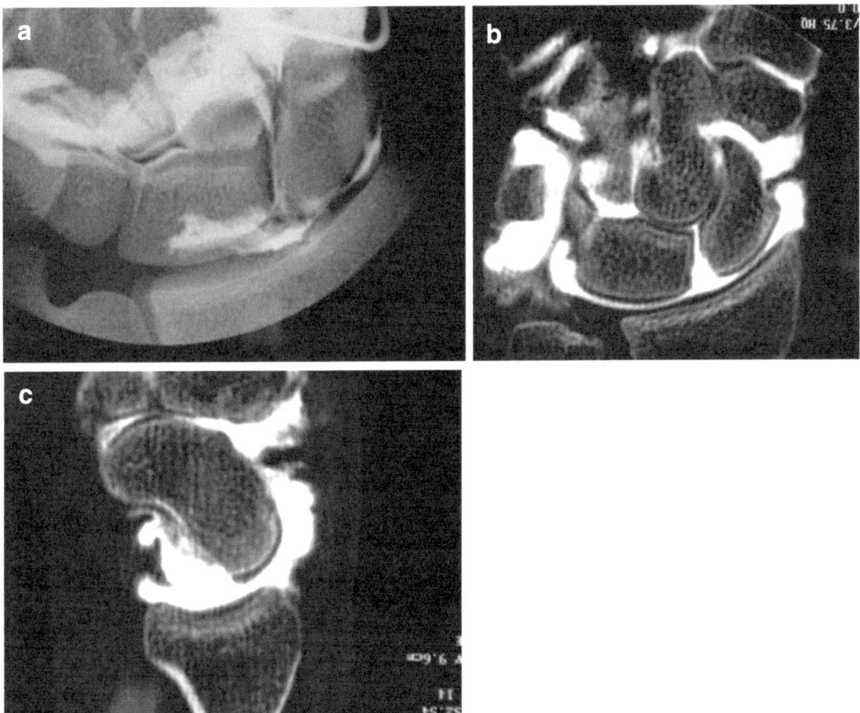

Fig. 6.2 Arthrography and arthro CT-scan showing an obvious SL tear. (**a**): arthography. (**b**) and (**c**): arthro CT scan

Dynamic examination of the scapholunate joint in the midcarpal space confirmed SL instability stage IV according to EWAS-Messina classification (Video 6.1).

No associated lesions were found: no lunotriquetral instability, no cartilaginous lesions.

Management Options

In this case of chronic scapholunate instability, a number of surgical options are possible, and there is no real current consensus on the optimal procedure:

Conventional Open Surgical Techniques

These techniques described elsewhere in this Casebook generally use screws or tendon grafts either for SL repair or reconstruction [3–6].

Arthroscopic Techniques

The arthroscopic dorsal capsulo-ligamentous repair (ADCLR). This technique enables SL space stabilization due to a capsule-to-ligament suturing. Some modifications have been described, according to intraoperative findings and EWAS stage (K-wires, large repair, anchors) [6–10].

Arthroscopic reconstructions [11, 12] are an alternative option in the more advanced SL instabilities.

Chosen Management

In this case, the surgical option chosen was the ADCLR. Moreover, it was decided intraoperatively to perform an additional scapholunate and scapho-capitate pinning to reduce the SL step-off that was found at the midcarpal assessment.

This decision was made based on the following basis:

- Arthroscopic management is less invasive than open procedures. With a minimal scarring and no extensive dissection of the tissues, it preserves crucial anatomical elements, especially the extrinsic ligaments, whose role in proximal carpal row stabilization is now well established.
- The injury was relatively recent. The "fresher" the lesions, the more effective this technique is.
- The established long-term satisfactory outcomes we have using this procedure for dynamic scapholunate instability.
- In this case, neither the preoperative imaging nor the arthroscopic assessment showed any degenerative changes of the radiocarpal or midcarpal joints. Of course, if the arthroscopy shows any cartilaginous degenerative lesions that were not obvious on the preoperative imaging, we will need to change the indications intraoperatively. It is mandatory to inform the patient of this possibility and obtain consent prior to surgery.

Surgical Technique (ADCLR) (Videos 6.1, 6.2, 6.3, 6.4, 6.5, 6.6, 6.7, 6.8, 6.9)

The principle of the technique is to achieve a dorsal capsule-to-ligament suture *to stabilize the scapholunate joint.*

The procedure is performed on an outpatient basis, under regional anesthesia and pneumatic tourniquet.

Standard dorsal arthroscopic portals are used: radiocarpal 3–4, 6U, midcarpal ulnar (MCU), and midcarpal radial (MCR).

The scapholunate interosseous ligament (SLIL) is directly visualized with the scope in 3–4 portal and a shaver is used to perform a synovectomy.

The scope is then placed in the 6R portal and the shaver in the 3–4 portal. The SLIL is visualized from its palmar to dorsal aspect. The origin of the ligament avulsion is checked with the probe and the quality of the remaining ligament stumps are assessed. Usually, the ligament is avulsed from its scaphoid insertion, and ligament remnants attached to the scaphoid and lunate are identified. The procedure can be performed only if good quality ligaments stumps remain attached.

A push test is performed to evaluate the Dorsal Capsulo-Scapholunate Septum (DCSS) status. If the probe can be pushed easily into the midcarpal joint, the test is positive and DCSS is considered torn (Fig. 6.3).

The next step is performed in the midcarpal joint. With the scope in the MCU and the shaver in the MCR, a meticulous synovectomy is performed, and SL joint instability is staged (Messina-EWAS and Geissler) [13]. The instability can also be more accurately evaluated with dynamic assessment (flexion-extension and radial-ulnar translation) after a slight traction release.

The arthroscope is then placed again in the 6R portal to control the exact location of the sutures and their passage across the ligament stumps. Two absorbable monofilament sutures are passed through two intramuscular needles (usually 3.0 or 4.0, depending on the patient's size). The first needle is inserted through the 3–4 radiocarpal portal, then shifted slightly distally so to cross the dorsal capsule up to 1 mm from the capsular hole. The needle is then pushed through the radial ligament stump attached to the scaphoid, oriented obliquely from dorsal to volar, and proximal to distal with an angulation close to 45°, to reach the midcarpal joint (Fig. 6.4).

Fig. 6.3 DCSS push test. The probe moves to midcarpal joint; the DCSS is torn

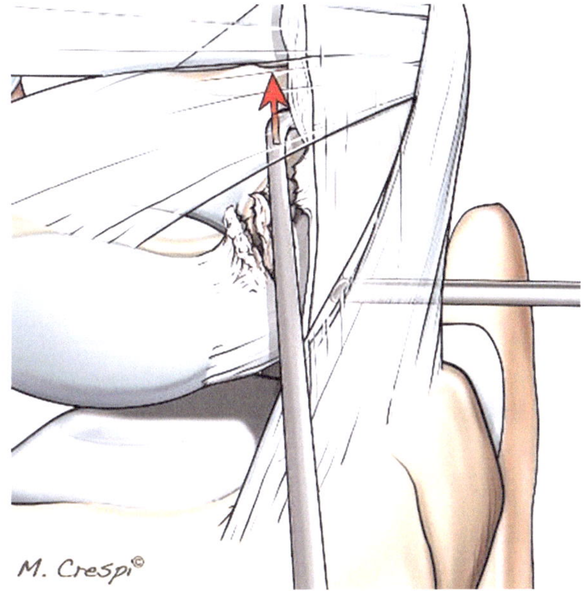

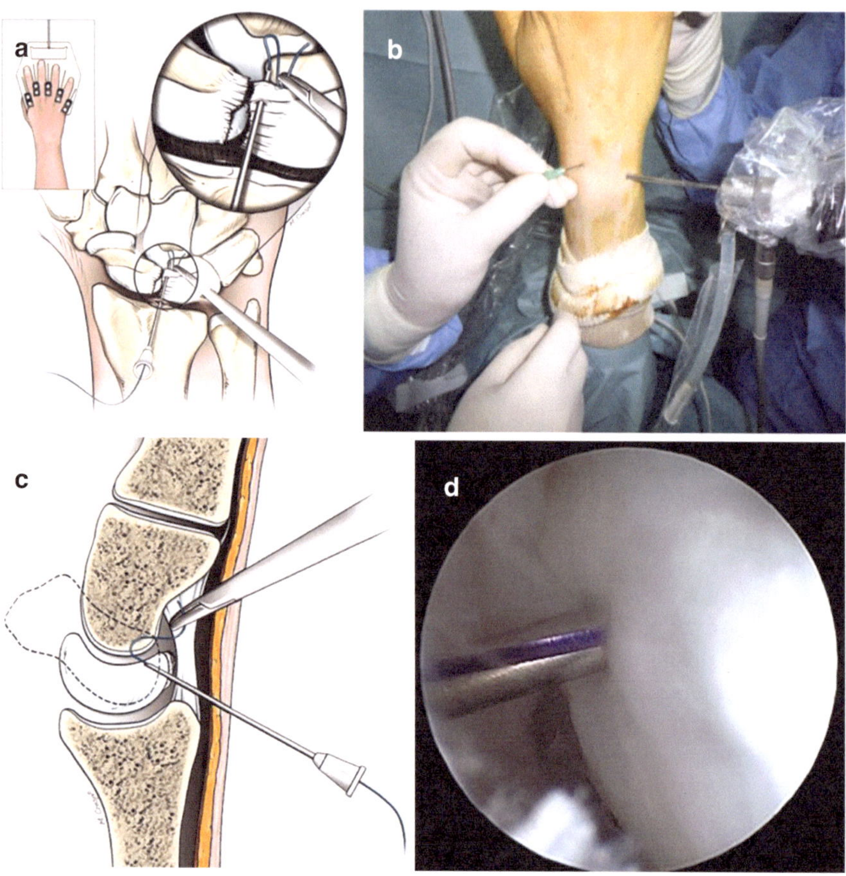

Fig. 6.4 Passage of the first suture. (**a**) and (**b**): passage of the first suture through the ulnar stump. (**c**): suture retrieved from the midcarpal joint. (**d**): arthroscopic view of the passage of the first suture

A second suture passed in the same way through a needle is inserted parallel to the first one, into the ulnar ligament remnant attached to the lunate (Fig. 6.5).

The principle of the next step is to fix the first knot in the midcarpal joint between the scaphoid and the lunate to reduce the SL space (Figs. 6.5, 6.6, 6.7). The arthroscope is switched once more to the MCU portal to visualize the sutures in the midcarpal joint. A forceps is used to externalize both sutures from the MCR portal and tie the first knot outside the joint. A proximal-distal traction is then applied to the sutures through the 3–4 radiocarpal portal to pull the midcarpal knot and place it between the scaphoid and the lunate and volar to the dorsal portion of the SLIL. The reduction is evaluated by maintaining a proximal tension on the sutures ends after a slight release of the traction. If reduction is satisfactory, the ligament is sutured to the dorsal capsule by tying the second knot in a subcutaneous position at the radiocarpal level. An open mosquito forceps can be used to protect the extensors while tying the knots in front of MCR and 3–4 portals.

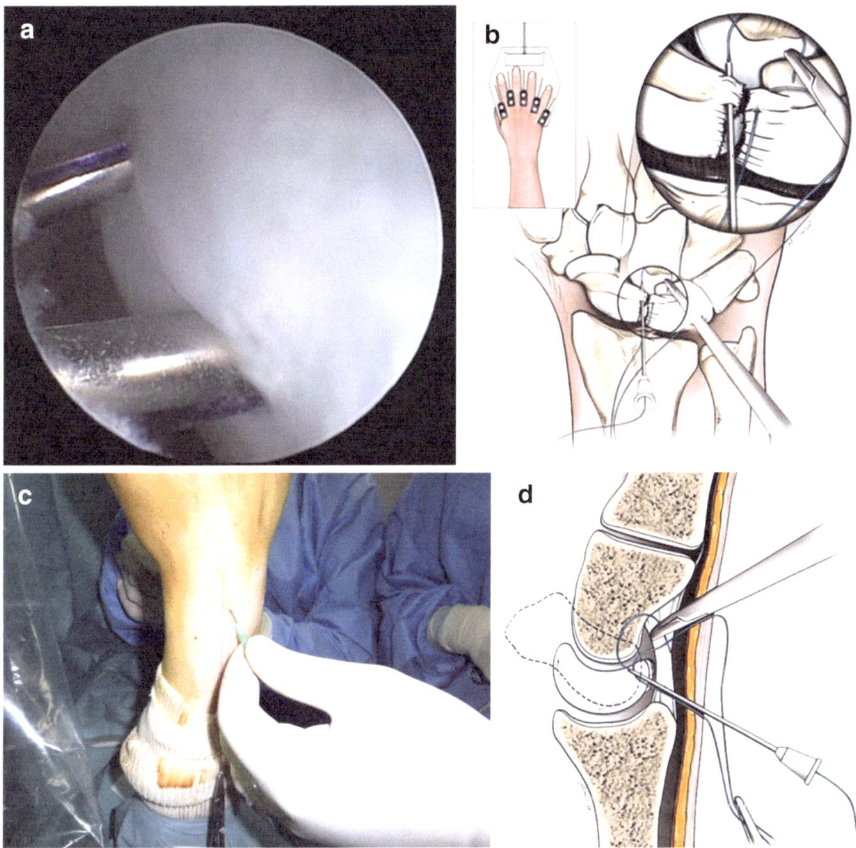

Fig. 6.5 Passage of the second suture

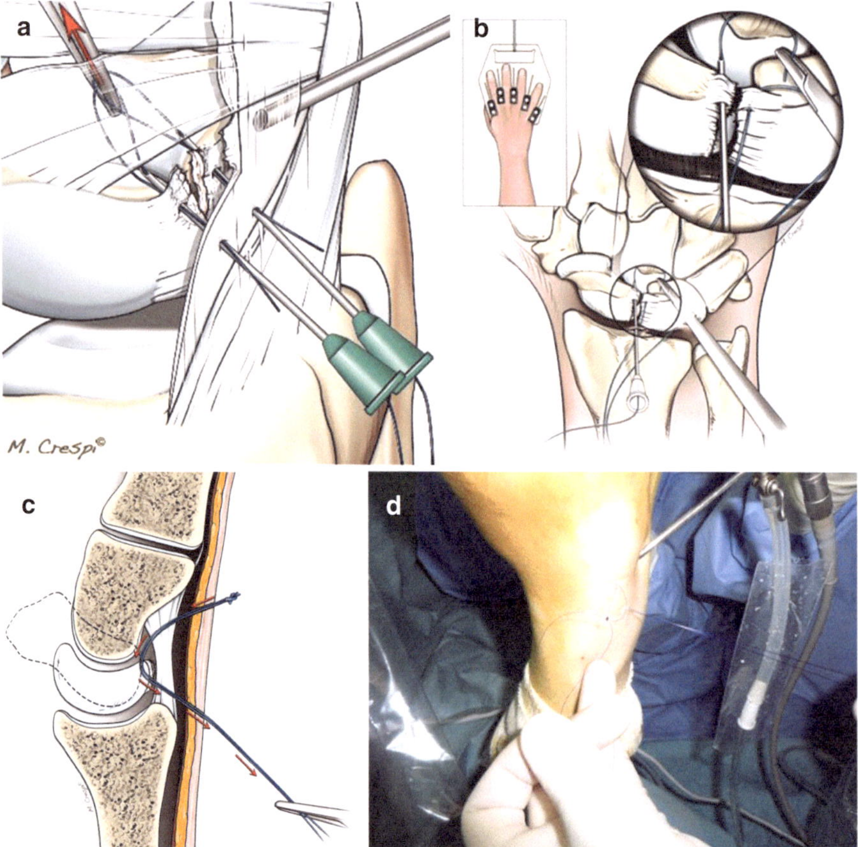

Fig. 6.6 Midcarpal knot is tied in the midcarpal joint. Proximal distal traction on the sutures

Modified Technique Using K-Wire Fixation

In this case, the scapholunate space had to be reduced by an additional step of pinning the carpal bones. Two scapholunate and an additional scapho-capitate K-wires are usually passed under fluoroscopic control. This reduction is performed before tying the second knot.

First, a blunt trocar is inserted through the MCR portal, positioned under the capitate and beyond the anterior edge of the proximal pole of the scaphoid. The scaphoid is reduced onto the lunate, using a lever action—tire iron-like maneuver (Fig. 6.7).

The K-wires are then introduced, while this reduced position is maintained. After the blunt trocar is removed, the scaphoid shifts back to its initial position and pulls the lunate back up (Fig. 6.8). The K-wires are removed generally at 8 weeks and the patient can start a specific rehabilitation protocol.

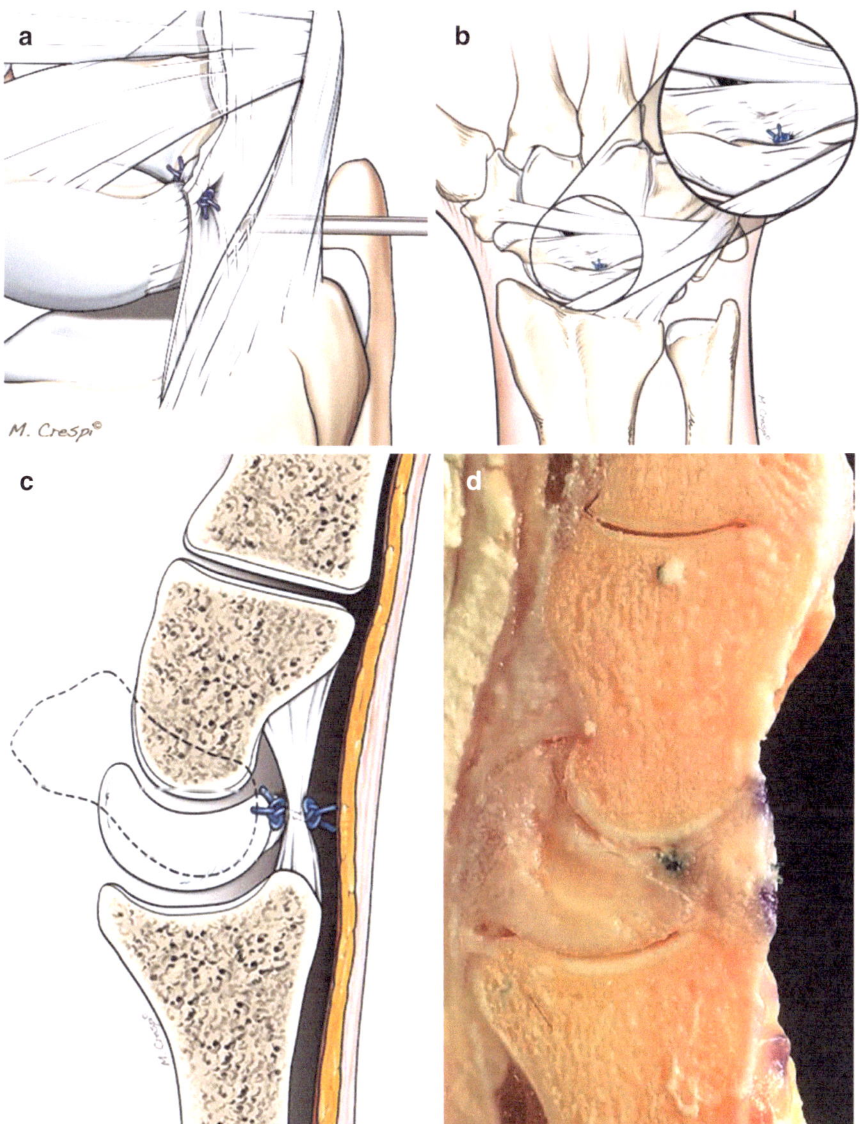

Fig. 6.7 The second knot is tied at the radiocarpal level

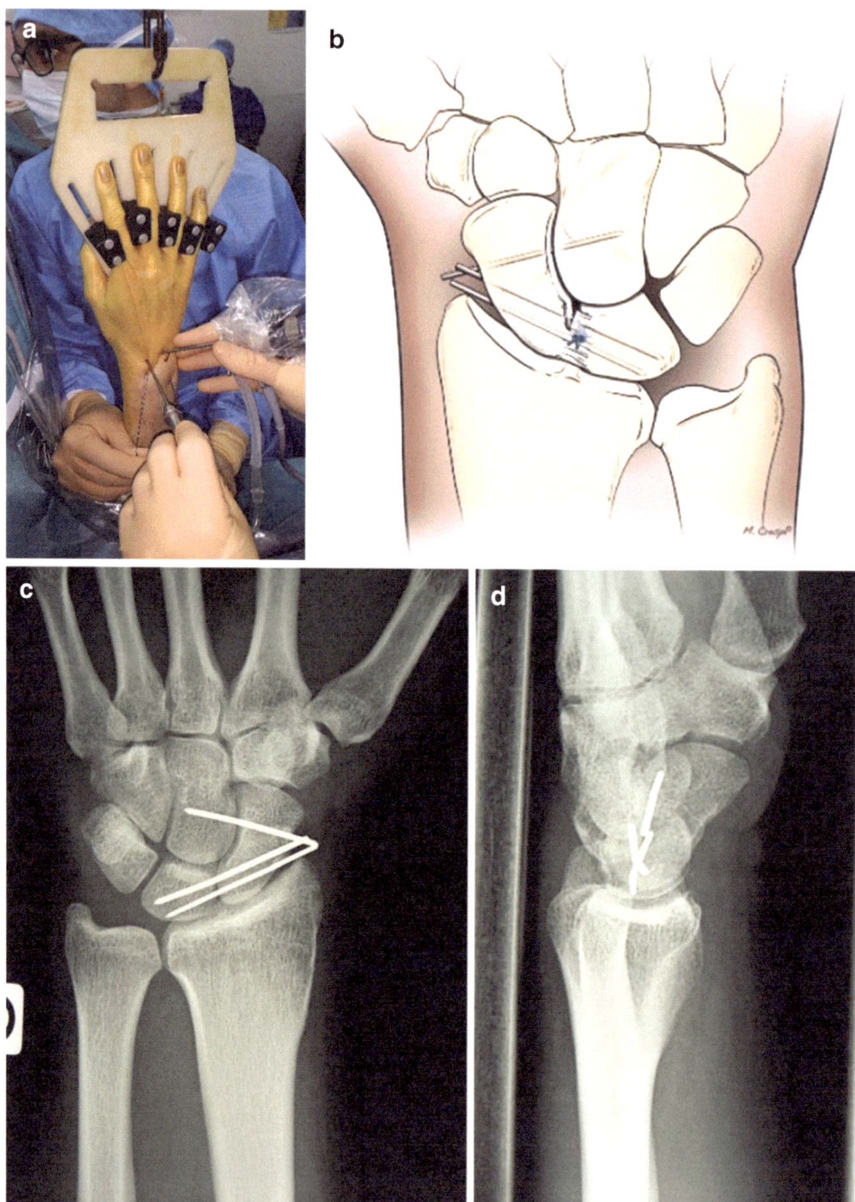

Fig. 6.8 K-wires are used for SL step-off reduction

Clinical Course and Outcome

The postoperative follow-up was carried out at 8 weeks, 3 months, 6 months, and once per year.

At 8 weeks, after pins removal, plain X-rays were ordered. The SL diastasis, the DISI, and the DST (dorsal scaphoid translation) were evaluated. The interest was mainly focused on the DST. The clinical examination showed that Watson test was normalized. The specific rehabilitation protocol was then started. The physiotherapy is focused initially on proprioception movements, especially Flexor Carpi Radialis proprioception. Stretching and clenched fist exercises were avoided for the first 3 weeks of physiotherapy.

The next follow-up consultations (at 3 months, 6 months, and once per year): we assessed for clinical instability recurrence (Watson and scaphoid shift test), the evolution of ROM and strength, and monitored pain especially on the radial compartment (SLAC occurrence).

The evolution was satisfactory with, at the last FU, at 3 years post-surgery, recovering good ROM and strength with a minimal residual pain in sports activities (Videos 6.6 and 6.7)

- Flexion: 65. Extension: 85. RD: 25. UD: 35
- Strength: 70 kg

There was no residual clinical SL instability (negative Watson and scaphoid shift tests).

X-rays were normal with no residual DST and partially corrected SL GAP and DISI (Fig. 6.9). The MRI showed a normal DCSS (Figs. 6.10)

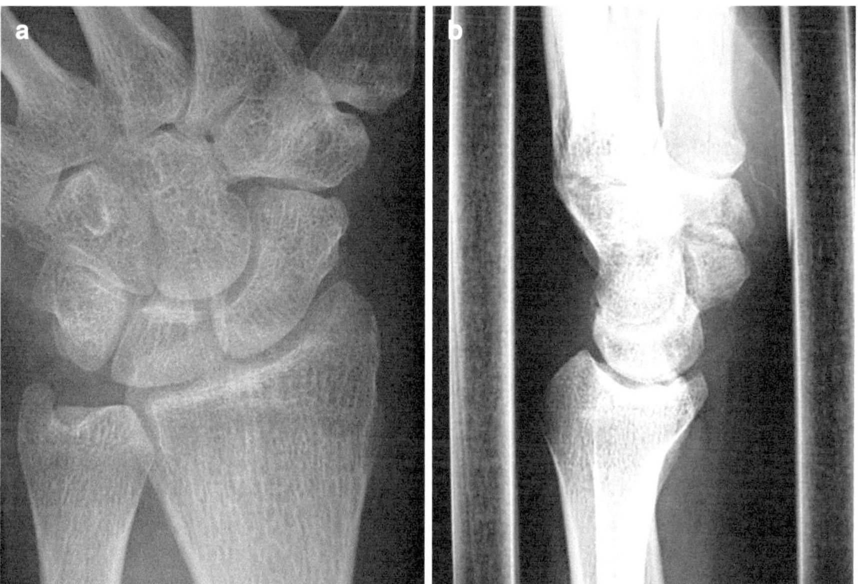

Fig. 6.9 Postoperative X-rays showing a corrected SL gap. (**a**): AP view. (**b**): The DISI is not corrected

  A. Arnaout and C. Mathoulin

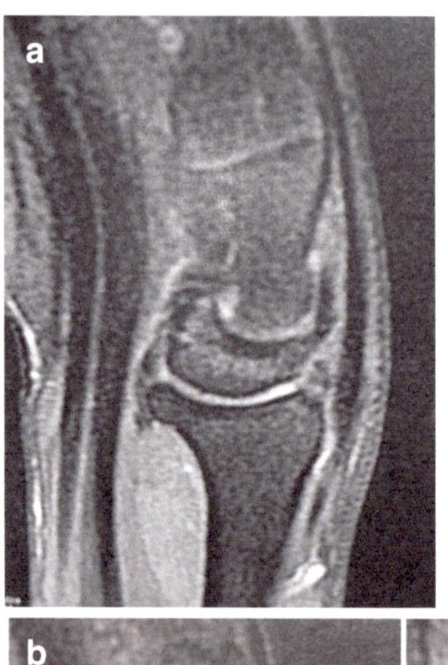

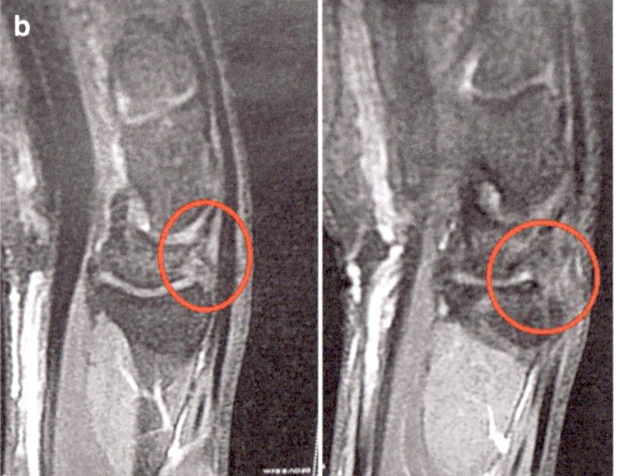

Fig. 6.10 Postoperative MRI showing a repaired DCSS. (**a**): preop torn DCSS. (**b**) and (**c**): repaired DCSS

Functional scores were good, and the patient returned to his professional tennis career at the same level as before his injury (Videos 6.4 and 6.5).

Bulleted Clinical Pearls/Pitfalls

- False negative is possible on the preoperative arthro CT-scan, especially in the chronic cases. If there are obvious clinical signs of instability, the indication of arthroscopy remains logical to confirm the diagnosis (diagnostic and therapeutic arthroscopy).
- The postoperative clinical examination at 6 weeks ensures the normalization of the Watson and scaphoid shift test. It is common at 6 weeks to find stiffness in wrist flexion that will progressively improve with rehabilitation, and it is necessary to reassure the patient.

Discussion

The preoperative diagnosis is based on a body of clinical and imaging elements. The association of a clinical instability with obvious abnormalities on the arthro CT-scan or the MRI advocate strongly for the diagnosis.

The relevant imaging parameters are [14, 15]:

- The bilateral and comparative X-rays. The dynamic views (ulnar deviation, radial deviation, clenched fist) are mandatory to assess a dynamic instability: an opening of the SL space and/or rupture of Gilula arcs are looked for.
- The arthro CT-scan, MRI, or arthro-MRI.
- An additional dynamic US or arthro US examination can help to diagnose preoperatively a dynamic SL instability.

The accurate arthroscopic assessment confirms the diagnosis by the dynamic examination of the scapholunate joint in the midcarpal joint. The instability is staged according to EWAS-Messina classification [13]. It also enables associated and differential diagnosis: associated lunotriquetral instability, cartilaginous lesions, etc.

The relevant parameters for postoperative assessment after scapholunate stabilization surgery are clinical and imaging parameters. The SL diastasis as well as the DISI, and the DST (dorsal scaphoid translation) are evaluated on the postoperative X-rays [16, 17]. The interest is mainly focused on the DST. The SL gap or the DISI are not necessarily corrected in the postoperative controls, and they are not relevant criteria to assess the permanent SL stabilization. Dorsal scaphoid translation measurement (MRI or X-rays) may be an accurate sign to assess the surgery effectiveness of SL stabilization.

The follow-up consultations assess a recurrence of clinical instability (Watson), the evolution of ROM and strength, and monitors pain (appearance of an SLAC).

Therapeutic Options for Scapholunate Instability Management

Open Techniques: Repair Or Reconstruction [2–5]

Many conventional open surgical techniques have been described for scapholunate joint stability; however, these procedures often result in stiffness, and this can be disabling especially for young and high-level athletes.

Arthroscopic Techniques [6–12]

In the last decades, wrist arthroscopy has dramatically changed the understanding of SL instability biomechanics and has led to development of less invasive and reproducible surgical repair techniques. Scapholunate joint stability is dependent not only on the SLIL, but also on a set of primary and secondary stabilizers that collectively form a complex. The crucial role of the DCSS and the extrinsic ligaments in SL stability, especially the dorsal intercarpal (DIC) ligament is now well established [18–23].

The ADCLR techniques (original and modified techniques) enable the stabilization and the repair of these structures by a capsule-to-ligament suturing and prevent the stiffness associated with open procedures. Moreover, the ADCLR techniques do not burn the bridges for secondary reconstruction techniques if necessary.

Other SLL arthroscopic reconstruction techniques are technically demanding and are indicated in the case of advanced SL instability. Some of these techniques target only SLL reconstruction, and they do not take into account the crucial role of extrinsic ligaments in SL stability. These limitations may partially explain some long-term poorer outcomes [24].

Our Therapeutic Decisional Tree Algorithm

We recommend the ADCLR technique in chronic SL instabilities, without any degenerative cartilaginous changes, in the stages up to EWAS IV. The sine qua none condition is a reducible SL joint, confirmed arthroscopically. A modified technique should be used if necessary (K-wires, anchors, or large ADCLR).

References

1. Lane LB. The scaphoid shift tests. J Hand Surg Am. 1993;18(2):366–8. https://doi.org/10.1016/0363-5023(93)90377-F.
2. Watson HK, Black DM. Instabilities of the wrist. Hand Clin. 1987;3(1):103–11.
3. Cuénod P. Osteoligamentoplasty and limited dorsal capsulodesis for chronic scapholunate dissociation. Ann Chir Main Memb Super. 1999;18:38–53.
4. Cognet JM, Levadoux M, Martinache X. The use of screws in the treatment of scapholunate instability. J Hand Surg Eur. 2011;36:690–3.
5. Sandow M, Fisher T. Anatomical anterior and posterior reconstruction for scapholunate dissociation: preliminary outcome in ten patients. J Hand Surg Eur. 2020;45(4):389–95. https://doi.org/10.1177/1753193419886536. Epub 2019 Nov 13.
6. Mathoulin CL. Indications, techniques, and outcomes of arthroscopic repair of scapholunate ligament and triangular fibrocartilage complex. J Hand Surg Eur. 2017;42(6):551–66.
7. Wahegaonkar AL, Mathoulin CL. Arthroscopic dorsal capsulo-ligamentous repair in the treatment of chronic scapho-lunate ligament tears. J Wrist Surg. 2013;2(2):141–8. https://doi.org/10.1055/s-0033-1341582.
8. Mathoulin C, Gras M. Role of wrist arthroscopy in scapholunate dissociation. Orthop Traumatol Surg Res. 2020;106(1S):S89–99. https://doi.org/10.1016/j.otsr.2019.07.008.
9. Arnaout A, Mathoulin C. Arthroscopic treatment of scapholunate instability. In: Arthroscopy and endoscopy of the elbow, wrist and hand; 2022. doi: https://doi.org/10.1007/978-3-030-79423-1_75.

10. Carratalá V, Lucas FJ, Miranda I, Sánchez Alepuz E, González JC. Arthroscopic scapholunate capsuloligamentous repair: suture with dorsal capsular reinforcement for scapholunate ligament lesion. Arthrosc Tech. 2017;6(1):e113–20. https://doi.org/10.1016/j.eats.2016.09.009.
11. Corella F, Del Cerro M, Ocampos M, Simon de Blas C, Larrainzar-Garijo R. Arthroscopic scapholunate ligament reconstruction, volar and dorsal reconstruction. Hand Clin. 2017;33(4):687–707. https://doi.org/10.1016/j.hcl.2017.07.019.
12. Ho PC. Arthroscopic-assisted box reconstruction of scapholunate ligament with tendon graft. In: Mathoulin C, editor. Wrist arthroscopy techniques. 2nd ed. Stuttgart: Thieme; 2019.
13. Messina JC, Van Overstraeten L, Luchetti R, Fairplay T, Mathoulin CL. The EWAS classification of scapholunate tears: an anatomical arthroscopic study. J Wrist Surg. 2013;2(2):105–9. https://doi.org/10.1055/s-0033-1345265.
14. Shahabpour M, Staelens B, Van Overstraeten L, et al. Advanced imaging of the scapholunate ligamentous complex. Skeletal Radiol. 2015;44(12):1709–25. https://doi.org/10.1007/s00256-015-2182-9.
15. Dietrich TJ, Toms AP, Cerezal L, Omoumi P, Boutin RD, Fritz J, Schmitt R, Shahabpour M, et al. Interdisciplinary consensus statements on imaging of scapholunate joint instability. Eur Radiol. 2021;31(12):9446–58. https://doi.org/10.1007/s00330-021-08073-8. Epub 2021 Jun 8.
16. Chan K, Vutescu ES, Wolfe SW, Lee SK. Radiographs detect dorsal scaphoid translation in scapholunate dissociation. J Wrist Surg. 2019;8(3):186–91. https://doi.org/10.1055/s-0038-1677536. Epub 2019 Jan 18.
17. Borrel F, Gras M, Arnaout A, Merlini L, Mathoulin C. Radiologic evolution after scapholunate dorsal capsulodesis for chronic tears. J Wrist Surg. 2023; https://doi.org/10.1055/s-0043-1764159.
18. Mathoulin CL. From scapholunate interosseus ligament to scapholunate ligament complex. J Wrist Surg. 2013;2(2):98. https://doi.org/10.1055/s-0033-1341961.
19. Branco JL. The scapholunate ligament complex. J Wrist Surg. 2013;2(3):282. https://doi.org/10.1055/s-0033-1353532.
20. Overstraeten LV, Camus EJ, Wahegaonkar A, et al. Anatomical description of the dorsal capsulo-scapholunate septum (DCSS)-arthroscopic staging of scapholunate instability after DCSS sectioning. J Wrist Surg. 2013;2(2):149–54. https://doi.org/10.1055/s-0033-1338256.
21. Carrara T, et al. The anatomy of the dorsal capsulo-scapholunate septum: a cadaveric study. J Wrist Surg. 2017;6(3):244–7.
22. Pérez AJ, al. Role of ligament stabilizers of the proximal carpal row in preventing dorsal intercalated segment instability: a cadaveric study. JBJS. 2019;101:1388.
23. Elsaidi GA, al. Dorsal wrist ligament insertions stabilize the scapholunate interval: cadaver study. Clin Orthop Relat Res. 2004;425:152.
24. Bain GI, Amasooriya M. Scapholunate instability: why are the surgical outcomes still so far from ideal? J Hand Surg Eur Vol. 2023; https://doi.org/10.1177/17531934221148009.

Suggested Reading

Bain GI, Amasooriya M. Scapholunate instability: why are the surgical outcomes still so far from ideal? J Hand Surg Eur Vol. 2023; https://doi.org/10.1177/17531934221148009.
Mathoulin CL. From scapholunate interosseus ligament to scapholunate ligament complex. J Wrist Surg. 2013;2(2):98. https://doi.org/10.1055/s-0033-1341961.
Overstraeten LV, et al. Anatomical description of the dorsal capsulo-scapholunate septum (DCSS)-arthroscopic staging of scapholunate instability after DCSS sectioning. J Wrist Surg.

2013;2(2):149–54. Wahegaonkar AL, Mathoulin CL. Arthroscopic dorsal capsulo-ligamentous repair in the treatment of chronic scapho-lunate ligament tears. J Wrist Surg. 2013;2(2):141–8. https://doi.org/10.1055/s-0033-1341582.

Wahegaonkar AL, Mathoulin CL. Arthroscopic dorsal capsulo-ligamentous repair in the treatment of chronic scapho-lunate ligament tears. J Wrist Surg. 2013;2(2):141–8. https://doi.org/10.1055/s-0033-1341582.

Chapter 7
Pre-dynamic Scapholunate Ligament Injury: Arthroscopic Thermal Shrinkage

Matthew B. Burn ⓘ and Alex Han

Case Presentation

Our patient is a 17-year-old right hand dominant male who presented for evaluation of right dorsal central wrist pain that had bothered him for the past 6 months. He noted that it mainly bothered him with wrist hyperextension and loading, such as push-ups or lifting weights at the gym. He denied any obvious inciting event or injury. Upon presentation, he was notably tender to palpation directly over the dorsal scapholunate (SL) ligament. On provocative testing, including scaphoid shift and scapholunate shear, he had no clinical instability, but these maneuvers did reproduce his pain. Wrist radiographs, including bilateral clenched fist and scaphoid views, did not demonstrate any widening at the scapholunate interval or carpal malalignment.

At his first visit, the patient was offered a course of immobilization, and he initially chose to wear a wrist brace. He re-presented a few weeks later noting that he was not able to comply with wearing the brace. Thus, he was placed into a short arm cast extending up to just below the elbow. He was treated with 6 weeks of casting and re-presented with improved examination including decreased tenderness and minimally positive provocative testing. He then re-presented 4 weeks later as the pain had returned. He elected for a corticosteroid injection to his wrist, which gave him temporary relief. He trialed a course of occupational therapy and further immobilization. Unfortunately, his pain continued. Thus, an MRI arthrogram of his wrist

M. B. Burn (✉)
Hand, Wrist, Elbow & Nerve Surgery, OrthoArkansas, Little Rock, AR, USA
e-mail: Matthew.burn@orthoarkansas.com

A. Han
Department of Orthopedics & Sports Medicine, Houston Methodist Hospital, Houston, TX, USA
e-mail: Ahan@houstonmethodist.org

was obtained. This demonstrated no obvious tearing of his scapholunate ligament but did show a small occult ganglion cyst at the most distal-dorsal extent of the scapholunate ligament. Due to his continued pain, inability to perform his previous activities, and ultimately the failure of non-operative management, he elected for wrist arthroscopy.

A standard diagnostic wrist arthroscopy was performed. However, in my practice, I tend to begin with midcarpal arthroscopy as I find the midcarpal joint is easier to gain access prior to distention and swelling from fluid. When probing the scapholunate interval, I was barely able to insert the tip of my probe into the interval. There was no obvious step-off. No other pathology was identified. I elected for thermal capsulorrhaphy given his mild instability (Geissler grade II). First, synovitis was debrided from the volar and dorsal portions of the scapholunate ligament within the midcarpal joint. Next, our electrothermal probe (Micro-TAC-S, Smith and Nephew, Andover, MA) was inserted into the midcarpal joint where both the volar and dorsal portions of the scapholunate ligament, including the portion of the radioscaphocapitate ligament adjacent to the volar scapholunate ligament, were treated. Next, through the radiocarpal joint, his dorsal scapholunate ligament was noted to have a convex appearance with mild fraying. This was also treated with debridement followed by thermal capsulorrhaphy. At the most distal-dorsal portion of the ligament, his small occult ganglion cyst was able to be removed with an arthroscopic shaver. After treatment, the arthroscope was re-inserted into the midcarpal joint. We were now unable to re-insert the probe into the scapholunate interval suggesting tightening or capsulorrhaphy of the scapholunate ligament.

Immediately post-operatively, he was placed into a plaster wrist splint. At 2 weeks post-operatively, he was placed into a short arm cast for an additional 4 weeks. From 6 weeks to 3 months, he used a wrist brace for protection but removed it frequently for gentle range of motion. At 3 months, he was allowed to return to all regular activities. At 6 months from surgery, he noted no pain, had returned to his prior activities and was pleased with his result. As of the writing of this chapter 1 year later, he has not received any additional treatment.

Diagnosis

History

Pre-dynamic SL ligament injuries are defined as injuries with clinical symptoms but no radiographic or advanced imaging changes. These injuries are generated by elevated tensile force across the ligament, classically with a fall onto an extended wrist in ulnar deviation and supination [1]. However, the patient may or may not remember an inciting injury or event.

Patients will often present with wrist pain aggravated by loading in wrist extension and will localize their pain mostly to the dorsal central wrist. However, it should be kept in mind that other co-existing wrist pathology can often be present, such as triangular fibrocartilage complex (TFCC) injuries, lunotriquetral ligament injuries, ganglion cysts, and dorsal capsular impingement. Classification of SL ligament injuries, including pre-dynamic instability, has been defined by Geissler, based on arthroscopic findings, and Garcia-Elias, based on clinical and radiographic parameters [2]. More recently, Messina and the European Wrist Arthroscopy Society (EWAS) developed the EWAS classification which is based on arthroscopic findings and classifies SL injuries based on the level of instability and the portion of the ligament involved based on corresponding anatomic-pathology findings in cadaver specimens [3]. SL ligament injuries amenable to thermal capsulorrhaphy or "shrinkage" tend to fall into Geissler grade I through III, Garcia-Elias stage 1, or EWAS stage I or II categories. Geissler grade I instability is defined by attenuation or hemorrhage of the SL ligament without incongruity at the midcarpal joint (being unable to insert a 2 mm arthroscopic probe), grade II by incongruity between the scaphoid and lunate viewed from the midcarpal joint (being able to insert a 2 mm arthroscopic probe but being unable to turn it), and grade III by incongruity between the scaphoid and lunate from both radiocarpal and midcarpal joint (being able to insert a 2 mm arthroscopic probe and turn it up to 90°) [4]. Garcia-Elias stage 1 instability (termed "pre-dynamic") is defined by a partial injury to the SL complex, with an intact dorsal ligament, and no gapping regardless of applied stress during arthroscopy [5]. EWAS stage I is defined by the inability to pass the probe into the SL interval from the midcarpal joint, while stage II is defined by the ability to pass the probe into the SL interval without widening and is believed to correspond to a tear of the proximal or membranous portion of the SL ligament [3].

Physical Examination

Examination often begins with palpation to identify the area(s) of maximal tenderness, which often includes the dorsal central wrist overlying the SL interval. Care should be taken to confirm the tenderness is reproducing their symptoms or typical pain. Again, co-existing ligament injuries or chondral lesions can be present that can cloud the exam. After palpation, there are various provocative maneuvers that can be performed. For SL pathology, these may include scapholunate shear/stress, and Watson shift testing. SL stress is produced by placing volar-to-dorsal pressure over the scaphoid tubercle with or without counterpressure on the dorsal lunate, while evaluating for reproduction of pain or instability. Instability is gauged by comparison to the contralateral side, and the accuracy/sensitivity of this is increased with experience. Watson shift testing involves placing pressure on the volar scaphoid tubercle before moving the wrist into flexion and radial deviation. In cases of instability, the dorsal scaphoid will subluxate out of the scaphoid facet. When this maneuver is released, a palpable clunk can be felt. Again, it is important to differentiate whether the patient had reproduction of their symptoms, the level of palpable instability, whether a clunk was felt, and whether this phenomenon also occurs on the contralateral/asymptomatic side. Finally, bilateral wrist and forearm motion and grip strength should be measured.

Radiographs

Plain radiographs should be the initial imaging studies obtained and should include standard 3 view wrist radiographs (anteroposterior, oblique, and lateral) and additionally scaphoid and clenched fist views. Special attention should be paid to the lateral view as dorsal subluxation of the scaphoid within the scaphoid facet may be visible, and this is often where the first signs of post-traumatic scapholunate advanced collapse (SLAC) occurs. The scaphoid view involves a posteroanterior (PA) radiograph of the wrist with full ulnar deviation of the wrist [6]. A number of techniques have been described for clenched fist views [1], but the pencil-grip technique described by Lee has been shown to produce a reliable view of the SL interval [7]. This view is obtained as a PA view of both forearms in pronation while clenching a pencil [7].

The clenched fist view is designed to exacerbate SL instability to better demonstrate whether any widening occurs at the SL interval.

Advanced Imaging

MRI is the next study of choice although the sensitivity for partial SL ligament injuries is variable. Meister described using a 3 T magnet with dedicated wrist coils to diagnose SL instability [8]. Dorsal subluxation of the scaphoid was measured on sagittal MRI cuts with the wrist in neutral position. In addition, the articular surfaces are able to be evaluated, which could help determine the most appropriate treatment. It may be beneficial to obtain an MRI arthrogram although some authors suggest that this may unnecessary if you have access to a 3 T or greater magnet [9–11].

Management

Initial management of pre-dynamic SL ligament injuries could include activity modification (avoiding exacerbating activities, such as wrist hyperextension with loading), oral anti-inflammatories/acetaminophen, bracing, therapy, corticosteroid injections, etc. Immobilization with activity restriction for a period of at least 6–8 weeks leads to improvement in many cases. Therapy could include exercises focusing on dart throwers motion (wrist extension/radial deviation to wrist flexion/ulnar deviation) in order to strengthen and train proprioception in the extensor carpi radialis longus (ECRL), flexor carpi ulnaris (FCU), and/or abductor pollicis longus (APL). Hagert and Garcia-Elias have described these muscles as being "friendly" (protective) to the scapholunate ligament in early/partial ligament injuries. They are believed to play a role in extension and supination of the scaphoid taking tension from the dorsal portion of the scapholunate ligament [12].

If non-surgical management fails and the patient elects for operative management of their symptomatic pre-dynamic scapholunate instability, then this will begin with arthroscopic evaluation. This evaluation determines the level of instability and plays a role in the choice of treatment. The length of non-surgical management is up to the surgeon's discretion but should generally be 3–6 months or longer for pre-dynamic SL injuries.

Arthroscopic thermal capsulorrhaphy is one method of treatment for pre-dynamic SL ligament instability. It involves treatment of the SL ligament, in both the midcarpal and radiocarpal joints, with a thermal probe as a form of tightening (often termed "shrinkage") and denervation for pain control. It can be used with debridement in Geissler grade I or II instability, while it could potentially also be used in Geissler grade III instability in combination with arthroscopic pinning. These pins would be placed across the SL and scaphocapitate (SC) joint, after reduction of the SL interval with slight volar-to-dorsal pressure over the scaphoid tubercle. Care should be taken not to subluxate the scaphoid out of its facet akin to the Watson shift test, but the goal is to correct any scaphoid flexion that may be present. The pins are generally left in place for 8 weeks before removal, and they are frequently buried to avoid pin site irritation. The timing of k-wire removal is also up to the surgeon's discretion as the time to SL ligament maturation after thermal treatment is not currently known but animal studies have shown return to pretreatment mechanical properties by 6 weeks after surgery and return to normalcy at 12 weeks [13]. The author leaves the wires in place for approximately 8 weeks before removal.

Careful attention must be paid to the temperature of the fluid within the wrist joint as higher temperatures could risk thermal damage to the cartilage. Monopolar probes have been found to cause less elevation in wrist joint temperature [14]. This procedure should not be performed using dry arthroscopy techniques as the arthroscopic fluid helps to cool the joint and decrease the risk of chondrolysis (seen when the fluid is over 60° Celsius). Some thermal ablation probes come equipped with a thermometer. If not, the probe should only be used in very short and staggered bursts. The tip of most probes can be gently angled or bent using a needle driver to allow access around corners or in tight spaces (Fig. 7.1).

After application of traction through your arthroscopy setup of choice, an PA image with fluoroscopy can help assess for potential intercarpal instability (Fig. 7.2a, b). Kwon et al. described this as the "modified carpal stretch test," which was a way to test for co-existing SL injuries during distal radius fracture surgery [15]. Approximately 5 kg (11 lbs) of traction is applied to the wrist either through manual pulling of traction or the use of a wrist arthroscopy tower for approximately 5 min. If fluoroscopy imaging (PA view) demonstrates disruption of Gilula's second arc, then an SL injury should be suspected. Through the midcarpal joint, the volar portion of the SL ligament is treated—as well as the distal portion of the radioscapho-capitate (RSC) ligament which is directly adjacent to the volar SL ligament (Fig. 7.3a, b). Through the radiocarpal joint, the dorsal portion of the SL ligament is treated. Care should be taken to visualize and treat the entire dorsal SL ligament including the most distal portion. This is done by placing your arthroscope in either the 4–5 or 6R portal, then passing it along the dorsal capsule to visualize the

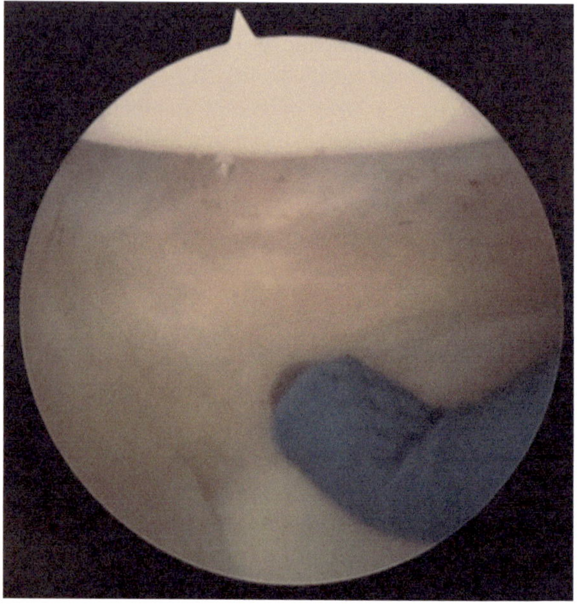

Fig. 7.1 Thermal probe with approximately 30° bent near the tip to allow for treatment of hard to reach areas

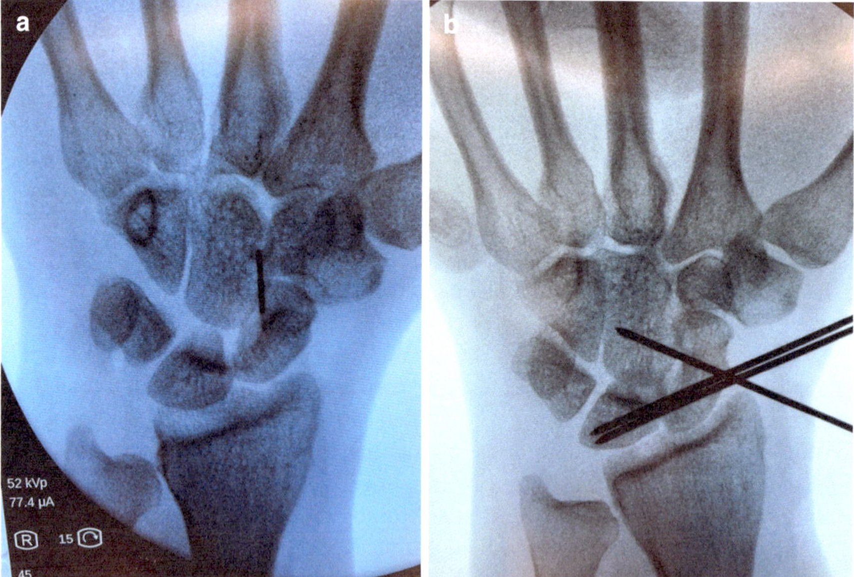

Fig. 7.2 (**a**) Traction view with the wrist in a traction tower. There is disruption of Gilula's lines at the scapholunate (SL) interval suggesting ligamentous injury. (**b**) Intercarpal pinning of the scaphocapitate and scapholunate joints for additional stability and immobilization after thermal capsulorrhaphy. These k-wires were maintained for 8–10 weeks before removal

scapholunate ligament. The thermal probe is inserted through the 3–4 portal. The most proximal portion may be treated and as the probe is then gradually moved distally to treat the portions of the SL ligament near the capsular reflection distally (Fig. 7.4a, b). This is often the site of origin for ganglion cysts which can be co-existing pathology. Post-operatively patients are immobilized for at least 6 weeks, followed by a 10-inch brace for protection from 6 weeks to 3 months. Patients are released to all activities at 3 months.

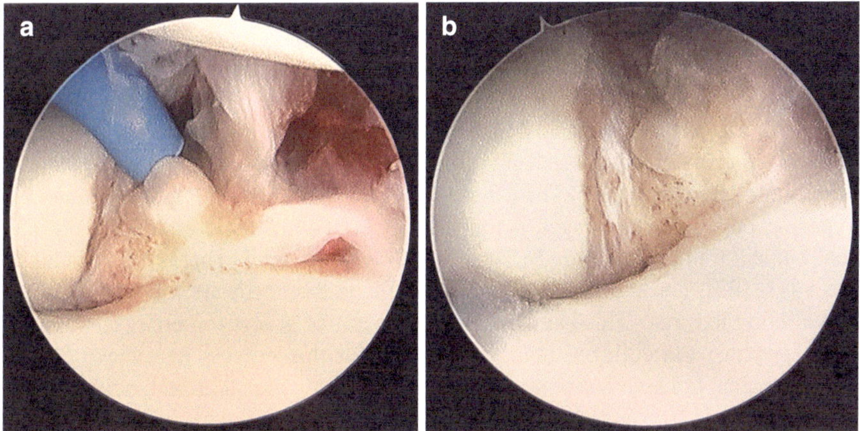

Fig. 7.3 (**a**) The volar scapholunate ligament visualizes through the midcarpal joint. The arthroscope is held in the midcarpal radial (MCR) portal, while the probe is inserted through the midcarpal ulnar (MCU) portal. (**b**) The volar scapholunate is pictured after treatment with debridement and thermal capsulorrhaphy

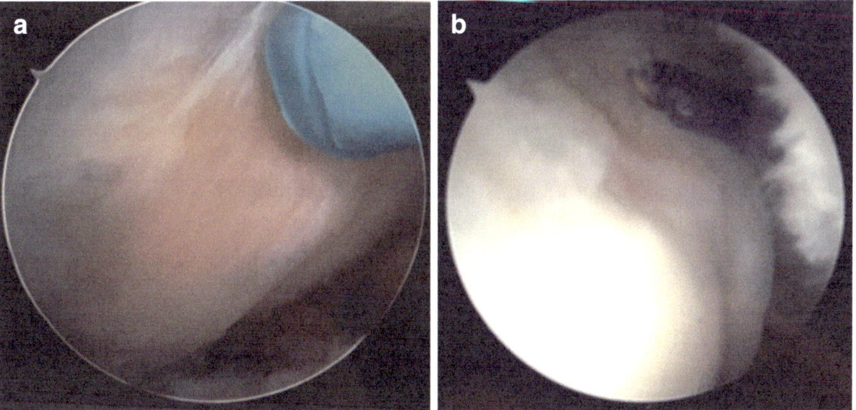

Fig. 7.4 (**a**) The proximal portion of the dorsal scapholunate ligament through the radiocarpal joint. The arthroscope is held in the 6R portal, while the probe is inserted through the 3,4 portal. (**b**) After treatment of the proximal portion of the scapholunate ligament, the probe is moved from distal-to-proximal traveling up the ligament. This allows for treatment of the entire dorsal ligament including the most distal portion near the capsular reflection

Outcomes

Few articles have looked specifically at isolated thermal capsulorrhaphy for the scapholunate ligament, and most of these studies are low level evidence or are confounded by the inclusion of other co-existing ligamentous injuries. However, these studies have shown clinical benefit at mid-term (1–2 years) follow-up [16–19]. A few studies have demonstrated good outcomes at long-term follow-up. Lee et al. looked at chondrolysis, based on prior issues with shoulder arthroscopic thermal capsulorrhaphy, and found no cases at 3–4 year follow-up [20]. We have demonstrated good long-term outcomes (5 year minimum, 7 year average follow-up) thermal capsulorrhaphy based on functional parameters (range of motion, grip strength) and standardized outcome scores [21].

Electrothermal therapy has been utilized in ophthalmologic and cardiac surgery procedures since the 1960s. The primary target of the treatment within ligament is Type 1 collagen. This collagen is made up of both heat-stable intermolecular and heat-labile intramolecular bonds. The heat-labile bonds tend to break between 60 °C and 80 °C [22]. Through electrothermal treatment, the fibrils are forced to contract into a shortened state. This is followed by a reparative process where reactive fibroblasts synthesize a collagen matrix. The time for this process to achieve normal biomechanical strength is not known but is thought to take approximately 6 weeks to mature [23]. It is also thought that thermal capsulorrhaphy offers benefit by decreasing pain through denervation. This denervation was demonstrated in a cadaver model using immunofluorescent staining [23].

This procedure was first utilized in shoulder instability surgery. However, there was a high failure rate with recurrent instability. In addition, there were reported cases of chondrolysis. However, these cases of chondrolysis were later attributed to other potential factors, such as a continuous intra-articular bupivacaine infusions [24, 25]. The poor results of thermal capsulorrhaphy in the shoulder does not translate to wrist surgery due to a number of different factors, The wrist and its ligaments are smaller than those in the shoulder, there is less mechanical stress, and perhaps most importantly, the wrist may tolerate prolonged post-operative immobilization (6 weeks and beyond) to allow for adequate maturation of the collagen whereas a shoulder should not be immobilized for that long without risking permanent stiffness. Finally, there is no evidence of chondrolysis in current studies.

Pearls and Pitfalls

- Careful attention should be paid to the intra-articular temperature to avoid cartilage injury or chondrolysis.
- Most 2 mm thermal probes can be bent to access hard to reach areas. To our knowledge, only one thermal frequency probe has been developed specifically for the purpose of thermal shrinkage of tissue in the wrist (Micro-TAC-S, Smith and Nephew, Andover, MA).

- The SL ligament should be treated through the midcarpal (volar and dorsal) and radiocarpal joints.
- The entire dorsal scapholunate ligament should be treated.
- There is also a denervation effect imparted by the thermal frequency probes, thereby decreasing dorsal wrist pain.
- Thermal capsulorrhaphy can be used in combination with pinning in more unstable or incongruent cases.
- This treatment is contraindicated if more severe instability is present.
- Immobilization post-operatively is required, but the optimal duration is not yet known (6–8 weeks).

References

1. Kitay A, Wolfe SW. Scapholunate instability: current concepts in diagnosis and management. J Hand Surg. 2012;37(10):2175–96. https://doi.org/10.1016/j.jhsa.2012.07.035.
2. Pappou IP, Basel J, Deal DN. Scapholunate ligament injuries: a review of current concepts. Hand N Y N. 2013;8(2):146–56. https://doi.org/10.1007/s11552-013-9499-4.
3. Messina JC, Van Overstraeten L, Luchetti R, Fairplay T, Mathoulin CL. The EWAS classification of scapholunate tears: an anatomical arthroscopic study. J Wrist Surg. 2013;2(2):105–9. https://doi.org/10.1055/s-0033-1345265.
4. Lee SK, Model Z, Desai H, Hsu P, Paksima N, Dhaliwal G. Association of lesions of the scapholunate interval with arthroscopic grading of scapholunate instability via the Geissler classification. J Hand Surg. 2015;40(6):1083–7. https://doi.org/10.1016/j.jhsa.2015.02.017.
5. Garcia-Elias M, Lluch AL, Stanley JK. Three-ligament tenodesis for the treatment of scapholunate dissociation. indications and surgical technique. J Hand Surg. 2006;31(1):125–34. https://doi.org/10.1016/j.jhsa.2005.10.011.
6. Kuo CE, Wolfe SW. Scapholunate instability: current concepts in diagnosis and management. J Hand Surg. 2008;33(6):998–1013. https://doi.org/10.1016/j.jhsa.2008.04.027.
7. Lee SK, Desai H, Silver B, Dhaliwal G, Paksima N. Comparison of radiographic stress views for scapholunate dynamic instability in a cadaver model. J Hand Surg. 2011;36(7):1149–57. https://doi.org/10.1016/j.jhsa.2011.05.009.
8. Meister DW, Hearns KA, Carlson MG. Dorsal scaphoid subluxation on sagittal magnetic resonance imaging as a marker for scapholunate ligament tear. J Hand Surg. 2017;42(9):717–21. https://doi.org/10.1016/j.jhsa.2017.06.015.
9. Sofka CM, Potter HG. Magnetic resonance imaging of the wrist. Semin Musculoskelet Radiol. 2001;05(3):217–26. https://doi.org/10.1055/s-2001-17545.
10. Kader N, Arshad MS, Chajed PK, et al. Evaluating accuracy of plain magnetic resonance imaging or arthrogram versus wrist arthroscopy in the diagnosis of scapholunate interosseous ligament injury. J Hand Microsurg. 2022;14(4):298–303. https://doi.org/10.1055/s-0040-1719231.
11. Schmitt R, Christopoulos G, Meier R, et al. Direct MR arthrography of the wrist in comparison with arthroscopy: a prospective study on 125 patients. ROFO Fortschr Geb Rontgenstr Nuklearmed. 2003;175(7):911–9. https://doi.org/10.1055/s-2003-40434.
12. Salva-Coll G, Garcia-Elias M, Hagert E. Scapholunate instability: proprioception and neuromuscular control. J Wrist Surg. 2013;2(2):136–40. https://doi.org/10.1055/s-0033-1341960.
13. Hayashi K, Markel MD. Thermal capsulorrhaphy treatment of shoulder instability: basic science. Clin Orthop. 2001;390:59–72. https://doi.org/10.1097/00003086-200109000-00009.
14. Huber M, Loibl M, Eder C, et al. Temperature in and around the scapholunate ligament during radiofrequency shrinkage: a cadaver study. J Hand Surg. 2015;40(2):259–65. https://doi.org/10.1016/j.jhsa.2014.10.030.

15. Kwon BC, Choi SJ, Song SY, Baek SH, Baek GH. Modified carpal stretch test as a screening test for detection of scapholunate interosseous ligament injuries associated with distal radial fractures. J Bone Joint Surg Am. 2011;93(9):855–62. https://doi.org/10.2106/JBJS.J.00361.
16. Hirsh L, Sodha S, Bozentka D, Monaghan B, Steinberg D, Beredjiklian PK. Arthroscopic electrothermal collagen shrinkage for symptomatic laxity of the scapholunate interosseous ligament. J Hand Surg Edinb Scotl. 2005;30(6):643–7. https://doi.org/10.1016/j.jhsb.2005.07.011.
17. Darlis NA, Weiser RW, Sotereanos DG. Partial scapholunate ligament injuries treated with arthroscopic debridement and thermal shrinkage. J Hand Surg. 2005;30(5):908–14. https://doi.org/10.1016/j.jhsa.2005.05.013.
18. Shih JT, Lee HM. Monopolar radiofrequency electrothermal shrinkage of the scapholunate ligament. Arthroscopy. 2006;22(5):553–7. https://doi.org/10.1016/j.arthro.2006.01.011.
19. Danoff JR, Karl JW, Birman MV, Rosenwasser MP. The use of thermal shrinkage for scapholunate instability. Hand Clin. 2011;27(3):309–17. https://doi.org/10.1016/j.hcl.2011.06.005.
20. Lee JIL, Nha KW, Lee GY, Kim BH, Kim JW, Park JW. Long-term outcomes of arthroscopic debridement and thermal shrinkage for isolated partial intercarpal ligament tears. Orthopedics. 2012;35(8):e1204–9. https://doi.org/10.3928/01477447-20120725-20.
21. Burn MB, Sarkissian EJ, Yao J. Long-term outcomes for arthroscopic thermal treatment for scapholunate ligament injuries. J Wrist Surg. 2020;9(1):22–8. https://doi.org/10.1055/s-0039-1693973.
22. Arnoczky SP, Aksan A. Thermal modification of connective tissues: basic science considerations and clinical implications. J Am Acad Orthop Surg. 2000;8(5):305–13. https://doi.org/10.5435/00124635-200009000-00004.
23. Pirolo JM, Le W, Yao J. Effect of electrothermal treatment on nerve tissue within the triangular fibrocartilage complex, scapholunate, and lunotriquetral interosseous ligaments. Arthroscopy. 2016;32(5):773–8. https://doi.org/10.1016/j.arthro.2015.11.050.
24. Good CR, Shindle MK, Kelly BT, Wanich T, Warren RF. Glenohumeral chondrolysis after shoulder arthroscopy with thermal capsulorrhaphy. Arthroscopy. 2007;23(7):797.e1–5. https://doi.org/10.1016/j.arthro.2007.03.092.
25. Lubowitz JH, Poehling GG. Glenohumeral thermal capsulorrhaphy is not recommended—shoulder chondrolysis requires additional research. Arthroscopy. 2007;23(7):687. https://doi.org/10.1016/j.arthro.2007.05.001.

Chapter 8
Dynamic Scapholunate Ligament Injury: Arthroscopic Volar Capsulodesis

Hayman Lui and Sanjeev Kakar

Case Presentation

A 36-year-old right hand dominant non-manual worker presented for evaluation regarding her left wrist and thumb 1 month after a fall. Her medical history was otherwise unremarkable. On examination, she reported pain over the dorsal radial and volar radial aspect of the wrist and also on the ulnar side of her thumb MCPJ joint. Clinically, she was point tender over the dorsal and volar scapholunate (SL) regions under stress testing. Otherwise, she was non-tender in her wrist. For her left thumb, she was tender over the ulnar collateral ligament (UCL) and demonstrated Grade 3 laxity without an endpoint compared to the uninjured side. No pain was elicited when palpating the radial collateral ligament. Extensor pollicis longus (EPL) and flexor pollicis longus (FPL) tendons were clinically intact.

Diagnosis

Hand X-rays demonstrated evidence of an SL injury as well as an avulsion fracture on the ulnar side of her thumb MCPJ. An axial view of her wrist MRI (Fig. 8.1) demonstrated a volar SL ligament injury and a Stener UCL injury on her thumb MRI scan (not shown).

H. Lui
School of Medicine and Dentistry, Griffith University, Gold Coast, QLD, Australia

Department of Orthopedic Surgery, Mayo Clinic, Rochester, MN, USA
e-mail: h.lui@griffith.edu.au

S. Kakar (✉)
Department of Orthopedic Surgery, Mayo Clinic, Rochester, MN, USA
e-mail: kakar.sanjeev@mayo.edu

J. Yao (ed.), *Carpal Instability*, https://doi.org/10.1007/978-3-031-55869-6_8

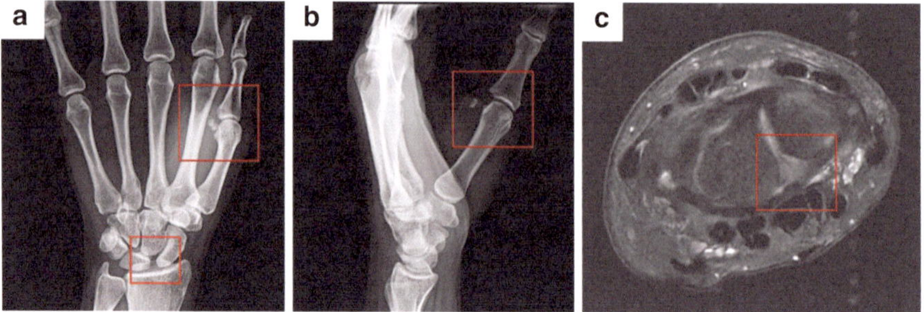

Fig. 8.1 Imaging of the left hand and wrist. (**a**) AP and (**b**) lateral radiographs show diastasis of the SL interval compared to the uninjured wrist and an avulsion fracture of UCL. (**c**) Axial MRI slice showing volar SL injury

Management Options

Management Chosen for this Case with Rationale [with Figures]

Given these constellation of findings, the patient elected for operative treatment which included thumb UCL ligament repair with synthetic tape augmentation and arthroscopic volar SL capsulodesis.

The arthroscopic volar SL ligament capsulodesis was repaired as previously described [1]. In brief, after performing a radiocarpal joint arthroscopy, midcarpal arthroscopy was performed to assess the location of the intercarpal ligament injury, its reducibility, the status of the cartilage and also to delineate any other injuries. After confirming a reducible, volar SL ligament injury (Fig. 8.2), we then addressed this using an "inside-out" technique [1] (Fig. 8.3). A palmar incision was made between the FCR and PL and the palmar cutaneous branch of the median nerve was identified. The median nerve and the digital flexor tendons were retracted ulnarly and the FCR tendon retracted radially. With the arthroscope positioned in the ulnar midcarpal portal, an 18-gauge spinal needle was loaded with a 2-0 FiberStick (Arthrex, Naples, FL) suture, with two suture tails positioned at the tip of the needle (Fig. 8.4). The needle was placed through the radial midcarpal portal and was first inserted through the capsule on the radial side of the volar SL ligament (Fig. 8.5a). One end of the suture was grasped in the palmar wound, with care taken to protect the volar structures. The needle was then retracted back into the midcarpal space prior to being advanced through the capsule on the ulnar side of the volar SL

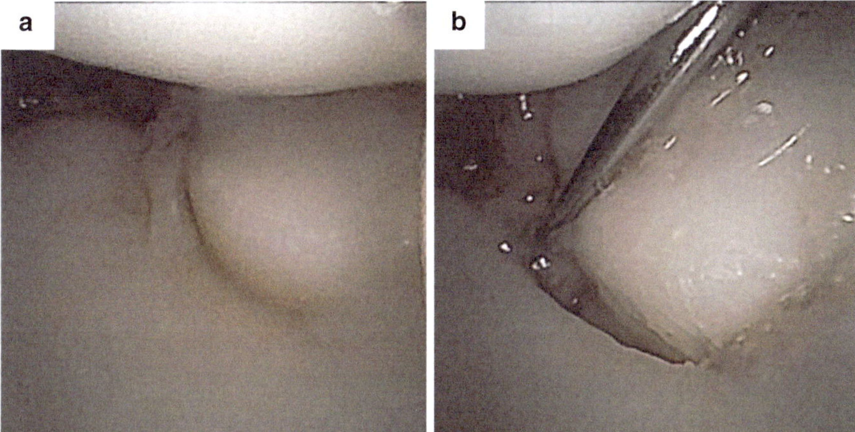

Fig. 8.2 Arthroscopic images through the ulnar midcarpal portal. (**a**) SL step-off. (**b**) Volar SL injury demonstrated upon probing

ligament (Fig. 8.5b). Care was taken not to withdraw the spinal needle out of the radial midcarpal space before passing the needle through the ulnar side of the volar capsule to prevent the formation of a soft tissue bridge. In tensioning the sutures, the diastasis and step-off of the volar SL region were reduced (Fig. 8.5c). Stability was confirmed arthroscopically (Fig. 8.5d) and no further carpal pinning was required. The dorsal SL ligament was stable to probing. The wrist was taken out of traction and the sutures tied down onto the volar capsule. Postoperatively, the patient was placed in a thumb spica AP splint.

Clinical Course and Outcome

The patient was reviewed in the outpatient clinic 2 weeks postoperatively where she was transitioned to a thumb spica cast with IP joint free for an additional 4 weeks. At 6 weeks after surgery, she was transitioned out of the cast and worked with a certified hand therapist on active range of motion of the wrist along a dart thrower's plane, FCR and ECRB strengthening, wrist proprioception and thumb exercises. At 12 weeks post surgery, she reported a visual analog scale score of 0, was non-tender over her SL joint and thumb and making continual functional improvements.

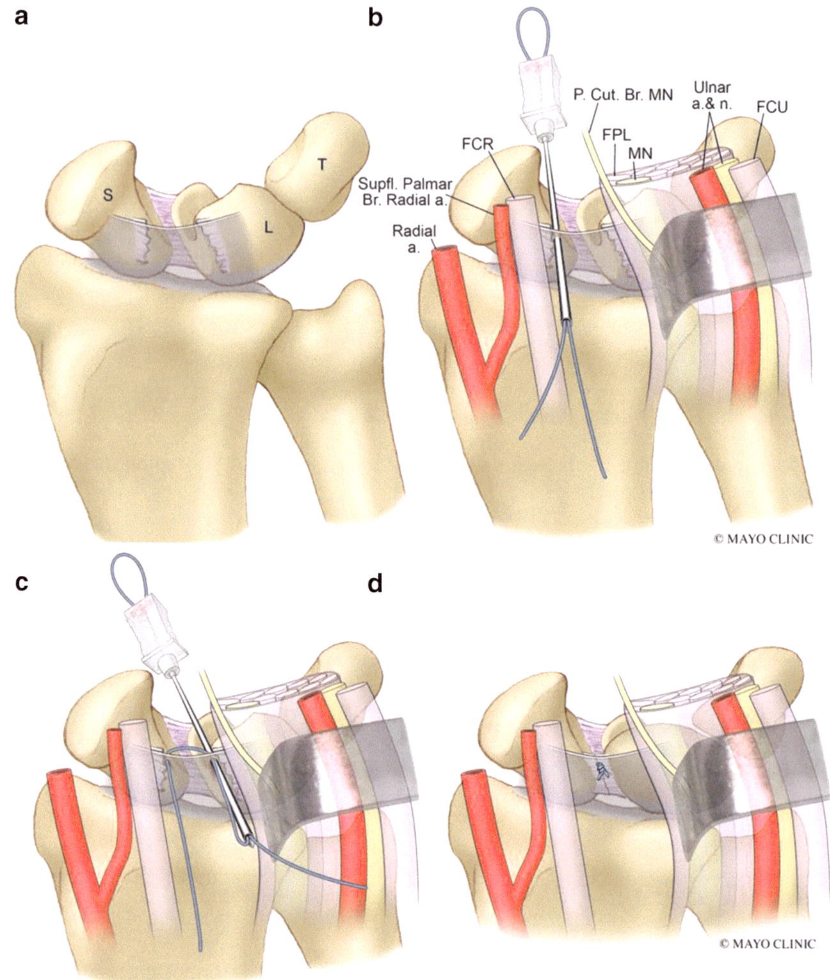

Fig. 8.3 Drawings depicting the procedure for arthroscopic-assisted volar SL capsulodesis previously published by Lui and Kakar [1] (http://creativecommons.org/licenses/by/4.0.). (**a**) Volar SL tear (S = scaphoid; L = lunate; T = triquetrum); (**b**) Insertion of 18G spinal needle from "inside-out" through radial aspect of the volar capsule; (**c**) Insertion of 18G spinal needle from "inside-out" through the ulnar limb of the volar capsule; (**d**) Suture tied over volar capsule to complete volar SL capsulodesis

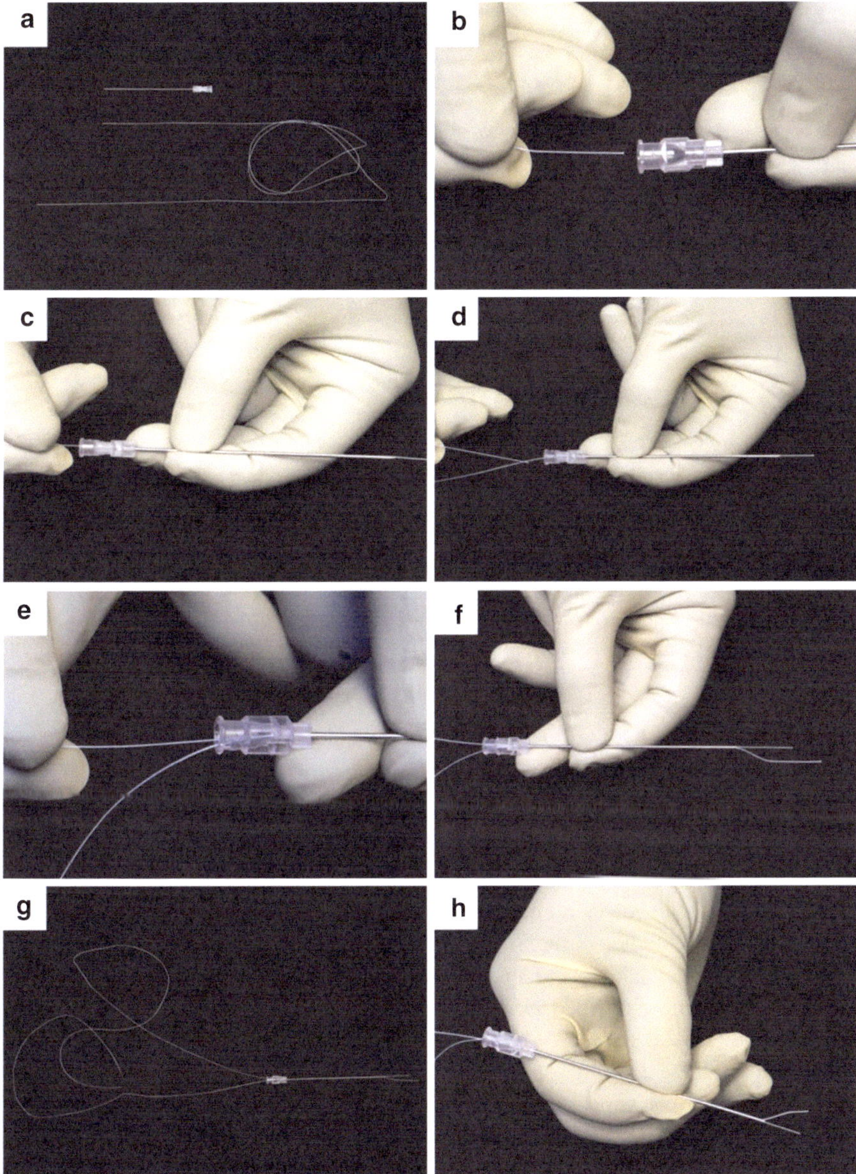

Fig. 8.4 Steps (**a–h**) demonstrate loading the suture into an 18G spinal needle for arthroscopic volar SL capsulodesis. (Figure previously published by Lui and Kakar [1], http://creativecommons.org/licenses/by/4.0)

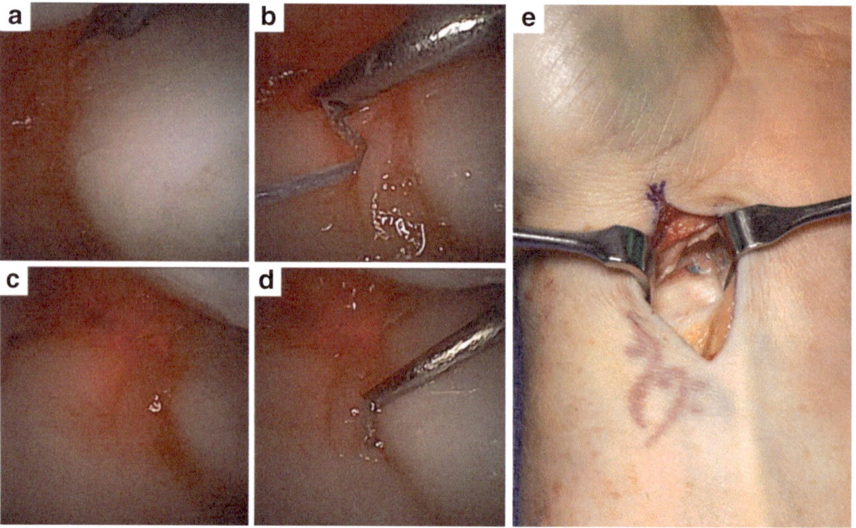

Fig. 8.5 Intra-operative arthroscopic images of the volar scapholunate ligament. (**a**) Placement of the suture through the capsule along the radial side of the volar SL. (**b**) Placement of the suture through the capsule along the ulnar side of the volar SL. (**c**) Volar capsulodesis post suture passage. (**d**) Stable volar SL joint upon probing after volar capsulodesis. (**e**) External view of volar capsulodesis after suture ends have been tied down over the volar capsule

Bulleted Clinical Pearls/Pitfalls [3–5, with Figures]

- SL ligament injuries can occur in concert with other hand injuries and can often be missed on initial presentation. A thorough history and examination is needed with supplemental imaging including stress radiographs and MRI, when appropriate, which can help with the assessment.
- Biomechanical studies of the SL have highlighted that the volar SL has an important role in carpal stability and repair should be considered when injury is confirmed.
- When using the described arthroscopic-assisted volar capsulodesis technique, care should be taken to avoid removing the spinal needle out of the radial midcarpal portal and creating a soft tissue bridge in the process of passing the sutures through the volar capsule from the ulnar aspect of the scaphoid to the radial border of the lunate.
- It is critical to protect the volar wrist structures such as the median nerve and flexor tendons by direct visualization when passing and tying the suture.

Literature Review and Discussion

Dynamic acute SL ligament injuries often occur after a fall involving supination and extension of the wrist and are frequently missed on initial presentation. Failure of repair in a timely manner can result in scapholunate advanced collapse (SLAC) heralded by altered carpal kinematics, dorsal intercalated segment instability and degenerative osteoarthritis [2–7].

The volar SL ligament has a biomechanical strength of approximately 45% of the dorsal SL ligament [8] and a recent 4D computed tomography study has demonstrated that it is particularly important in preventing SL diastasis during wrist flexion [9]. Histological analysis of the volar SL ligament has also found a high number of proprioceptors and this further suggests that it has an important role in wrist proprioception [10]. Despite its important function in wrist kinematics, there remains a paucity of surgical techniques available to address volar SL ligament instability. Access to the palmar portion of the SL ligament during surgery can be difficult due to the anatomical location of the extrinsic carpal ligaments, flexor tendons, and median nerve. An open approach to reconstruct the volar SL ligament using a strip of the long radiolunate ligament has been previously described by Van Kampen and colleagues [11] and the case example provided in a collegiate football player, demonstrated good clinical outcomes 3 years postoperatively.

With the recent advances in wrist arthroscopy, this has permitted repair of volar SL ligament injuries. Del Pinal [12] reported using an outside-to-inside arthroscopic approach to repair volar SL ligament injuries. The outcomes of 8 patients (6 also requiring arthroscopic dorsal capsular plication) were reported [12].

The described arthroscopic-assisted volar SL ligament capsulodesis technique in this chapter presents an alternative method to address volar SL ligament pathology and can be combined with other dorsal SL ligament repair procedures. Given its simplicity, it is our preferred technique for addressing volar SL ligament injury and utilizes an open palmar incision to allow for visualization and protection of key anatomical structures in the volar wrist [13]. Indications for this procedure includes patients with a symptomatic, reducible volar SL ligament instability (European Wrist Arthroscopy Society (EWAS) stages IIA, IIC, IIIA, IIIC, and IV) without concurrent posttraumatic arthritis irrespective of chronicity. Contraindications include patients with chronic static, irreducible SLIL instability, and/or posttraumatic arthritis.

A case series of six patients (4 male and 2 female) with a mean duration of follow-up of 41 ± 17 weeks has demonstrated positive clinical outcomes [14]. Specifically, we noted improvements in pain, functional outcome scores, grip strength, SL gap, SL, and radiolunate angles [14].

Further studies with longer clinical follow-up are underway to ascertain this technique's clinical efficacy over time. Given these encouraging results, arthroscopic-assisted volar SL ligament capsulodesis may be considered in the treatment algorithm for acute or chronic dynamic SL ligament injuries.

References

1. Lui H, Kakar S. Arthroscopic-assisted volar scapholunate capsulodesis: a new technique. J Hand Surg Am. 2022;47(11):1124.e1121–6. https://doi.org/10.1016/j.jhsa.2022.05.018.
2. Johnson JE, Lee P, McIff TE, Toby EB, Fischer KJ. Scapholunate ligament injury adversely alters in vivo wrist joint mechanics: an MRI-based modeling study. J Orthop Res. 2013;31(9):1455–60. https://doi.org/10.1002/jor.22365.

3. Kauer JM. The interdependence of carpal articulation chains. Acta Anat (Basel). 1974;88(4):481–501. https://doi.org/10.1159/000144254.
4. Padmore CE, Stoesser H, Langohr GDG, Johnson JA, Suh N. Carpal kinematics following sequential scapholunate ligament sectioning. J Wrist Surg. 2019;8(2):124–31. https://doi.org/10.1055/s-0038-1676865.
5. Pappou I, Basel J, Deal DN. Scapholunate ligament injuries: a review of current concepts. Hand. 2013;8:146–56.
6. Rajan P, Day C. Scapholunate interosseous ligament anatomy and biomechanics. J Hand Surg Am. 2015;40(8):1692–702.
7. Rohman E, Agel J, Putnam M, Adams J. Scapholunate interosseous ligament injuries: a retrospective review of treatment and outcomes in 82 wrists. J Hand Surg Am. 2014;39(10):2020–6.
8. Berger RA, Imeada T, Berglund L, An KN. Constraint and material properties of the subregions of the scapholunate interosseous ligament. J Hand Surg Am. 1999;24(5):953–62. https://doi.org/10.1053/jhsu.1999.0953.
9. de Roo MGA, Muurling M, Dobbe JGG, Brinkhorst ME, Streekstra GJ, Strackee SD. A four-dimensional-CT study of in vivo scapholunate rotation axes: possible implications for scapholunate ligament reconstruction. J Hand Surg Eur. 2019;44(5):479–87. https://doi.org/10.1177/1753193419830924.
10. Berger RA. The gross and histologic anatomy of the scapholunate interosseous ligament. J Hand Surg Am. 1996;21(2):170–8. https://doi.org/10.1016/s0363-5023(96)80096-7.
11. van Kampen RJ, Bayne CO, Moran SL. A new technique for volar Capsulodesis for isolated palmar Scapholunate interosseous ligament injuries: a cadaveric study and case report. J Wrist Surg. 2015;4(4):239–45. https://doi.org/10.1055/s-0035-1556854.
12. Del Piñal F. Arthroscopic volar capsuloligamentous repair. J Wrist Surg. 2013;2(2):126–8. https://doi.org/10.1055/s-0033-1343016.
13. Gillis JA, Kakar S. Volar midcarpal portals in wrist arthroscopy. J Hand Surg Am. 2019;44(12):1094.e1091–6. https://doi.org/10.1016/j.jhsa.2019.02.006.
14. Kakar S, Lui H. Clinical outcomes of arthroscopic-assisted volar scapholunate capsulodesis: a case series. J Wrist Surg. 2023;12:428. https://doi.org/10.1055/s-0043-1762930.

Suggested Reading

Del Piñal F. Arthroscopic volar capsuloligamentous repair. J Wrist Surg. 2013;2(2):126–8.
Kakar S, Lui H. Clinical outcomes of arthroscopic-assisted volar scapholunate capsulodesis: a case series. J Wrist Surg. 2023;12:428–32.
Lui H, Kakar S. Arthroscopic-assisted volar scapholunate capsulodesis: a new technique. J Hand Surg Am. 2022;47:1124.e1.
van Kampen RJ, Bayne CO, Moran SL. A new technique for volar capsulodesis for isolated palmar scapholunate interosseous ligament injuries: a cadaveric study and case report. J Wrist Surg. 2015;4(4):239–45.
Wahegaonkar AL, Mathoulin CL. Arthroscopic dorsal capsulo-ligamentous repair in the treatment of chronic scapho-lunate ligament tears. J Wrist Surg. 2013;2(2):141–8.

Chapter 9
Acute SL Instability: Arthroscopic Treatment

Vicente Carratalá Baixauli and Francisco Lucas García

Clinical Case

A 32-year-old male professional sportsman. Right wrist pain after wrist hyperextension lifting weights 3 weeks before. Pain, swelling, and difficulty in mobility and activities of daily living. Without improvement with rest, immobilization with a splint and medical treatment with anti-inflammatories. The patient reports pain when extending the wrist. Limited range of motion and weakness in the wrist.

Physical Exam Findings

On physical examination, the patient presented with pain on the dorsal aspect of the wrist, with pain on flexion and extension. The Watson maneuver is painful and with a sensation of dorsal translation of the scaphoid, compared to the contralateral wrist, but the pain makes examination difficult.

Imaging and Diagnosis

Plain radiographs did not demonstrate any fractures or malalignment.

Due to the diagnostic suspicion of a scapholunate lesion, dynamic X-rays were performed.

In supinated radiographs with clenched grip, an increase in the scapholunate space was observed compared to the contralateral wrist (Fig. 9.1). An MRI study

V. C. Baixauli (✉) · F. L. García
Hand Surgery Unit, Quironsalud Hospital Valencia, Valencia, Spain

J. Yao (ed.), *Carpal Instability*, https://doi.org/10.1007/978-3-031-55869-6_9

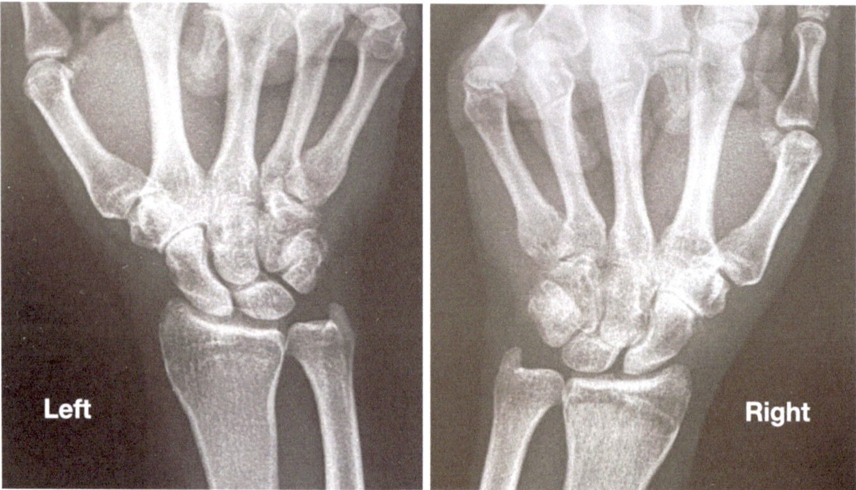

Fig. 9.1 Dynamic X-rays. In supinated radiographs with clenched grip, an increase in the scapholunate space is observed compared to the contralateral wrist

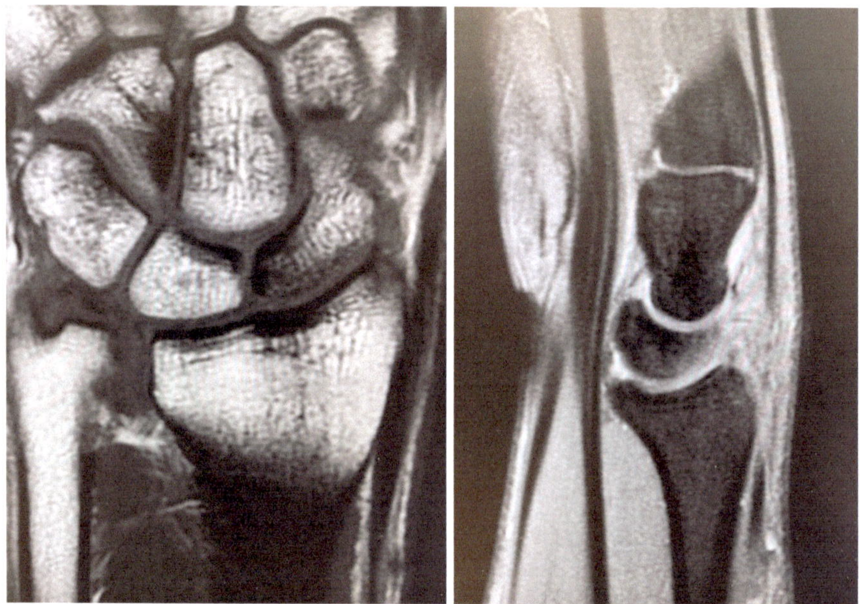

Fig. 9.2 MRI study showed a slight DISI deformity and edema in the proximal pole of the scaphoid. No clear image of scapholunate tear

showed a slight DISI deformity and edema in the proximal pole of the scaphoid. No clear evidence of a scapholunate tear (Fig. 9.2). The clinical evolution, physical examination, and imaging test suggested a possible SL injury. Wrist arthroscopy was indicated to confirm the diagnosis and treat the potential acute injury of the SL ligament.

Arthroscopy

Wrist arthroscopy was performed. Complete dorsal and volar SL (IWAS III C) detachment was confirmed, with SL complete instability tested in the midcarpal space (Fig. 9.3).

Since the injury was acute and the quality of the tissue was good, an arthroscopic volar and dorsal and volar capsuloligamentous repair was performed.

The technique can be performed through the standard wrist arthroscopy portals: 3–4, 6R, midcarpal radial (MCR), and midcarpal ulnar (MCU).

With the arthroscope in the 6R portal, the 3–4 portal is used as a working portal to introduce a suture anchor into the dorsal and proximal edge of the scaphoid or lunate bone, depending on where the SLL has been detached (Fig. 9.4a).

A TFCC SutureLasso 70°® (Arthrex, Naples, FL) is used from the 3–4 portal to pass through the dorsal portion of the SLL and recover the Nitinol loop through the same portal (Fig. 9.4b). Using the loop, one of the suture ends of the implant is passed through the detached edge of the ligament and is pulled out again through the 3–4 portal.

Occasionally, as was the case in this case, more than one anchor is needed to repair the dorsal portion of the SLL. The position of the implants in the scaphoid, the lunate, or both will depend on the location and characteristics of the injury. Using a knot pusher, we tie both sutures with a sliding knot over the implant (Fig. 9.4c), leaving a simple stitch through the SLL with the sutures tied but not cut.

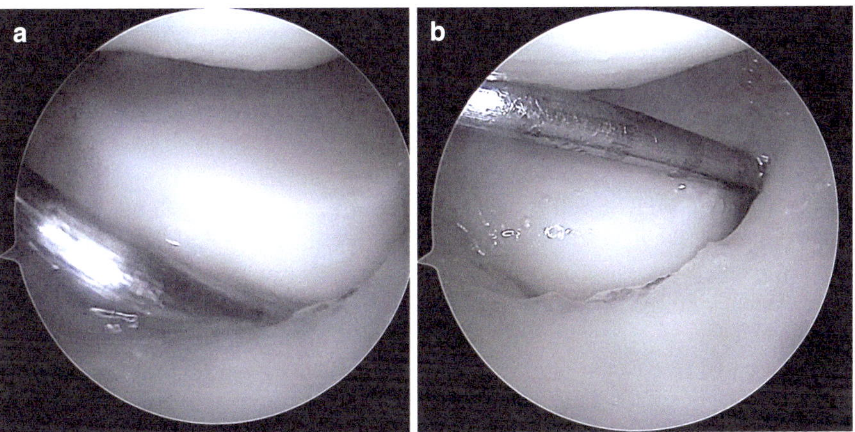

Fig. 9.3 Arthroscopic evaluation from midcarpal portals. SL instability in both parts, dorsal (**a**) and volar (**b**) of the SL joint. Ewas IIIC

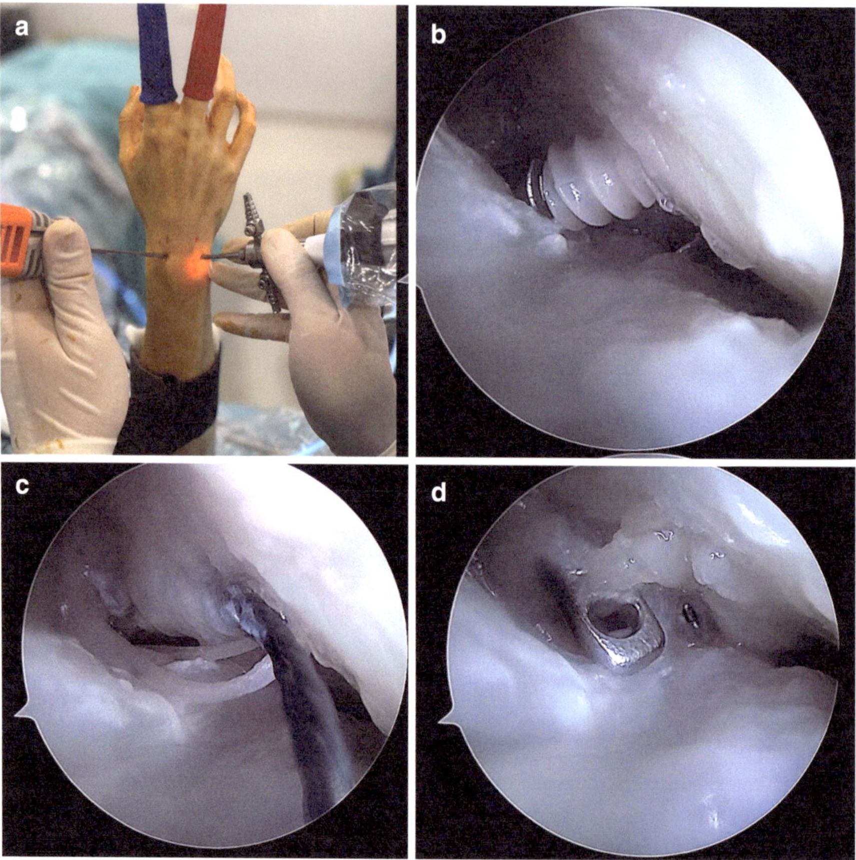

Fig. 9.4 Arthroscopic dorsal reinsertion of the SL ligament. (**a**) Bone anchor is introduced through the 3–4 portal and placed in the most dorsal part of the lunate or scaphoid, depending on where the SLL has been detached (**b**) with the scope in 6R portal, the bone anchor is introduced through the 3–4 portal. (**c**) A TFCC SutureLasso 70°® (Arthrex, Naples, FL) is used from the 3–4 portal to pass through the dorsal part of the SLL. (**d**) Using a knot pusher, we tie both sutures in a sliding knot over the implant

Using these sutures, a dorsal capsuloligamentous plication is performed. An 18G needle is introduced with one of the implants' sutures inside through the 3–4 portal, passing through the ligament's tissue towards the midcarpal joint. The suture introduced through the needle is recovered, using a grasper, through the MCR portal and is recovered from the 3–4 portal incision through the space in between the dorsal capsule and the extensor tendons. With the arthroscope in the 6R portal, the implant sutures are tied again, after releasing the traction. This completes the closure of the dorsal interval of the SL with the capsular plication performed by reconstructing the dorsal capsuloligamentous union of the scapholunate ligament.

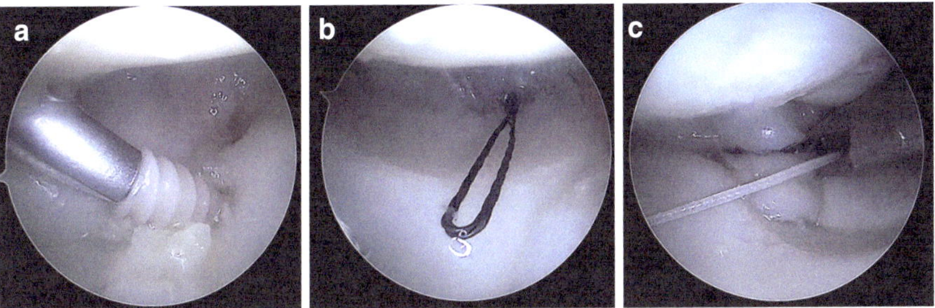

Fig. 9.5 Volar SLL capsuloligamentous repair using dorsal portals. (**a**) Bone anchor is introduced through the MCR portal and placed in the most volar part of the lunate. (**b**) A TFCC SutureLasso 70°® (Arthrex, Naples, FL) is used from MCR portal to pass through the volar part of the SLL and the volar capsular attachments. (**c**) Using the nitinol loop of the TFCC SutureLasso 70°® (Arthrex, Naples, FL) to pass the suture through the volar capsuloligamentous tissue. After that using a knot pusher, we tie both sutures in a sliding knot over the implant

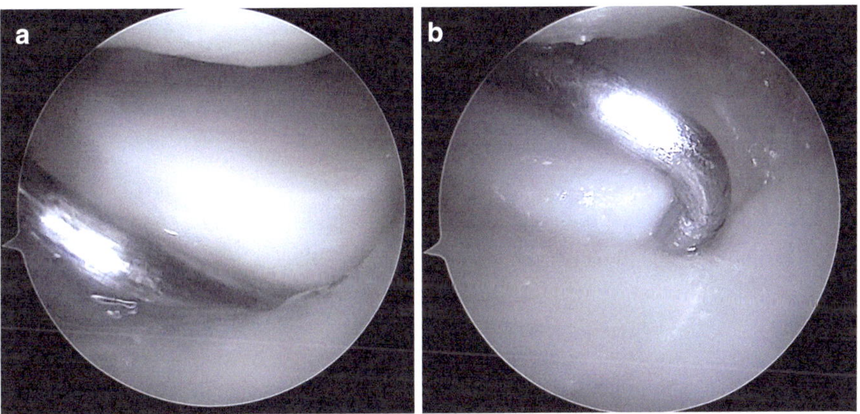

Fig. 9.6 Comparison between previous SL instability (**a**) and after the arthroscopic volar and dorsal suture (**b**)

Sometimes, there is not enough ligament tissue to complete the reinsertion. In that situation, the anchor can be placed in the midcarpal space, performing a Mathoulin-like [1] capsuloligamentous plication but using a bone anchor to strengthen the reconstruction.

The volar capsuloligamentous repair can be performed through the dorsal portals, using a.

SutureLasso 70°® (Arthrex, Naples, FL) from the MCR portal with the scope in the MCU portal (Fig. 9.5). This repair can also be performed using the volar radial portal (VR) as described by Slutsky [2].

After the suture, the SL stability must be confirmed using the probe through the midcarpal portals (Fig. 9.6).

Table 9.1 Rehabilitation protocol

Immobilization	Extension, ulnar deviation and supination
2 weeks post immobilization	Active and assisted exercises in F/E and P/S. Active Dart Throwing Motion (DTM) Isometric exercises for the ECRL Aponeurotic muscle massage Start of propioceptive reeducation: Mirror Therapy, Joint position sense (JPS)
4 weeks post immobilization	Passive exercises in F/E and P/S are allowed. Active DTM Isometrics exercises for secondary stabilisers: ECRL, APL and FCR Propioception: Close kinetic chain exercises
6 weeks onwards	Progressive strengthening of ECRL, FCR and APL with theraband and forearm in neutral position Propioception: Open kinetic chain exercises, perturbation, exercises, powerball and reeducation palmar support

A forearm splint is placed, allowing the patient to move fingers and elbow. After 2 weeks, the stitches are removed, maintaining the forearm splint up to 4 weeks. Four weeks postoperatively, after removing the forearm splint, the patient starts a specific rehabilitation treatment (Table 9.1).

Discussion

SL dissociation is the most common cause of acquired carpal instability. The natural course of SL dissociation without treatment is still unclear [3]. The dorsal aspect of the SLL is the thickest and most resistant and plays the most important role in SL stability, mainly due to its attachment to the dorsal capsule [4]. The dorsal capsulo-ligamentous scapholunate septum (DCSS) is also part of the SL complex, joining the ligament to the dorsal capsule and the dorsal intercarpal ligament, and it has been demonstrated that it plays an important role in SL stability [5].

Reattachment of the SLL is indicated in acute injuries. Unfortunately, early diagnosis is uncommon because most of the patients are diagnosed with a wrist "sprain" and further diagnosis (MRI and/or arthroscopy) and treatment is often delayed for more than 6–8 weeks. However, this condition can be found frequently associated to other lesions such as fractures (scaphoid, distal radius, etc.) and perilunate injuries.

Recently, a new radiologic test (Bilateral Ulnar Deviation Supination Stress Test) has been described to assess the integrity of the scapholunate ligament in dynamic scapholunate dysfunction[6.] SLL injuries are reportedly common with distal radius fractures (16–40%) [6] but also associated to scaphoid fractures [7, 8]. The use of arthroscopy in the treatment of the distal radius fractures and carpal fractures allows us to make this diagnosis, among other advantages. The healing potential of SL injuries is limited, and treatment must be performed during the acute phase of the injury to achieve better results [9]. The ideal time for performing a repair in the acute phase is not well defined. However, the intercarpal ligaments degenerate rapidly in the first 2–6 weeks, after which primary repair or reinsertion may be difficult, and with an often-poor result due to poor tissue quality and poor healing capacity.

Several arthroscopic techniques have been described for the treatment of acute scapholunate ligament injuries such as thermal shrinkage, debridement, and reduction and Kirschner wire fixation [10] The preferred open surgery method for treating acute injuries is direct repair of the ligament using bone anchors or transosseous tunnels, sometimes in combination with dorsal capsulodesis and fixation with Kirschner wires [11, 12].

The dorsal wrist approach increases the damage to the soft tissues and the fibrosis and joint rigidity. This approach also almost always injures the posterior interosseous nerve (PIN), which is involved in the proprioception of the SLL [13] and may be instrumental for dynamic stability and functional recovery. Moreover, during the approach and the dorsal and volar capsulotomy, there is also a significant injury to the vascular supply to the SLL, which impairs its healing capacity. Finally, the secondary stabilizers are also affected by this surgical approach [14].

After publication of their studies, Mathoulin [1] demonstrated that arthroscopic-guided dorsal capsuloplasty gave promising results in the short term with regard to improving pain, mobility of the wrist, strength, and reduction of the SL angle. With the development of arthroscopic techniques, it is now possible to perform a treatment similar to that described for open surgery, with reinsertion of the dorsal portion of the SL ligament [15, 16] and to add dorsal capsular reinforcement over the repair performed [16, 17], thereby reproducing the dorsal capsuloligamentous union (DCSS). A volar SLL capsuloligamentous reattachment has been recently described using dorsal and volar portals [18].

The different imaging tests used for diagnosing SL dissociation, including magnetic resonance imaging (MRI) and arthrography, have a high percentage of false negatives [19, 20].

The gold standard for diagnosing scapholunate injuries is wrist arthroscopy, which also allows for in situ treatment of the lesion [21].

Acute injuries of the SLL usually fall into the García Elías type II category [22], a complete tear with a repairable dorsal ligament and good carpal alignment. Moreover, the injury occurs more frequently at the insertion on the scaphoid, in approximately 40% of cases [23].

The results published on SL reinsertion using open surgery have been satisfactory regarding SL stability when the treatment was performed in the acute phase of the lesion [24, 25, 26, 27]. However, the treatment has been linked to greater joint stiffness and restricted motion due to the surgical approach, scarring, and association of the dorsal capsulodesis [25, 26].

The authors studied 19 patients with acute SLL injury treated with this technique [17]. Prospective follow-up of the patients was performed with systematic collection of data preoperatively and at 6 and 12 months with good functional and clinical results. The reduction in range of motion was markedly lower than that published after open surgery.

Arthroscopy is the gold standard for diagnosing scapholunate injuries and allows to perform a repair/reattachment of the SLL with dorsal and volar capsular reinforcement reproducing the treatment conducted by open surgery but avoiding the damage of the soft tissues and blood supply that is inherent to the open approach [28].

Conclusions

The arthroscopic technique for repair/reattachment of the volar and dorsal SLL with dorsal capsular reinforcement allows a reliable and stable primary repair of the dorsal and volar aspects of the ligament in acute or subacute SL injuries where there is tissue that can potentially be repaired, thus achieving an anatomical repair similar to that obtained with open surgery, but without the complications and stiffness secondary to the injury of the soft tissues that is inherent to the open dorsal and volar approach.

References

1. Mathoulin CL, Dauphin N, Wahegaonkar AL. Arthroscopic dorsal capsuloligamentous repair in chronic scapholunate ligament tears. Hand Clin. 2011;27:563–72.
2. Slutsky DJ. Wrist Arthroscopy Through a Volar Radial Portal. Anthroscopy. 2002;18(6):624–30.
3. Manuel J, Moran SL. The diagnosis and treatment of scapholunate instability. Hand Clin. 2010;26(1):129–44.
4. Bednar JM. Acute scapholunate ligament injuries: arthroscopic treatment. Hand Clin. 2015;31(3):417–23.
5. Carrara T, de Sambuy M, Burgess TM, Cambon-Binder A, Mathoulin CL. The anatomy of the dorsal Capsulo- Scapholunate septum: a cadaveric study. J Wrist Surg. 2017;6(3):244–7.
6. Puig de la Bellacasa I, Salva-Coll G, Esplugas M, Quintas S, Lluch A, Garcia-Elias M. Bilateral ulnar deviation supination stress test to assess dynamic Scapholunate instability. J Hand Surg Am. 2022 Jul;47(7):639–44.
7. Jørgsholm P, Thomsen NO, Björkman A, Besjakov J, Abrahamsson SO. The incidence of intrinsic and extrinsic ligament injuries in scaphoid waist fractures. J Hand Surg Am. 2010 Mar;35(3):368–74.
8. Kastenberger T, Kaiser P, Schmidle G, Schwendinger P, Gabl M, Arora R. Arthroscopic assisted treatment of distal radius fractures and concomitant injuries. Arch Orthop Trauma Surg. 2020 May;140(5):623–38.
9. Garcia-Elias M. Carpal instability. In: Wolfe SW, Hotchkiss RN, Pederson WC, Kozin SH, editors. Green's operative hand surgery, vol. 1. 6th ed. New York: Elsevier Churchill Livingstone; 2011. p. 465–522.
10. Rohman EM, Agel J, Putnam MD, Adams JE. Scapholunate interosseous ligament injuries: a retrospective review of treatment and outcomes in 82 wrists. J Hand Surg Am. 2014;39(10):2020–6.
11. Swanstrom MM, Lee SK. Open treatment of acute Scapholunate instability. Hand Clin. 2015;31(3):425–36.
12. Zarkadas PC, Gropper PT, White NJ, Perey BH. A survey of the surgical management of acute and chronic scapholunate instability. J Hand Surg Am. 2004;29(5):848–57.

13. Hagert E, Persson JK. Desensitizing the posterior interosseous nerve alters wrist proprioceptive reflexes. J Hand Surg Am. 2010;35:1059–66.
14. Elsaidi GA, Ruch DS, Kuzma GR, Smith BP. Dorsal wrist ligament insertions stabilize the scapholunate interval: cadaver study. Clin Orthop Relat Res. 2004;425:152–7.
15. Stuffmann ES, McAdams TR, Shah RP, Yao J. Arthroscopic repair of the scapholunate interosseous ligament. Tech Hand Up Extrem Surg. 2010 Dec;14(4):204–8.
16. Carratalá V, Lucas FJ, Miranda I, Sánchez Alepuz E, González JC. Arthroscopic Scapholunate Capsuloligamentous repair: suture with dorsal capsular reinforcement for Scapholunate ligament lesion. Arthrosc Tech. 2017;6(1):e113–20.
17. Carratalá V, Lucas FJ, Miranda I, Prada A, Guisasola E, Miranda FJ. Arthroscopic reinsertion of acute injuries of the Scapholunate ligament technique and results. J Wrist Surg. 2020 Aug;9(4):328–37.
18. Carratalá V, Corella F, Lucas FJ, Gisasola E, Martínez C, editors. Carpal Ligament injuries and instability. FESSH Instructional Course Book. Thieme; 2023.
19. Weiss AP, Akelman E, Lambiase R. Comparison of the findings of triple-injection cinearthrography of the wrist with those of arthroscopy. J Bone Joint Surg Am. 1996;78(3):348–56.
20. Hobby JL, Tom BD, Bearcroft PW, et al. Magnetic resonance imaging of the wrist: diagnostic performance statistics. Clin Radiol. 2001;56(1):50–7.
21. Geissler WB. Arthroscopic management of scapholunate instability. J Wrist Surg. 2013;2:129–35.
22. Garcia-Elias M, Lluch AL, Stanley JK. Three-ligament tenodesis for the treatment of scapholunate dissociation: indications and surgical technique. J Hand Surg Am. 2006;31(1):125–34.
23. Andersson JK, García EM. Dorsal Scapholunate ligament injury: a classification of clinical forms. J Hand Surg Eur. 2013;38(2):165–9.
24. Pomerance J. Outcome after repair of the scapholunate interosseous ligament and dorsal capsulodesis for dynamic scapholunate instability due to trauma. J Hand Surg Am. 2006;31(8):1380–6.
25. Bickert B, Sauerbier M, Germann G. Scapholunate ligament repair using the Mitek bone anchor. J Hand Surg Br. 2000;25(2):188–92.
26. Rosati M, Parchi P, Cacianti M, Poggetti A, Lisanti M. Treatment of acute scapholunate ligament injuries with bone anchor. Musculoskelet Surg. 2010;94:25–32.
27. Minami A, Kato H, Iwasaki N. Treatment of scapholunate dissociation: ligamentous repair associated with modified dorsal capsulodesis. Hand Surg 2003;8(1):1–6.
28. Luchetti R, Atzei A, Cozzolino R, Fairplay T. Current role of open reconstruction of the scapholunate ligament. J Wrist Surg. 2013;2:116–25.

Chapter 10
Static Acute Scapholunate Ligament Injury: Arthroscopic RADiCL (Repair/Augmentation Dorsal Capsular Ligaments)

Mark Ross and Greg Couzens

Case Presentation

A 61-year-old male electrician sustained an acute wrist injury in a heavy fall 8 weeks previously. He had no prior history of wrist injury or symptoms.

He had initial symptomatic management but complained of ongoing pain, weakness, and difficulty working.

Diagnosis

Physical Examination

There was swelling over the dorsal central carpus with associated tenderness. Wrist flexion was 60° and extension 50° and grip strength was 7.2 kg compared to 42 kg on the opposite side. His scaphoid shift test was markedly positive with pain and a clunk. Lunotriquetral ballottement was normal.

M. Ross (✉)
Department of Orthopaedic Surgery, University of Queensland, Brisbane Hand and Upper Limb Research Institute, Brisbane, QLD, Australia
e-mail: markross@upperlimb.com

G. Couzens
Queensland University of Technology, Brisbane Hand and Upper Limb Research Institute, Brisbane, QLD, Australia
e-mail: greg.couzens@upperlimb.com

© The Author(s), under exclusive license to Springer Nature Switzerland AG 2024
J. Yao (ed.), *Carpal Instability*, https://doi.org/10.1007/978-3-031-55869-6_10

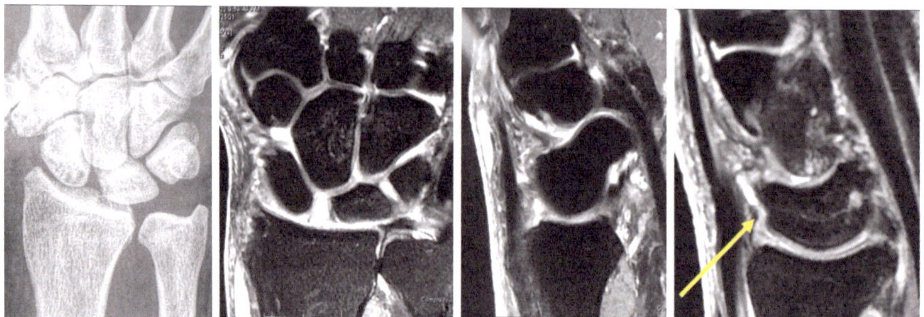

Fig. 10.1 Imaging. Plain radiograph shows static SL gap. MRI scan demonstrates a complete rupture of the SLIL with complete stripping of the dorsal capsule from the dorsal lunate—yellow arrow—(lunate "bare area"), an intact LRL, no dorsal translation of the proximal scaphoid and a Type 2 lunate

Imaging

Static plain radiographs showed an increased scapholunate interval with a slightly increased angle. Radio-lunate and capito-lunate angles were within normal limits.

MRI scan demonstrated a complete rupture of the SLIL with complete stripping of the dorsal capsule from the dorsal lunate (lunate "bare area" [1]), an intact LRL, no dorsal translation of the proximal scaphoid and a Type 2 lunate (Fig. 10.1).

Management

Management Options

Options were discussed including ongoing non-operative management, reconstruction using trans-osseous tendon graft [2], or arthroscopic tightening and anchor reinsertion of the dorsal capsular ligaments to the proximal row (RADiCL [3]) . The patient elected to proceed with arthroscopic treatment.

Operative Management

Arthroscopic assessment confirmed complete rupture of the SLIL with intact articular cartilage, and extensive capsular stripping from the dorsal lunate ("Bare Area," Fig. 10.2).

The dorsal surface of the lunate between the articular cartilage margins was debrided with a shaver and the deep surface of the capsule (DICL and DRCL) was

Fig. 10.2 Lunate bare area. Scope in 6R portal and probe in 3–4 portal. Acute stripping of dorsal capsule with exposed bone on dorsal lunate

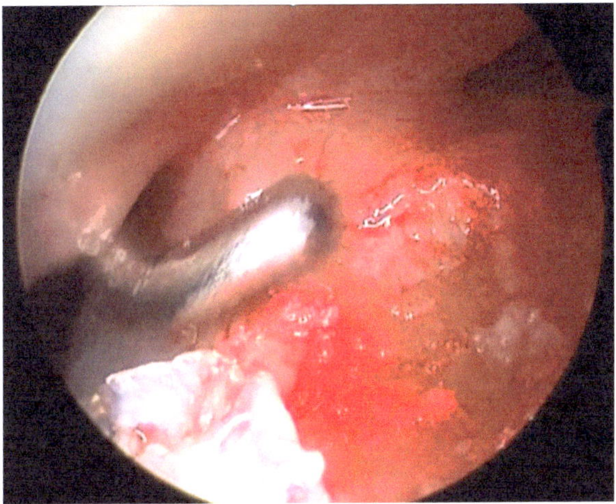

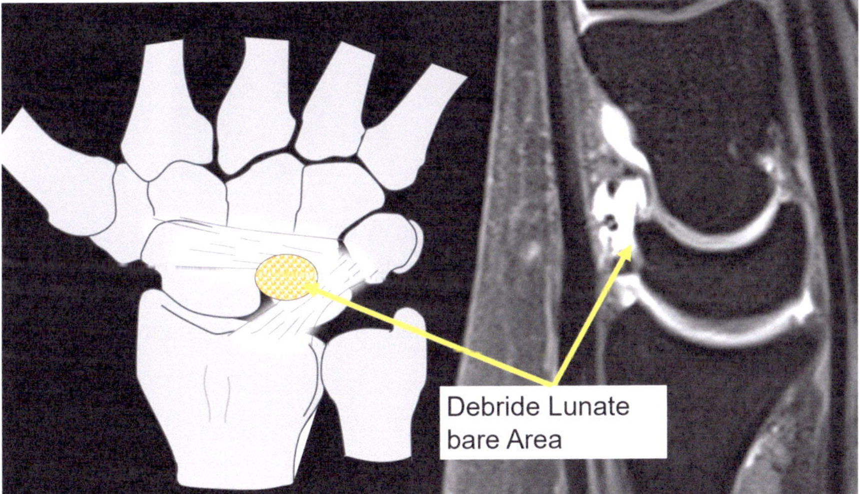

Fig. 10.3 Debride lunate bare area

freshened (Fig. 10.3). With the arthroscope in the 1–2 or 6R portal and all suture anchor was placed through the 3–4 portal into the center of the non-articular portion of the dorsal lunate (Fig. 10.4). Using 21 gauge needles, 2–0 PDS as suture shuttles were placed percutaneously through the DICL, distally and radially to the anchor, through the DRCL proximally and ulnar to the anchor, and one end of each was retrieved through the 3–4 portal beside the sutures from the anchor (Fig. 10.5).

A small skin incision was then made to identify the shuttle sutures exiting the dorsal capsule within the fourth extensor compartment to bring them together in the

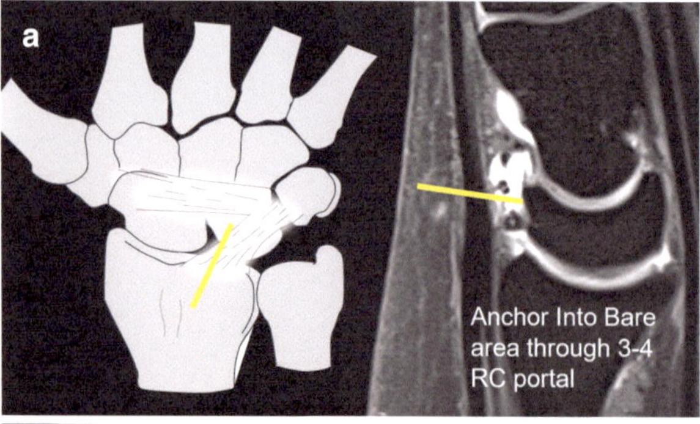

Fig. 10.4 (**a**, **b**) Anchor placed in bare area

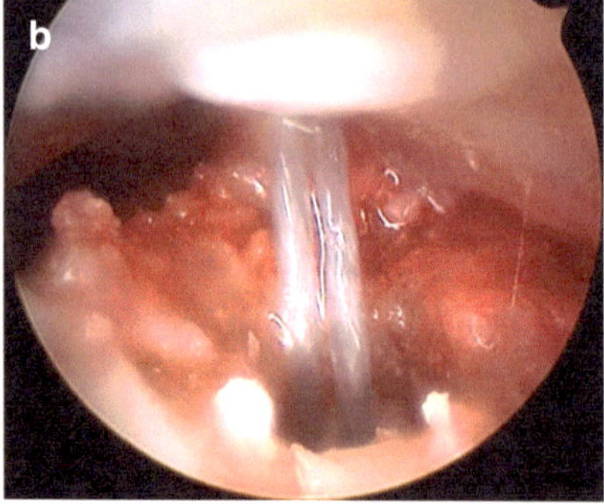

same gap between extensor tendons (Fig. 10.6). The PDS was then used to shuttle the braided anchor sutures from the 3–4 portal out through the capsule for tying. After releasing the traction, a sliding knot was used to tighten the ligaments and reapproximate the capsule to the dorsal lunate (Fig. 10.7). No temporary K-Wires were used.

Postoperative Management

Postoperatively, the patient was immobilized in a temporary volar slab and changed to a removable thermoplastic splint with the thumb MCPJ free the following day. Intermittent removal of the splint to commence inner range active motion was commenced allowing flexion to 10° and extension to 30° in both orthogonal and dart throwing planes. This was increased to flexion 20° and extension 40° at 4 weeks and the splint removed at 6 weeks. Isometric strengthening focusing on SL protective muscles commenced at 8 weeks. Garcia-Elias and Hagert have demonstrated in a

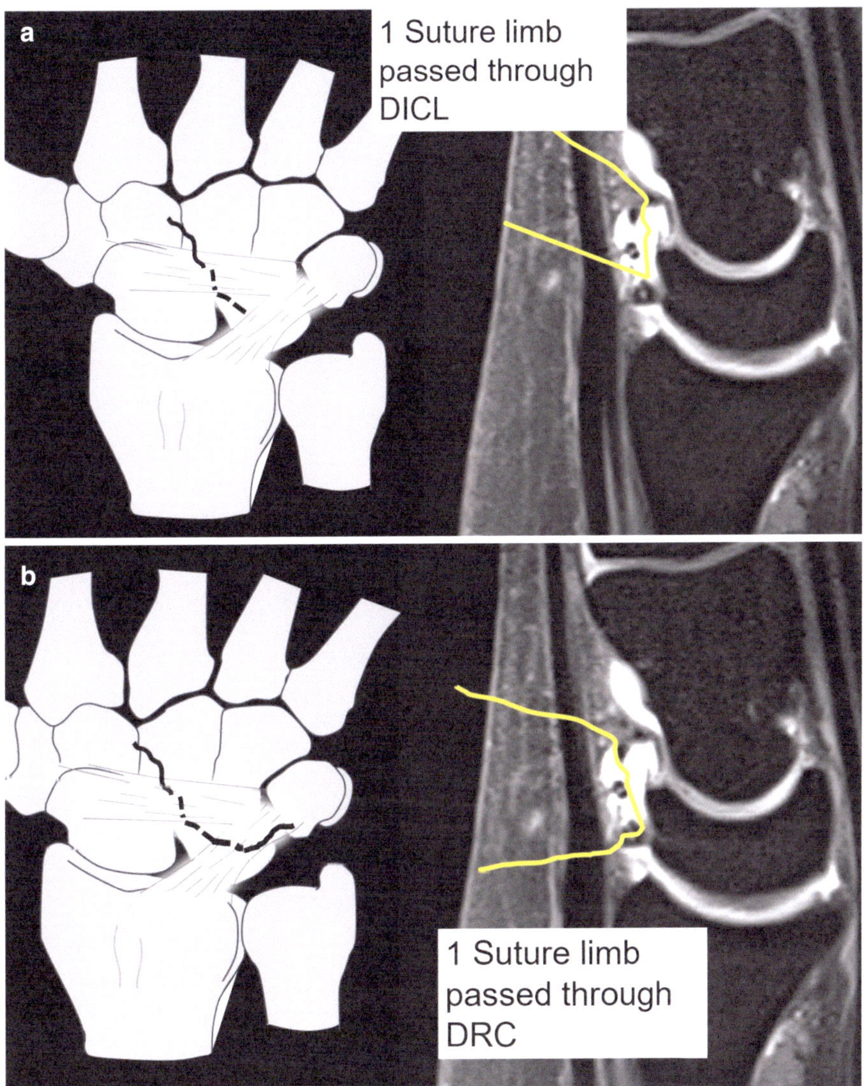

Fig. 10.5 (**a**, **b**) Sutures shuttled through DICL and DRCL

cadaver model that the Abductor Pollicis Longus (APL), the extensor carpi radialis longus (ECRL), and the FCU are intracarpal supinators and protect the carpus from excessive pronation (which can put stress on the dorsal SLIL) [4, 5].

The patient returned to light duties at 6 weeks and normal duties at 12 weeks.

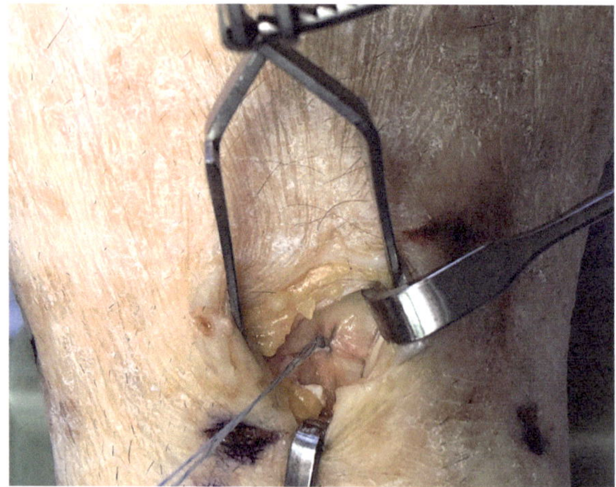

Fig. 10.6 A small incision was made to separate the sutures from the extensor tendons bringing suture both limbs into the same interval. The PDS shuttle was then used to pass the anchor sutures through the capsular ligaments

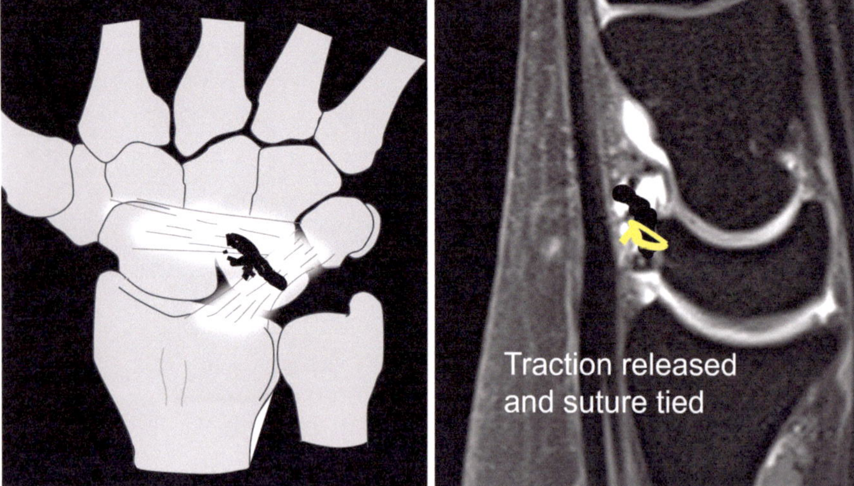

Fig. 10.7 After release of the traction a sliding knot was used to plicate the ligaments and reapproximate the capsule to the dorsal lunate

Outcomes

The patient was extremely satisfied and managed to return to his normal duties and demonstrated excellent objective and subjective outcome measures maintained at 2 years post-surgery (Table 10.1). His radiographs at 2 years demonstrated satisfactory carpal alignment with maintained decrease in the static gap (Fig. 10.8).

Table 10.1 Pre-op and 2-year post-op scores

	Pre-op	6 months	1 year	2 year
Pain with normal activities	60	23	5	6
Satisfaction	0	90	92	93
GRC symptoms (± 7point scale)		+5	+6	+7
GRC function (± 7point scale)		+4	+6	+7
PRWE	82.5	20	14	12
QuickDASH	75	10	9	7
Flexion—Right wrist	60	45	50	60
Extension—Right wrist	50	55	60	70
Grip strength	7.2 kg	15 kg	23.6 kg	39 kg

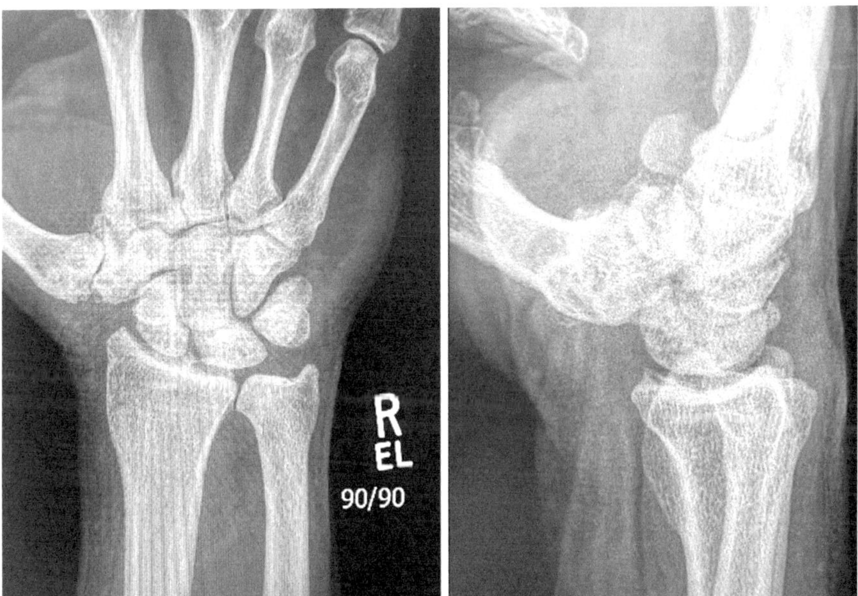

Fig. 10.8 Two-year post-op radiographs

Pearls and Pitfalls

- The 1–2 and/or 6R portals are essential for viewing and debriding the dorsal lunate bare area, inserting the anchor, and passing the sutures.
- It is important to exercise extreme care to ensure the capsular sutures are clear of the extensor tendons under direct vision before tying.
- Care should be taken to carefully assess the capsular attachments to the proximal row. On occasion, the capsule may be dissociated from the scaphoid instead of, or as well as, the lunate. This may require an additional anchor in the scaphoid.

- We also use the Arthroscopic RADiCL repair for lower grades of injury and have found it particularly useful in those patients with partial injuries to the SLIL (Geissler 2/Ewas 2 / 3a and b) and a demonstrated lunate bare area who have failed an adequate trial of non-operative management [4, 5].
- The extent to which this technique can be pushed for higher grades of instability remains unclear. In cases such as this where there is an absence of dorsal scaphoid translation combined with an intact LRL and a Type 2 lunate, we have been prepared to utilize this technique.

In higher grades of instability with more features of static deformity including dorsal translation of the proximal pole, scaphoid flexion, and larger SL gaps, the RADiCL technique may be combined with other arthroscopic / minimally invasive techniques such as a modified Mathoulin ADCLR [6–8], Smith volar STT mini open reconstruction [8], and volar suture of SL/capsule [9, 10] as part of a "modular" ligament-specific approach to carpal instability [1, 8, 11].

References

1. Raja S, Williams D, Wolfe S, Couzens G, Ross M. In: Geissler WB, editor. New concepts in carpal instability In Wrist and elbow arthroscopy with selected open procedures; 2022.
2. Ross M, Loveridge J, Cutbush K, Couzens G. Scapholunate ligament reconstruction. J Wrist Surg. 2013;2(2):110–5. https://doi.org/10.1055/s-0033-1341962.
3. Salva-Coll G, Garcia-Elias M, Hagert E. Scapholunate instability: proprioception and neuromuscular control. J Wrist Surg. 2013;2:136–40. https://doi.org/10.1055/s-0033-1341960.
4. Salvà-Coll G, Garcia-Elias M, Llusá-Pérez M, Rodríguez-Baeza A. The role of the flexor carpi radialis muscle in scapholunate instability. J Hand Surg Am. 2011;36(01):31–6.
5. Mathoulin C, Dauphin N, Sallen V. Arthroscopic dorsal capsuloplasty in chronic scapholunate ligament tears: a new procedure; preliminary report. Chir Main. 2011;30(03):188–97.
6. Williams D, Raja S, Ross M. In: Geissler WB, editor. The RADICL procedure: repair/augmentation of dorsal intercarpal ligament In Wrist and elbow arthroscopy with selected open procedures; 2022.
7. Wahegaonkar AL, Mathoulin CL. Arthroscopic dorsal capsuloligamentous repair in the treatment of chronic scapho-lunate ligament tears. J Wrist Surg. 2013;2(02):141–8.
8. Smith NC, Yates SE, Mettyas T. Open Volar STT Ligament reconstruction to augment the mathoulin's arthroscopic dorsal capsuloligamentous reconstruction: technique description and case reports. J Wrist Surg. 2023;13(1):1–9. https://doi.org/10.1055/s-0043-1768931.
9. del Piñal F, Studer A, Thams C, Glasberg A. An All-Inside Technique for Arthroscopic Suturing of the Volar Scapholunate Ligament J Hand Surg. 2011;36A:2044–6. https://doi.org/10.1016/j.jhsa.2011.09.021.
10. Lui H, Kakar S. Arthroscopic-Assisted Volar Scapholunate Capsulodesis: A new technique. J Hand Surg Am. 2022;47(1124):e1–1124.e6. https://doi.org/10.1016/j.jhsa.2022.05.018.
11. Loisel F, Orr S, Ross M, Couzens G, Leo AJ, Wolfe S. Traumatic nondissociative carpal instability: a case series. J Hand Surg Am. 2022;47(3):285.e1–285.e11. https://doi.org/10.1016/j.jhsa.2021.04.024.

Chapter 11
Static Acute Scapholunate Ligament Injury: Open Suture Anchor Repair

Leah R. F. Demetri and Lauren M. Shapiro

Case Presentation

The patient was a 35-year-old man with no prior medical history, surgical history, or prior wrist injury who fell rollerblading. He noted immediate wrist pain and presented to the emergency room on the day of his injury.

Physical Assessment

Physical exam demonstrated a mild wrist deformity. There was no evidence of open injury. He was neurovascularly intact. The patient had notable tenderness to palpation about the distal radius and ulnar styloid. Given the acuity of the injury and difficulty obtaining a reliable physical examination due to pain, we did not perform a Watson shift test, a scapholunate ballottement test, nor an evaluation of distal radial ulnar joint (DRUJ) stability.

L. R. F. Demetri (✉)
Department of Orthopedic Surgery, Brigham and Women's Hospital, Boston, MA, USA
e-mail: ldemetri@bwh.harvard.edu

L. M. Shapiro
Department of Orthopedic Surgery, University of California, San Francisco,
San Francisco, CA, USA

J. Yao (ed.), *Carpal Instability*, https://doi.org/10.1007/978-3-031-55869-6_11

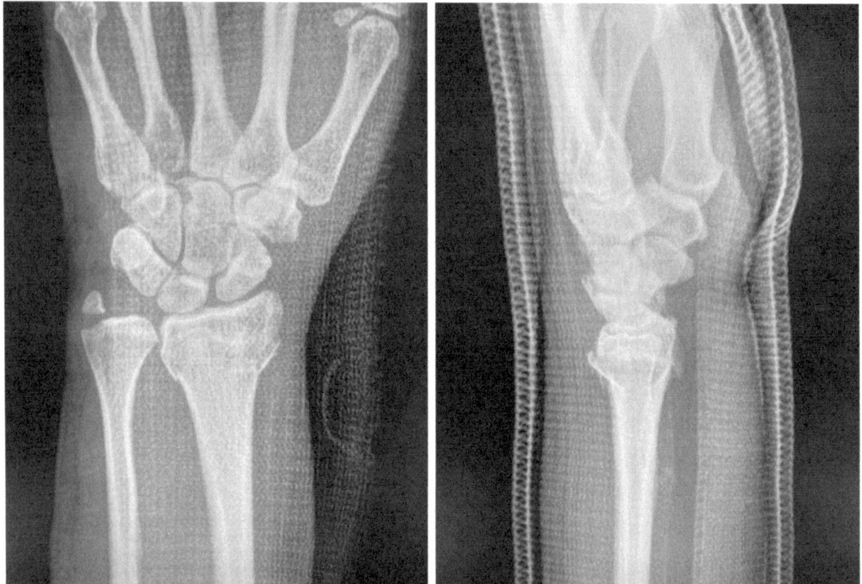

Fig. 11.1 AP and lateral radiographs of the wrist. The AP view demonstrates an acute, extra-articular, dorsally angulated distal radius fracture with loss of radial height and inclination as well as widening of the scapholunate interval. The lateral view demonstrates DISI deformity with an increased SL angle

Diagnostic Studies

Plain radiographs demonstrated an extra-articular distal radius fracture with widening of the scapholunate (SL) interval (Fig. 11.1). There was also a displaced ulnar styloid fracture. The authors do not routinely obtain a pre-operative MRI or other advanced imaging in this setting and instead rely on intra-operative physical examination and fluoroscopy to guide the care of injuries associated with acute distal radius fractures. Arthroscopy is a common method for diagnosing and staging SL injury, however in this case, this patient had notable static instability and we did not feel an arthroscopy would have changed our management.

Diagnosis

Based upon the clinical exam and pre—and intra-op imaging findings, this patient was diagnosed an acute SL tear as well as a distal radius and ulnar styloid fractures.

Management Options

Early recognition and treatment of SL injuries is critical as chronic scapholunate instability may lead to the development of degenerative wrist arthritis, known as scapholunate advanced collapse (SLAC) [1]. Furthermore, treatment in the acute setting yields better outcomes than delayed treatment. Rohman et al. performed a retrospective review comparing outcomes of patients treated in the acute (<6 weeks post injury) or chronic (>6 weeks post injury) setting and found that injuries treated acutely had significantly lower failure rate (4% vs. 18%, $p = 0.034$) and a trend toward superior radiographic and QuickDASH scores [2].

When performing open SL ligament repair, there are several options regarding approach, fixation technique, and associated procedures. Cadaveric studies suggest the dorsal SL ligament is the strongest portion of the ligament and as such, the dorsal SL ligament has been the structure that has received the most focus [3–5]. Several different dorsal approaches to the wrist have been described. The more traditional fiber-splitting capsulotomy was introduced by Berger in 1995 [6–8], with the intent of preserving the dorsal ligaments of the proximal carpal row. While this approach preserves the triquetral insertions of the dorsal intercarpal ligament (DIC) and dorsal radiocarpal ligament (DRC), it may disrupt their critical insertions on the lunate and scaphoid [9]. In 1999, a cadaveric study by Viegas et al. described the importance of the lunate and scaphoid attachments of the DIC and DRC [10]. Building upon this work, a recent cadaveric study by Loisel and colleagues found that in scapholunate-deficient wrists, a fiber-splitting capsulotomy leads to iatrogenic carpal instability, even after the DIC and DRC are repaired to the scaphoid and lunate with suture anchors. As an alternative technique, they suggest a "window" approach in which two separate capsulotomies are made to expose the proximal row at the radiocarpal and midcarpal joints. This technique preserves the scaphoid and lunate insertions of the DIC and DRC [11].

Regarding fixation techniques for open repair, the two main options are using transosseus tunnels verses suture anchors. Melone and colleagues report the outcome of transosseus fixation in 18 professional basketball players presenting with acute, static SL injuries. Their technique involves making small drill holes for the SL repair as well as performing a dorsal capsulodesis in the proximal edge of the DIC to augment the dorsal SL ligament. They found that at an average of 5 years follow-up, all patients demonstrated good or excellent outcomes based on the Mayo wrist score and an average SL angle of 62 degrees and SL interval of 2.5 mm. 83% of patients had no radiographic evidence of degenerative changes at final follow-up [12].

Despite these excellent clinical outcomes with transosseus repair, biomechanical data supports the use of suture anchors over transosseus techniques. A cadaveric biomechanical study performed by Kang and colleagues found that primary SL repair using double-loaded suture anchors demonstrated significantly higher strength compared with single-loaded anchors and transosseus repairs, and transosseus repairs demonstrated the greatest gap formation with cyclic loading [13].

Incorporating a dorsal capsulodesis to augment the SL repair has also become common practice. In 2003, Minami and colleagues suggested incorporating a modified dorsal capsulodesis to SL repair and/or reconstruction as they found that after SL repair or reconstruction, SL angles worsened from 50 degrees to 60 degrees when patients were followed post-operatively [14]. Although this radiographic progression was not associated with deteriorating clinical outcomes, they began performing a modified dorsal capsulodesis in addition to SL repair or reconstruction and found that the SL angle averaged 49 degrees at 4 years follow-up, suggesting that the dorsal capsulodesis added stability to the repair [14].

There are several different techniques for dorsal capsulodesis. Swanstrom and Lee describe a "double-dorsal" capsulodesis in which an ulnar-based capsulotomy flap is raised, bisected, and then repaired with the distal limb attaching to the distal pole of the scaphoid and the proximal limb attaching to the dorsal aspect of the scaphoid and lunate as the reinforcing portion of the capsulodesis [1].

The decision to conduct an open versus arthroscopic repair is also debated. Advocates for arthroscopic repair cite that this technique allows for arthroscopic visualization and classification of the injury, as well as visualization of the reduction and implant placement [15, 16]. Authors further cite that by avoiding a large dorsal approach, arthroscopic repair may lead to less stiffness, lower risk of damage to the posterior interosseus nerve, and preservation of the dorsal blood supply and secondary dynamic ligamentous stabilizers. While these benefits and their subsequent impact on clinical and radiographic outcomes are not fully demonstrated in the literature, early reports of arthroscopic SL repair demonstrate fairly reliable and satisfactory outcomes. For example, Carratalá et al. performed an arthroscopic SL reinsertion with a dorsal capsulodesis in 19 patients [16]. The authors note patients had a mean age of 44 years and that 37% of patients also had a distal radius fracture. At a minimum follow-up of 12 months, 79% of patients noted good to excellent results according to functional outcome scores. Grip strength was significantly improved from pre-operative measures yet about 13% decreased from the contralateral side. While the results from small studies are encouraging, arthroscopic repair techniques have a notable learning curve and require additional operative setup if the surgeon is not already performing wrist arthroscopy.

Lastly, there is also debate regarding the treatment of soft tissue injuries (e.g., SL tears) associated with distal radius fractures. While associated soft tissue injuries with acute distal radius fractures are reported with a high incidence, there are no high-quality studies that provide evidence in support of improved outcomes with concomitant arthroscopy and/or treatment. Notably, one study evaluated the differences in outcomes of 82 patients with a radiographically apparent SL ligament tear (SL angle >70) and 110 patients without radiographic evidence of an SL ligament tear (SL angle <70) [17]. At 12 and 24 months follow-up, the authors demonstrate no difference in patient-reported outcomes between these two cohorts.

To summarize, the literature available to guide the care of acute scapholunate injuries with or without a concomitant distal radius fracture is heterogenous and does not support one approach. As such, we detail the management approach chosen for this case with the rationale utilized to guide our care and recommend that surgeons select an approach in a systematic manner in accordance with their clinical experience and technical skill.

Management Chosen for this Case with Rationale [with Figures]

Requirements for primary SL repair include a robust repairable ligament, a reducible carpus, and the absence of degenerative changes [1, 18]. In this case, after reduction and fixation of the distal radius, there was notable static diastasis of the SL interval of this young patient. Although there is no clear consensus in the literature, we perform an open SL repair if a static deformity persists after reduction and fixation of a distal radius fracture in a young patient. Given static deformities are visible on intra-operative fluoroscopy, and there is limited evidence to support the arthroscopy during distal radius fixation [19] nor arthroscopic SL repair, we do not routinely utilize arthroscopy for diagnosis nor treatment. If there is no evidence of static instability after fixation of the distal radius fracture, we recommend intra-operative stress testing of the carpus using PA, lateral, ulnar deviated, and traction views to determine whether there is dynamic instability. If the stress testing is equivocal, we recommend arthroscopy to evaluate the intercarpal ligaments [20]. Given the natural history of SL tears associated with distal radius fractures, we recommend non-operative treatment for partial (grade 1–2) SL tears and operative management of complete (grade 3–4) SL tears or tears with evidence of dynamic instability on stress testing [20, 21]. Regarding the ulnar styloid fracture, in this case, it was treated non-operatively as the DRUJ was stable in pronation, supination, and neutral following fixation of the distal radius.

The patient was treated with an acute, open SL repair with sutures anchors. A dorsal "window" approach to the wrist, as described by Loisel et al. [11], was performed. The SL ligament was noted to be avulsed from the scaphoid and was associated with an acute hematoma. There was no significant cartilage damage. Two 0.045 k-wires were placed into the scaphoid and lunate and used a joystick to reduce the deformity (Fig. 11.2). We recommend placing the k-wires at oblique angles to maximize the utility of the joystick. Furthermore, placing the k-wires away from the planned location of definitive fixation is advised. After reduction, intercarpal (scaphocapitate and scapholunate) 0.045 k-wires were placed to protect the SL repair (Fig. 11.3). The SL ligament was repaired with a small suture anchor [a 1.0 mm juggernaut anchor (ZimmerBiomet, Warsaw, IN)]. Lastly, a capsulodesis was performed.

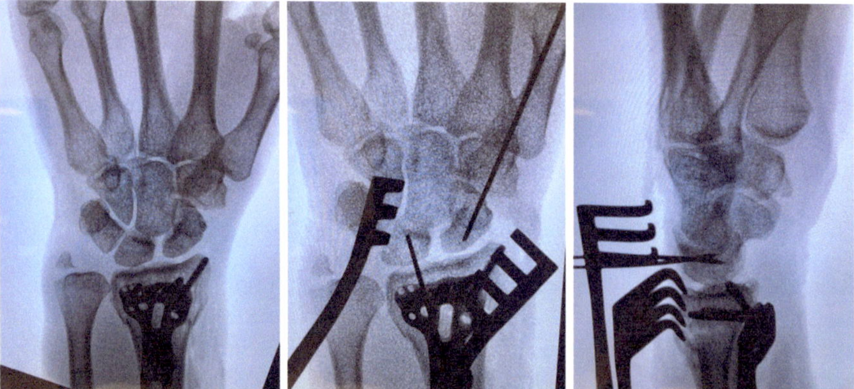

Fig. 11.2 Intra-operative fluoroscopy images demonstrate the wide SL interval after distal radius ORIF followed by k-wire joysticks in the lunate and scaphoid with reduction of the DISI deformity on the lateral view

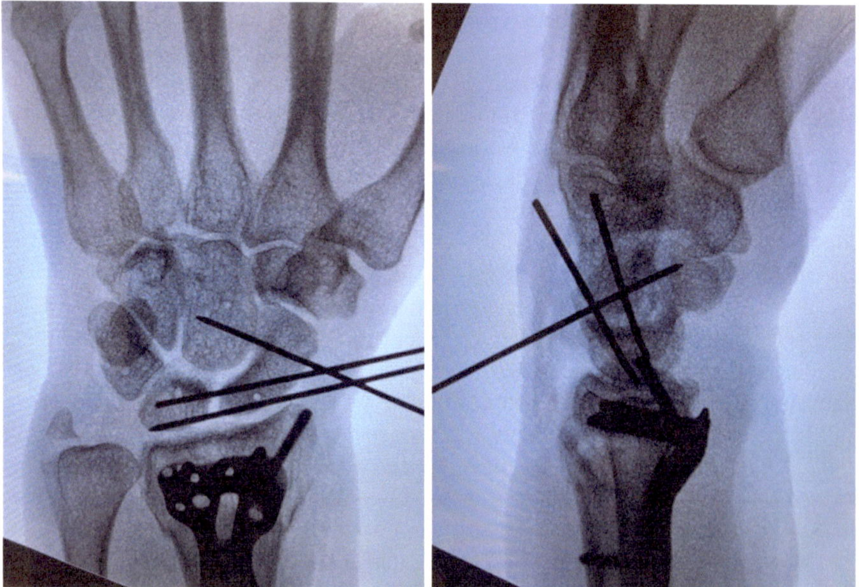

Fig. 11.3 Intra-operative fluoroscopy at the end of the case demonstrates k-wires between the scaphoid and lunate as well as a k-wire between the scaphoid and capitate to protect the SL repair

Clinical Course and Outcome [with Figures]

Post-operatively, the patient was placed in a short arm splint and was encouraged to avoid weight bearing through the hand and wrist. Active digital and elbow range of motion were encouraged. At 2 weeks, the patient's sutures were removed, the patient was transitioned into a short arm cast. At 6 weeks, the pins were removed, the short arm cast was removed, and the patient was transitioned to a removable wrist brace. Hand therapy was prescribed for range of motion exercises, and the patient is instructed to gently increase weight bearing and gradually wean out of the removable wrist brace.

Clinically, this patient did well post-operatively. At his most recent clinic visit (approximately 3 months post-operative), his range of motion was 75′ flexion, 80′ extension. His pronosupination was symmetric to the contralateral side. His grip strength is about 80% that of his contralateral side. Radiographically, there is no evidence of scapholunate instability (Fig. 11.4).

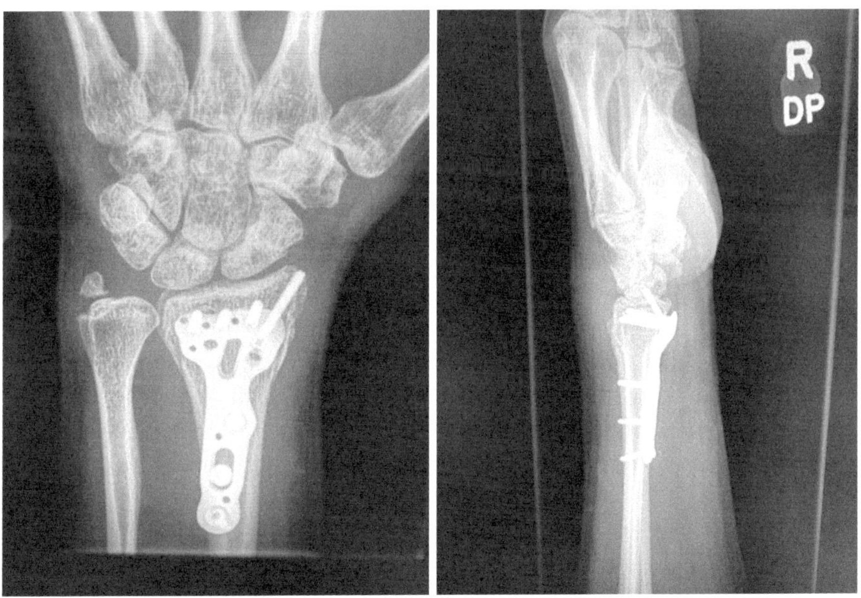

Fig. 11.4 AP and lateral XR obtained at 3 months post-operatively demonstrating maintained reduction of the SL interval and no recurrence of the DISI deformity

Clinical Pearls/Pitfalls [3–5, with Figures]

- A dorsal "window" approach as described by Loisel et al. avoids detachment of the DIC and DRC from the scaphoid and lunate, thereby theoretically reducing the risk of iatrogenic SL instability.
- K-wire joysticks may be placed in the lunate and scaphoid to assist with reduction of the SL interval and DISI deformity.
- Adding a dorsal capsulodesis may augment the SL repair and prevent recurrence of a DISI deformity.
- Arthroscopic treatment of acute SL injuries, which may improve visualization and notably avoids the relatively large dorsal approach, has demonstrated satisfactory clinical results, yet is associated with a steep learning curve.

Literature Review and Discussion

There are several studies in the literature demonstrating good outcomes with suture anchor repair in the acute setting. Rosati et al. found that in 18 patients with acute SL injuries treated with mini-Mitek suture anchor repair, 88% had excellent or good functional outcomes based on the Mayo Wrist score with an average follow-up of 32 months. Of note, only 44% (8/18) of patients in these series had static injuries with abnormal static radiographs; the rest of the patients had dynamic instability diagnosed with either dynamic fluoroscopic evaluation or MRI arthrography [22]. Bickert and colleagues reported the results of 12 patients treated with acute SL repair with mini-Mitek suture anchors and found excellent or good results in 67% of patients with only one patient developing recurrent dissociation of the SL radiographically (despite excellent functional outcomes) [23]. It was not reported whether these patients were presenting with acute or chronic, or static or dynamic instability. In sum, isolated, acute SL repairs are relatively uncommon, and there is notable heterogeneity in the literature that informs the care of these injuries. Identifying and treating isolated, acute SL tears in a timely manner likely improves outcomes and possibly reduces the risk of development of long-term arthritic change. The authors utilize an open "window" approach with a suture anchor repair and k-wire stabilization based upon the available literature; however, we recognize that long-term clinical outcome studies are lacking to guide the specific nuances of treatment. Lastly, the authors perform a capsulodesis when conducting an SL repair, particularly in the presence of a DISI deformity (as this may help serve as a checkrein for sagittal plane instability and augment the repair). While multiple capsulodesis techniques exist, none has proven superior and the addition of a capsulodesis to an SL repair has demonstrated satisfactory outcomes.

References

1. Swanstrom MM, Lee SK. Open treatment of acute Scapholunate instability. Hand Clin. 2015;31:425–36. https://doi.org/10.1016/j.hcl.2015.04.008.
2. Rohman EM, Agel J, Putnam MD, Adams JE. Scapholunate interosseous ligament injuries: a retrospective review of treatment and outcomes in 82 wrists. J Hand Surg Am. 2014;39:2020–6. https://doi.org/10.1016/j.jhsa.2014.06.139.
3. Berger RA. The ligaments of the wrist. A current overview of anatomy with considerations of their potential functions. Hand Clin. 1997;13:63–82.
4. Berger RA, Imeada T, Berglund L, An KN. Constraint and material properties of the subregions of the scapholunate interosseous ligament. J Hand Surg Am. 1999;24:953–62. https://doi.org/10.1053/jhsu.1999.0953.
5. Sokolow C, Saffar P. Anatomy and histology of the scapholunate ligament. Hand Clin. 2001;17:77–81.
6. Berger RA. A method of defining palpable landmarks for the ligament-splitting dorsal wrist capsulotomy. J Hand Surg Am. 2007;32:1291–5. https://doi.org/10.1016/j.jhsa.2007.07.023.
7. Berger RA, Bishop AT. A fiber-splitting capsulotomy technique for dorsal exposure of the wrist. Tech Hand Up Extrem Surg. 1997;1:2–10. https://doi.org/10.1097/00130911-199703000-00002.
8. Berger RA, Bishop AT, Bettinger PC. New dorsal capsulotomy for the surgical exposure of the wrist. Ann Plast Surg. 1995;35:54–9. https://doi.org/10.1097/00000637-199507000-00011.
9. Nagao S, Patterson RM, Buford WLJ, et al. Three-dimensional description of ligamentous attachments around the lunate. J Hand Surg Am. 2005;30:685–92. https://doi.org/10.1016/j.jhsa.2005.03.002.
10. Viegas SF, Yamaguchi S, Boyd NL, Patterson RM. The dorsal ligaments of the wrist: anatomy, mechanical properties, and function. J Hand Surg Am. 1999;24:456–68. https://doi.org/10.1053/jhsu.1999.0456.
11. Loisel F, Wessel LE, Morse KW, et al. Is the dorsal fiber-splitting approach to the wrist safe? A kinematic analysis and introduction of the "window" approach. J Hand Surg Am. 2021;46:1079–87. https://doi.org/10.1016/j.jhsa.2021.05.029.
12. Melone CP, Polatsch DB, Flink G, et al. Scapholunate interosseous ligament disruption in professional basketball players: treatment by direct repair and dorsal Ligamentoplasty. Hand Clin. 2012;28:253–60. https://doi.org/10.1016/j.hcl.2012.05.002.
13. Kang L, Ek ET, Wei MT, et al. Biomechanical analysis of Scapholunate ligament repair techniques. J Hand Surg Am. 2015;40:1534–9. https://doi.org/10.1016/j.jhsa.2015.03.031.
14. Minami A, Kato H, Iwasaki N. Treatment of scapholunate dissociation: ligamentous repair associated with modified dorsal capsulodesis. Hand Surg. 2003;8:1–6. https://doi.org/10.1142/s0218810403001443.
15. Suárez B, de Puga D, Cebrián Gómez R, Sanz-Reig J, et al. Indirect Scapholunate ligament repair: all arthroscopic. Arthrosc Tech. 2018;7:e423–8. https://doi.org/10.1016/j.eats.2017.11.001.
16. Carratalá V, Lucas FJ, Miranda I, et al. Arthroscopic reinsertion of acute injuries of the Scapholunate ligament technique and results. J Wrist Surg. 2020;9:328–37. https://doi.org/10.1055/s-0040-1710502.
17. Klifto KM, Hein RE, Klifto CS, et al. Outcomes associated with Scapholunate ligament injury following intra-articular distal radius fractures. J Hand Surg Am. 2021;46:309–18. https://doi.org/10.1016/j.jhsa.2020.12.005.
18. Garcia-Elias M, Lluch AL, Stanley JK. Three-ligament tenodesis for the treatment of scapholunate dissociation: indications and surgical technique. J Hand Surg Am. 2006;31:125–34. https://doi.org/10.1016/j.jhsa.2005.10.011.
19. Kamal RN, Shapiro LM. Practical application of the 2020 distal radius fracture AAOS/ASSH clinical practice guideline: a clinical case. J Am Acad Orthop Surg. 2022;30:e714–20. https://doi.org/10.5435/JAAOS-D-21-01194.

20. Desai MJ, Kamal RN, Richard MJ. Management of Intercarpal Ligament Injuries Associated with distal radius fractures. Hand Clin. 2015;31:409–16. https://doi.org/10.1016/j.hcl. 2015.04.009.
21. Mrkonjic A, Lindau T, Geijer M, Tägil M. Arthroscopically diagnosed scapholunate ligament injuries associated with distal radial fractures: a 13- to 15-year follow-up. J Hand Surg Am. 2015;40:1077–82. https://doi.org/10.1016/j.jhsa.2015.03.017.
22. Rosati M, Parchi P, Cacianti M, et al. Treatment of acute scapholunate ligament injuries with bone anchor. Musculoskelet Surg. 2010;94:25–32. https://doi.org/10.1007/s12306-010-0057-8.
23. Bickert B, Sauerbier M, Germann G. Scapholunate ligament repair using the Mitek bone anchor. J Hand Surg Br. 2000;25:188–92. https://doi.org/10.1054/jhsb.1999.0340.

Further Reading

Minami A, Kato H, Iwasaki N. Treatment of scapholunate dissociation: ligamentous repair associated with modified dorsal capsulodesis. Hand Surg. 2003;8(1):1–6. https://doi.org/10.1142/s0218810403001443.
Rosati M, Parchi P, Cacianti M, Poggetti A, Lisanti M. Treatment of acute scapholunate ligament injuries with bone anchor. Musculoskelet Surg. 2010;94(1):25–32. https://doi.org/10.1007/s12306-010-0057-8.
Swanstrom MM, Lee SK. Open treatment of acute Scapholunate instability. Hand Clin. 2015;31(3):425–36. https://doi.org/10.1016/j.hcl.2015.04.008.

Chapter 12
Capsulodesis with Internal Brace Augmentation for Treatment of Static Scapholunate Instability

H. B. Parikh and S. S. Shin

Introduction

Scapholunate instability is the most common cause of carpal instability [12]. As the scapholunate (SL) ligament fails in terminal wrist extension with ulnar deviation and supination, a common mechanism of injury includes a fall with impact onto the hypothenar aspect of the hand [14]. In the acute setting, patients commonly report pain at the dorsal and radial aspect of the wrist and generalized wrist swelling due to bleeding from the ligament injury [1]. As the swelling subsides, patients may begin to notice more focal painful popping/clicking at the SL interval and decreased grip strength [1].

As illustrated by Geissler, the degree of SL ligament injury can vary from ligament attenuation and partial sprain to complete rupture resulting in gross instability [7]. The degree of instability may depend on the level of SL injury and chronicity of symptoms and can be categorized as occult, dynamic, or fixed [12]. Occult instability occurs with partial SL ligament injuries that only cause pain during mechanical loading. These injuries are not apparent on resting or stress radiographs [1]. Patients with dynamic instability have disruption of all components of the SL ligament, and this can only be seen on stress radiographs [2]. Patients with fixed deformity, or static instability, demonstrate a widened SL interval on static anteroposterior radiographs and scaphoid flexion with lunate extension on lateral radiographs, characteristic of dorsal intercalated segment instability.

The authors have no financial disclosures or conflicts of interest.

H. B. Parikh (✉) · S. S. Shin
Department of Orthopaedics, Cedars-Sinai Medical Center, Los Angeles, CA, USA
e-mail: harin.parikh@cshs.org

J. Yao (ed.), *Carpal Instability*, https://doi.org/10.1007/978-3-031-55869-6_12

Treatment goals of static SL instability includes the reduction of both coronal and sagittal instability and the restoration of native SL joint kinematics. Many different surgical techniques have been described, including direct ligament repair using drill holes or anchors, pinning, screw fixation, bone-retinaculum-bone or bone-ligament-bone autograft, and reconstruction through various techniques using a tendon transfer or free tendon autograft [8, 22, 28]. These techniques function to restore SL ligament function and coronal plane instability.

Despite the multitude of options outlined in the literature for the treatment of static SL ligament instability, no superior treatment exists. It has been established that the optimal treatment strategy is some form of SL repair or reconstruction [13]. This allows the maintenance of SL joint stability while fostering an optimal healing environment. In this chapter, we present a novel technique for treating static SL instability: capsulodesis with internal brace augmentation (CIBA). This method utilizes the "internal brace" concept for SL reconstruction. We review preoperative planning, technical pearls, postoperative rehabilitation, technique rationale, and pearls and pitfalls.

Preoperative Planning/Indications for CIBA

For surgical planning, standard postero-anterior (PA), lateral, and oblique radiographs of the injured wrist are obtained. On the PA view, a gap of >3 mm is suggestive of static SL ligament injury [1]. Other indicators of static SL instability include visualization of the scaphoid "ring sign" or disruption of the contour of the proximal and distal carpal rows. On the lateral view, the angle between the long axis of the scaphoid and long axis of the lunate is measured. If this is greater than 70°, a dorsal intercalated segment instability (DISI) deformity and SL injury is suspected [1]. Comparison of radiographs of the opposite wrist should also be obtained. Magnetic resonance imaging (MRI) can be helpful in confirming disruption of the SL ligament and further defining the extent of ligamentous injury (Figs. 12.1a, b).

Based on the above work-up, patients who are found to have high-grade partial SL tear or complete SL tear with a reducible SL interval are indicated for the CIBA procedure. Patients with degenerative changes, non-reducible deformity, pediatric patients, or suspected infection are not candidates for this procedure. For patients who have had prior surgery, further advanced imaging including computed tomography may be needed to assess the location of pre-existing hardware and bony architecture which may preclude the CIBA procedure.

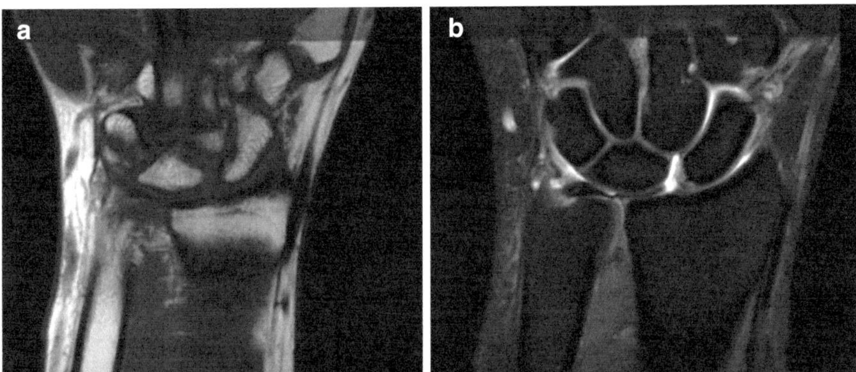

Fig. 12.1 (**a** and **b**) Coronal magnetic resonance imaging (MRI) images of a patient's left wrist demonstrating scapholunate rupture with scapholunate interval widening on T1 (**a**) and proton density (**b**) sequences

Surgical Technique

Exposure

After the affected upper extremity is prepped and draped and the tourniquet inflated, a 5 cm mid-dorsal longitudinal incision is made over the wrist slightly ulnar to Lister's tubercle.

A distally based capsulotomy is made by elevating the capsule off of the dorsal distal radius. This reveals the underlying complete SL ligament tear and gapping at the SL joint (Fig. 12.2). Care is taken to avoid further injury to the dorsal capsular scapholunate septum (DCSS) as this provides additional stability to the SL joint. Because the capsule is elevated at the level of the radiocarpal joint and reflected distally, the DCSS can be spared from further injury. Soft-tissue elevation off of the dorsal scaphoid is limited to only critical areas requiring exposure for anchor placement in order to avoid compromising vascularity the proximal pole.

Joint Reduction and Scapholunate Ligament Reconstruction

With fluoroscopic guidance, a guidewire for the Arthrex 3.5 mm SwiveLock (Arthrex, Naples, FL) is inserted dorsally into mid-body of the lunate from dorsal to palmar. This is then over-drilled with a 3.0 mm cannulated drill bit with a drill guide to avoid injury to surrounding extensor tendons. The drill bit and wire are removed and a 3.5 mm SwiveLock anchor is inserted into the lunate, securing FiberTape and 3–0 mm FiberWire suture. Secure fixation of the anchor is confirmed by pulling tightly on the tape and suture tails.

A second guidewire is then placed into the dorsal proximal scaphoid and over-drilled with a 3.0 mm drill bit. One of the tails of the FiberTape and a second 3–0 FiberWire suture is subsequently secured in this hole with a second 3.5 mm SwiveLock anchor. Care is taken to leave at least 3 mm of bone intact between the hole and the most proximal aspect of the scaphoid. The remaining FiberTape tail from the Lunate is then passed over the dorsal SL joint and secured with a third SwiveLock anchor in the dorsal distal scaphoid, again with at least 3 mm of intact bone between the anchor and the most distal aspect of the scaphoid (Fig. 12.3). The extraneous ends of the FiberTape are cut.

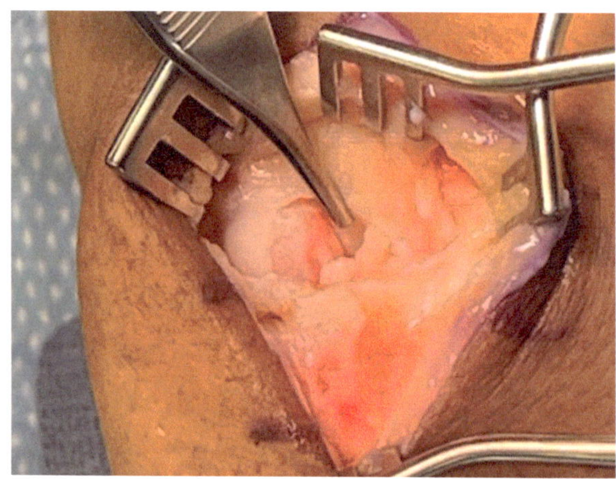

Fig. 12.2 Dorsal approach to the wrist revealing a scapholunate ligament tear and gapping at the scapholunate interval

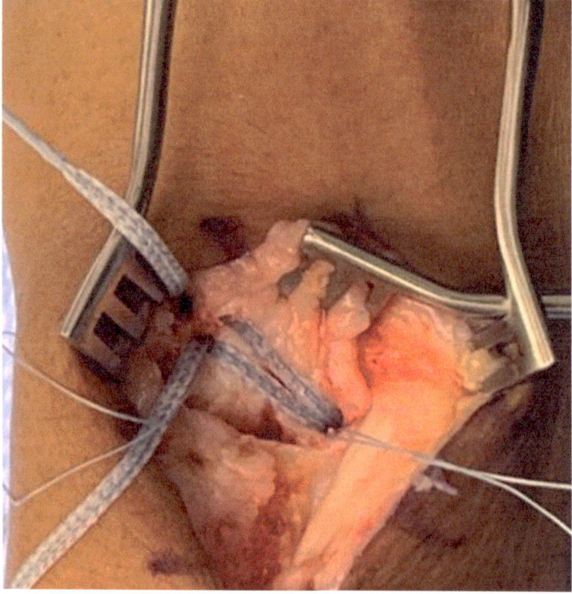

Fig. 12.3 SwiveLock anchor placement. Note that two anchors are placed in the proximal and distal aspect of the scaphoid, and the third centrally in the lunate

Capsulodesis and Wound Closure

The capsulodesis is then performed by passing the FiberWire sutures from the lunate and proximal scaphoid through the dorsal capsuloligamentous complex and tying them to each other, bringing down the tissue to the dorsal scapholunate joint (Fig. 12.4). Final fluoroscopic PA and lateral images are taken to confirm narrowing of the SL joint space and improvement in the SL angle. The wound is closed in a layered fashion. Following closure of the skin, a short-arm dorsal plaster splint with the thumb free is applied with the wrist in neutral position.

Postoperative Rehabilitation

Sutures are removed 7–10 days following surgery. At that time, a custom brace is applied for another 5 weeks. Though the wrist is immobilized, active range of motion of the fingers is encouraged to prevent stiffness. At 6 weeks postop, therapy is initiated with a focus on range of motion exercises. Gentle active and active-assisted range of motion exercises are permitted; passive motion exercises are not. Brace wear is reduced at this point for comfort only.

Grip strengthening is initiated a 2 months postoperative. Gradual weight bearing is also initiated. We expect eventual unrestricted return to activities around 3–4 months postoperative after achieving favorable range of motion, grip strength, ability to bear weight, and ability to perform sports-specific skills (in athletes). Figs. 12.5a, b are PA and lateral radiographs of a patient who is 4 months postoperative from the CIBA procedure—demonstrating maintained scapholunate reduction.

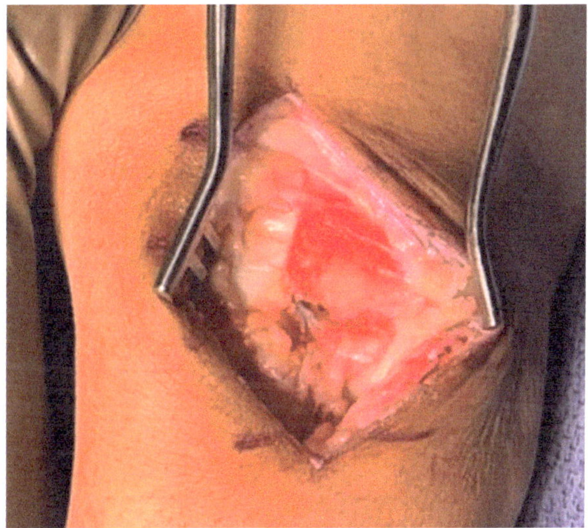

Fig. 12.4 Dorsal capsulodesis using FiberWire suture passed through the dorsal capsuloligamentous complex from the lunate and proximal scaphoid

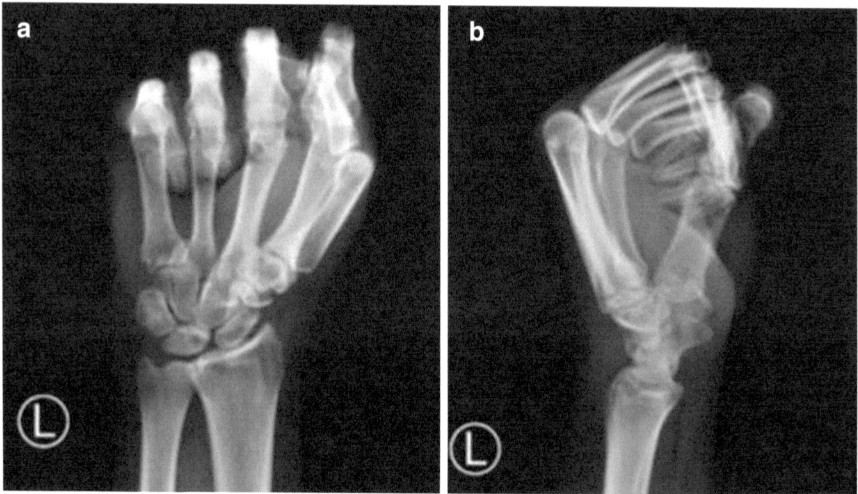

Fig. 12.5 (**a** and **b**). Postero-anterior (PA) and lateral clenched fist radiographs demonstrating reduction of the scapholunate interval and correction of scaphoid flexion 4 months following the CIBA procedure

Technique Rationale

Scapholunate repair using suture anchors or transosseous drill holes has previously been discussed in the literature and is the method of choice for many surgeons due to its technical ease [3, 11]. The CIBA technique utilizes the internal brace concept using a form of suture tape. This tape consists of a ultra-high-molecular-weight polyethylene (UHMWPE) core with a braided jacket of polyester and UHMWPE [23]. Because of these properties, suture tape has been increasingly used in orthopedic applications such as rotator cuff and ankle ligament repairs [4, 5].

Prior literature demonstrates the efficacy of suture tape augmentation in SL ligament repair. Thompson et al. demonstrate an increased load to failure (135 N versus 68 N for suture tape vs. repair-only, respectively) in patients undergoing SL ligament repair using suture tape augmentation and suture anchors from an all-dorsal approach [25]. A subsequent biomechanical study demonstrated similar findings, with patients undergoing suture tape augmentation having a higher load to failure compared to repair alone (98.5 N versus 37.7 N, respectively) [17]. Of note, neither of these methods compared to the biomechanical strength of the native intact SL ligament, found to have a load to failure of 211.8 N [17]. In terms of suture tape configuration, a V-shaped construct (including a short transverse suture tape from the lunate to the proximal scaphoid and a long oblique suture tape from the lunate to the distal scaphoid) confers the highest stability to the SL interval [16].

The CIBA technique utilizes high-tensile suture tape material in a V-configuration to allow for the strongest biomechanical support possible. This technique, incorporating the principles outlined above, allows for both joint space closure and reduction of scaphoid flexion with the goal of restoring native carpal biomechanics. In addition, the dorsal capsulodesis has also been previously shown to provide sagittal stability and resist rotatory subluxation of the scaphoid [19, 24]. Outcomes of both SL reduction and capsulodesis performed together are superior to either procedure performed alone [13, 15]. We believe the capsulodesis provides for extrinsic healing (i.e., scarring) around the scapholunate interval and also longer term stability of the SL joint when supported by the underlying internal brace augmentation.

Two other techniques described in the literature also utilize suture tape ligament reconstruction: SL interosseous reconstruction and SL ligament intrinsic brace 360° tenodesis (SLITT) reconstruction [9, 29]. However, neither technique has demonstrated long-term superiority over others. Advantages of the CIBA technique over more traditional techniques include an all-dorsal approach, superior biomechanical fixation, reproducibility with readily available materials and implants, and less soft-tissue dissection compared to more involved techniques. As K-wires are not used in this technique, potential risks of pin-site infection or loosening are also avoided.

Pearls and Pitfalls

When performing the CIBA technique, the treating surgeon should keep a few principles in mind. When making the drill holes for the SwiveLock anchors with the 3.0 mm drill bit, it is important to leave at least a 3 mm distance between the outer edge of the hole and the proximal or distal end of the scaphoid. Anchor placement too close to the periphery may lead to increased risk of peri-implant fracture and anchor pull-out. Thus, it is recommended to account for this distance during initial placement of the guidewire.

In the case of a difficult reduction, additional K-wires may be used. K-wires can be used outside of proposed anchor placement sites to facilitate joystick reduction of the SL interval and can be clamped together to maintain the reduction. Care should also be taken to ensure that the anchors are fully seated and not proud. During anchor insertion, the anchor body should be sitting on the cortex and perpendicular to the bone prior to advancing the anchor. The laser line on the driver should be at least level with the bone before being disengaged from the anchor. Care should also be taken to ensure that the tape lay as flat as possible when creating each limb of the V-construct outlined above.

Outcomes

Given the variability in degree of injury, chronicity, and patient-related factors, outcomes following SL repair/reconstruction are not well-defined. However, untreated SL instability is known to lead to increased risk of degenerative changes seen in SLAC wrist deformity [27]. This can develop within 3–15 years after initial injury

[1]. Patients undergoing a modified three-ligament tenodesis reported by Garcia-Elias et al. demonstrated that 75% of patients were able to return to work following injury and had 65% of grip strength relative to the non-injured side at mean follow-up of approximately 4 years [6]. This cohort was found to only have a 5% recurrence of carpal collapse. Another cohort of patients undergoing SL ligament repair using suture anchors and dorsal capsulodesis demonstrated improvement in patient reported outcomes, SL interval of 2.1 mm, and scapholunate angle of 71.3° at approximately 8.1 years following surgery [21]. Of note, two out of five patients in this cohort demonstrated osteoarthritis changes at final follow-up [21].

Though biomechanical studies demonstrate the strength of suture tape repair for SL instability, a paucity of outcomes data using these techniques remains. A nine-patient cohort was investigated after undergoing SLITT [10]. At a mean of 33 months postoperative, this cohort demonstrated 50% grip strength compared to the contralateral side, mean SL gap of 2.1 mm, mean SL angle of 50°, and improved patient reported outcomes following this procedure [10]. To our knowledge, no other outcome data using an all-dorsal SL reconstruction or intraosseous reconstruction has been reported in the literature and thus should be included in future investigations.

Complications of Scapholunate Injury and Treatment

Missed diagnosis: A high index of suspicion is required to diagnose scapholunate injury as this condition is frequently missed. Approximately 19% of patients who received a diagnosis of wrist sprain are found to have SL interval widening [26]. Furthermore, SL ligament injury can be missed when additional work-up for dynamic SL instability is not performed. A study found that 43% of SL ligament injuries can be missed when only plain films were obtained [18]. In addition, SL injury may be associated with other traumatic injuries; for example, they are found to occur in as high as 54% of patients sustaining fractures of the distal radius [26]. Timely diagnosis is critical in maximizing patient outcomes and minimizing progression towards disabling post-traumatic wrist arthritis as seen in the SLAC wrist.

Stiffness: As a result of scar formation and prolonged immobilization, stiffness is a common complication of surgical treatment of SL injury. Risks of allowing range of motion very soon following surgery include disruption of the construct (leading to chronic instability) and compromise of the overall healing environment. Thus, a difficult challenge for the treating surgeon is to balance this with the risk of long-term stiffness postoperatively. Patients should thus be counseled that some loss of range of motion can be expected following operative treatment of SL injury [24].

Persistent Pain: An obvious goal of surgical treatment of SL instability is improvement in pain; however, complete pain relief may not be attainable. Thus, providers may consider anterior and/or posterior interosseous neurectomy in their treatment algorithm. A small subset of patients may also develop post-traumatic complex regional pain syndrome.

Arthritis: Patients sustaining SL ligament tears are at inherently increased risk of post-traumatic arthritis due to both the possibility of traumatic articular cartilage damage at the time of injury and the subsequent altered kinematics without (or even with) surgical treatment. Missed diagnosis, malreduction, or failure of fixation can result in SL widening, scaphoid flexion, and thus increased risk of disease progression. In a retrospective review of 82 patients undergoing surgical treatment for scapholunate injury, Rohman et al. reported progression in 11% of cases requiring proximal row carpectomy, four-corner arthrodesis, or total wrist arthrodesis [20]. Of note, worker's compensation status was reported to have increased association with treatment failure [20].

Conclusion

Scapholunate injury represents a spectrum of disease, ranging from partial to complete injuries of varying chronicity. These injuries can cause a level of pain that can prevent one's ability to meaningfully engage in work, athletics, or other activities of daily living. In this chapter, we outline a novel technique for the treatment of static scapholunate instability with reducible deformity: Capsulodesis with Internal Brace Augmentation (CIBA). Except for cases of SLAC where a salvage procedure would be required, we use this technique for all cases of static SLIL instability patterns. This technique utilizes the internal brace concept using a V-construct through an all-dorsal approach. We believe that a dorsal capsulodesis supported by a strong underlying internal brace maximizes the chance of successful healing of the injured scapholunate ligament. Though further outcome data is needed, this technique may be a promising treatment option for the treatment of static scapholunate instability in the future.

References

1. Andersson JK. Treatment of scapholunate ligament injury: current concepts. EFORT Open Rev. 2017;2(9):382–93.
2. Berger RA, Imeada T, Berglund L, An KN. Constraint and material properties of the subregions of the scapholunate interosseous ligament. J Hand Surg Am. 1999;24(5):953–62.
3. Bickert B, Sauerbier M, Germann G. Scapholunate ligament repair using the Mitek bone anchor. J Hand Surg Br. 2000;25(2):188–92.
4. Borbas P, Fischer L, Ernstbrunner L, Hoch A, Bachmann E, Bouaicha S, et al. High-strength suture tapes are biomechanically stronger than high-strength sutures used in rotator cuff repair. Arthrosc Sports Med Rehabil. 2021;3(3):e873–e80.
5. Cho BK, Park KJ, Kim SW, Lee HJ, Choi SM. Minimal invasive suture-tape augmentation for chronic ankle instability. Foot Ankle Int. 2015;36(11):1330–8.
6. Garcia-Elias M, Lluch AL, Stanley JK. Three-ligament tenodesis for the treatment of scapholunate dissociation: indications and surgical technique. J Hand Surg Am. 2006;31(1):125–34.

7. Geissler WB, Freeland AE, Savoie FH, McIntyre LW, Whipple TL. Intracarpal soft-tissue lesions associated with an intra-articular fracture of the distal end of the radius. J Bone Joint Surg Am. 1996;78(3):357–65.

8. Harvey EJ, Hanel D, Knight JB, Tencer AF. Autograft replacements for the scapholunate ligament: a biomechanical comparison of hand-based autografts. J Hand Surg Am. 1999;24(5):963–7.

9. Kakar S, Greene RM, Denbeigh J, Van Wijnen A. Scapholunate ligament internal brace 360 Tenodesis (SLITT) procedure: a biomechanical study. J Wrist Surg. 2019;8(3):250–4.

10. Kakar S, Logli AL, Ramazanian T, Gaston RG, Fowler JR. Scapholunate ligament 360 degrees procedure. Bone Joint J. 2021;103-B(5):939–45.

11. Kang L, Ek ET, Wei MT, Meyers KN, Hearns KA, Carlson MG. Biomechanical analysis of Scapholunate ligament repair techniques. J Hand Surg Am. 2015;40(8):1534–9.

12. Kitay A, Wolfe SW. Scapholunate instability: current concepts in diagnosis and management. J Hand Surg Am. 2012;37(10):2175–96.

13. Lavernia CJ, Cohen MS, Taleisnik J. Treatment of scapholunate dissociation by ligamentous repair and capsulodesis. J Hand Surg Am. 1992;17(2):354–9.

14. Manuel J, Moran SL. The diagnosis and treatment of scapholunate instability. Hand Clin. 2010;26(1):129–44.

15. Minami A, Kato H, Iwasaki N. Treatment of scapholunate dissociation: ligamentous repair associated with modified dorsal capsulodesis. Hand Surg. 2003;8(1):1–6.

16. Park IJ, Lim D, Maniglio M, Shin SS, Chae S, Truong V, et al. Comparison of three different internal brace augmentation techniques for Scapholunate dissociation: a cadaveric biomechanical study. J Clin Med. 2021;10(7):1482.

17. Park IJ, Maniglio M, Shin SS, Lim D, McGarry MH, Lee TQ. Internal bracing augmentation for Scapholunate interosseous ligament repair: a cadaveric biomechanical study. J Hand Surg Am. 2020;45:985.e1–9.

18. Pliefke J, Stengel D, Rademacher G, Mutze S, Ekkernkamp A, Eisenschenk A. Diagnostic accuracy of plain radiographs and cineradiography in diagnosing traumatic scapholunate dissociation. Skeletal Radiol. 2008;37(2):139–45.

19. Pomerance J. Outcome after repair of the scapholunate interosseous ligament and dorsal capsulodesis for dynamic scapholunate instability due to trauma. J Hand Surg Am. 2006;31(8):1380–6.

20. Rohman EM, Agel J, Putnam MD, Adams JE. Scapholunate interosseous ligament injuries: a retrospective review of treatment and outcomes in 82 wrists. J Hand Surg Am. 2014;39(10):2020–6.

21. Shibayama H, Matsui Y, Kawamura D, Momma D, Endo T, Iwasaki N. Minimum 5-year outcomes of dorsal Intercarpal ligament Capsulodesis with Scapholunate interosseous ligament repair for subacute and chronic static Scapholunate instability: a clinical series of 5 patients. J Hand Surg Glob Online. 2022;4(3):162–5.

22. Shin SS, Moore DC, McGovern RD, Weiss AP. Scapholunate ligament reconstruction using a bone-retinaculum-bone autograft: a biomechanic and histologic study. J Hand Surg Am. 1998;23(2):216–21.

23. Soreide E, Denbeigh JM, Lewallen EA, Thaler R, Xu W, Berglund L, et al. In vivo assessment of high-molecular-weight polyethylene core suture tape for intra-articular ligament reconstruction: an animal study. Bone Joint J. 2019;101-B(10):1238–47.

24. Szabo RM. Scapholunate ligament repair with capsulodesis reinforcement. J Hand Surg Am. 2008;33(9):1645–54.

25. Thompson RG, Dustin JA, Roper DK, Kane SM, Lourie GM. Suture tape augmentation for Scapholunate ligament repair: a biomechanical study. J Hand Surg Am. 2021;46(1):36–42.

26. Ward PJ, Fowler JR. Scapholunate ligament tears: acute reconstructive options. Orthop Clin North Am. 2015;46(4):551–9.

27. Watson HK, Ballet FL. The SLAC wrist: scapholunate advanced collapse pattern of degenerative arthritis. J Hand Surg Am. 1984;9(3):358–65.
28. Weiss AP. Scapholunate ligament reconstruction using a bone-retinaculum-bone autograft. J Hand Surg Am. 1998;23(2):205–15.
29. Zbeda RM, Lee SJ. Internal brace for carpal instability. Wrist and Elbow Arthroscopy with Selected Open Procedures: Springer; 2022. p. 203–15.

Chapter 13
Chronic, Reducible Scapholunate Ligament Injury: Arthroscopic Supercapsuloplasty

Gustavo Mantovani Ruggiero and Marcio Aurelio Aita

Introduction

Scapholunate ligament (SL) injuries pose a challenging dilemma in hand surgery, requiring precise diagnosis and prompt intervention to restore optimal hand function. Over the past two decades, numerous advancements have been made in the management of scapholunate injuries, with a particular focus on arthroscopic techniques [3, 8, 9, 13]. This chapter aims to provide a comprehensive overview of a new surgical technique based on the principles of arthroscopic capsuloplasty for the treatment of chronic and reducible scapholunate ligament injuries.

The scapholunate ligament, a critical stabilizer of the wrist joint, is frequently implicated in traumatic injuries, such as falls on an outstretched hand or high-energy trauma [11, 16, 18]. Untreated scapholunate ligament injuries can result in chronic pain, restricted range of motion, and ultimately, wrist instability [4]. Early recognition and appropriate management of these injuries are vital to prevent long-term sequelae [11, 18].

Recent understanding of wrist anatomy and biomechanics has shown that the SL joint is stabilized by a complex of ligaments and capsular insertions, including the SL intrinsic ligament (SLIL), the Dorsal Intercarpal Ligament (DICL), Dorsal Radiocarpal Ligament (DRCL), Radioscaphocapitate Ligament (RSCL), Long

G. M. Ruggiero (✉)
Hospital Beneficencia Portuguesa de São Paulo, São Paulo Hand Center, Sao Paulo, SP, Brazil

Universita Degli Studi di Milano, Milano, MI, Italy
e-mail: dr.mantovani@redeopera.com

M. A. Aita
Centro Universitário FMABC (ABC Medical School) ABC Hand Center, Santo André, SP, Brazil

J. Yao (ed.), *Carpal Instability*, https://doi.org/10.1007/978-3-031-55869-6_13

Radiolunate Ligament (LRLL), Scaphotrapezium-Trapezoid volar ligaments (STTL), and all the capsular insertions between those structures which include a very important connection recently described as Dorsal Capsular Scapholunate Septum (DCSS) [3, 4, 14, 19]. The capsule also plays a paramount function in vascular supply for the bones and ligaments and proprioception and innervation, responsible for the action of the dynamic stabilizers of the SL joint [3, 5, 18]. In this new context, arthroscopic techniques, by sparing the capsule and the extrinsic ligamentous components of the SL complex, may provide a more reliable result and avoid the frequent complications involved in the technically complex traditional open reconstruction techniques, often focused mainly on the SLIL reconstruction, neglecting the relevance of the other accessory stabilizers of the SL joint [3, 5, 13].

Several techniques using flaps from the dorsal capsule and extrinsic ligaments to reinforce the SLIL were described and the literature reports satisfactory results [15, 17, 20]. Lately, arthroscopic capsuloplasty has emerged as an effective option for treating scapholunate ligament injuries [13, 18]. These procedures offer several advantages by employing minimally invasive techniques including: improved visualization, reduced soft tissue disruption, and decreased postoperative morbidity [6, 7, 10, 12]. However, the literature advocates the use of capsuloplasty techniques for partial injuries and less severe presentations of instability [1, 8, 9].

The cornerstone of arthroscopic capsuloplasty involves thorough debridement of the injured ligament, followed by the reconstruction or augmentation of the scapholunate interosseous ligament using the adjacent capsule insertions. To perform it properly and effectively, minimal soft tissue conditions involving the SLIL and adjacent capsule are necessary [6, 7, 10, 12]. For the patients classified in the worst stages in the different classification methods only tenoplasty techniques using bone tunnels and tendon grafts could be applied. These injuries include those with non-repairable SLIL, chronic injuries, with no proper remnants of the SL or capsular attachments [1, 8, 9, 13, 16].

This chapter introduces a technique that expands the indications for arthroscopic capsuloplasty. This technique capitalizes on sutures anchored in the stronger portions of the DICL within the midcarpal joint, combined with attachments of the DRCL and dorsal capsule. It promotes a stronger shortening effect of the DICL and the DRCL besides a capsulodesis effect on the SL joint, effectively recreating the function of the DCSS [3, 12, 14]. The robust mechanical effect of this technique, validated through cadaveric specimens (Fig. 13.1) and subsequent clinical application, contributes to the restoration of SL joint stability. The proposed technique enhances the traditional indications and effectiveness of arthroscopic capsuloplasties, thus earning our designation of "Supercapsuloplasty."

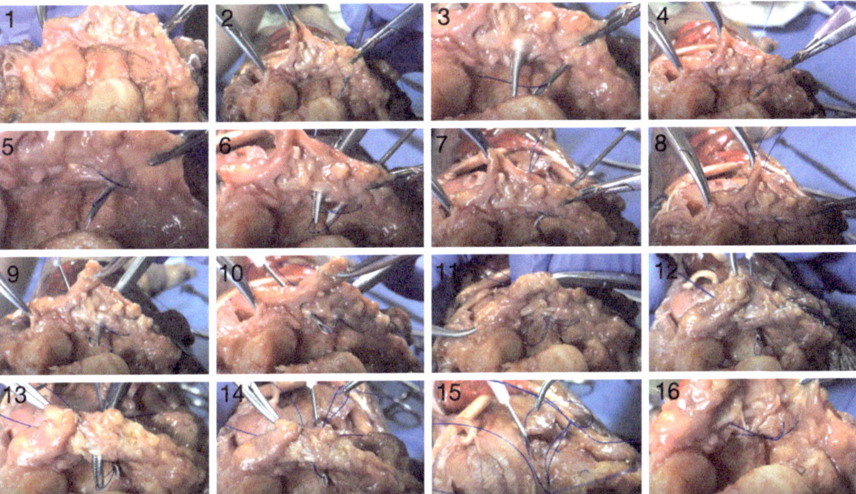

Fig. 13.1 Cadaver specimen validation of the Supercapsuloplasty, showing a strong mechanical effect reducing a provoked SL instability Grade 4, with complete resection of the SLIL and the adjacent attachments to the dorsal aspect of the SL joint of the capsule (DCSS). The figure shows the main sutures on the DICL through a direct vision of the midcarpal joint step by step

Indications

The indications for arthroscopic capsuloplasty techniques, as well as other alternative techniques, are influenced by the degree of instability and the combination of anatomic conditions affecting the various stabilizers of the scapholunate (SL) joint. Arthroscopy provides a comprehensive evaluation of the joint, enabling the identification of specific lesions and guiding the most appropriate surgical intervention [8, 9, 13, 18].

The literature suggests that arthroscopic capsuloplasty is effective in treating mild to moderate SL instabilities. These instabilities typically involve ligamentous laxity, subluxation, or partial disruption of the SL complex. Arthroscopic techniques offer the advantage of minimal invasiveness, allowing for precise repair or reconstruction of damaged ligaments while preserving the surrounding structures [5].

In cases of more severe instabilities, such as Geissler stage 3 or 4, alternative techniques may be necessary. The malalignment of carpal bones observed in static images (X-ray, CT, MRI) serves as a negative prognostic factor, indicating more severe instability known as static SL instability. For such cases, the current literature does not recommend capsuloplasty techniques but instead suggests ligament reconstruction techniques using tendon grafts and bone tunnels, performed either arthroscopically or through open surgery. Intraoperatively, other important factors to consider when determining the appropriate treatment include the reducibility of the malalignment and the status of the cartilage [9]. In instances where the chronicity of the injury may lead to unmanageable stiffness or cartilage damage (Scapho-Lunate Advanced Collapse—SLAC wrist), salvage procedures and bone fusions may be necessary [2, 9].

Furthermore, the combination of anatomic conditions affecting the different stabilizers of the SL joint is a crucial aspect to consider when selecting the appropriate technique. The literature emphasizes the importance of evaluating not only the SL ligament but also other supporting structures, such as the DICL, lunotriquetral ligament, and volar and dorsal radiocarpal ligaments. Depending on the specific combination of injuries and the integrity of these stabilizers, the choice of technique may vary. Since the main effect of the supercapsuloplasty depends on the shortening of the DICL and its action on the scaphoid and triquetrum, it is indispensable to have the integrity of the DICL insertions on both bones. If the DICL insertions are compromised, techniques that specifically address this structure, such use of bone anchors to reinsert this ligament, may be preferred to provide optimal stability and prevent a recurrence [9, 13, 16].

It is important to note that individual patient factors, including age, activity level, and associated wrist pathologies, should also be taken into account when determining the most appropriate technique. A comprehensive evaluation and a tailored treatment approach are paramount to achieving better outcomes [9, 13, 16].

In summary, the literature highlights the indications for arthroscopic capsuloplasty techniques, as well as alternative techniques, depending on the degree of instability and the combination of anatomic conditions affecting the different stabilizers of the SL joint. Mild to moderate instabilities can often be effectively managed with arthroscopic capsuloplasty, while more severe instabilities may require combined procedures or alternative techniques. The selection of the most suitable technique should be based on a thorough assessment of the specific injury pattern, the integrity of the supporting structures, and the individual characteristics of the patient [5, 9].

Additionally, we emphasize the paramount importance of arthroscopic assessment in treating SL instabilities. Without arthroscopic evaluation, it is challenging and inaccurate to diagnose the exact pattern of combined injuries involving the different components of the SL complex. Relying solely on preoperative imaging exams for open technique selection may be one of the factors that explain the actual failure rates on those techniques [3, 10].

Regarding the supercapsuloplasty technique, as previously mentioned, it represents an advancement in the current capsuloplasty techniques, expanding their indications before considering more aggressive, complex, and risky ligament reconstructions using tendon grafts. The details of this technique will be thoroughly described in this chapter, highlighting its reliance on the integrity of the attachments of the dorsal intercarpal ligament (DICL). Recent understanding has shed light on the DICL as a major stabilizer of the scapholunate (SL) joint, serving as a secondary stabilizer also to the lunotriquetral (LT) joint. This ligament exhibits strength and is easily identifiable during midcarpal joint arthroscopy [3, 4].

The key aspect of the supercapsuloplasty technique involves anchoring the capsuloplasty sutures on the DICL, which provides a significantly stronger and more reliable mechanical effect in reducing and stabilizing the SL joint. This anchoring not only involves fibers from the DICL but also incorporates those from the dorsal radiocarpal ligament (DRCL), thus recreating the dorsal capsular shift and sling effect, maximizing the strength of the reconstruction, and recovering the mechanical effect of the DCSS [3, 14, 19].

As a result, the indications for the supercapsuloplasty technique encompass both dynamic and static SL instabilities, including chronic cases ranging from stage 3 to 4 (Geissler). The requisite conditions for achieving favorable outcomes with this technique are the reducibility of the SL joint and the integrity of the DICL insertions on both the scaphoid and triquetrum [4, 16, 19].

By incorporating the supercapsuloplasty technique into the treatment algorithm for SL instabilities, surgeons can broaden the scope of indications for capsuloplasty procedures. This innovative approach offers a valuable alternative to more extensive ligament reconstructions, allowing for improved outcomes while minimizing the inherent risks associated with complex tendon graft procedures. The subsequent sections of this chapter will provide a comprehensive description of the supercapsuloplasty technique, including its surgical nuances, outcomes, and potential complications.

Technique Description

The arthroscopic supercapsuloplasty technique is performed using conventional wrist arthroscopy portals (3–4; 6R; MCR; MCU). The procedure starts with a thorough joint inventory and diagnostic evaluation. Diagnostic criteria include assessing SL dissociation, instability stage (based on EWAS or Geissler classification), and cartilage condition (to rule out SLAC wrist). The integrity of the DICL insertions on the dorsum of the scaphoid and triquetrum is assessed using an arthroscopic maneuver that our team baptized the "Tug of War" sign, where the probe is used to evaluate the movement of the bones (scaphoid and triquetrum) when pulled by the dorsal capsule and DICL attachments.

Once the necessary conditions for supercapsuloplasty are confirmed, joint debridement and synovectomy are performed. Bone scarring on the dorsal aspect of the proximal pole of the scaphoid and lunate may be done in chronic cases to promote stronger scar adhesions between the imbricated DICL, capsule, and SL joint (Figs. 13.2.1 and 13.3c, d).

The supercapsuloplasty step-by-step technique is summarized in Fig. 13.2. This technique involves creating two "lassos" anchored on the DICL, one on the middle part of the scaphoid insertions and the other on the dorsum of the lunotriquetral joint

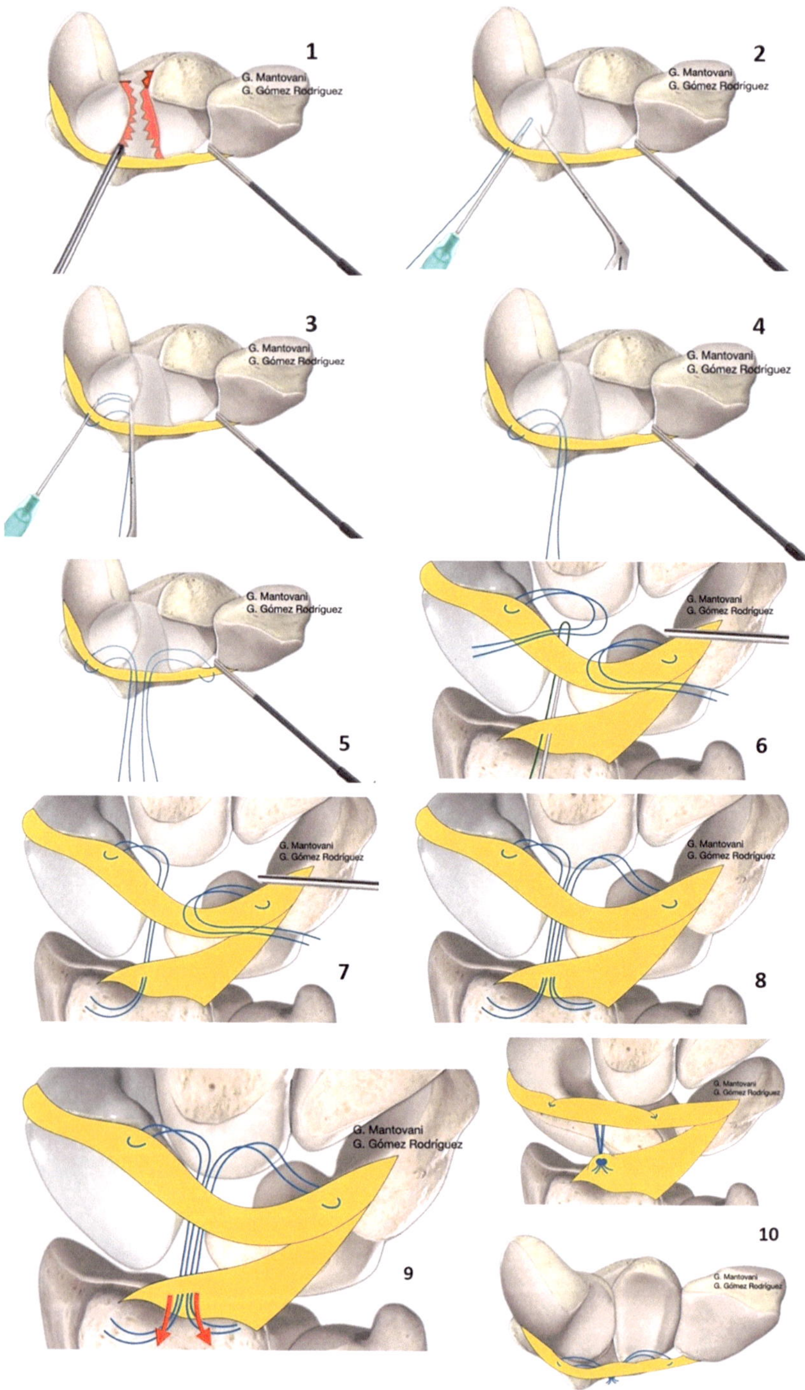

Fig. 13.2 Supercapsuloplasty suture step-by-step schematic

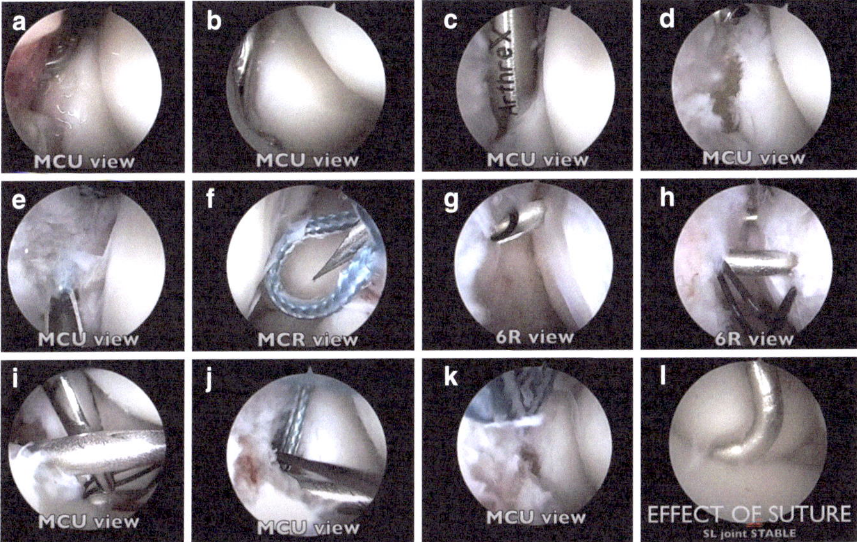

Fig. 13.3 Arthroscopic step-by-step procedure performed on the clinical case

(Figs. 13.2.2, 13.2.3, 13.2.4, 13.2.5, and 13.3e, f). The lasso sutures are retrieved through midcarpal portals. Two new sutures are passed through the dorsal capsule close to the 3–4 portal in a similar manner to Mathoulin's described capsuloplasty [12], using looped sutures instead of single sutures (Figs. 13.2.6 and 13.3g, h). These loops are retrieved through midcarpal portals, and the double sutures from the supercapsuloplasty are passed through the SL joint back to the radiocarpal joint, exiting through the 3–4 Skin Portal (Figs. 13.2.7, 13.2.8, 13.2.9, and 13.3i–k). This configuration results in a four-point anchored suture on the DICL, dorsal capsule, and dorsal radiocarpal ligament (DRCL), which provides a shortening effect on the DICL, re-tensioning of the DRCL and capsule, and a bulky tissue over the SL joint, recreating the labrum-like effect of the DICL and DCSS [3, 14] (Figs. 13.2.10 and 13.3l).

Technique Variations

If the DICL insertions are found to be ruptured from the scaphoid or triquetrum, a bone anchor can be used to restore these attachments. The technique remains the same, using the anchor threads after a first knot to the capsule, as one of the two "lasso" sutures.

Postoperative Care

Considering that the supercapsuloplasty technique is indicated for reducible SL joint situations, where intraoperative reduction and significant stability are achieved and confirmed arthroscopically, K-wire fixation is not recommended. Following the surgery, postoperative care involves the use of a palmar removable splint set in a slightly extended position (20°) for 6 weeks, which is sufficient to prevent suture stress. Active and passive mobilization of the wrist, ranging from 0° of flexion to full extension, is initiated as early as the first week after the operation. Weight-bearing activities are strictly prohibited during the initial 6-week period.

After 6 weeks, a natural gain of flexion is encouraged over 2 weeks (from 6 to 8 weeks postoperatively). Subsequently, hand therapy is initiated to facilitate complete flexion and extension without any restrictions on force or exercises. Contact sports are permissible after 12 weeks of postoperative recovery.

Case Report

An illustrative case report is presented of a male patient, 34 years old, who sustained a traumatic injury on his right (dominant) hand, during a soccer game 8 months before the consultation. The patient did not receive any specific orthopedic treatment initially but complained of pain on the dorsal aspect of the wrist and limited wrist flexion and extension. X-rays revealed a slight increase in the scapholunate (SL) angle and SL space, while MRI showed a complete rupture of the SL ligament without any associated injuries.

Arthroscopy was performed, revealing good cartilage condition. Complete avulsion of the SL ligament from the proximal pole of the scaphoid, as well as avulsion of the capsule and dorsal intercarpal ligament (DIC) from the proximal part of the scaphoid, were observed (Fig. 13.3a). The SL joint instability was classified as stage 4 according to the Geissler classification and stage 5 on the EWAS classification (Figs. 13.3a, b). The "Tug of War" sign was positive on both the scaphoid and triquetrum, indicating the integrity of the DIC attachments and dorsal capsule on both bones. Accordingly, a supercapsuloplasty procedure was performed using a high-resistance number 2 suture (Figs. 13.3e–k). Intraoperatively, the stability increased to stage 2 of the Geissler/EWAS classification upon tying the sutures (Fig. 13.3l). A standard postoperative protocol was followed.

At 6-month postoperative follow-up, the patient exhibited a grip strength of 50 kgF in the left hand and 45 kgF in the right hand, with a mild restriction of flexion (−20° compared to the opposite side) but a normal extension and full prono-supination. The patient was able to return to sports and regular activities without experiencing pain or restrictions. Subsequent MRI evaluations demonstrated a favorable SL angle, improved relationships, and good congruency between the proximal pole of the scaphoid and the radius scaphoid fossa, suggesting resolution of the SL dissociation (Figs. 13.4 and 13.5).

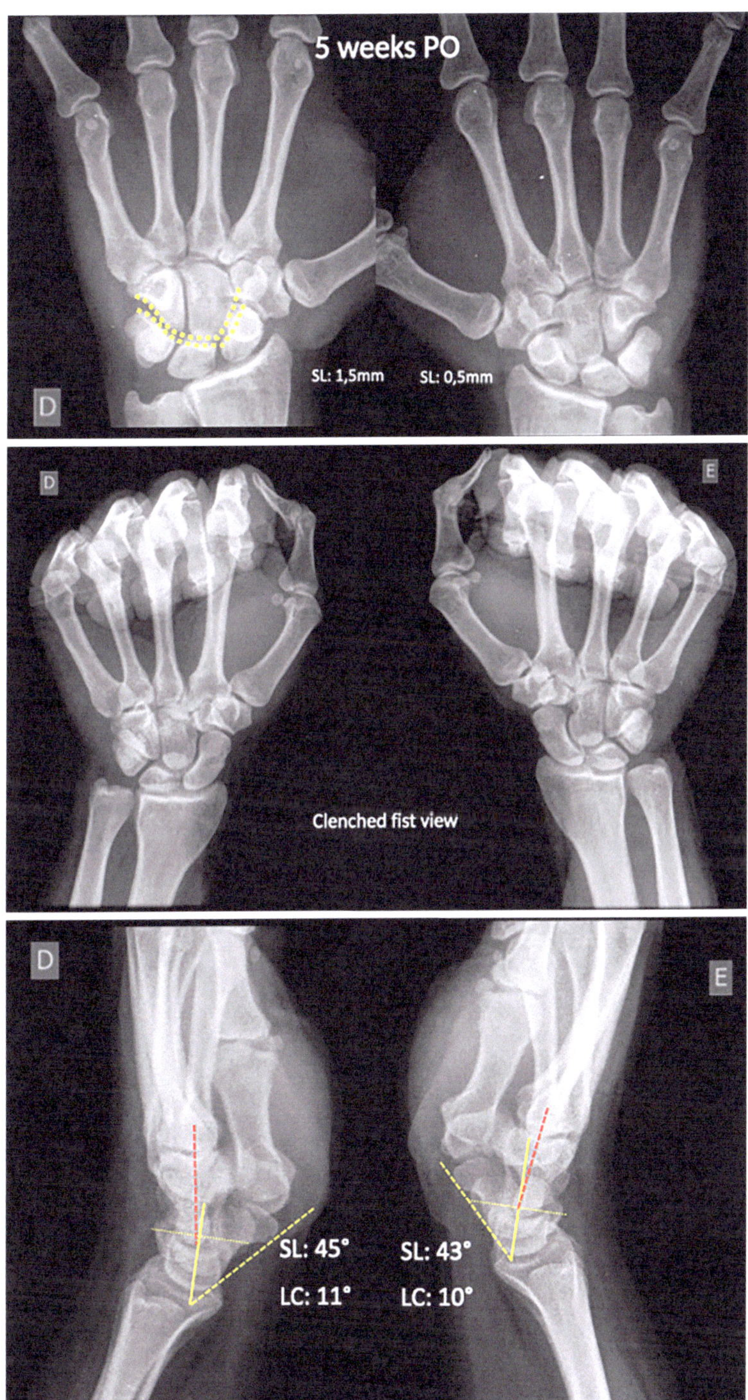

Fig. 13.4 Preoperative and postoperative imaging exams of the patient

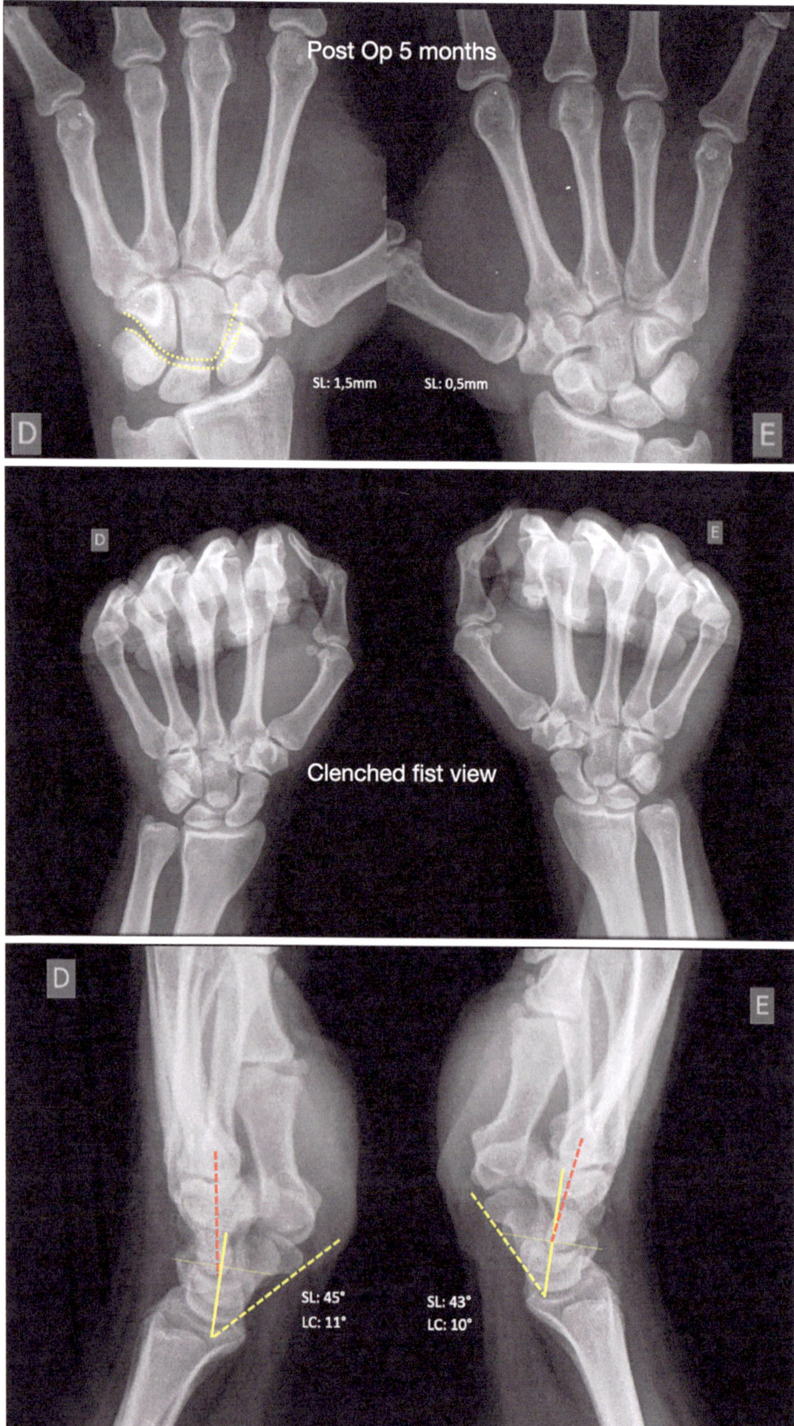

Fig. 13.4 (continued)

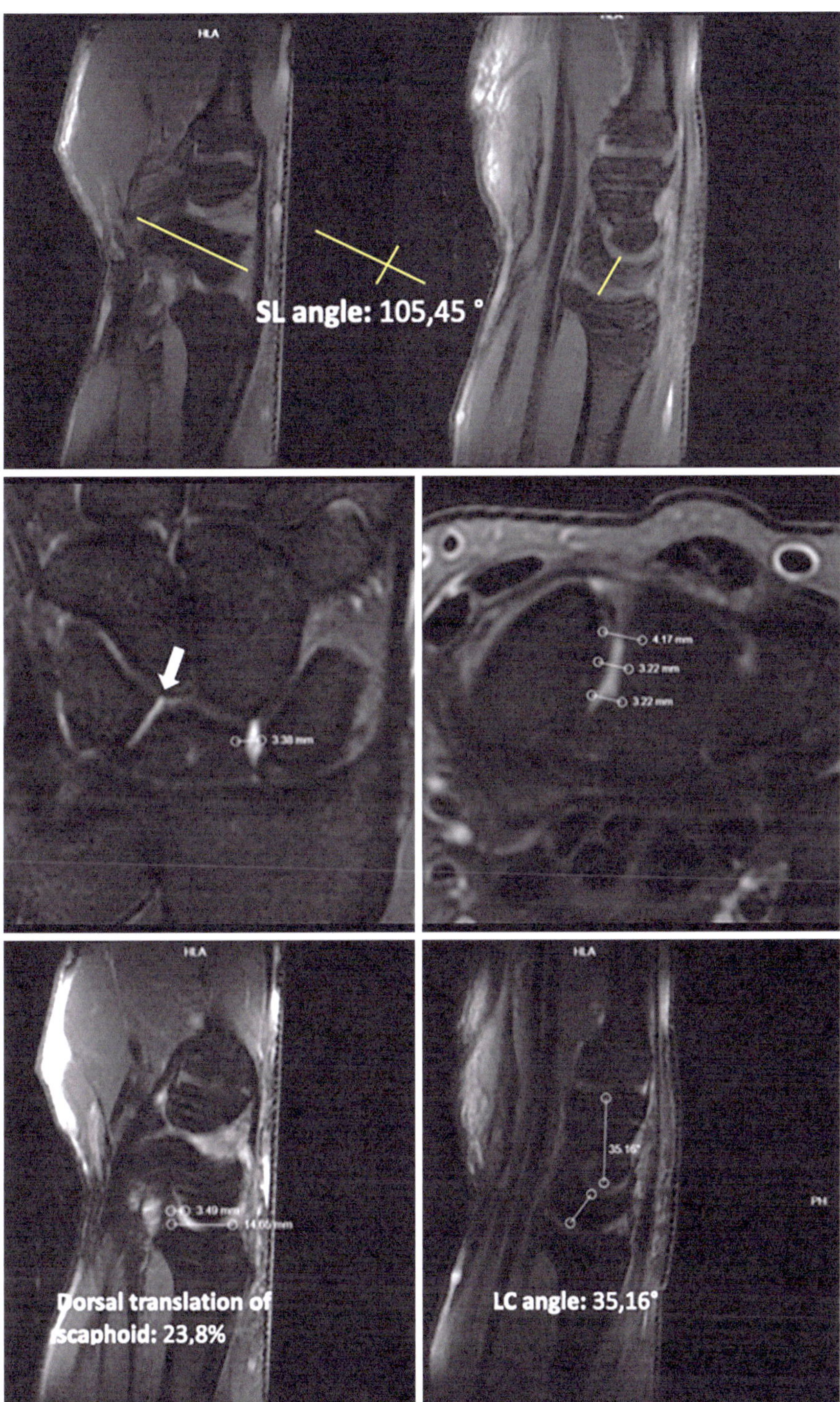

Fig. 13.4 (continued)

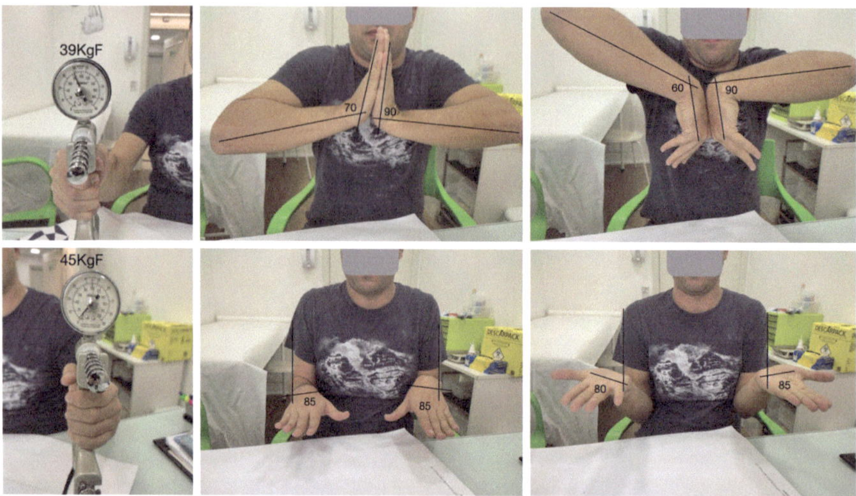

Fig. 13.5 Post op clinical results of the patient

Risks and Complications

Since this is a recent technical variation, no longer follow-up and revised series are yet available to understand the specific long-term complications involved with this option. However, some special steps of the procedure raise specific concerns and attention.

During the creation of the anchoring "lassos" through the "back and forward" maneuver, there is a risk of tendon entrapment. When the needle is first retracted out of the capsule, the surgeon must have the delicate sensitive haptic feedback to perceive the tip of the needle exactly on the level of the superficial dorsal aspect of the articular capsule and move the needle more superficial than that (extensor tendon layer) under the risk of inadvertently capturing tendinous structures during the second entrance of the needle. This technique of creating the capsular "lasso" (back and forward), if properly performed using the aforementioned care, can be applied through an intact skin entry point since the final "lasso" stays only at the capsule layer, not affecting the surrounding tissues (nerves and tendons) even if they were in the trajectory of the needle.

An important step to prevent tendon entrapment relies on testing passive flexion and extension of the fingers and tenodesis effect, out of the traction just before performing the final knot of the supercapsuloplasty. In case of non-symmetric tenodesis motion found in any of the fingers, or some resistance is present during the passive flexion, there is a high probability of having an extensor tendon entrapment in the supercapsuloplasty suture, and thus removing the suture and repeating the procedure is recommended.

Discussion

Arthroscopic capsuloplasty has demonstrated promising results in the treatment of chronic scapholunate ligament tears [6, 7, 10, 12]. Providing a less invasive alternative to open exposure techniques, it offers a viable option for patients who may benefit from a reduced surgical burden. Furthermore, the procedure has proven effective in addressing dorsal wrist capsular avulsions associated with scapholunate instability, thereby aiming to enhance stability and restore wrist function [10, 12]. Additionally, arthroscopic capsuloplasty has been employed in pre-dynamic, dynamic instability, and DCSS lesions, offering a surgical avenue to manage these conditions [10, 12, 14].

However, it is crucial to consider the restrictions associated with arthroscopic capsuloplasty. Not all cases of scapholunate injuries are suitable for this technique, particularly certain clinical forms of dorsal scapholunate ligament injury [1, 9]. The choice of surgical technique should be tailored to the individual characteristics and needs of the patient. Skill and experience also play a significant role in the successful execution of arthroscopic capsuloplasty. Given the specialized nature of wrist arthroscopy, proficiency in this technique is paramount to ensuring optimal outcomes and minimizing potential complications.

While the literature results of different arthroscopic and open capsuloplasty techniques appear promising, the long-term outcomes and durability of the procedure warrant further investigation [3, 6, 7, 10, 12, 15, 17, 20]. It is also important to note that the literature specifically addresses earlier stages of scapholunate (SL) instabilities, and few to no detailed information on the treatment and good outcome of more severe cases (stage 4) using arthroscopic capsuloplasty can be found [6, 7, 10, 12]. Stage 4 SL instabilities typically entail complete disruption of the SL ligament and other extrinsic ligaments part of the SL complex, accompanied by significant carpal instability. In such instances, treatment options often necessitate more extensive procedures, such as ligament reconstruction or salvage procedures like wrist partial fusions [1, 2, 8, 9].

The novel arthroscopic supercapsuloplasty technique described in this chapter introduces several notable advantages over existing techniques. One of its key benefits lies in its ability to effectively reduce and constrain even more severe instabilities, including stage 4 SL injuries [1, 8, 9, 15]. While traditional techniques may yield suboptimal outcomes for advanced-stage instabilities, the new technique demonstrates improved results, even in cases of combined instabilities with concurrent lunotriquetral dissociation and DICL insufficiency, effectively addressed by the supercapsuloplasty procedure [3, 4].

Furthermore, the new technique offers the advantage of reinforcing and shortening the Dorsal Intercarpal Ligament (DICL), a component from the SL complex considered pivotal for restoring normal wrist biomechanics in SL instabilities [3]. By addressing this crucial component, the new technique enhances long-term stability and mitigates the risk of degenerative changes to an SLAC wrist [19].

Simplicity and ease of execution also distinguish the new technique from its counterparts. Complex procedures described in the literature often involve intricate steps, bone tunnels, or implants, which can present technical challenges and protracted surgical durations [9]. In contrast, the new technique's streamlined approach simplifies its execution and facilitates teaching, thereby reducing the learning curve for surgeons and potentially broadening its accessibility to a wider range of practitioners [3, 9, 18].

The cost-effectiveness of the new technique merits consideration as well. Traditional techniques often entail the use of implants, contributing to increased expenses [9, 13, 15]. The absence of implants in the new technique reduces costs, rendering it a more economically viable option for patients and healthcare systems alike.

Additionally, the reduced use of radiation distinguishes the new technique as a safer alternative. Traditional approaches frequently necessitate imaging guidance due to bone tunnels or implants, thereby increasing radiation exposure [9]. In contrast, the new technique circumvents these requirements, minimizing radiation usage and enhancing the safety of both patients and the surgical team while concurrently reducing procedural time.

The new technique also offers advantages in terms of surgical efficiency. Compared to techniques proposed in the literature for the more severe indications, the new approach enables faster surgeries [9]. Traditional methods often involve intricate steps and lengthier operative times, whereas the streamlined nature of the new technique saves valuable operating room time, affording more efficient surgical procedures.

Finally, the new arthroscopic supercapsuloplasty technique exhibits superior biomechanical strength when compared to previously described capsuloplasties techniques, showing a clinical perception of efficiency when closing the SL space and stabilizing the SL joint. Through its anchoring of the sutures in a strong ligament like the DICL, the new technique provides the necessary biomechanical strength to ensure its effectiveness even in more severe SL instabilities presentations, where the usual surgical option was the tenoplasties reconstructions [9].

In conclusion, the new arthroscopic supercapsuloplasty technique presented in this chapter represents a significant advancement in the treatment of scapholunate (SL) injuries. With its capacity to address severe instabilities, reinforce the DICL, its simplicity of execution, cost-effectiveness, reduced use of radiation, faster surgery, and improved biomechanical strength, this technique holds great promise for achieving favorable clinical outcomes and enhancing the quality of life for patients with SL injuries. However, it is important to acknowledge that as a novel technique, long-term clinical follow-up data is currently unavailable. Further studies will be required to establish this technique as a routine practice option, providing a comprehensive understanding of its long-term efficacy and potential complications.

References

1. Andersson JK, Garcia-Elias M. Dorsal scapholunate ligament injury: classification of clinical forms. J Hand Surg. 2013;38(2):165–9. https://doi.org/10.1177/1753193412441124.
2. Atzei A, Luchetti R. Treatment of scapholunate advanced collapse wrist with an original technique of arthroscopic debridement and limited intercarpal fusion: preliminary report. Tech Hand Up Extrem Surg. 2017;21(1):7–14. https://doi.org/10.1097/BTH.0000000000000152.
3. Bain GI, Amarasooriya M. Scapholunate instability: why are the surgical outcomes still so far from ideal? J Hand Surg. 2023;48(3):257–68. https://doi.org/10.1177/17531934221148009.
4. Bain GI, Overstraten L. Anatomy of wrist ligaments. In: Scapholunate ligament injuries. Cham: Springer; 2018. p. 3–9.
5. Berger RA, Bishop AT, Bettinger PC. New dorsal capsulotomy for the surgical exposure of the wrist. Tech Hand Upper Extrem Surg. 1996;1(2):70–8. https://doi.org/10.1097/00130911-199601020-00001.
6. Degeorge B, Coulomb R, Kouyoumdjian P, Mares O. Arthroscopic dorsal Capsuloplasty in Scapholunate tears EWAS 3: preliminary results after a minimum follow-up of 1 year. J Wrist Surg. 2018;7(4):324–30. https://doi.org/10.1055/s-0038-1660446.
7. Del Pinal F, Garcia-Bernal FJ, Regalado J, Studer A. Arthroscopic dorsal capsuloligamentous repair for the treatment of scapholunate dissociation. J Hand Surg. 2012;37(4):343–51. https://doi.org/10.1177/1753193411434410.
8. Garcia-Elias M, Lluch A. Diagnostic arthroscopy of wrist instability. Arthroscopy: the journal of Arthroscopic & Related. Surgery. 1992;8(2):204–11. https://doi.org/10.1016/0749-8063(92)90085-R.
9. Garcia-Elias M, Lluch AL, Stanley JK. Three-ligament tenodesis for the treatment of scapholunate dissociation: indications and surgical technique. J Hand Surg Am. 2006 Jan;31(1):125–34. https://doi.org/10.1016/j.jhsa.2005.10.011.
10. Haerle M, Schmelzer-Schmied N, Lampert FM. Arthroscopic Capsulodesis for the treatment of dynamic Scapholunate dissociations. Tech Hand Up Extrem Surg. 2022;27:95. https://doi.org/10.1097/BTH.0000000000000418.
11. Jørgsholm P, Thomsen NO, Björkman A, Besjakov I, Abrahamsson SO, Englund M. Wrist arthroscopy versus magnetic resonance imaging for the diagnosis of scapholunate ligament tears: a systematic review. Arthroscopy: the journal of Arthroscopic & Related. Surgery. 2016;32(12):2568–74. https://doi.org/10.1016/j.arthro.2016.05.019.
12. Mathoulin C, Dauphin N, Sallen V. Arthroscopic dorsal capsuloplasty in chronic scapholunate ligament tears: a new procedure; preliminary report. Chir Main. 2011;30(3):188–97. https://doi.org/10.1016/j.main.2011.04.007.
13. Mathoulin C, Gras M. Role of wrist arthroscopy in scapholunate dissociation. Orthop Traumatol Surg Res. 2020;106(1S):S89–99. https://doi.org/10.1016/j.otsr.2019.07.008.
14. Overstraeten LV, Camus EJ, Wahegaonkar A, Messina J, Tandara AA, Binder AC, Mathoulin CL. Anatomical description of the dorsal Capsulo-Scapholunate septum (DCSS)-arthroscopic staging of Scapholunate instability after DCSS sectioning. J Wrist Surg. 2013 May;2(2):149–54. https://doi.org/10.1055/s-0033-1338256.
15. Rosa ND, Sapino G, Vita F, di Summa PG, Adani R. Modified Viegas dorsal capsuloplasty for chronic partial injury of the scapholunate ligament in young athletes: outcomes at 24 months. J Hand Surg. 2020;45(9):945–51. https://doi.org/10.1177/1753193420939490.
16. Ruch DS, An KN. The interosseous ligament of the wrist. J Hand Surg Am. 2006;31(5):849–58. https://doi.org/10.1016/j.jhsa.2006.02.021.
17. Ruch DS, Yang CC, Smith BP, Kuzma GR, Bishop AT. Open dorsal capsulodesis for treatment of scapholunate instability. Tech Hand Up Extrem Surg. 2004;8(4):225–31. https://doi.org/10.1097/01.bth.0000131242.69459.7b.
18. Slutsky DJ, Osterman AL. Management of scapholunate instability. J Hand Surg. 2008;33(6):998–1013. https://doi.org/10.1016/j.jhsa.2008.03.017.

19. Taleisnik J. The ligaments of the wrist. J Hand Surg. 1976;1(2):110–8. https://doi.org/10.1016/S0363-5023(76)80024-8.
20. Watanabe T, Sasaki K, Tsunoda K, Otsuka T, Nishio J, Takeuchi E. Dynamic scapholunate ligamentoplasty using the dorsal cut of the radius. Tech Hand Up Extrem Surg. 2019;23(1):33–8. https://doi.org/10.1097/BTH.0000000000000219.

Chapter 14
Chronic, Reducible Scapholunate Ligament Injury: Arthroscopic Box Reconstruction

Pak-Cheong Ho

Case Presentation

A 39-year-old gentleman, right-handed banker presented to our clinic for his left wrist injury sustained 9 weeks previously. His left wrist was hit by a basketball from the volar aspect during a basketball competition. He denied any pain or injury to the left wrist before the episode. He developed central wrist pain acutely which was progressively worsening. He received no treatment initially and then went overseas for a medical consultation at around 1 month after the injury. Magnetic resonance imaging and computed topography revealed a complete tear of the scapholunate (SL) interosseous ligament and a wide dissociation of the SL joint with dorsal intercalated segmental instability (DISI) deformity of the left wrist. He underwent surgery there consisting of an arthroscopic-assisted reduction and percutaneous pinning of the SL joint, followed by below-elbow plaster cast immobilization. He came to seek our medical advice for post-operative care. The cast was removed for examination. The arthroscopic portal wounds had healed, and the pins were exposed with no evidence of pin track infection. There was no sign of chronic regional pain syndrome though considerable swelling in the wrist with limited finger movement noted. The palmaris longus (PL) tendon was present.

P.-C. Ho (✉)
Department of Orthopaedic and Traumatology, Prince of Wales Hospital, Hong Kong SAR, China
e-mail: pcho@cuhk.edu.hk

J. Yao (ed.), *Carpal Instability*, https://doi.org/10.1007/978-3-031-55869-6_14

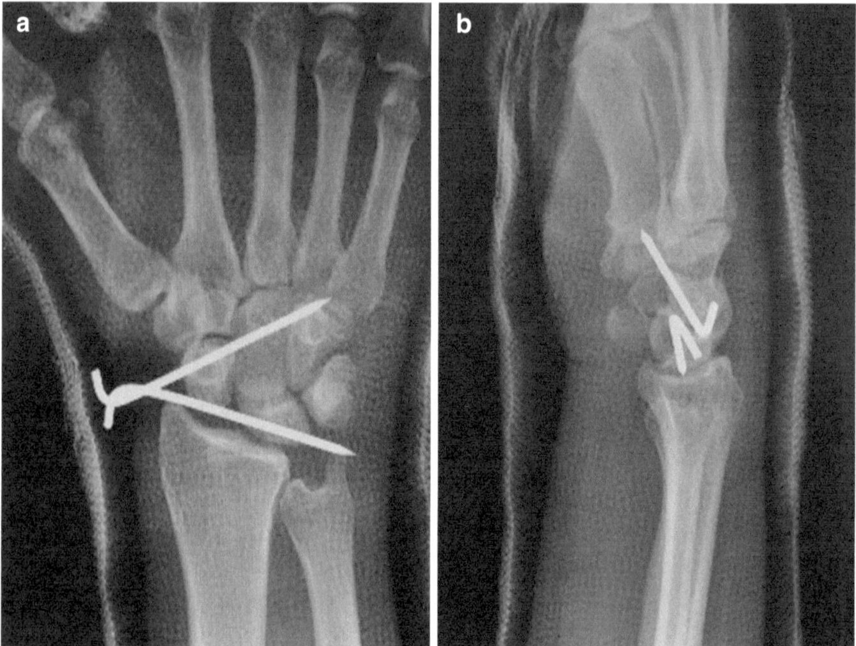

Fig. 14.1 X-ray of the left wrist after the operation overseas. (**a**) Posterior-anterior view. (**b**) Lateral view

Diagnosis

The plain radiographs were reviewed. Pinning was noted across the SL joint and the scapho-capitate joint. However, there was persistently wide gap of 4 mm between the scaphoid and lunate bone and the scaphoid was grossly malrotated. There was no sign of ongoing arthritis (Fig. 14.1). Radiograph of the opposite wrist was shown to be normal, indicating the unilaterality of the injury. The wrist was further assessed dynamically under a mobile mini-C arm by the author. The SL gap measured 6 mm compared to the 2 mm gap in the uninjured right wrist. Marked DISI deformity was noted, with no obvious dorsal subluxation of the scaphoid. There was no ulnar translocation of the lunate and the luno-triquetral joint interval was normal.

Management Options and Management Chosen for this Case with Rationale

In this patient with a severe SL dissociation of 9 weeks old, with the high likelihood of persistent pain, dysfunction, and progressive degeneration of the wrist, we offered a revision surgery to the patient. We discussed the treatment options thoroughly with the patient which included revision surgical repair of the SL ligament complex, tendon reconstruction, RASL procedure, proximal row carpectomy, and partial wrist fusion. We concluded to proceed to arthroscopic-assisted box reconstruction of the SL ligament with the PL tendon graft to restore the carpal alignment as much as possible. Informed consent was obtained, with the mutual understanding that open surgery might be required in case the dissociation was not possible to be reduced by percutaneous and/or arthroscopic means. If significant articular cartilage damage was found, a salvage procedure might need to be initiated.

Surgical Treatment

The pins were removed in the clinic and the revision surgery was scheduled in 2 weeks' time to enable a complete healing of the pin sites before the surgery to minimize risk of infection. The wrist was protected with a thermoplastic splint and the patient was referred to the physiotherapist to undergo mobilization exercise for the fingers and wrist.

The surgery was performed 2 weeks later under general anesthesia. The patient lied supine on the operating table. The wrist was stiff with 35° extension and 25° flexion. The range improved to 55° extension and 65° flexion after gentle manipulation. The wrist was first assessed fluoroscopically under a mini-C arm to evaluate the dissociation status and its passive reducibility. Posterior-anterior views were taken both in neutral and radial-deviated positions. It was noted that the wide SL joint gap of 7 mm in the neutral position only reduced by 2 mm even in a maximally radial-deviated position, signifying the non-reducibility of the SL dissociation. There was DISI deformity with a large SL angle of 84.8° without dorsal subluxation of the scaphoid (Fig. 14.2).

Wrist arthroscopy was conducted. The left hand was suspended in a sterilizable wrist traction tower through three plastic finger traps applied to the index, middle, and ring fingers. A traction force of 5 kg was applied with counter-traction provided by a broad Velcro band on the brachium. The arm and forearm of the patient were well padded to avoid pressure injury. A pneumatic tourniquet was placed on the arm loosely but was not inflated in the initial procedure. Under traction, the various standard arthroscopic portals in the radiocarpal and midcarpal joint were marked on the skin through thumb tip palpation. Lignocaine solution of 2% admixed with 1:200,000 adrenaline was injected into the skin and capsule of each portal using a 25G needle. The anesthetic mixture provided effective local hemostasis in the joint capsule and synovium, rendering the routine use of tourniquet unnecessary. The radiocarpal joint was then distended by injecting a few milliliters of saline through the 3–4 portal. Transverse skin incision was performed following the old scars wherever appropriate. An arthroscopic trocar and cannula for a 1.9 mm arthroscope was inserted gently through the portal. Extreme care was exercised to avoid inadvertent injury to the articular cartilage. The arthroscope was inserted, and the cannula

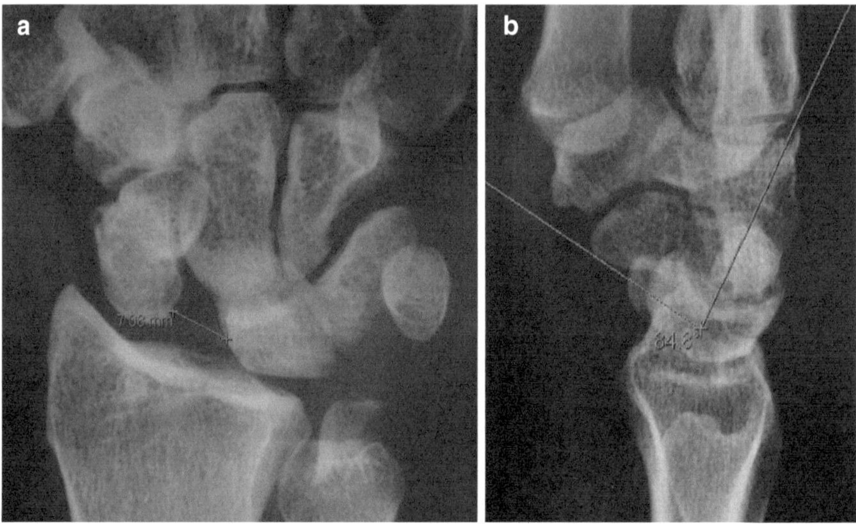

Fig. 14.2 X-ray of the left wrist after removing the K wires. (**a**) Posterior-anterior view, showing wide SL gap of 7.08 mm. (**b**) Lateral view, showing DISI deformity with SL angle of 84.8°

was connected by long tubing to a 3-L saline bag placed 1.5 m above the patient using a drip post.

It was anticipated that the surgery would not be straightforward due to prevailing scar and adhesions related to the index surgical procedure some 6 weeks before. Plenty of scar tissue was encountered in the radiocarpal joint, obliterating the view to assess intra-articular structures critically. With the help of an 18-G needle, the ideal site and trajectory of the 4–5 portal was established with confidence. The portal was gradually dilated to accommodate a 2 mm full radius shaver to start resecting the fibrous tissue inside the radiocarpal joint. Intra-articular structures were progressively exposed, showing the preservation of most articular cartilage except in a small area over the inter-condylar ridge of the distal radius just opposite to the radio-scapho-lunate ligament with full-thickness cartilage loss, likely due to previous surgical intervention. There was no sign of ongoing SLAC wrist changes. The SL interosseous ligament was completely torn with remnants retracted, but the opposing articular surfaces of scaphoid and lunate couldn't be reviewed readily. The volar and dorsal extrinsic ligaments were structurally intact though appeared markedly scarred and fibrotic. The scar tissue was cleared using the shaver and radiofrequency ablation. The debridement of the ligaments during the process helped to stress relax the contracted ligaments to regain motion.

The midcarpal joint was then viewed through the midcarpal radial (MCR) portal. Again, plenty of scar was noted and this was cleared with a 2 mm shaver and radiofrequency ablation. No cartilage lesion was noted. The luno-triquetral joint was normal, but the SL joint was markedly widened. The space was completely occupied with dense fibrous tissue, rendering drive-through sign invalid and the dissociation non-reducible (Fig. 14.3). All the scar tissues were resected carefully, with preservation of articular cartilage and functioning extrinsic ligaments.

After the arthroscopic arthrolysis procedure, the wrist was lifted off from the traction tower and subjected to evaluation under fluoroscopic assessment on a hand table. It was then noted that the wide gap of the SL joint could now be reduced in the maximally radial-deviated position, signifying a much-improved reducibility of the SL dissociation (Fig. 14.4). It was decided to proceed to arthroscopic-assisted box reconstruction of the SL ligament complex.

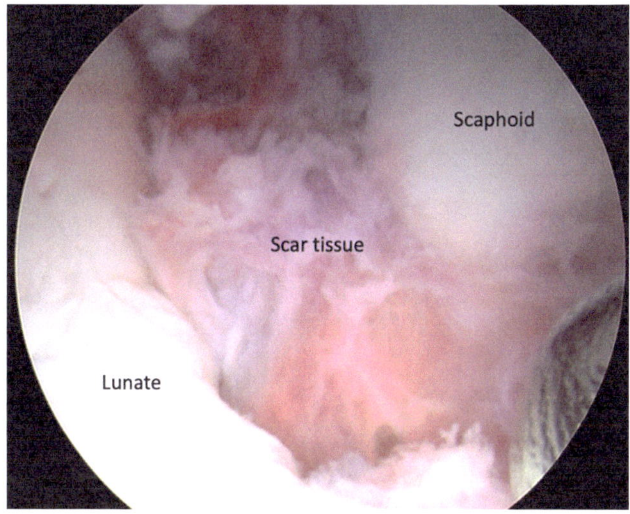

Fig. 14.3 Arthroscopic view at midcarpal joint, showing the wide gap at the scapholunate joint occupied with dense scar tissues, preventing its passive reducibility

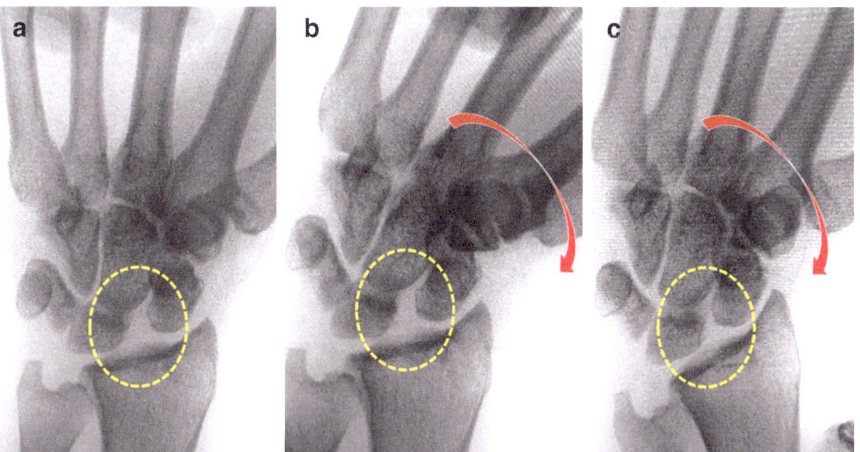

Fig. 14.4 Posterior-anterior X-ray view of the left wrist; (**a**) at neutral position, showing the wide SL gap; (**b**) at maximal radially deviated position before arthroscopic arthrolysis, showing that the SL gap did not change significantly from that at neutral position; (**c**) at maximal radially deviated position after arthroscopic arthrolysis. Noted that the SL gap had been largely reduced to near normal

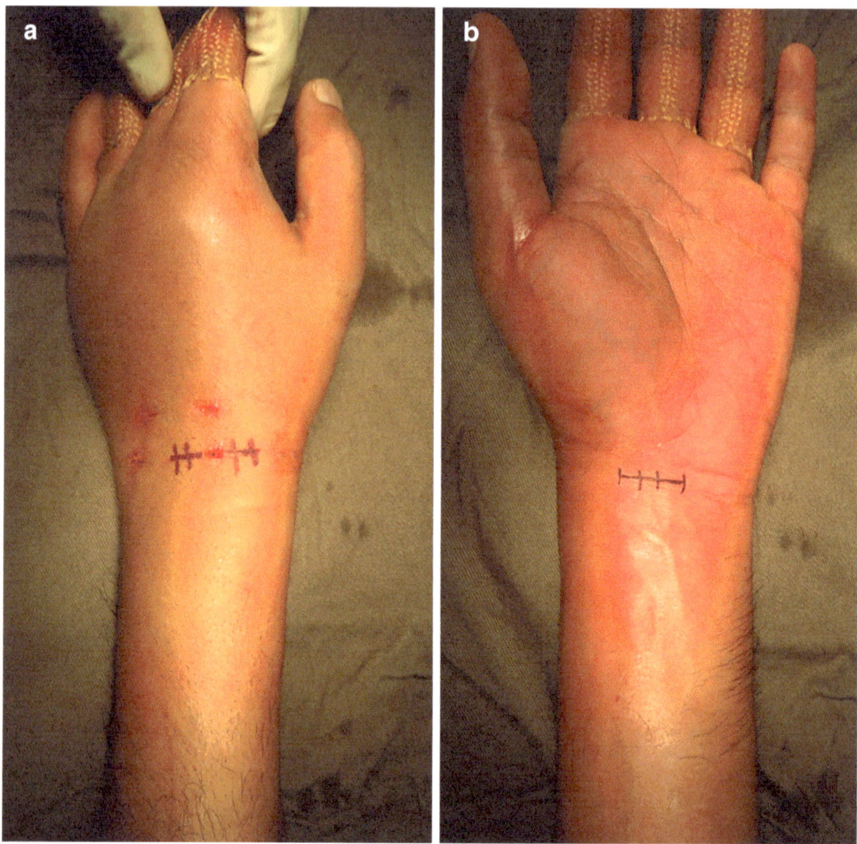

Fig. 14.5 Surgical incisions. (**a**) Dorsal incision, 2 cm transverse incision centering at 3–4 portal. (**b**) Volar incision along proximal wrist crease, extended from interval of FCR tendon to PL tendon

The arm tourniquet was inflated after limb exsanguination. A 2 cm transverse incision was extended from the 3–4 portal 1 cm radial and 1 cm ulnar to it (Fig. 14.5). Radially, the interval between the extensor carpi radialis brevis (ECRB) tendon and the extensor carpi radialis longus (ECRL) tendon just distal to the extensor retinaculum was identified. This interval usually corresponds well to the ideal position of the scaphoid tunnel (Fig. 14.6). The lunate was exposed by entering into the interval between the extensor digitorum communis tendons after splitting the extensor retinaculum along its oblique fibers. A transverse palmar incision of 2 cm was made along the proximal wrist crease from the radial border of the PL tendon to the ulnar border of the flexor carpi radialis (FCR) tendon, exactly at the same level of the dorsal incision. The palmar cutaneous branch of the median nerve was identified and protected with a silicone sling. Using a tendon stripper, a full length of the palmaris longus free graft was obtained. The tendon graft was stretched with a graft

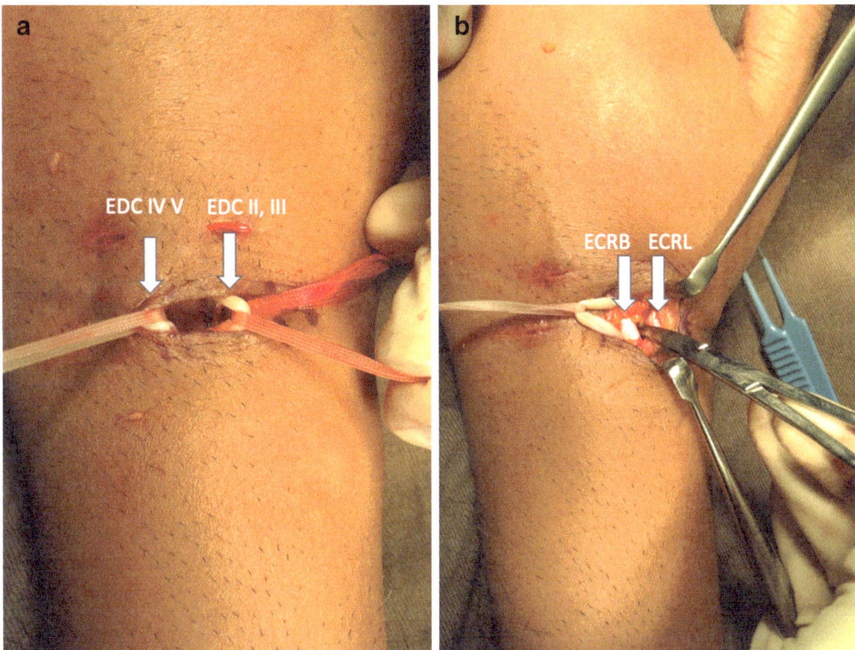

Fig. 14.6 Landmarks to establish bone tunnels. (**a**) Retracting between EDC tendon interval to expose dorsal central lunate. (**b**) Retracting between ECRL and ECRB tendon to expose dorsal proximal scaphoid

tensioner. The anterior forearm fascia was then incised. The interval between the FCR tendon, and the finger flexor tendons and median nerve was entered to reach the volar wrist joint capsule and its palmar extrinsic ligaments. The volar and dorsal wrist joint capsule were not violated (Fig. 14.7). The soft tissue dissection was kept to a minimum to maximally preserve the vascular supply and innervation. The wrist was then ready for bone tunnel preparation.

The hand was turned to the dorsal side. While the chief surgeon was operating on the dorsal side of the wrist, a reliable assistant surgeon should sit opposite the operating surgeon to help manage the structures in the volar wound area. Under fluoroscopic guidance, a 1.1 mm guide pin was inserted via a protective sheath into the proximal scaphoid, through the dorsal capsule at the interval between ECRB and ECRL tendons, aiming at a site more distal to the guide pin entry site of the lunate, and was directed proximally and volarly, to provide a better counter-rotational force on the scaphoid to correct the typical flexion and pronation deformity (Fig. 14.8). The drill hole should be made at least 2–3 mm from all the surrounding articular margins to avoid iatrogenic fracture. Copious fluid irrigation was performed to prevent over-heating during the drilling process. Onto the volar side, with the FCR tendon retracted radially, the scaphoid pin exited through the volar wound. Back to

Fig. 14.7 Through the volar incision, the volar wrist capsule is exposed by retracting the FCR tendon to the radial side, and the finger flexor tendons and median nerve to the ulnar side. Noted that the palmar cutaneous branch of the median nerve is safeguarded by a silicone loop

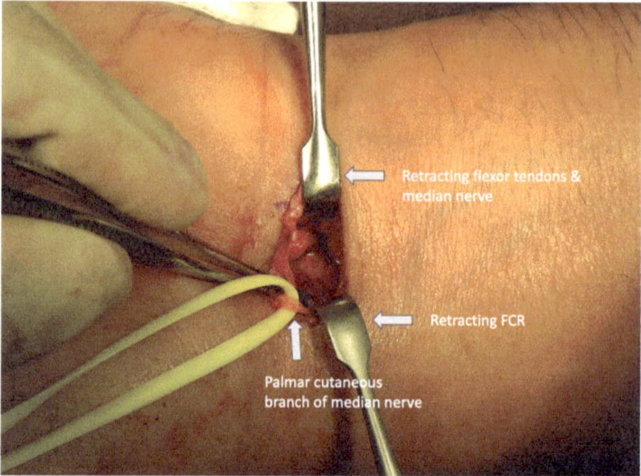

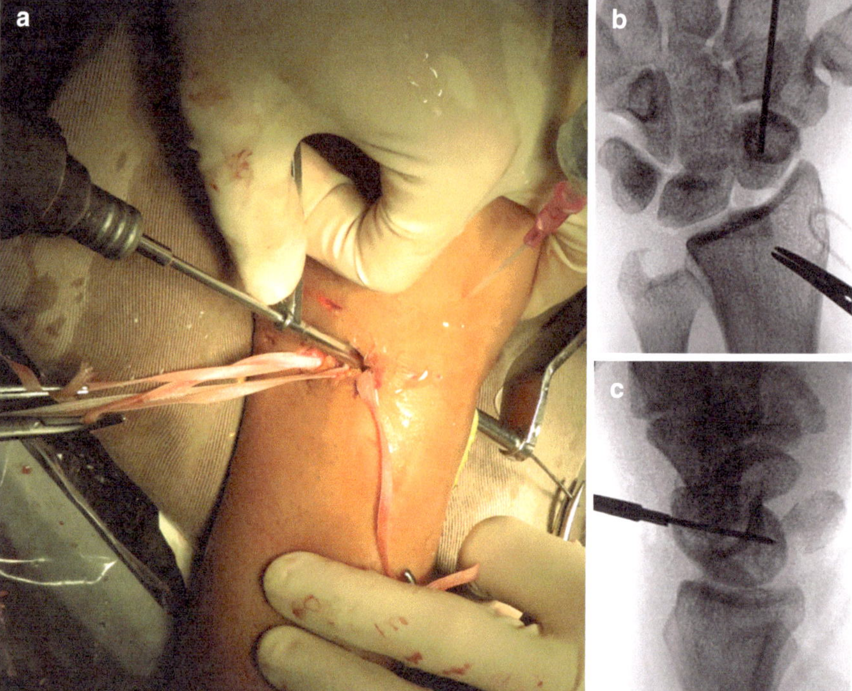

Fig. 14.8 (**a**) Drilling of the scaphoid bone tunnel through the tendon interval. (**b**) Posterior-anterior view of X-ray showing the position of the guide pin over proximal scaphoid. (**c**) Lateral view of X-ray showing the position of the guide pin and cannulated drill on the dorsal proximal scaphoid. Noted the sufficient safety margins from the articular surfaces

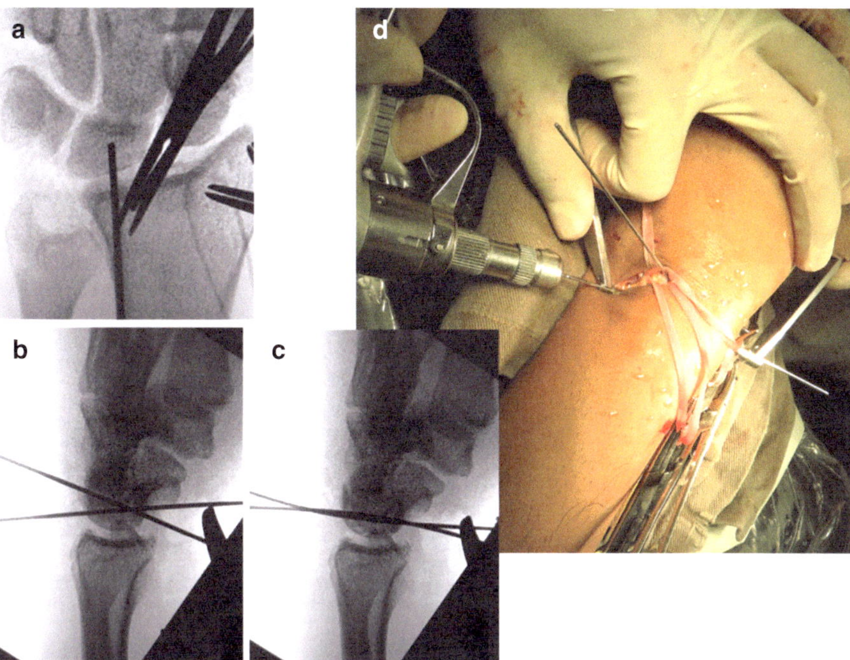

Fig. 14.9 (**a**) Posterior-anterior view of X-ray showing the position of the guide pin over central lunate. (**b**) Drilling of the lunate bone tunnel through the tendon interval. (**c**) Position of the two guide pins over the scaphoid and lunate on lateral view of X-ray at rest. Noted their convergent orientation. (**d**) When the two pins are pulled together, the extension stance of the lunate and the flexion stance of the scaphoid can be corrected to reduce the DISI deformity

the dorsum, the EDC tendons were retracted radially (or alternatively by passing between the EDC tendon intervals) and a 1.1 mm guide pin was inserted into the lunate, aiming at the center of the bone. The guide pin should be targeted in a trajectory of slightly proximal dorsal to distal volar direction, so that the scaphoid and lunate pins could form a convergent angle in both sagittal and axial plane (Fig. 14.9). The angle of convergence varied depending on the severity of the DISI deformity. Again the drill hole should be at least 2–3 mm from all the articular margins. The guide pin was advanced volarly to perforate the volar cortex and exit through the volar wound, while the flexor tendons and median nerve were carefully protected by the assistant. Sequentially expanding the lunate and scaphoid tunnel with cannulated drill bits from 2.0 mm to 2.4 mm was performed through a large protective sheath under copious fluid irrigation. The free tendon graft was delivered through the two bone tunnels with a 2 mm arthroscopic grasper, both from the volar side to the dorsal side. The tendon graft was passed outside the capsule on the volar and

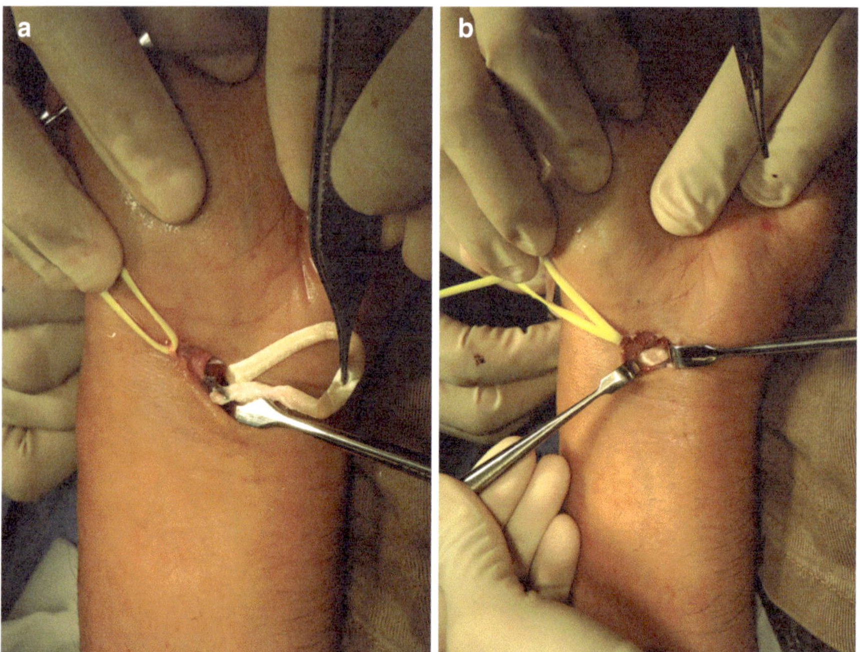

Fig. 14.10 (**a**) A 2 mm mini-grasper inserted through the lunate tunnel from dorsal to volar to grab onto the end of the tendon graft, which had been passed through the scaphoid tunnel on its other end. (**b**) After the tendon was being delivered to the dorsal side of the lunate tunnel, the volar part of the box reconstruction was completed and secured right over the volar capsule of the wrist

dorsal wrist forming a loop to cross the SL interval so that the reconstruction also helped to tighten the capsule and the extrinsic ligaments, which conferred added stability to the SL joint (Fig. 14.10). It is important to minimize the potential risk of inducing ischemic necrosis in the carpal bones by vigorously preserving soft issue and its blood supply, use of small-sized bone tunnels and inclusion of the capsule at the reconstruction site. It was also important to avoid the entrapment of any tendon or nerve during the tendon delivery process.

The wrist was put back on the traction tower with minimal traction. The midcarpal joint was inspected through the MCR portal. With manual traction of the two ends of the tendon graft by an assistant, the SL gapping and step off were corrected. The reduction was also confirmed fluoroscopically (Fig. 14.11). The hand was put back on the hand table. The ends of the tendons graft were carried underneath all the extensor tendons on the surface of the dorsal capsule to meet at the SL joint area. The tendon graft was maximally tensioned and tied in a shoe-lace manner (or half of a square knot) over the dorsal capsule and secured with 2–0 nonabsorbable

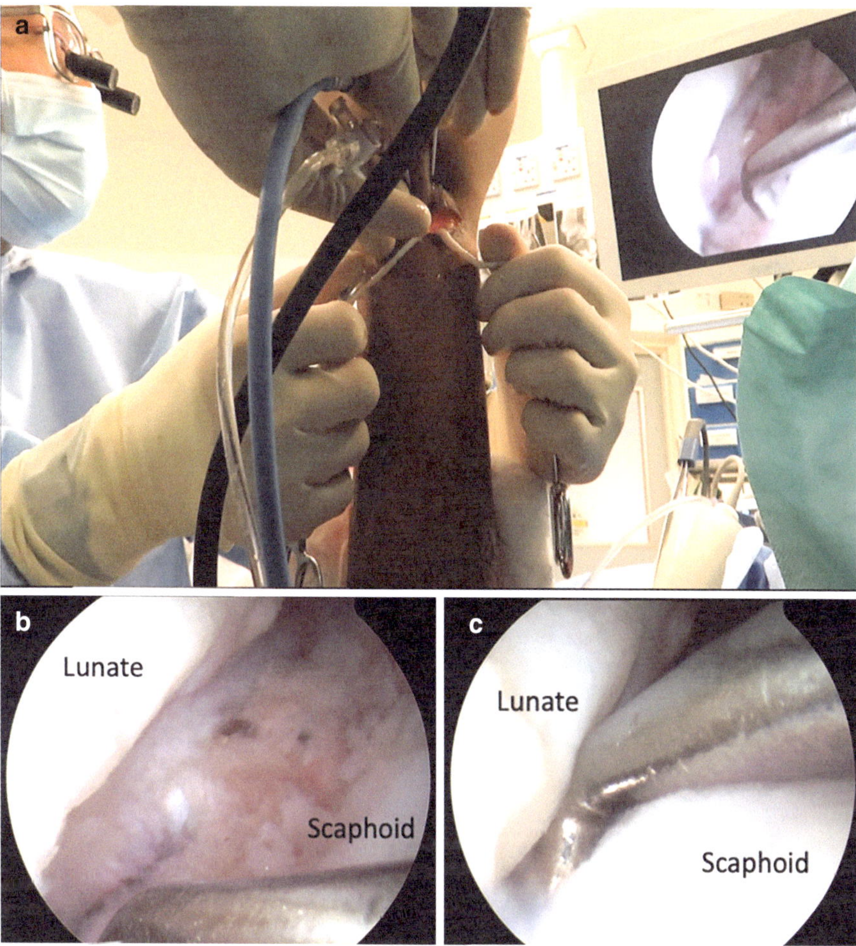

Fig. 14.11 (**a**) While the wrist was suspended in the traction tower with minimal traction force, the surgeon could check the reducibility of the SL joint at the midcarpal joint through the arthroscope while an assistant held to pull the two ends of the tendon graft together to approximate the bones. (**b**) The SL joint was wide open before tendon pulling. (**c**) The SL joint was reduced when the ends of the tendon graft were pulled together

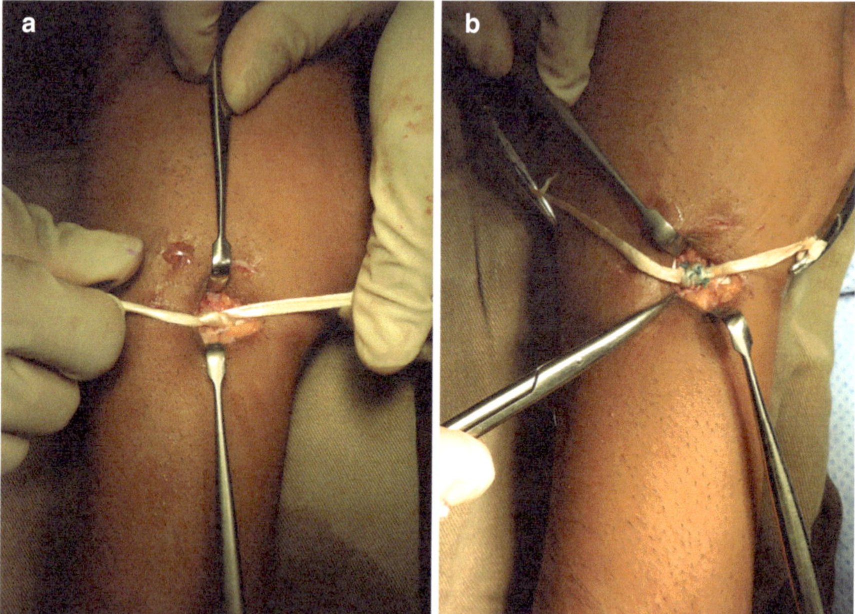

Fig. 14.12 (**a**) The tendon graft was tied in a shoe-lace manner in maximal tension; (**b**) the tendon knot was sutured with 2′0 nonabsorbable braided suture. Additional sutures were also placed to the adjacent capsular structures for augmentation

sutures using non-cutting needle. The tendon graft was tied once more and sutured, completing the box reconstruction of the SL ligament complex (Fig. 14.12). Additional sutures were placed to the adjacent capsule for reinforcement. The reconstruction was stable and no pinning was needed. The extensor retinaculum split was repaired. Satisfactory reduction was confirmed again with fluoroscopy (Fig. 14.13). The tourniquet was released for hemostasis and the wound was closed with absorbable subcuticular sutures. A bulky dressing and a scaphoid plaster slab were applied with wrist in a neutral position and the thumb in neutral palmar abduction.

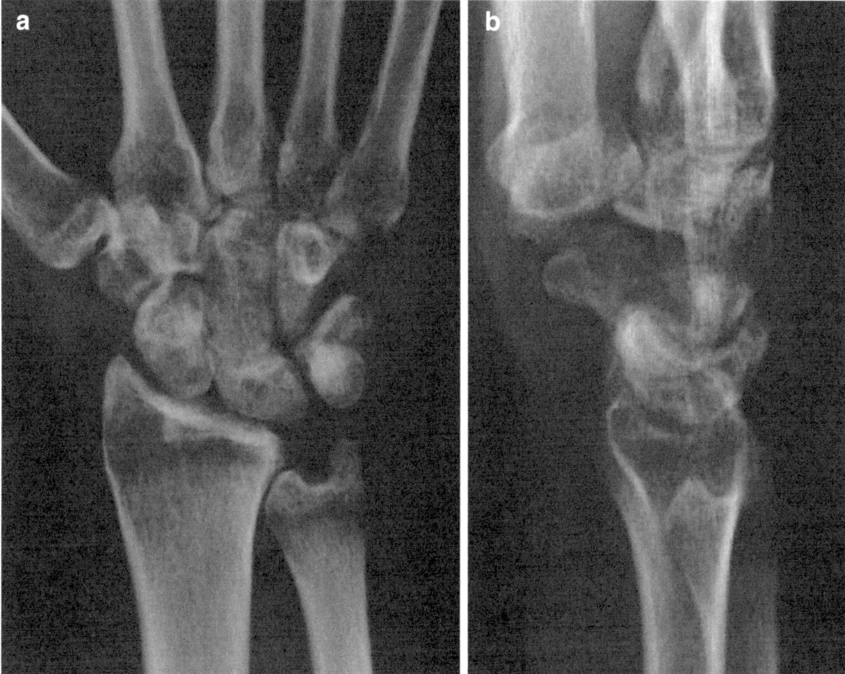

Fig. 14.13 X-ray of the left wrist immediately after the operation showing the good reduction of SL dissociation. (**a**) Posterior-anterior view. (**b**) Lateral view

Clinical Course and Outcome

The wrist was immobilized for 6 weeks and then changed to a thumb spica splint for an additional 2 weeks after which gentle wrist mobilization was performed under supervision of a physiotherapist. At the 11th week post-operatively, he had restricted ROM of the wrist. Vigorous passive mobilization exercises and a turnbuckle splint were prescribed to increase the ROM. Strengthening exercises were conducted by 14th week post-op. He resumed playing basketball 6 months after the surgery and experienced no pain or restriction in daily life.

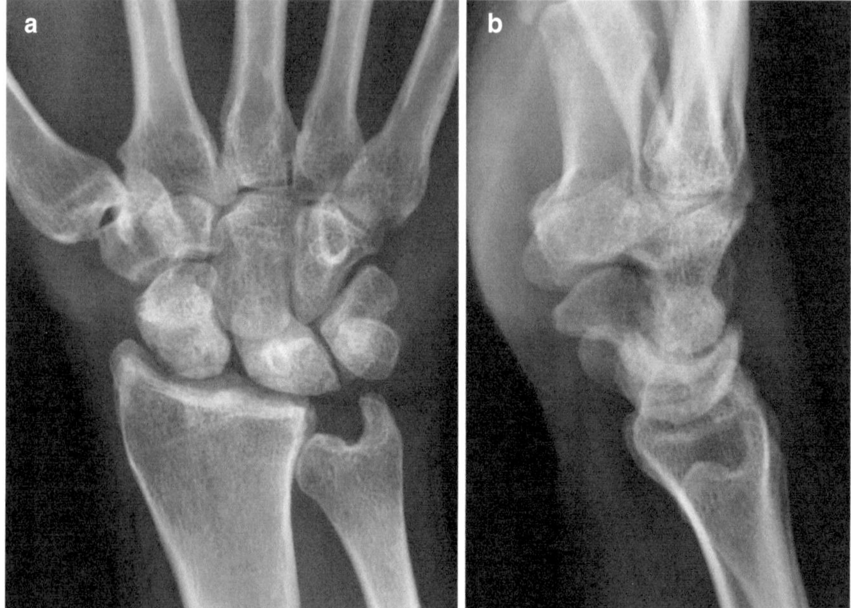

Fig. 14.14 X-ray of the left wrist at 4 years 10 months after the operation showing the maintenance of satisfactory carpal alignment with no degenerative changes noted. (**a**) Posterior-anterior view. (**b**) Lateral view

At the final follow-up of 4 years and 10 months post-operation, he was pain free, enjoyed normal life and was highly satisfied. Wrist examination revealed no tenderness, smooth and painless wrist grinding, negative Watson sign and strong resisted prono-supination. The wrist extension and flexion range were 60° and 50°, respectively. Radial and ulnar deviation were 25° and 30°, respectively. Grip power was 26.1 Kgf or 78.6% of the opposite side. DASH score was 7.5% and PRWE 10/100. The PWH Wrist Performance score was 40/40 and pain score 0/20. The SL interval was 3 mm and SL angle 64°. There was no dorsal scaphoid translation or arthritic change. The bone tunnels remained small with no blow out phenomenon (Fig. 14.14).

Clinical Pearls/Pitfalls

- Keep Bone Tunnels Away from Articular Margins of Scaphoid and Lunate both in PA and Lateral Views to Avoid Iatrogenic Fracture
- Keep Bone Tunnels Small (≤ 2.5 Mm) and Capsule Intact to Prevent Ischemic Insult to Carpal Bones

- Do Not Use Cutting Needle to Suture the Tendon Graft Knot as it May Rupture the Graft
- Do Not Pin across SL Joint to Avoid Iatrogenic Injury to the Tendon Graft; Pin the SC Joint Instead if more Stable Construct Is Needed

Literature Review and Discussion

Reconstruction of the SL joint complex has a long history starting from the initial work of Palmer, Dobyns, and Linsheid at the Mayo Clinic reported as early as in 1978 [1]. Bone tunnels were designed on the surface of scaphoid and lunate to be connected with a split graft of the ECRL tendon to simulate the dorsal SLIL, and the graft was fixed at the dorsal triquetrum to replicate the function of the DIC. A series of 30 patients had been reported all with improvement in pain. However, the surgical method was complicated resulting in difficulties in tendon passing, breakage of drill holes, fracturing, and avascular necrosis. The popularity of this method waned as limited intercarpal fusion became popular as advocated by Watson and Rotman [2, 3]. Intercarpal fusion aimed to overcome the rotational moments imposed on the scaphoid and to resist carpal collapse and had predictable clinical outcomes. However, the normal intercarpal kinematics were distorted, [4] normal cartilage destroyed, and complications of progressive arthrosis, carpal translation, reflex sympathetic dystrophy, stiffness, and non-union of the fusion sites were not uncommonly reported [2, 5–7]. The capsulodesis techniques were developed to control scaphoid flexion but the non-anatomical vertical tether across the radiocarpal joint inevitably limited the wrist motion. 78% had radiographic progression of arthritis on long-term follow-up [8]. Various tenodesis and anatomical reconstruction solutions focusing on dorsal ligament reconstruction emerged again with attempts to control both scaphoid flexion and diastasis. Ligament reconstructions using tendon weaves with ECRB/ECRL or FCR reconstruct the dorsal SL ligament and created a tether to hold the scaphoid in position. Bone-retinaculum-bone techniques reproduced the dorsal SL ligament. Recent systemic reviews on clinical outcome of various SL reconstruction techniques however indicated similar results across different methods. In general, tenodesis had a greater impact on coronal and sagittal plane abnormalities than capsulodesis, but both did not restore normal dorsal SLIL anatomy [9]. Better radiological outcome could be seen in tenodesis group with 1 mm less in SL gap and 12° less in SL angle [10]. Improvement in SL gap and SL angle tended to lose with time though still better than preoperative level [11]. Both methods resulted in loss of flexion by 10–15% and extension 10% [10]. In another study, tenodesis group lost more flexion-extension arc (−32%) than capsulodesis group (−22%) [12]. Tenodesis also appeared to be more technically demanding and risk prone. Some benefit of bone-tissue-bone reconstruction in pain control and function improvement was shown but not in radiological outcome [9]. Unfortunately, almost all studies were of low evidence level of IV to V [13]. There was often no correlation between radiological and clinical outcome. Thus, there was clearly insufficient evidence to suggest efficacy of one over the other in clinical practice [12–14].

While older techniques mainly focused on the dorsal ligament reconstruction and correction of scaphoid deformity, a better understanding of the role of various intrinsic and extrinsic ligaments helped to develop more anatomical reconstruction techniques. It is increasingly notable on the importance of the volar part of the SLIL and the extrinsic ligaments contributing to the stability of the SL joint and the wrist kinematic [15]. David Slutsky coined the term "SL Ligament Complex" to signify the complexity of the ligament connections around the SL joint and the relative contribution [16]. Isolated sectioning of the SL interosseous ligament would not cause diastasis of the joint. The rotational instability of the scaphoid with respect to the lunate and distal radius would result if the "critical stabilizers," including the DIC, DRC, DCSS on the dorsal side, and the LRL on the volar side were also violated or attenuated with cyclical loading [17, 18]. Within the interosseous components, the contribution of the volar portion of the ligament got increasing attention [19–22]. The failure force could be variable from 62 to 270 N for the dorsal ligament and from 86 to 125 N for the palmar ligament. Different studies measured different forces across the SLIL. The variation could be due to the difference in the loading rate as it is now clear that a greater force is required to cause failure of volar SLIL at higher testing rate which simulates the situation during a fall [23]. Based on these biomechanical studies, it is logical and more ideal to restore both the dorsal and volar components of the SL ligament. Yi and Zdero worked on cadaveric specimens to confirm the biomechanical advantages of this. Yi used palmaris longus tendon which passed through drill holes in the AP plane of the scaphoid and the lunate [24]. The SL diastasis was effectively reduced to normal, and the scaphoid and lunate contact pressure on the radius and the scaphoid-to-lunate contact ratio were significantly improved after the reconstruction. Zdero used bovine tendons passing through double bone tunnels of the scaphoid and lunate in 19 cadaveric wrists [25]. There was no difference in the mechanical properties from the normal wrists except a lower linear stiffness. In a recent biomechanical analysis of three reconstruction techniques comparing 360° SLIL reconstruction, double dorsal limb only and modified Brunelli tenodesis in eight cadavers, it was noted that while the dorsal SLG could be restored in all techniques, the volar SLG in extended position could only be normalized after the 360° reconstruction, and DDL SL reconstruction tended to over-correct the deformity [26].

Being inspired by the study of Yi, we first developed the technique of arthroscopic-assisted box reconstruction of the SL ligament in 2002 [27]. The initial indication was subacute and chronic SL dissociation of 6 weeks or beyond. Both dynamic and static instabilities were appropriate, as long as the SL diastasis and DISI deformity were reducible, as confirmed arthroscopically and radiologically. There should be no ulnar translocation of the lunate. The use of arthroscopy helped to evaluate the articular status of the affected wrist, the aetiology, degree and chronicity of the SL dissociation, the reducibility of the dissociation and deformity, and the confirmation of the reduction status after the tendon graft fixation, without the need to widely open and dissect the wrist structures. This is beneficial in preserving the vascularity of the carpal bones thus minimizing the chance of avascular necrosis. The disruption of the mechanoreceptors and hence proprioceptive function of the wrist joint is minimized [28]. The tendon looping reconstruction through the bone tunnels is extra-capsular and therefore also includes the important dorsal capsular ligaments, namely the DIC and DRC, and the volar ligaments, namely the RSC and LRL to be imbricated and tightened underneath the tendon graft. By adjusting the position of the scaphoid and lunate bone tunnels in a convergent manner both in coronal and sagittal planes, the flexion-pronation and extension-supination tendency of the scaphoid and lunate, respectively, can be automatically corrected when the tendon graft is tightened. Using this technique, the SL ligament remnant is preserved to be incorporated into the ultimate capsular-ligament-tendon graft healing mass. The potential benefit of remnant integration into the reconstructed ligament has been discussed [29]. There is high density of Pacini and Ruffini receptors, especially in the palmer band. The preservation of this remnant aids to improve vascularity and mechanoreceptor regeneration during the ligamentization of the graft. There is evidence showing a trend toward earlier ligamentization in grafts with remnant stumps, i.e., accelerated and enhanced healing, and faster return to activities.

From October 2002 to June 2012, this treatment method was applied in 17 patients of mean age 42 (range 26–60) with chronic SL instability of average duration of 9.5 months (range 1.5–18). There were three Geissler grade 3 and 14 grade 4 instability cases. The average pre-op SL interval was 4.9 mm (range 3–9). DISI deformity was present in 13 patients and the average SL angle was 85° (range 52–102). The average follow-up was 48.3 months (range 11–132). Thirteen were able to return to their pre-injury job level, four had some restrictions at work. Eleven patients had no wrist pain at all and six had some pain on either maximum exertion or at the extreme of motion. The average total pain score was 1.7/20 in performing the 10 ADL tasks, compared with the preoperative score of 8.3/20. Visual analog scale of pain at daily maximum exertion averaged 1.8/10 (preoperative 6.2/10). The average extension range improved 13%, flexion range 16%, radial deviation 13%, and ulnar deviation 27%. Postoperative average total wrist performance score was 37.8/40, with improvement of 35%. Mean grip strength was 32.8 kg, which was 120% of the preoperative status, and was 84% of the contralateral side. Radiographs showed the average SL interval of 2.9 mm (range 1.6–5.5). Recurrence of DISI deformity was noted in four patients without symptoms. Ischemic change of the proximal scaphoid was noted in one case without symptoms or progression. There were no major complications. All patients were satisfied with the procedure and treatment outcome. In the systemic review of Naqui et al., the current technique had better pain reduction than others (63% vs. 50% in capsulodesis and 52% in tendodesis). Flexion-extension arc improved for 15% in our series while tendodesis and capsulodesis universally had decreased motion range [12].

References

1. Palmer AK, Dobyns JH, Linsheid RL. Management of post-traumatic ligament reconstruction for treatment of chronic complete scapholunate separation. J Hand Surg Am. 1978;396:507–32.
2. Watson HK, Belniak R, Garcia-Elias M. Treatment of scapholunate dissociation: preferred treatment - STT fusion vs. other methods. Orthopedics. 1991;14:365–70.
3. Rotman MB, Manske PR, Pruitt DL, et al. Scaphocapitolunate arthrodesis. J Hand Surg Am. 1993;18(1):26–33.
4. Ambrose L, Posner MA, Green SM, Stuchin S. The effects of scaphoid intercarpal stabilization on wrist mechanics: an experimental study. J Hand Surg Am. 1992;17:429–37.
5. Kleinman WB. Long-term study of chronic scapho-lunate instability treated by scapho-trapezio-trapezoid arthrodesis. J Hand Surg Am. 1989;14:429–45.
6. Rogers WD, Watson HK. Radial styloid impingement after triscaphe arthrodesis. J Hand Surg Am. 1989;14:297–301.
7. Hom S, Ruby LK. Attempted scapholunate arthrodesis for chronic scapholunate dissociation. J Hand Surg Am. 1991;16(2):334–9.
8. Megerle K, Bertel D, Germann G, et al. Long-term results of dorsal intercarpal ligament capsulodesis for the treatment of chronic scapholunate instability. J Bone Joint Surg Br. 2012;94(12):1660–5.
9. Wu M, Ilyas A. Comparison of outcomes of scapholunate ligament reconstruction techniques. J Wrist Surg. 2022;12:558. https://doi.org/10.1055/s-0042-1757442.
10. Daly LT, Daly MC, Mohamadi A, et al. Chronic scapholunate interosseous ligament disruption: a systematic review and meta-analysis of surgical treatments. Hand (N Y). 2020;15(1):27–34.
11. Montgomery SJ, Rollick NJ, Kubik JF, et al. Surgical outcomes of chronic isolated scapholunate interosseous ligament injuries: a systematic review of 805 wrists. Can J Surg. 2019;62(03):1–12.
12. Naqui Z, Khor WS, Mishra A, et al. The management of chronic non-arthritic scapholunate dissociation: a systematic review. J Hand Surg Eu. 2018;43(4):394–401.
13. Anderson JK, Rööser B, Karlsson J. Level of evidence in wrist ligament repair and reconstruction research: a systematic review. J Exp Orthop. 2018;5(1):15.
14. Imada AO, Eldredge J, Wells L, et al. Review of surgical treatment for chronic scapholunate ligament reconstruction: a long-term study. Eur J Orthop Surg Traumatol. 2023;33(4):787–93.
15. Badida R, Akhbari B, Vutescu E, et al. The role of scapholunate interosseous, dorsal intercarpal, and radiolunate ligaments in wrist biomechanics. J Biomech. 2021;125:110567.
16. Slutsky DJ. The scapholunate ligament complex (SLLC). J Wrist Surg. 2013;2:97.
17. Elsaidi M, Wang J, Ronga M, et al. Dorsal wrist ligament insertions stabilize the scapholunate interval: cadaver study. Clin Orthop Relat Res. 2004;425:152–7.
18. Pérez AJ, Jethanandani RG, Vutescu ES, et al. Role of ligament stabilizers of the proximal carpal pow in preventing dorsal intercalated segment instability: a cadaveric study. J Bone Joint Surg Am. 2019;101(15):1388–96.
19. Berger RA, Imeada T, Berglund L, et al. Constraint and material properties of the subregions of the scapholunate interosseous ligament. J Hand Surg Am. 1999;24(5):953–62.
20. Fotios VN, Emmanuel PA, Apostolos DP, et al. Biomechanical properties of the scapholunate ligament and the importance of its portions in the capitate intrusion injury. Clin Biomech. 2011;26:819–23.
21. Veigas SF, Yamaguchi S, Boyd NL, et al. The dorsal ligaments of the wrist: anatomy, mechanical properties, and function. J Hand Surg Am. 1999;24:456–68.
22. Logan SE, Nowak MD, Gould PL. Biomechanical behavior of the scapholunate ligament. Biomed Sci Instrum. 1986;22:81–5.
23. Werner FW. Design requirements for scapholunate interosseous ligament reconstruction. J Wrist Surg. 2021;10(6):484–91.
24. Yi IS, Firoozbakhsh K, Racca J, et al. Treatment of scapholunate dissociation with palmaris longus tendon graft: a biomechanical study. UPOJ. 2000;13:53–9.

25. Zdero R, Olsen M, Elfatori S, et al. Linear and torsional mechanical characteristics of intact and reconstructed scapholunate ligaments. J Biomech Eng. 2009;131(4):041009.
26. Chae S, Nam J, Park IJ, et al. Biomechanical analysis of three different reconstruction techniques for scapholunate instability: a cadaveric study. Clin Orthop Surg. 2022;14(4):613–21.
27. Ho PC, Wong CWY, Tse WL. Arthroscopic-assisted combined dorsal and volar scapholunate ligament reconstruction with tendon graft for chronic SL instability. J Wrist Surg. 2015;4:252–63.
28. Mathoulin C, Gras M. Role of wrist arthroscopy in scapholunate dissociation. Orthop Traumatol Surg Res. 2020;106(1S):S89–99.
29. Lindsay TAJ, Myers HR, Tham S. Ligamentization and remnant integration: review and analysis of current evidence and implications for scapholunate reconstruction. J Wrist Surg. 2020;10(6):476–83.

Further Reading

Ho PC, Wong CWY, Tse WL. Arthroscopic-assisted combined dorsal and volar scapholunate ligament reconstruction with tendon graft for chronic SL instability. J Wrist Surg. 2015;4:252–63.
Naqui Z, Khor WS, Mishra A, et al. The management of chronic non-arthritic scapholunate dissociation: a systematic review. J Hand Surg Eu. 2018;43(4):394–440.
Yi IS, Firoozbakhsh K, Racca J, et al. Treatment of scapholunate dissociation with palmaris longus tendon graft: a biomechanical study. UPOJ. 2000;13:53–9.
Zdero R, Olsen M, Elfatori S, et al. Linear and torsional mechanical characteristics of intact and reconstructed scapholunate ligaments. J Biomech Eng. 2009;131(4):041009.

Chapter 15
Chronic, Reducible Scapholunate Ligament Injury: Double Circle Arthroscopic Ligamentoplasty

Fernando Corella, Montserrat Ocampos, Rafal Laredo, José Tabuenca, and Ricardo Larrainzar-Garijo

Case Presentation

The case used to illustrate this double circle arthroscopic ligamentoplasty is that of a 49-year-old, right hand dominant man who had right wrist pain after a trauma 2 years ago.

F. Corella (✉)
Orthopedic and Trauma Department, Hospital Universitario Infanta Leonor, Madrid, Spain

Orthopedic and Trauma Department, Hospital Universitario Quironsalud Madrid, Madrid, Spain

Surgery Department, School of Medicine, Universidad Complutense de Madrid, Madrid, Spain

M. Ocampos
Orthopedic and Trauma Department, Hospital Universitario Infanta Leonor, Madrid, Spain

Orthopedic and Trauma Department, Hospital Universitario Quironsalud Madrid, Madrid, Spain

R. Laredo
Orthopedic and Trauma Department, Hospital Universitario Quironsalud Madrid, Madrid, Spain

Orthopedic and Trauma Department, Hospital Universitario Quironsalud Toledo, Toledo, Spain

J. Tabuenca
Orthopedic and Trauma Department, Hospital Universitario Quironsalud Madrid, Madrid, Spain

R. Larrainzar-Garijo
Orthopedic and Trauma Department, Hospital Universitario Infanta Leonor, Madrid, Spain

Surgery Department, School of Medicine, Universidad Complutense de Madrid, Madrid, Spain

J. Yao (ed.), *Carpal Instability*, https://doi.org/10.1007/978-3-031-55869-6_15

At the moment of the trauma, he went to the emergency department, no fractures were identified, and he was diagnosed with wrist sprain. Since then, he had pain in the wrist, but it worsened in the last few months. An MRI was performed showing a scapholunate rupture, and he was referred to our center.

Diagnosis

Physical Assessment/Relevant Maneuvers

Patients with SL dysfunction may complain of pain on the dorsal aspect of the scapholunate (SL) joint, especially with wrist hyperextension. They may also report weakness, clicking or even episodes of "giving way" of the wrist.

The classic clinical test for scapholunate instability is the scaphoid shift test described by Watson et al. This test demonstrates proximal scaphoid subluxation from the dorsal edge of the radius while pressure is exerted on the distal pole of the scaphoid as the wrist moves from ulnar to radial deviation, preventing its flexion. Relief of pressure on the distal pole will allow the scaphoid to spontaneously reduce, often with an audible or palpable clunk [1]. The contralateral wrist must also be assessed for idiopathic ligamentous laxity due to the prevalence among the uninjured population of up to 32% [2].

An adjunctive test for SL instability is the scaphoid ballottement test. This test is positive when there is pain, crepitus, and excessive mobility of the scaphoid when it is moved dorsally and palmarly with a fixed lunate. This is a variation of the scaphoid shift maneuver and has also been called the scaphoid thrust test [3].

The finger extension test is useful in patients with minor SL instability and chronic wrist pain. They will experience pain extending the fingers maximally with the wrist flexed. This maneuver drives the head of the capitate between the scaphoid and lunate and increases the tension on the SL interval [4].

Furthermore, as in many other carpal injuries, the range of motion, the degree of pain, the grip strength, and patient-reported outcome measures should be measured in every patient.

The range of motion of this patient was 80° of extension (90° contralateral) and 90° of wrist flexion (90° contralateral) with full pronosupination. Grip strength was 50 kg (57 kg contralateral), with a visual analog score of 7.6 and a Disabilities of the Arm, Shoulder and Hand score of 58.3.

Diagnostic Studies

Image Studies

Plain radiographs are essential when evaluating a patient for suspected scapholunate (SL) instability. Posteroanterior (PA) and lateral films, PA in radial and ulnar deviations and clenched fist or pencil views are obtained to evaluate static and dynamic instability patterns. In a static injury, there is an SL interval greater than 3 mm (Terry Thomas sign) and a scaphoid ring sign (the scaphoid is viewed along its long axis, and its two poles overlap). Lateral X-rays will show the dorsal intercalated segment instability (DISI) deformity due to scaphoid flexion and lunate extension [5, 6]. However, subtle changes in the X-ray may suggest incomplete injuries of the SL ligament. The X-rays of the patient in the current case are shown in Fig. 15.1.

Magnetic resonance imaging (MRI) can be a useful adjunct study in an examination suspicious for scapholunate ligament injury. Recent studies have shown that 3-T magnetic resonance imaging (MRI) and minimally invasive magnetic resonance arthrography (MRA) have sensitivities of 75.7% (66.8–83.2) and 82.1% (76.1–87.2), respectively, and specificities of 97.1% (89.8–99.6) and 92.8% (90.2–94.9), respectively, for the detection of SL ligament injuries [7]. Images of the MRI of the patient are shown in Fig. 15.2.

Arthroscopic Evaluation

We included arthroscopic evaluation as a diagnostic study because it is the gold standard tool to evaluate SL dysfunction and to ensure that the indication for arthroscopic ligamentoplasty is correct.

We have previously published a 7-item arthroscopic exploration for scapholunate dysfunction. These seven items include the following [8]:

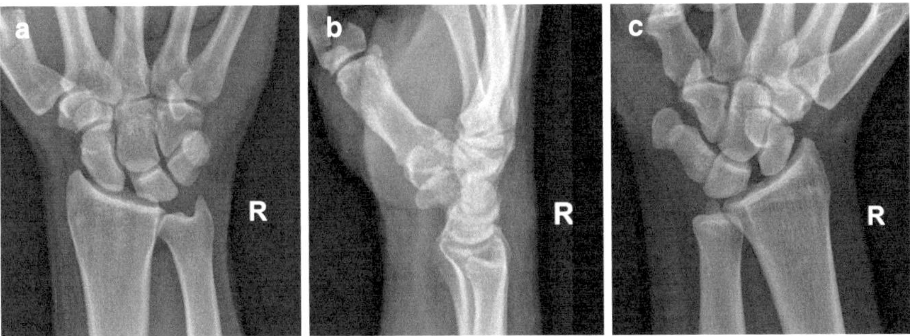

Fig. 15.1 Preoperative X-rays. (**a**) PA view. (**b**) Lateral view. (**c**) Clench fist X-ray

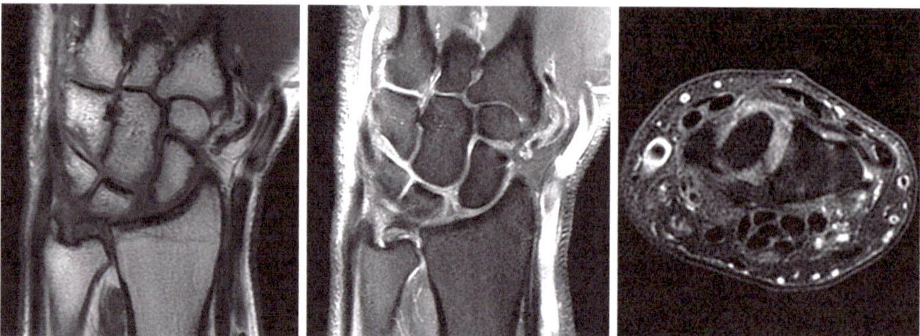

Fig. 15.2 Preoperative MRI images

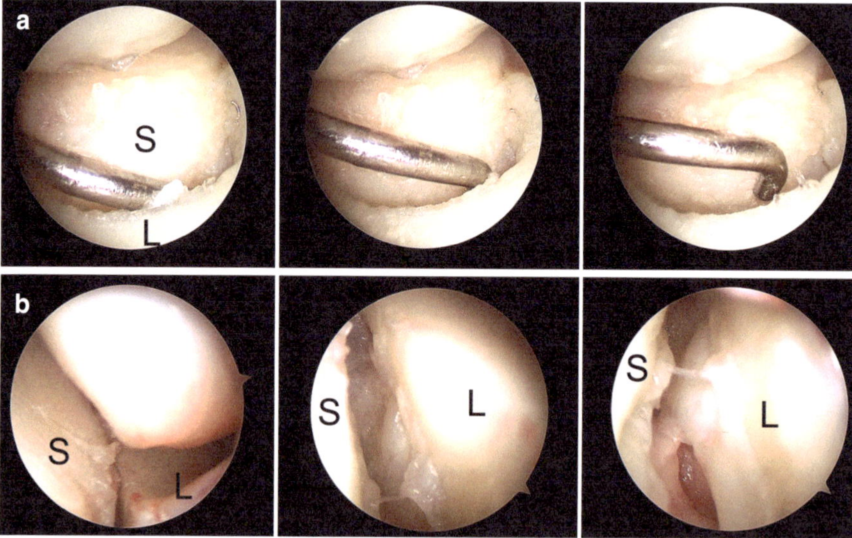

Fig. 15.3 Grade V instability. (**a**) Wide SL gap. (**b**) Passage of the arthroscope from midcarpal to radiocarpal joint Sl. Radiological signs of chronic SL instability are added to these arthroscopic findings

Gap between the Bones

The probe enters through the RMC portal, and the degree of instability is evaluated considering the passage of the tip and the grade of twisting of the probe, EWAS classification [9].

The patient had grade V instability, as shown in Fig. 15.3.

Acute vs. Chronic

Most of the time, the suspicion of an acute or chronic injury is not in doubt, when knowing when the trauma has occurred. However, there can be doubts when evaluating injuries associated with distal radius fractures or carpal bone fractures. In these cases, old and chronic injuries can be found, and no specific treatment is needed. Therefore, it is important to look for signs of acute injury, that is, a hemorrhagic ligament along with freshly torn stumps.

In the present case, it was a chronic lesion, and no fresh injury was found.

Quality of the Ligament Remnant

This is one of the most important items to explore in order to decide between a reinforcement technique of the ligament and a reconstruction. A complete injury with no remnant or a poor-quality remnant of the ligament will lead to the need for a reconstruction technique.

To evaluate the quality and attachments of the dorsal portion of the SL ligament, a "Hook test" can be performed. The probe is introduced in the SL joint, and dorsal traction is placed, capturing the dorsal portion of the ligament. If there is a competent ligament, the probe is caught in the dorsal SL ligament (positive Hook test); if not, there will be no capture (negative Hook test) (Fig. 15.4).

In the arthroscopic exploration, we found a negative Hook test, so we found no indication for a reinforcement technique (Fig. 15.5).

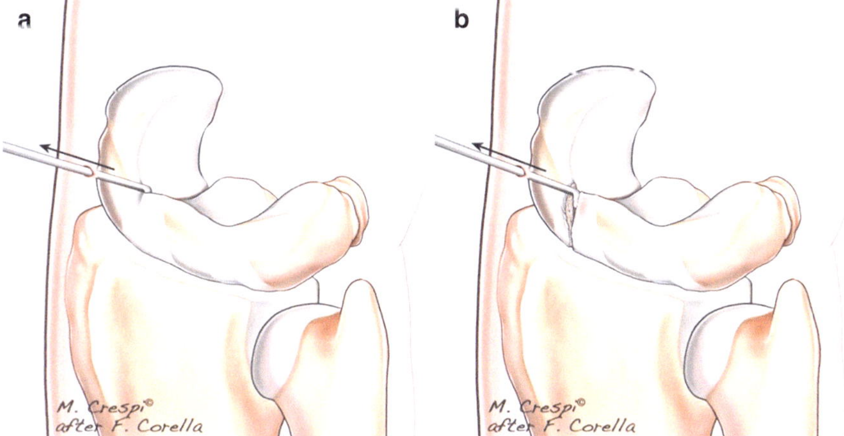

Fig. 15.4 Hook test. (**a**) Positive Hook test: the probe is caught in the dorsal SL ligament. (**b**) Negative Hook test: there is no capture. Reproduced from Heras-Palou, Corella, Luchetti. Carpal Ligament Injuries and Instability: FESSH Instructional Course Book 2023. Stuttgart: Thieme; 2023

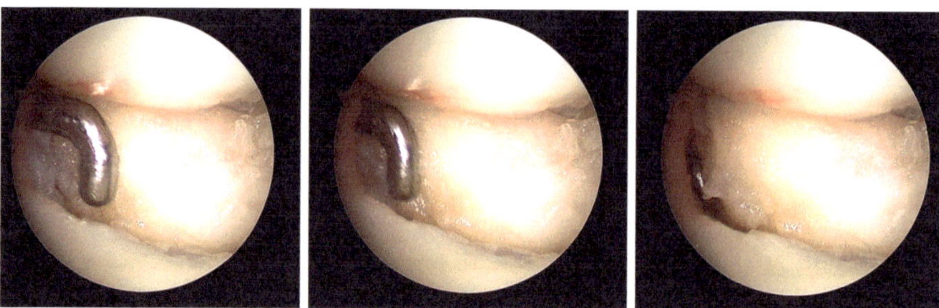

Fig. 15.5 Vision from the UMC portal. Negative Hook test

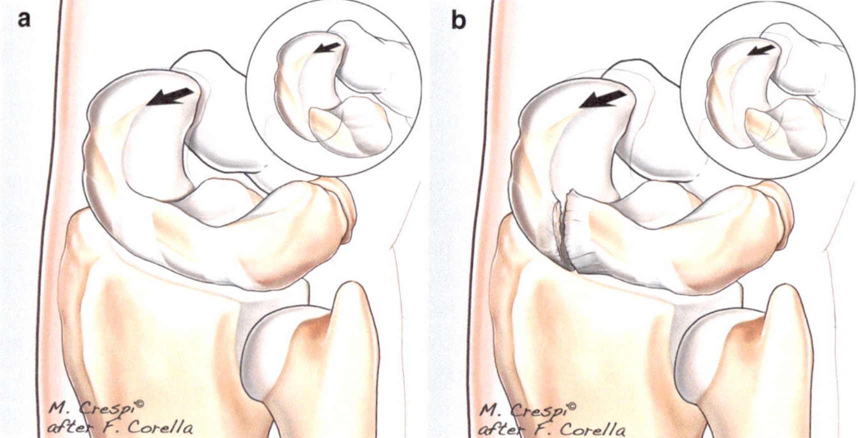

Fig. 15.6 3D test. (**a**) Negative test: all proximal rows move together. (**b**) Positive test: the scaphoid moves dorsally while the lunate remains in the same position. Reproduced from Heras-Palou, Corella, Luchetti. Carpal Ligament Injuries and Instability: FESSH Instructional Course Book 2023. Stuttgart: Thieme; 2023

Dorsal Displacement of the Scaphoid

Patients usually complain of pain on the dorsal side of the wrist. This occurs due to the dorsal displacement of the proximal pole of the scaphoid over the dorsal edge of the radius when it is detached from the lunate.

This dorsal displacement can be arthroscopically explored with the "arthroscopic scaphoid 3D (dorsal, dynamic, displacement) test" [14] (Fig. 15.6). If there is a positive 3D test with an important dorsal displacement of the scaphoid, we encourage the use of stronger reconstruction techniques, such as the one explained in this chapter.

This patient had a positive 3D test, and it was observed how the scaphoid moved dorsally while the lunate remained in the same position (Fig. 15.7).

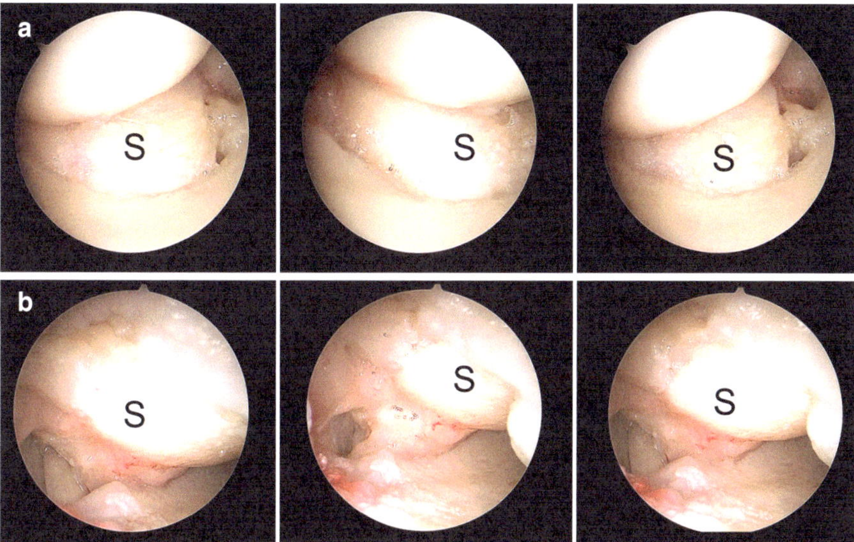

Fig. 15.7 Vision from the UMC portal. Positive 3D test. Dorsal displacement of the scaphoid in the midcarpal joint (**a**) and radiocarpal joint (**b**). *S* scaphoid

Reducibility

This is another key point when deciding the performance of this arthroscopic ligamentoplasty because if the scaphoid cannot be easily reduced to its normal position, this reconstruction technique is not indicated, and a salvage procedure should be considered.

In an easily reducible instability, the scaphoid should be reduced and positioned to the height of the lunate only by pushing with the arthroscopic probe (Fig. 15.8).

This patient had reducible instability (Fig. 15.9).

Associated Ligament Injuries

The concurrence of tears of the SL and LT ligaments is not unusual and can also occur without an apparent perilunate dislocation, which is called a perilunate injury not dislocated (PLIND) [10].

To discard this combined injury, a "Rocking Chair Sign" [11] can be performed (Fig. 15.10).

This patient did not have an LT injury (Fig. 15.11).

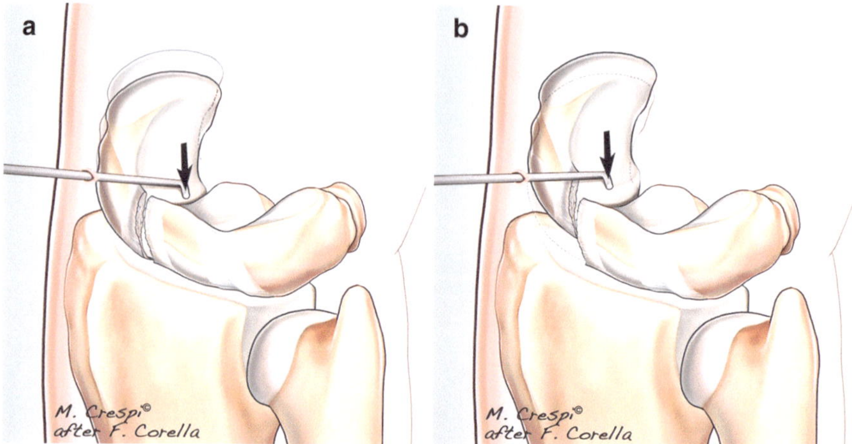

Fig. 15.8 (**a**) Reducible instability. The scaphoid is easily reduced and positioned to the height of the lunate by pushing with the arthroscopic probe. (**b**) Nonreducible instability. The scaphoid cannot be positioned to the height of the lunate. Reproduced from Heras-Palou, Corella, Luchetti. Carpal Ligament Injuries and Instability: FESSH Instructional Course Book 2023. Stuttgart: Thieme; 2023

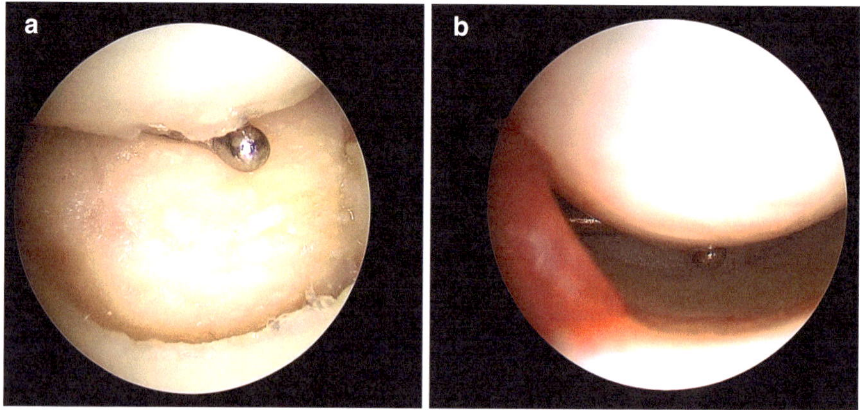

Fig. 15.9 (**a, b**) Vision from the UMC portal. The scaphoid is reduced by pushing with the probe

Degenerative Changes

As a nonreducible instability precludes the performance of this ligamentoplasty, the presence of cartilage damage will also lead to the contraindication of this procedure.

The degenerative process of an SL ligament injury has been called scapholunate advanced collapse (SLAC) of the wrist [12]. Both radiocarpal and midcarpal joints should be explored, keeping in mind that the first degenerative lesions (Stage 1) appear on the dorsal side of the radiocarpal joint and not in the radial styloid.

The patient did not have an important degenerative lesion (Fig. 15.12).

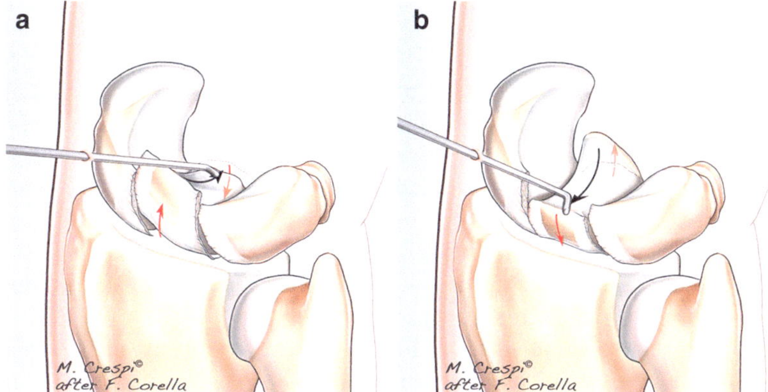

Fig. 15.10 The "Rocking Chair Sign." (**a, b**) If there is combined injury of the SL and LT ligaments, the lunate performs a "rocking chair"-like motion. Reproduced from Heras-Palou, Corella, Luchetti. Carpal Ligament Injuries and Instability: FESSH Instructional Course Book 2023. Stuttgart: Thieme; 2023

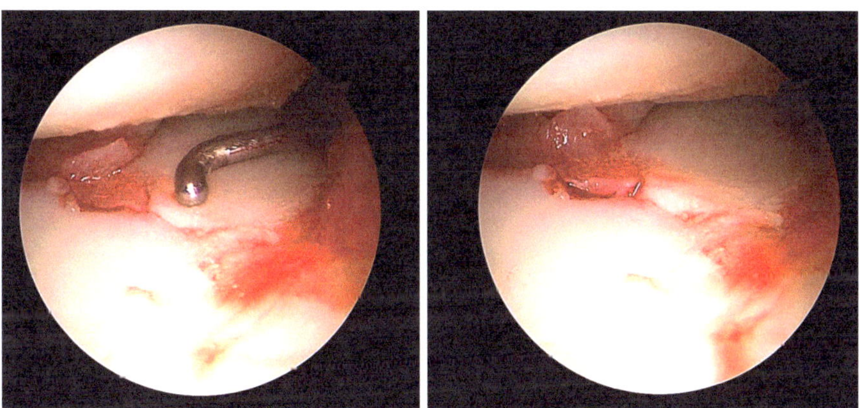

Fig. 15.11 Vision from the RMC portal. There was no LT injury

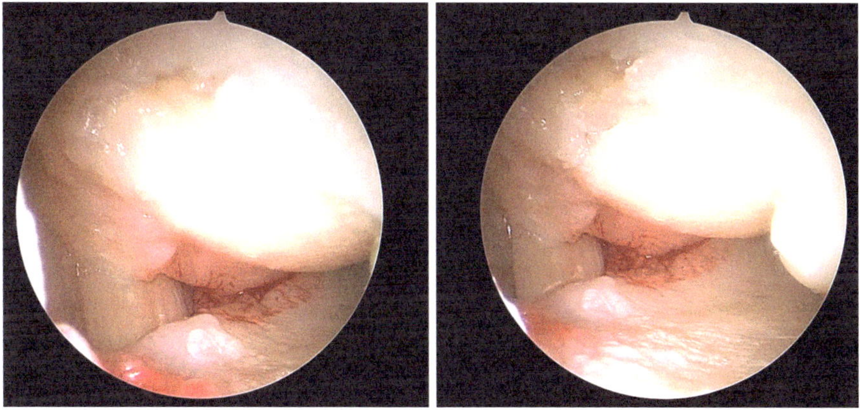

Fig. 15.12 Vision from the 6R portal. Minimal degenerative lesion on the dorsal edge of the radius

Management Options

Scapholunate (SL) dysfunction is not a unique injury but a spectrum of multiple injuries, including acute and chronic injuries, partial and complete tears, reducible and nonreducible instabilities, etc. This spectrum of injuries can be treated with a myriad of techniques, both open and arthroscopic. We recently described how to merge all these techniques into four major groups called "the 4R" [13]. These groups are repair, reinforcement, reconstruction, and resection techniques.

In a previous heading, we explained how arthroscopic exploration could guide use to decide between these four groups.

Reinforcement vs. Reconstruction: Reinforcement techniques include capsulo-ligamentous sutures used to reinforce an SL ligament and the soft tissue around it. Reconstruction techniques replace an injured ligament with a new tissue (usually a tendon graft) that resembles its function. It could be challenging to decide between these two techniques, especially in grade IIIC or IV. Therefore, we made this decision based on the quality of the ligament remnant (SL Hook test) and the dorsal dynamic displacement (3D test) [14]. If there is no ligament remnant of enough quality attached to the bones and there is an important dorsal displacement, we prefer to perform a complete ligament reconstruction. This has been decided and carried out in this case.

Reconstruction vs. Resection: Resection techniques include salvage procedures used when the SL injury evolves into a fixed and collapsed carpus with or without arthritic changes. Again, sometimes it could be challenging to decide between a reconstruction technique and a salvage procedure. We make this decision based on the presence of degenerative lesions (SLAC 1 or 2) and on the reducibility of the scaphoid. As explained before, even in the absence of degenerative lesions, if the instability is not easily reducible, the performance of this technique is avoided.

In conclusion, the indications for this arthroscopic ligamentoplasty are as follows:

1. Complete SL ligament tear, grade IIIC, IV, or V SL lesions [9].
2. No remnant of the ligament of sufficient quality (negative SL Hook Test).
3. Dorsal Dynamic Displacement of the Scaphoid (Positive Arthroscopic 3D Test) [14]

The contraindications are as follows:

1. Not Easily Reducible Instability. The Scaphoid Is Not Easily Reduced and Positioned to the Height of the Lunate by Pushing with the Arthroscopic Probe
2. Presence of Degenerative Lesions
3. The Presence of Associated Ligament Injuries, Especially Lunotriquetral (LT) Injury (PLND Injury) [10]

The present case fulfills all these criteria.

Management Chosen for this Case with Rationale [with Figures]

In this case, we have chosen to perform a modified form of our previously published arthroscopic SL ligamentoplasty called the double circle technique.

Preparation and Patient Positioning

The operation is performed under regional anesthesia (axillary block) or general anesthesia with a pneumatic tourniquet placed at the upper arm closest to the armpit.

The patient is placed supine with the affected arm on a hand table. The wrist is maintained in vertical traction during the entire procedure. The traction tower commonly used is the Arc Wrist Tower™ (Acumed, Hillsboro, OR), which maintains vertical traction and leaves the volar side of the wrist free.

The C-arm is entered parallel to the floor from the volar side of the wrist so that suspended hand pronation or supination, PA or lateral views are easily obtained.

Step 1: Bone Tunnels

Two blind tunnels will be made in the scaphoid. The first one from dorsal to volar and the second one from volar to dorsal.

The dorsal tunnel is placed centered on the scaphoid from the insertion of the dorsal portion of the SL to the insertion of the volar portion of the SL. As it is a blinded tunnel, only the tip of the 1.0 mm k wire will cross the volar cortex of the scaphoid.

The volar tunnel is placed distal to the volar exit of the K-wire of the dorsal tunnel, with a slight inclination from proximal to distal. Again, as it is a blind tunnel, only the tip of the K-wire will cross the dorsal cortex of the scaphoid exiting distally and radially to the dorsal tunnel (Fig. 15.13).

Scaphoid K-Wire Placement

The placement of the two K-wires of the dorsal and volar tunnels of the scaphoid is the first step. Both K-wires will be introduced from the dorsal side.

To introduce the K-wire of the dorsal tunnel, a 14-G Abbocath is used as a guide. It is introduced through the 3/4 portal and slid distally until the insertion of the dorsal portion of the SL is reached. The K-wire is introduced from the dorsal side and exits on the volar side at the level of the insertion of the volar portion of the SL ligament (Fig. 15.14).

Fig. 15.13 Schematic representation of two blinded 2.7 mm (dorsal) and 2.5 mm (volar) tunnels in the scaphoid. Printed with permission of Crespi and Corella

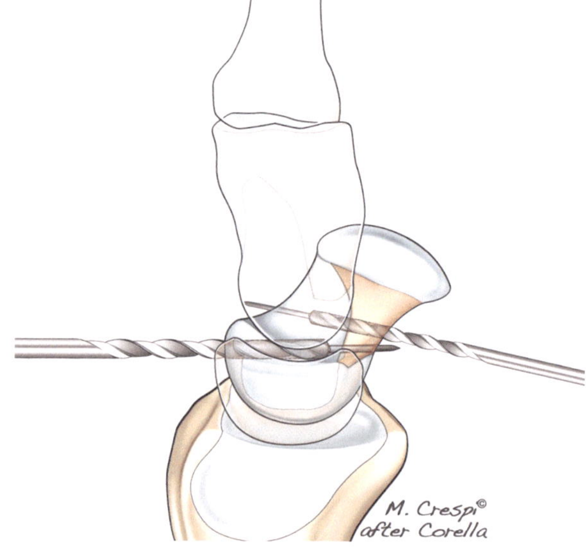

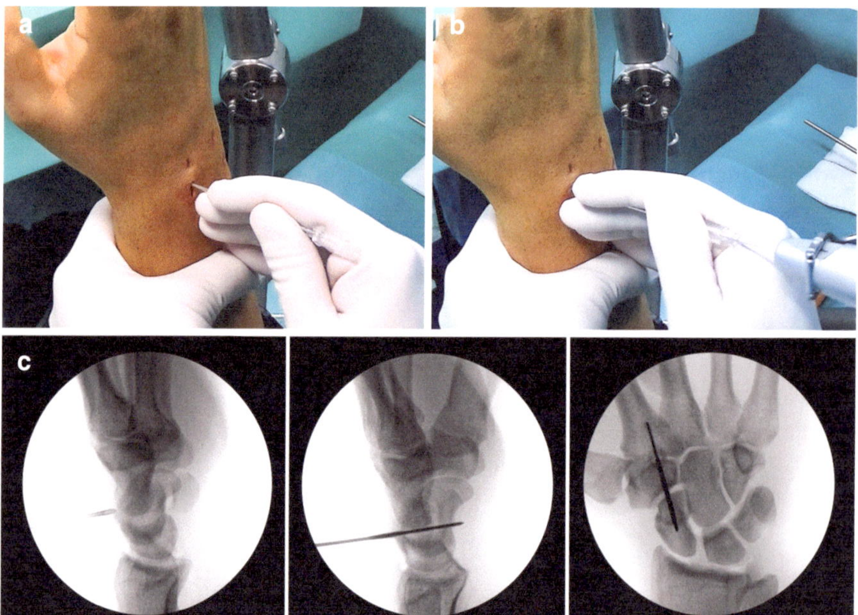

Fig. 15.14 K-wire placement for the dorsal tunnel. (**a, b**) The K-wire is placed through the 3/4 portal using a 14-G Abbocath as a guide. C. X-ray of the K-wire position

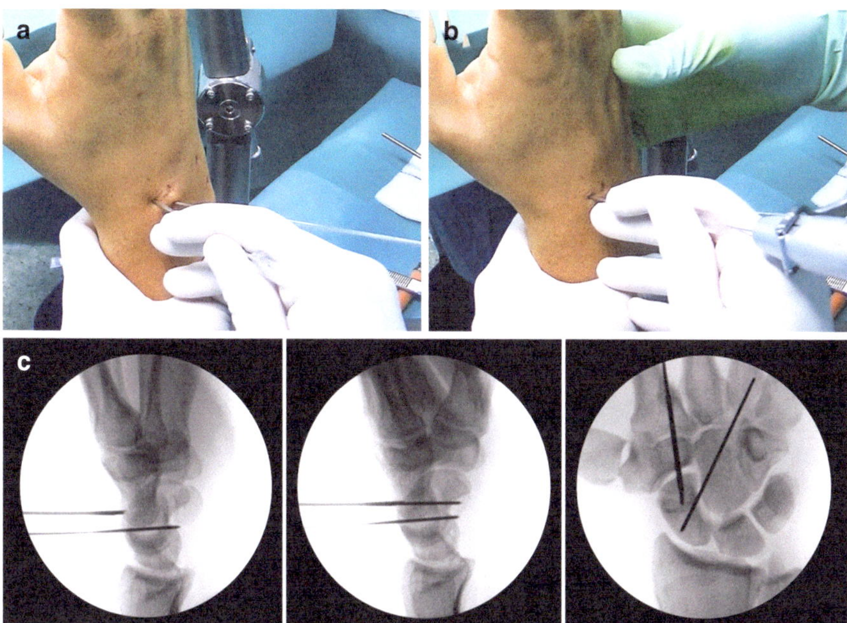

Fig. 15.15 K-wire placement for the volar tunnel. (**a, b**) Placement of the K-wire through an incision distal and radial to 3/4. (**c**) X-ray of the K-wire position

The insertion of the K-wire of the volar tunnel is introduced distally and radially to the 3/4 portal at the same level as the radial midcarpal (RMC) portal. It can be introduced directly through the skin or after making a small skin incision. Care should be taken not to damage or cross the extensor carpi radialis tendons. This K-wire should be placed with a slight volar inclination and should exist on the volar side distal to the dorsal tunnel K-wire (Fig. 15.15).

Scaphoid Dorsal Tunnel

After the insertion of the K-wire, a 2.7-mm tunnel should be created using a cannulated drill bit. The depth of the tunnel should be at least 1 cm, as the screw is 8 mm long but should not go close to the volar side to avoid the risk of a bone fracture.

After drilling, a small red canula (that can be found in the biotenodesis set) is placed inside the tunnel to make it easier to locate in the next steps. The K-wire is removed (Fig. 15.16).

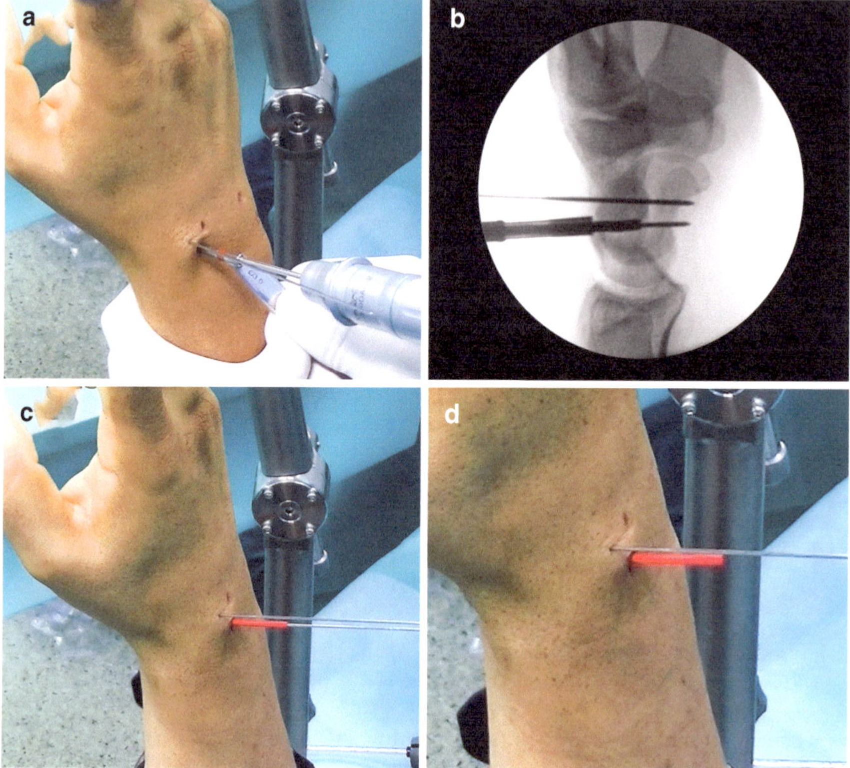

Fig. 15.16 (**a, b**) Dorsal tunnel in the scaphoid (2.7 mm). (**c, d**) A small red cannula is placed inside the tunnel following the K-wire

Lunate K-Wire Placement and Tunnel

A 1.5 cm longitudinal dorsal central (DC) incision is made overlying the fourth extensor tendon compartment and the lunate. The extensor retinaculum is opened longitudinally, and the tendons of the fourth compartment are retracted toward the radial side, exposing the articular capsule (Fig. 15.17).

Once the capsule is exposed, the Abbocath is used again as a guide. The K-wire is placed centered in the lunate in the posteroanterior view and parallel to its surface on the lateral view (Fig. 15.18).

The tunnel at this step is performed with a 2.5-mm drill bit, but its final size will be 3 mm. The final drilling of this size will be performed in a further step when the volar central portal is performed and not now to avoid overdrilling if the 3 mm drill bit is used twice. The red canula is introduced in the tunnel, and the K-wire is removed (Fig. 15.19).

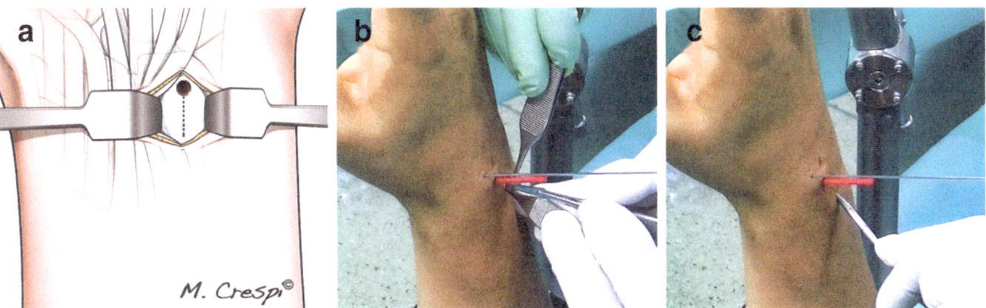

Fig. 15.17 (**a**) Dorsal central (DC) incision overlying the lunate. (**b**) The extensor retinaculum is opened longitudinally (**c**) Tendons of the fourth compartment are retracted toward the radial side.

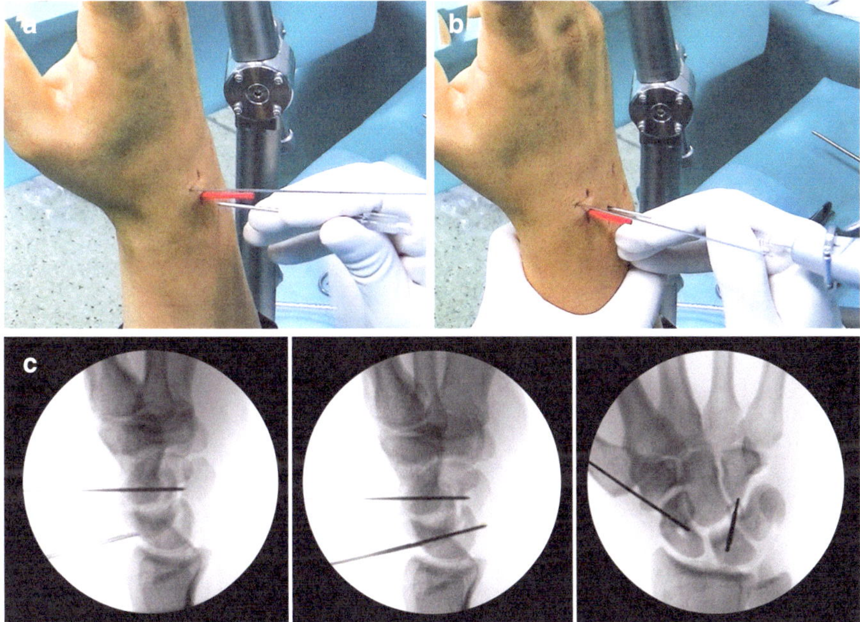

Fig. 15.18 K-wire placement for the lunate tunnel. (**a**, **b**) Placement of the K-wire through the DC incision. (**c**) X-ray of the K-wire

Scaphoid Volar Tunnel

On the volar size, the 1.5 cm approach of a volar radial (VR) portal is performed. The flexor carpi radialis (FCR) tendon is retracted to the ulnar size, and the volar sheath of the tendon is opened until the volar capsule is reached, and the volar exit of the K-wire is seen. It is useful to perform this step with the arthroscope inserted through the ulnar midcarpal (UMC) portal; in this way, the light inside the joint and the transillumination will help with the visualization of the K-wire.

The K-wire is advanced from dorsal, and the volar tunnel is performed with a 2.5 mm cannulated drill bit. The depth of the tunnel should be 1 cm, but again, it

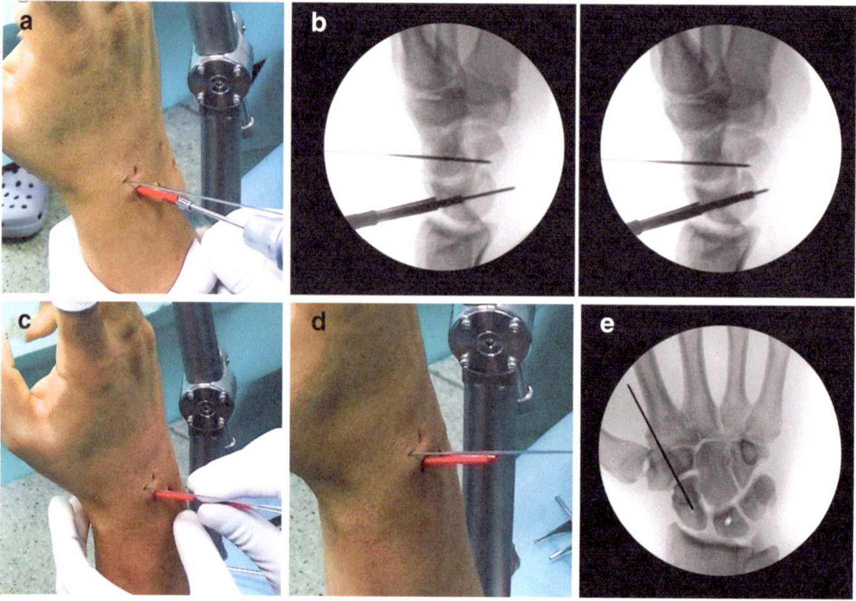

Fig. 15.19 (**a, b**) Lunate tunnel (2.5 mm). (**c, d**) A small red cannula is placed inside the tunnel. (**e**) PA X-ray of the lunate tunnel

should not go too close to the dorsal side to avoid the risk of a bone fracture Fig. 15.20.

Step 2: Graft Harvesting and Preparation for Recovering the Graft

Graft Harvesting

The graft is obtained from the palmaris longus (PL) tendon (or if not possible from the radial side of the FCR tendon). The width of the graft should be 2.5 cm.

The graft is harvested through the 1.5 cm incision of the volar central portal. A 2O' monofilament suture is passed around the PL. An incision is performed 12–15 cm proximally over the tendon. A passing wire is introduced from this incision to the volar central (VC) portal. The threads of the 2O' monofilament suture are loaded into the passing wire and brought to the proximal incision. By pulling the threads, the tendon graft is separated from the surrounding soft tissues. Finally, the graft is cut proximally and retrieved in the VC portal (Fig. 15.21).

The graft is pretensed in a bone graft preparation station (Fig. 15.22).

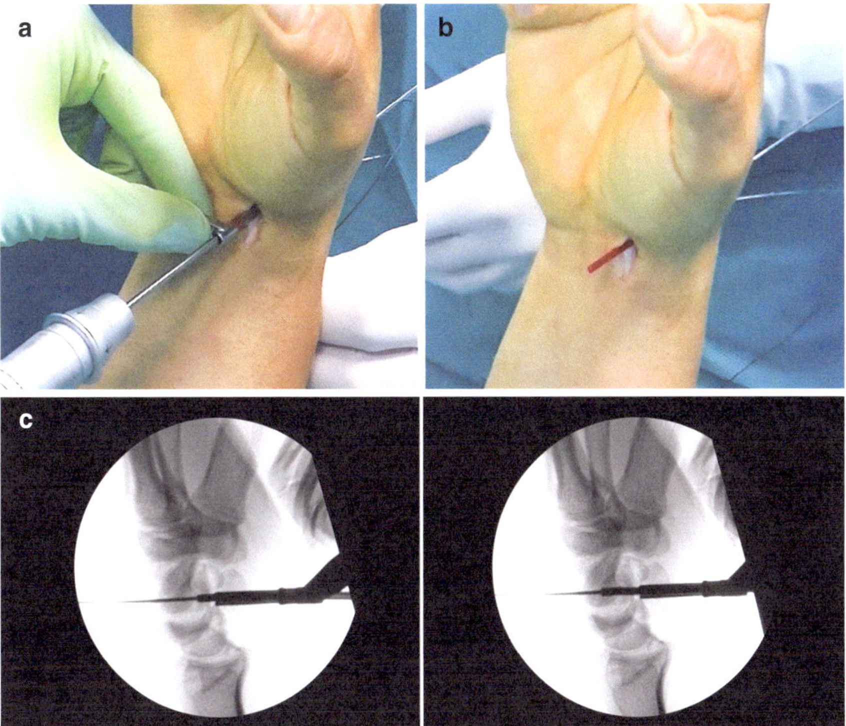

Fig. 15.20 (**a**) Volar tunnel in the scaphoid (2.5 mm). (**b**) A small red cannula is placed inside the tunnel. (**c**) X-ray of the drilling

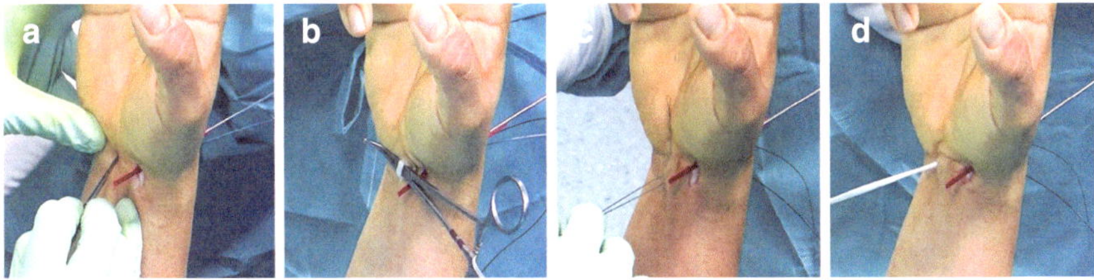

Fig. 15.21 (**a–d**) Palmaris longus graft harvest through the incision of the VC portal

Volar Central Portal and Redrill of the Lunate Tunnel

The volar central portal approach is performed until the volar capsule is reached. To make this approach easier, it is useful again to introduce the arthroscope and use transillumination to improve vision.

Once the approach is performed, a K-wire is introduced through the red cannula and advanced inside the VC portal. Now, the final 3 mm drilling is performed. The

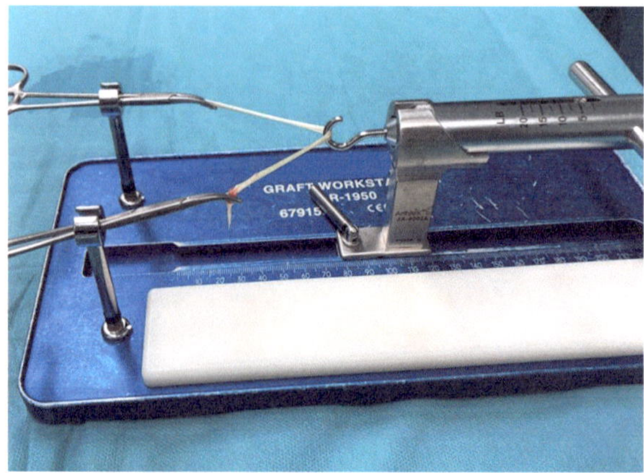

Fig. 15.22 Graft pretensing in a graft preparation station

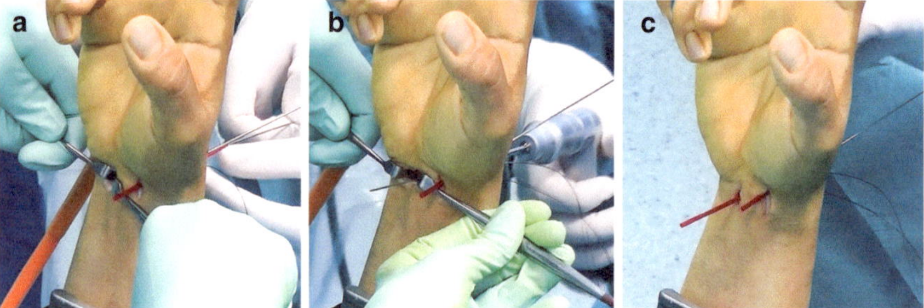

Fig. 15.23 (**a, b**) Second drilling of the lunate (3 mm). (**c**) A small red cannula is placed inside the tunnel

drill bit is advanced until the volar capsule is pierced through. Once more, the red canula is introduced and advanced inside the VC portal (Fig. 15.23).

Preparation for Recovering the Graft Volar Side

A dissector is passed over the capsule underlying the flexor tendons from the VC portal to the VR portal. A nitinol loop is captured in the VR portal and taken to the VC portal (Fig. 15.24).

To ensure that there is no tendon capture or between the loop and capsule, the arthroscope can be introduced in the VR portal and advanced under the tendons (Fig. 15.25).

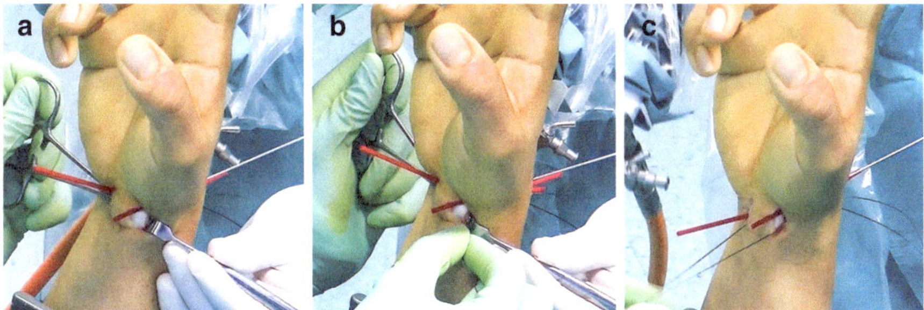

Fig. 15.24 Placement of a nitinol loop underlying the flexor tendons from the VC portal to the VR portal. (**a**) A dissector is passed over the capsule underlying the flexor tendons from the VC portal to the VR portal. (**b**) A nitinol loop is captured. (**c**) The nitinol loop is taken to the VC portal

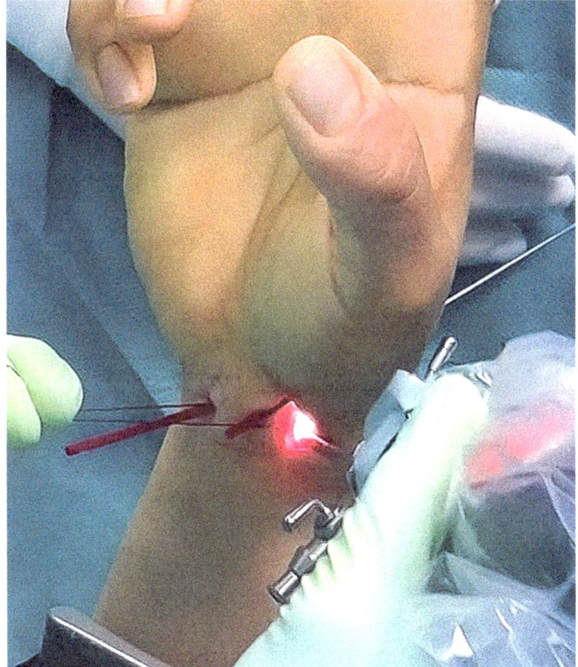

Fig. 15.25 The correct position of the nitinol loop can be checked with the arthroscope through the VR portal to ensure that there are no tendons captured

Preparation for Recovering the Graft Dorsal Side

The arthroscope is located in the 6R portal. Under arthroscopic control, a small incision is made in the capsule through the DC incision, uniting the entrance of the lunate tunnel (red cannula) with the radiocarpal joint (Figs. 15.26, 15.27). This detail ensures that the graft will pass from inside the joint to the tunnel without wedging in the capsule.

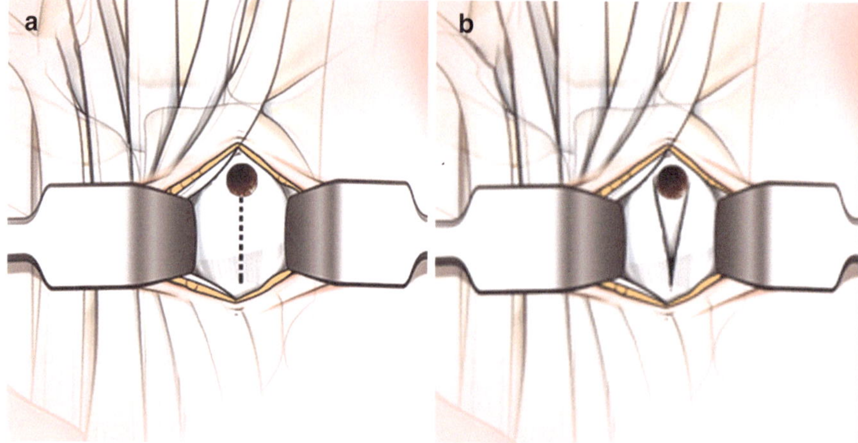

Fig. 15.26 (**a**) Schematic representation showing how the lunate tunnel needs to be united with the joint. (**b**) Size of the opening in the joint capsule

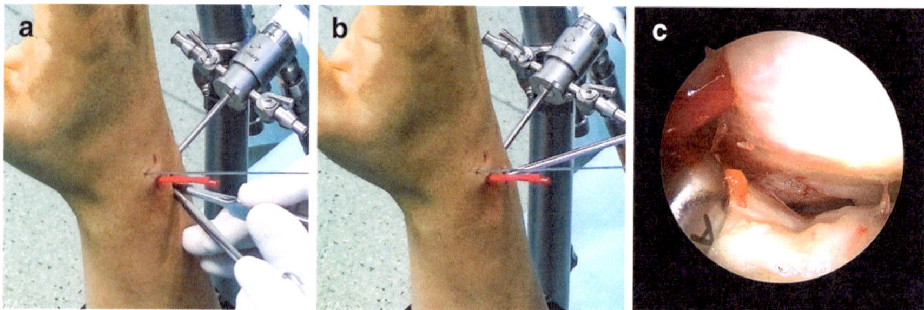

Fig. 15.27 (**a**) An incision in the capsule is performed to unite the lunate and the radiocarpal joint. (**b, c**) Soft tissues are removed around the red cannula to ensure that the graft will not be caught

The arthroscope is advanced until the red canula of the dorsal tunnel is found. The soft tissue around the canula is removed to ensure that there is no tissue between the canula and the 3/4 portal (Fig. 15.28). Again, it is extremely important to ensure that the graft will pass intraarticularly from the scaphoid tunnel to the lunate tunnel without wedging with the capsule.

Now, the nitinol loop is introduced through the DC incision and retrieved from the 3/4 portal with a mosquito clamp (Figs. 15.28, 15.29).

Step 3: Graft Passage and Fixation

SutureTape® (Arthrex, Naples, FL, USA) is used both to improve the resistance and fixation strength of the graft and for the final step of reinforcement.

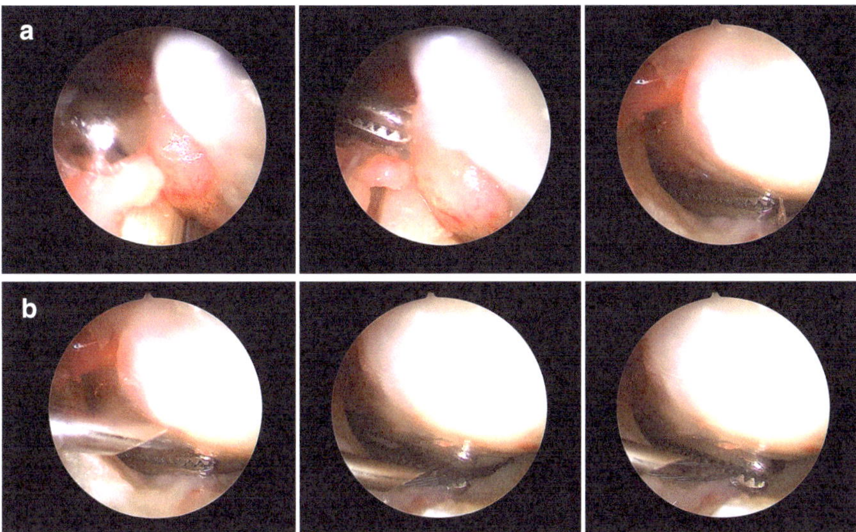

Fig. 15.28 (**a**) A mosquito is introduced through the 3/4 portal. (**b**) A SutureLasso introduced through the DC incision. Its loop is captured with the mosquito

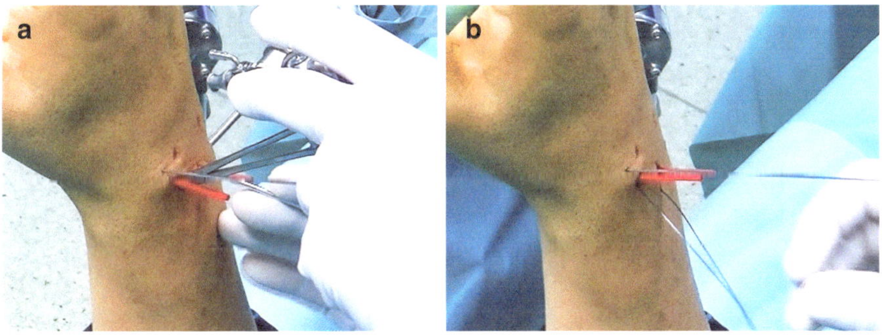

Fig. 15.29 (**a**) The mosquito enters through the 3/4 portal and the SutureLasso through the DC incision. (**b**) Placement of the nitinol loop

Graft Passage and Fixation in the Scaphoid Dorsal Tunnel

A speed whip-stitch technique with a 4/0 fiber loop is performed in one tail of the graft.

A 1.0 passing wire is introduced through the red canula from dorsal to the VR portal. The canula is removed, and the threads of the graft plus the SutureTape are captured and taken to the VR portal until the graft is introduced inside the scaphoid dorsal tunnel.

Under arthroscopic visualization, a 3x8 mm BioTenodesis screw→ (Arthrex, Naples, FL) was used to fix the graft and SutureTape. It is introduced from dorsal while tension is placed on the threads from volar (Fig. 15.30).

Graft Passage and Fixation in the Lunate Tunnel

The graft is now captured by the loop that was prepared before and taken to the DC incision over the lunate.

It can be checked under arthroscopy visualization that the graft is intraarticular, and no capsule or soft tissues are captured (Fig. 15.31).

A Straight SutureLasso® (Arthrex, Naples, FL, USA) is introduced from the VC portal to the DC incision following the red cannula. The graft and SutureTape are captured and taken to the VC portal. The tail of the SutureTape is retained on the dorsal side; in this way, there is a loop of SutureTape on the volar side. This loop is cut, leaving 2 pieces of tape inside the tunnel. One of them will run along with the graft, and the other one will be used afterwards to create the reinforcement (Fig. 15.32).

The reduction in instability is visualized with the arthroscope located in the UMC portal. Tension is applied to the graft from the volar side, and the reduction of instability (SL step-off, SL gap, and dorsal extension of the lunate) is checked (Fig. 15.33).

Finally, while maintaining the correct tension, the BioTenodesis screw is inserted into the lunate tunnel from dorsal (Fig. 15.34). Its insertion can be visualized and checked, either under fluoroscopic or arthroscopic control with the scope entering through the 6R portal (Fig. 15.35).

Graft Passage and Fixation in the Scaphoid Volar Tunnel

For this last fixation, the graft and SutureTape will be fixed in the volar tunnel with a 2. × 6 mm BioTenodesis screw® (Arthrex, Naples, FL, USA) (Fig. 15.36).

The graft and both tails of the SutureTape are passed in an extraarticular manner. They are captured by the previously placed loop and brought to the VR portal (Fig. 15.37).

A mark is made where the tendon will enter the volar tunnel. This exact point can be better visualized with the help of the arthroscope. A crossing suture is performed with the 4/0 fiber loop, and the excess tendon is cut away from the graft (Fig. 15.38). A passing wire is introduced in the volar tunnel, and the threads of the fiber loop and one SutureTape are captured and taken to dorsal (Fig. 15.39).

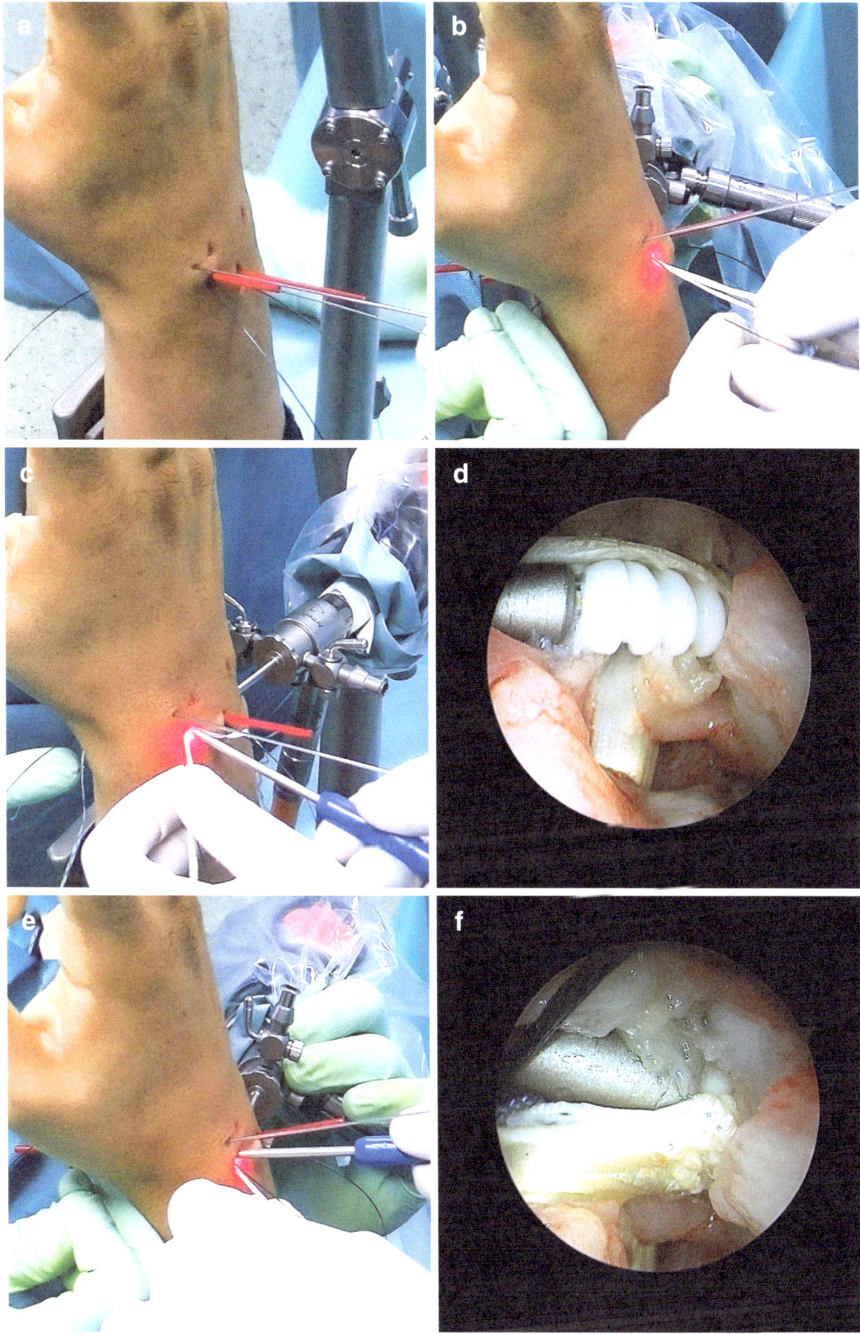

Fig. 15.30 (**a**, **b**) The graft and tape are captured with a passing wire and taken inside the dorsal scaphoid tunnel. (**c-f**) Fixation of the graft and suture tape with a 3x8 mm BioTenodesis screw® (Arthrex, Naples, FL) was performed under arthroscopic control from the 6R portal

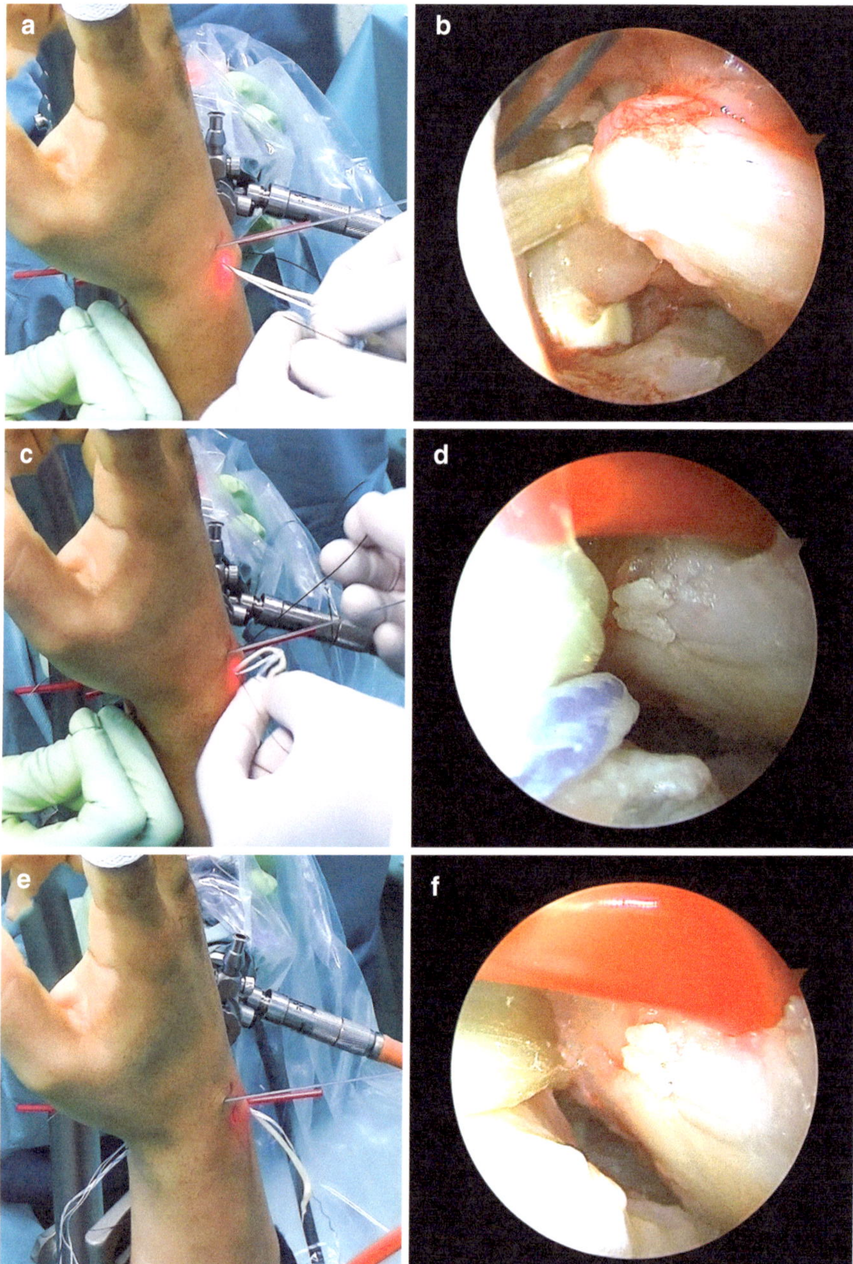

Fig. 15.31 The graft and tape are captured with the nitinol loop (**a**) The graft and tape are captured with the nitinol loop. (**b**) they are passed inside the joint under the capsule. (**c**) Finbally taken to the DC incision

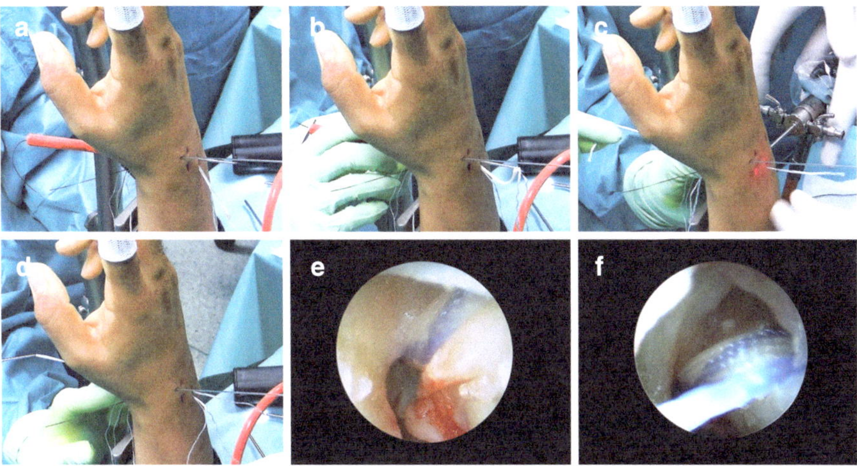

Fig. 15.32 (**a-c**) Passage of the graft and suture tape through the tunnel in the lunate. A tail of the tape should be maintained in the dorsal side (**d**) The loop of suture tape is cut on the volar side. (**e, f**) There are two pieces of tape inside the lunate tunnel. One follows the graft, and the other remains in the DC incision

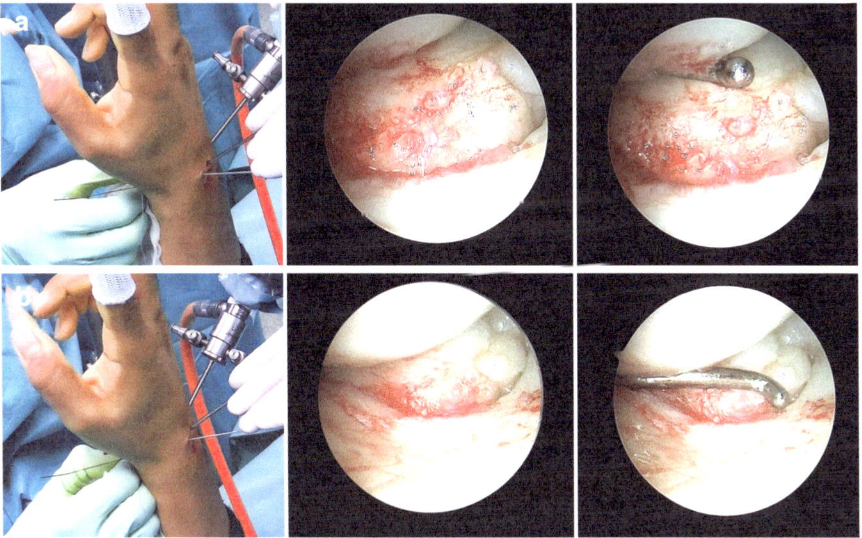

Fig. 15.33 (**a**) Without traction, there is a large step-off between the scaphoid and lunate and a DISI deformity. (**b**) The step-off and the DISI deformity are corrected while traction from the tape and graft is applied from volar

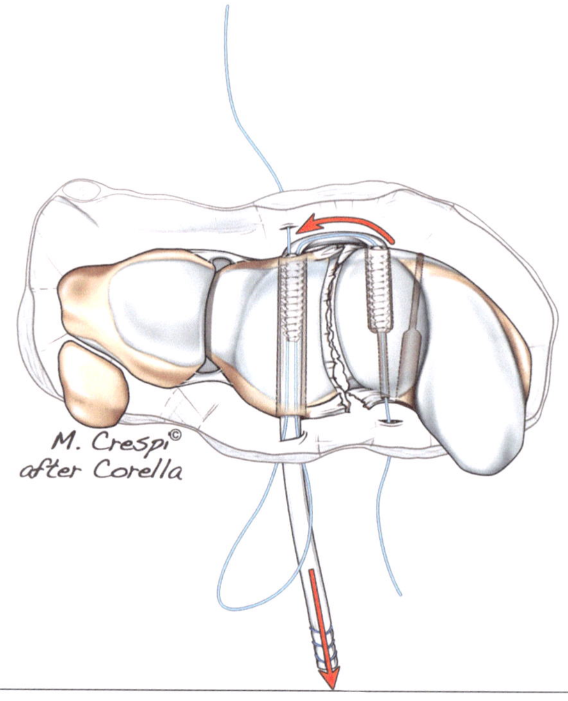

Fig. 15.34 Schematic representation of the fixation of the graft with a 3 mm BioTenodesis screw in the lunate while traction is applied from the volar side. Printed with permission of Crespi and Corella

Now, while traction is applied to the threads and SutureTape from dorsal, the BioTenodesis screw is introduced from volar. Again, this can be performed under fluoroscopic or arthroscopic visualization (Fig. 15.40).

Step 4: Extrinsic Ligament Reinforcement

The last step is the reinforcement of the extrinsic ligaments on both the dorsal and volar sides (Fig. 15.41).

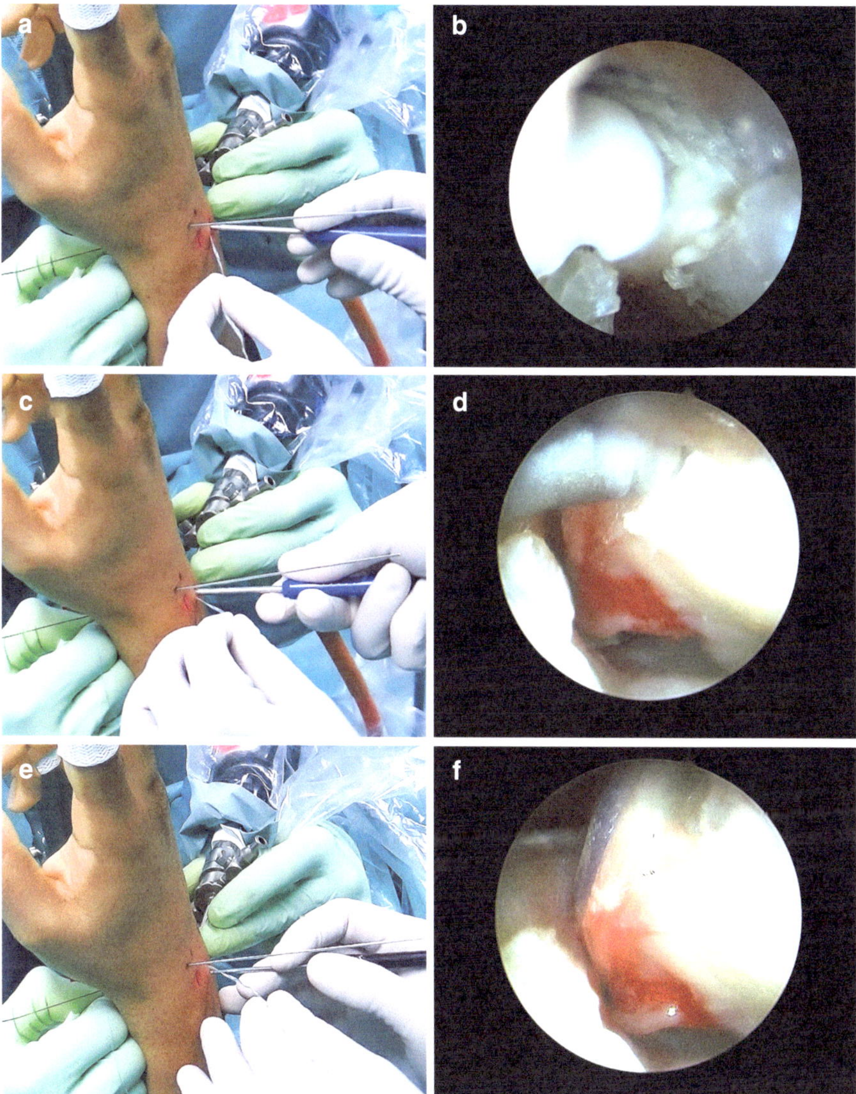

Fig. 15.35 (**a-d**) Fixation of the graft and tape with a 3x8 mm BioTenodesis screw under arthroscopic control from the 6R portal. (**e, f**) Testing of the graft tension

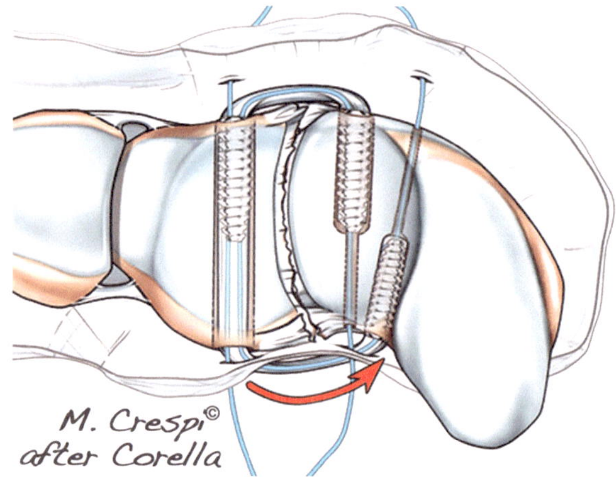

Fig. 15.36 Schematic representation of the fixation of the graft and suture tape in the volar scaphoid tunnel with a 2.5 × 6 mm BioTenodesis screw. Printed with permission of Crespi and Corella

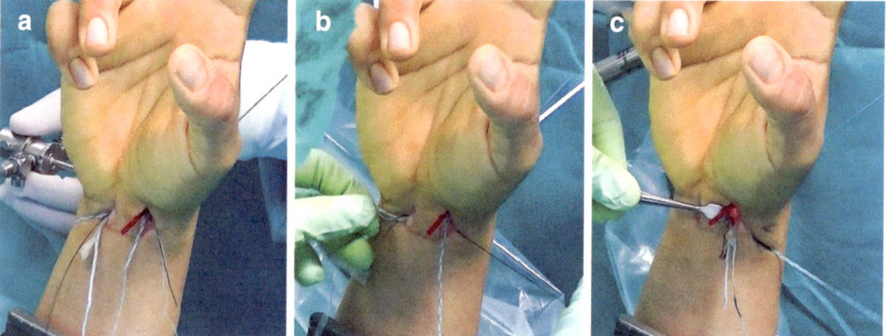

Fig. 15.37 Passage of the graft and the two tails of the suture tape under the flexor tendons from the VC portal to the VR portal. (**a**) Graft and Tape in the VC portal. (**b**) They are carpture with the nitinol loop. (**c**) And taken to the VR portal

Volar Reinforcement

Inside the VR portal, the portion of the SutureTape that exits from the scaphoid tunnel is sutured to the portion that exits from the lunate tunnel (Fig. 15.42).

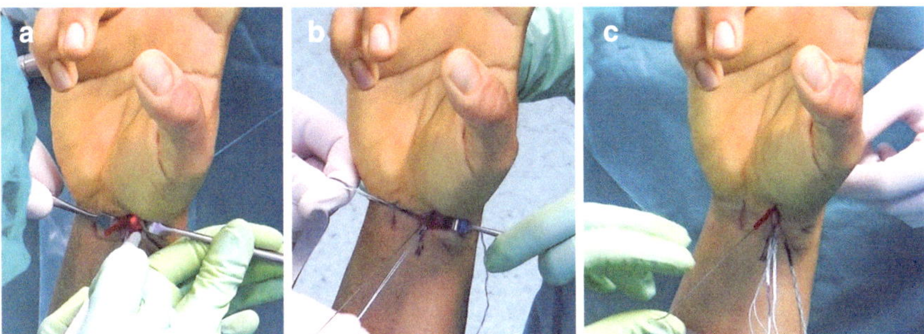

Fig. 15.38 (**a**) (a) A mark is made where the tendon will enter the volar tunnel (**b**) A 4/0 cross suture is performed and the rest of the graft is cut. (**c**) A passing wire is introduced inside the red canula and retrieved from the dorsal side

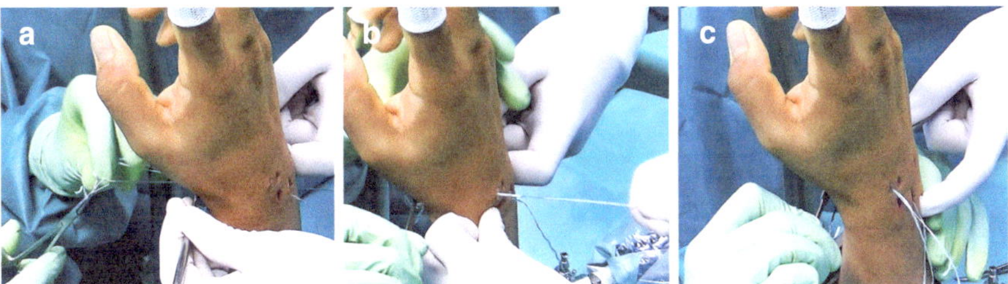

Fig. 15.39 (**a**) The threads and one tape are captured with a passing wire (**b**), taken through the scaphoid tunnel (**c**) and exit on the dorsal side

Dorsal Reinforcement

The knot of the two dorsal SutureTapes is performed in the 3/4 portal. The suture tape of the radial side is taken to the 3/4 portal, ensuring that it goes under the extensor radialis tendons (Fig. 15.43). Finally, the tape that is located in the DC incision is passed under the extensor tendons and over the capsule to the 3/4 portal. The knot is performed, and the technique is completed (Fig. 15.44).

The final arthroscopic result can be seen in (Fig. 15.45).

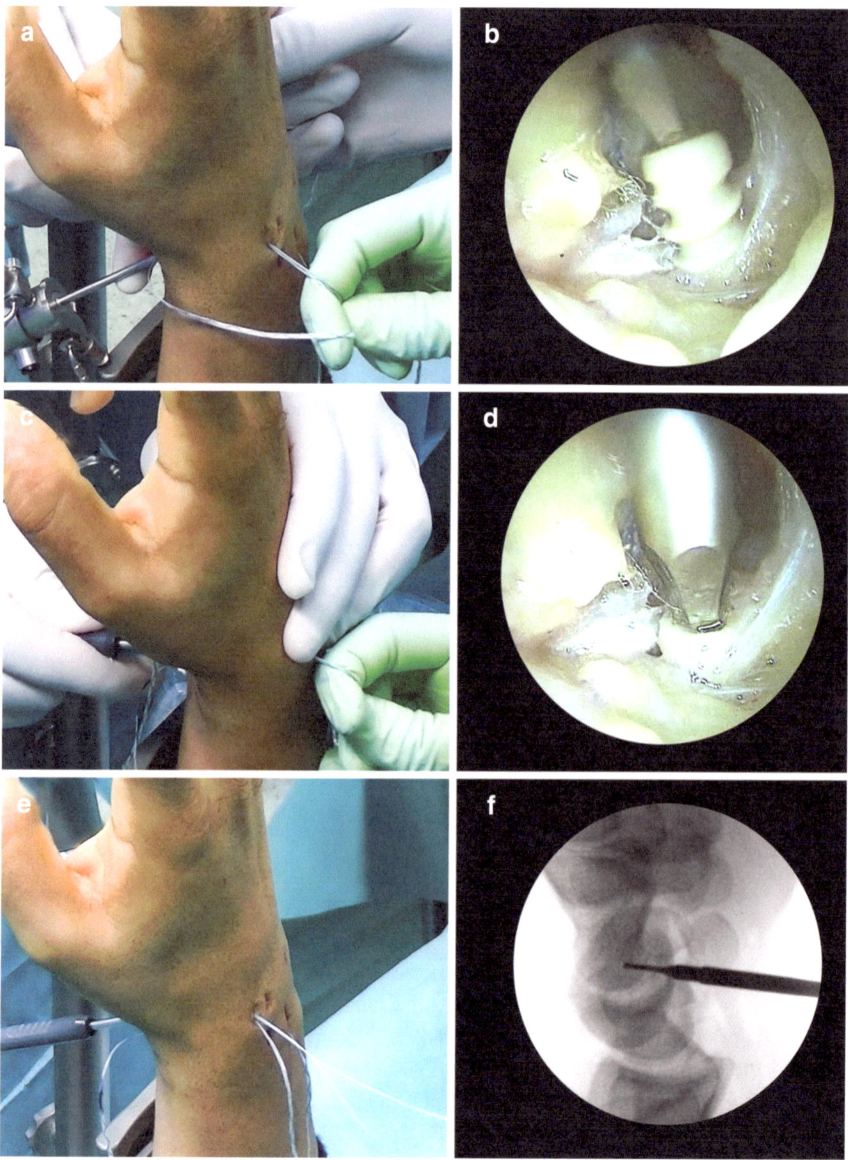

Fig. 15.40 (**a-e**). Fixation of the tape and graft in the scaphoid volar tunnel with a 2.5 × 6 mm. BioTenodesis screw under arthroscopic control. (**f**). X-ray control

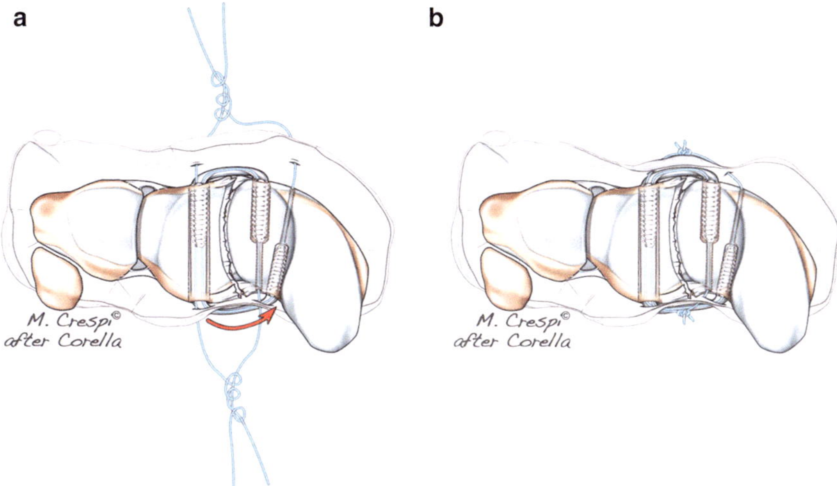

Fig. 15.41 (**a, b**) Schematic representation of the reinforcement of the extrinsic ligaments on both dorsal and volar sides

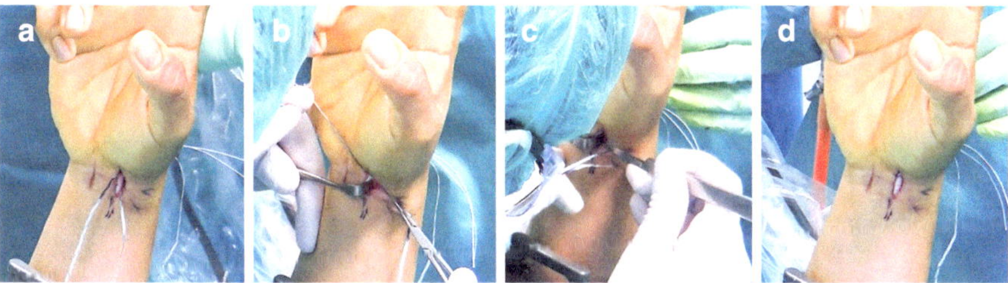

Fig. 15.42 (**a-d**) Volar reinforcement. The SutureTape that exits from the scaphoid (the one that comes from the dorsal scaphoid tunnel) is sutured to the tail that exits from the lunate tunnel

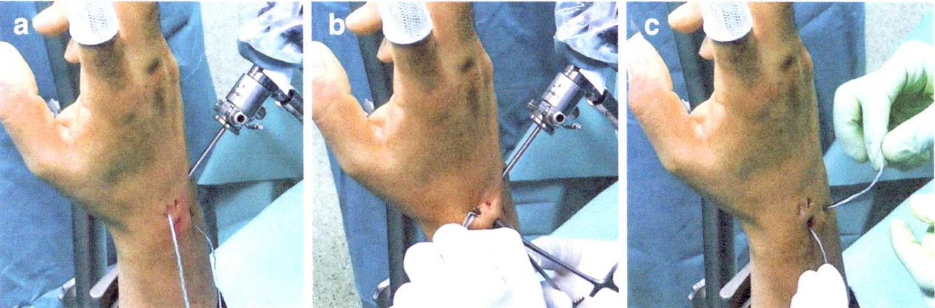

Fig. 15.43 (**a-c**) The tape that exits from the volar tunnel of the scaphoid is taken to the 3/4 portal under the extensor radialis tendons

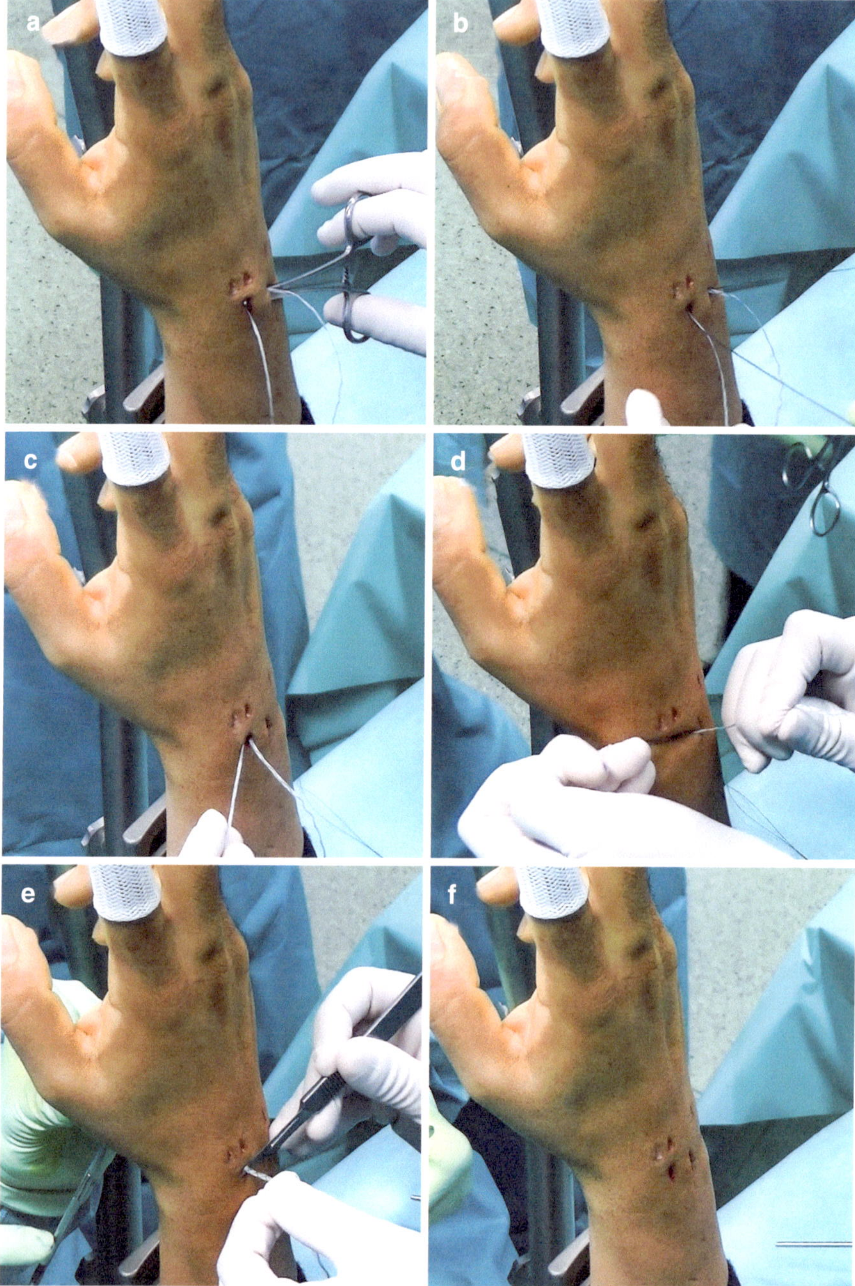

Fig. 15.44 (**a**) A mosquito is passed from the DC incision under the extensor tendons and over the capsule to the 3/4 portal. (**b**) A loop is placed in this location and is used to pass the tape that exists from the lunate tunnel to the 3/4 portal. (**c**, **d**) Both tails of the tape are sutured (**e**, **f**) The Tapes are cut, and the technique is completed

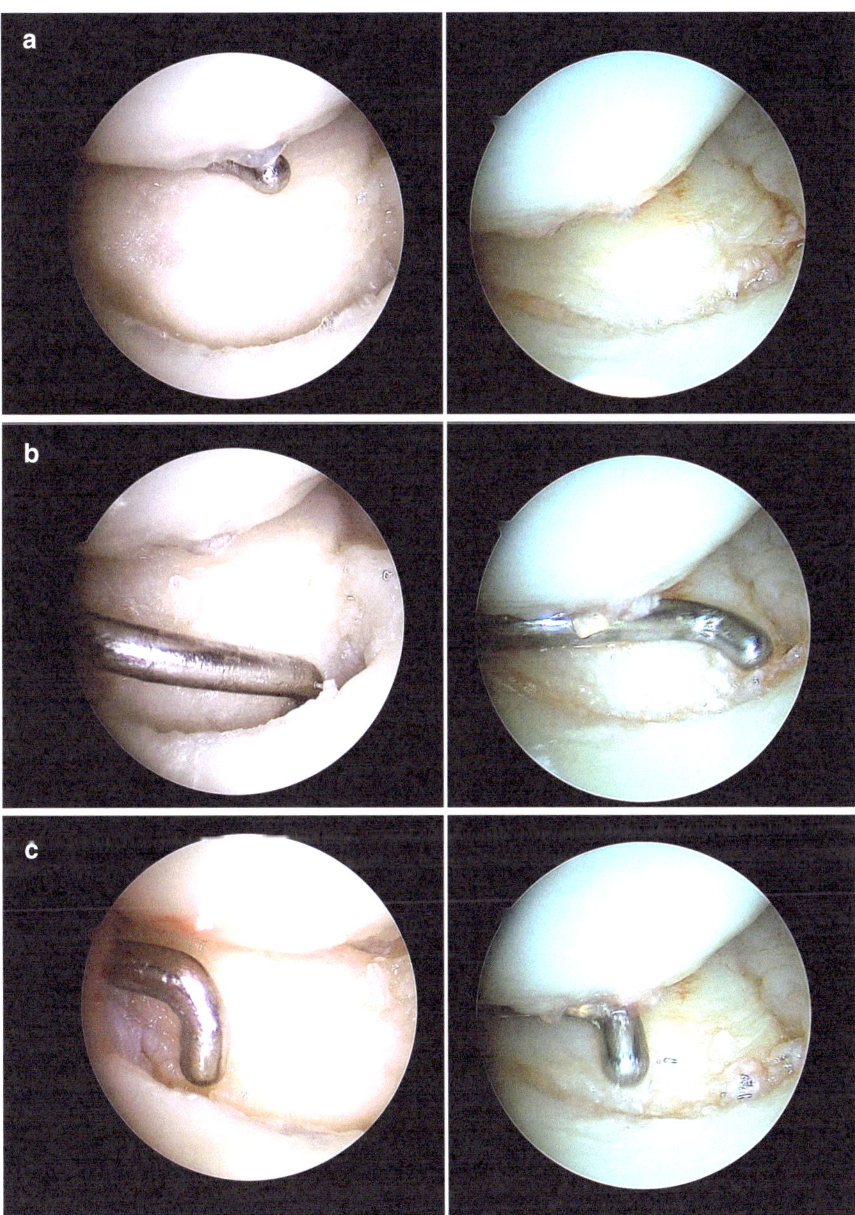

Fig. 15.45 (**a-c**) Arthroscopic comparison before reconstruction on the left and after reconstruction on the right. The correction of the step-off, gap, and DISI can be observed

Clinical Course and Outcome [with Figures]

The patient followed an early mobilization protocol (as the reinforcement of the extrinsic ligaments was performed in this technique, the motion begins at the third week compared with the previous technique in which the protocol begins at the second week).

At 1 month, the range of motion of the patient was 35° of wrist extension and 45° of wrist flexion. At 3 months, the range of motion was 50° of wrist extension, 65° of wrist flexion, and a grip force of 41 kg.

The last follow-up was performed at the sixth month. The range of motion was 75° of wrist extension and 80° of wrist flexion with complete pronosupination. Grip strength was 55 kg, with a visual analog scale of 1.4 and a Disabilities of the Arm, Shoulder and Hand score of 5.8.

In Figs. 15.46, 15.47, the clinical evolution and final X-ray are shown.

In our previous publication, there was a significant improvement in these parameters between 6 months and 1 year, so it is probable that the patient will continue improving in grip strength and range of motion.

The satisfaction of the patient in the last visit quantified using a visual analog scale was 8.9.

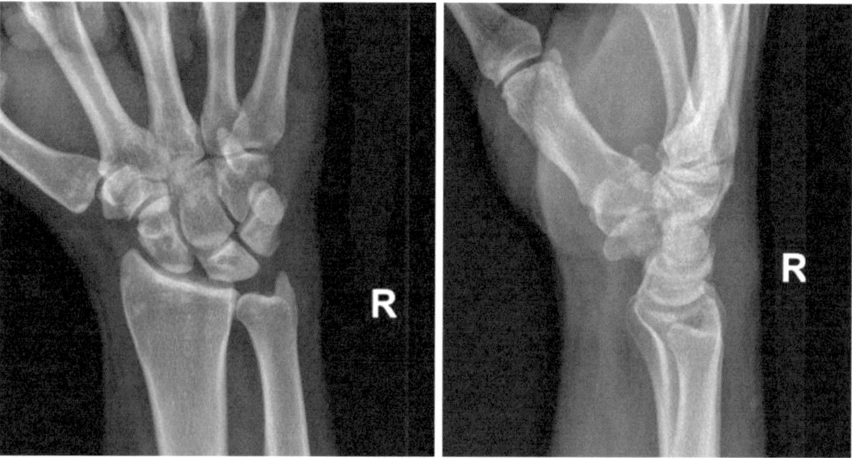

Fig. 15.46 X-rays 6 months after surgery

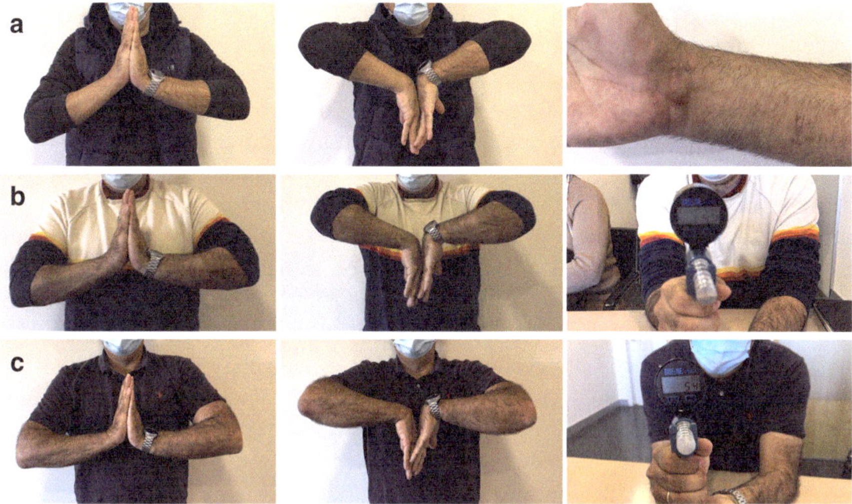

Fig. 15.47 Evolution of the clinical result. (**a**) One month after surgery. (**b**) Three months after surgery. (**c**) Six months after surgery

Bulleted Clinical Pearls/Pitfalls [3–5, with Figures]

- To perform an accurate indication between the different 4R techniques, utilize the 7-item arthroscopic exploration.
- To indicate this arthroscopic ligamentoplasty, the patient should have a complete and chronic injury, with no remnant of the ligament of sufficient quality (negative SL Hook Test) and important dorsal dynamic displacement (positive 3D test) but a reducible instability without degenerative changes.
- To reduce the surgical time, the surgeon should perform the four steps of the technique in the specific order.
- Be extremely accurate in the position of the tunnels to avoid any fracture.

Literature Review and Discussion

The management of chronic injuries to the scapholunate ligament is a challenge for hand surgeons. Many reconstructive procedures have been described to address chronic SL instability although none has come forward to be superior to others [15]. One of the options includes the use of tendon weaves. Multiple tendon weaves with the use of different tendons and patterns have been proposed to tether scaphoid motion. Brunelli and Brunelli first developed a tendon weave procedure in which a slip of the flexor carpi radialis (FCR) tendon was passed through a tunnel in the scaphoid from volar to dorsal and was fixed to the dorsoulnar side of the radius. They intended to reduce scaphoid flexion, which in turn induced reduction of the dorsal subluxation of the proximal pole and correction of the SL dissociation [16]. This technique was modified to avoid crossing the radiocarpal joint so that the tendon was fixed on the lunate or the scaphoid [17]. Several different modifications have been carried out since its original description with the purpose of reconstructing the dorsal portion of the scapholunate ligament and the secondary stabilizers of the scapholunate joint [18–20]. Chee et al. went further and modified this technique for the treatment of chronic perilunar instabilities with the reconstruction of the antipronation ligamentous complex (including the palmar lunotriquetral ligament) [21].

Historically, the different forms of reconstruction of the scapholunate ligament were focused on the dorsal portion since it is the thickest and the strongest. The palmar portion is the second strongest part, and it is an important constraint to rotation of the Sl joint [22, 23]. Reconstruction with only one dorsal fixation point between the two bones cannot preclude volar widening and sagittal rotation. With an additional reconstruction on the volar side, the second strongest portion is also restored. Therefore, recreating both the dorsal and volar Sl portions becomes logical biomechanically and is gaining attention in recent years combined or not with reconstruction of the secondary stabilizers [24–30]. The SLAM technique is another procedure in which a tendon graft is placed in the central axis of the SL joint and anchored with a graft anchor.

While most of the procedures described are performed open, some authors have proposed arthroscopic ligament reconstruction to preserve capsuloligamentous structures [24, 25, 27, 31].

Arthroscopic ligamentoplasty of the dorsal and volar portions of the scapholunate ligament was described in 2013 and combined the advantages of arthroscopic (minimally invasive surgery) and open techniques (reconstruction of the ligament) [24]. It serves the three-fold purpose of anatomic reconstruction, avoidance of open surgery, and reliable and sturdy reconstruction for early mobilization [24].

Anatomic Reconstruction

This technique restores the dorsal and volar portions of the SL ligament and reinforces the dorsal intercarpal (DIC) ligament. In addition, it also restores scaphoid alignment. Short and colleagues demonstrated that the scaphoid bone was not only flexed but also pronated in SL instability [32, 33]. Scaphoid pronation creates static stress at the dorsum of the wrist. It also produces dynamic stress as the scaphoid is dorsally translated over the dorsal rim of the radius at wrist extension and radial deviation. This technique supinates the scaphoid and prevents dorsal translation of the scaphoid over the scaphoid fossa.

In the original description, the authors used a strip of FCR tendon; however, in this modification, the palmaris longus graft is used. Thus, a potential scaphoid stabilizer is not endangered [34].

The fixation of the graft to the scaphoid has also been modified by means of two blind transosseous tunnels and tenodesis screws, which provides a more robust fixation. Now, all tails of the graft are fixed inside the bone with a screw instead of suturing the volar side with an anchor.

Avoidance of Open Surgery and Detachment of the Joint Capsule

Arthroscopic SL reconstruction is a minimally invasive technique that obviates the need for extensive open dissection and capsulotomy. Postoperative fibrosis, scarring, and stiffness are minimized in this way. The dorsal intercarpal ligament is not detached from the bones and is one of the most important SL secondary stabilizers [35]. In addition, with this technique, the posterior interosseous nerve (PIN) is preserved, so the function of important dynamic stabilizers such as the abductor pollicis longus, extensor carpi radialis, FCR, and flexor carpi ulnaris is also preserved [36–38].

Reinforcement of Extrinsic Ligaments

In recent years, numerous papers have focused on the importance of the dorsal intercarpal (DIC) ligament in SL instability. With this evolved technique, not only is the ligament reconstructed, but the DIC is reinforced to the bone as the dorsal suture tape goes over the capsule and under the extensor tendons.

Reliable and Sturdy Reconstruction for Early Mobilization

In this technique, the graft is fixed directly onto the bone with interference screws. A K-wire is not used. This allows midcarpal motion in 3 weeks and a full range of motion in 4 weeks.

Double Circle Technique Justification

As explained in the chapter, this technique reconstructs the scapholunate dorsal and volar portions with a free tendon graft that is fixed inside the bone with three interference screws. This is the first circle of a "biological circle."

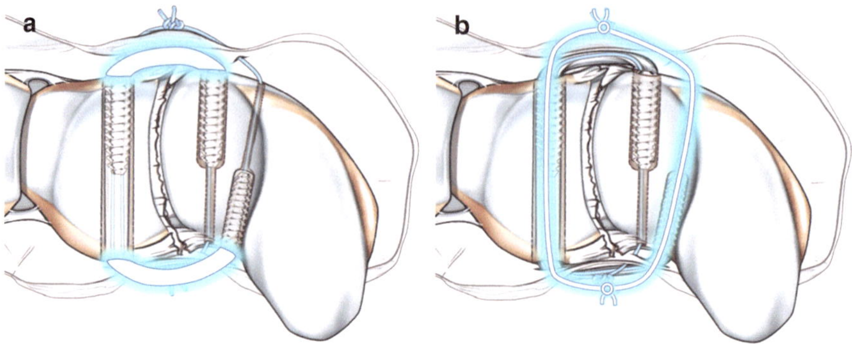

Fig. 15.48 (**a**) First "biological circle." (**b**) Second "reinforcement circle"

Furthermore, the extrinsic ligaments are reinforced by using a SutureTape over the capsule, which improves the strength of the reconstruction and secures the extrinsic ligaments to the bone. This is the second circle is termed the "reinforcement circle" (Fig. 15.48).

References

1. Kirk Watson H, Ashmead D, Vincent MM. Examination of the scaphoid. J Hand Surg. 1988;13(5):657–60.
2. Easterling KJ, Wolfe SW. Scaphoid shift in the uninjured wrist. J Hand Surg. 1994;19(4):604–6.
3. Garcia-Elias MLAL. Wrist Instabilities, Misalignments, and Dislocation. In: HRKSPWCM WSW, editor. Green's operative hand surgery. 7th ed. Churchill Livingstone: Elsevier; 2017.
4. Kleinman WB. Physical examination of the wrist: Useful provocative maneuvers. J Hand Surg. 2015;40(7):1486–500.
5. Caggiano N, Matullo KS. Carpal instability of the wrist. Orthop Clin North Am. 2014;45(1):129–40.
6. Michelotti BF, Adkinson JM, Chung KC. Chronic scapholunate ligament injury: techniques in repair and reconstruction. Hand Clin. 2015;31(3):437–49.
7. Hafezi-Nejad N, Carrino JA, Eng J, Blackmore C, Shores J, Lifchez SD, et al. Scapholunate Interosseous Ligament Tears: Diagnostic Performance of 1.5 T, 3 T MRI, and MR Arthrography—A Systematic Review and Meta-analysis. Acad Radiol. 2016;23(9):1091–103.
8. Corella F, Messina J, Ocampos M, Ranelli P. Arthroscopic Examination of the Wrist. In: Corella F, Heras-Palou C, Luchetti R, editors. Carpal ligament injuries and instability. First. Stuttgart, Germany: Thieme; 2023. p. 59–79.
9. Messina JC, Van Overstraeten L, Luchetti R, Fairplay T, Mathoulin CL. The EWAS Classification of Scapholunate Tears: An Anatomical Arthroscopic Study. J Wrist Surg. 2013;2(2):105–9.
10. Herzberg G. Perilunate Injuries, Not Dislocated (PLIND). J Wrist Surg. 2013;02(04):337–45.
11. Corella F, Del Cerro M, Ocampos M, Larrainzar-Garijo R. The "Rocking Chair Sign" for Floating Lunate. J Hand Surg Am. 2015;40(11):2318–9. http://linkinghub.elsevier.com/retrieve/pii/S0363502315010965.
12. Watson HK, Ballet FL. The SLAC wrist: Scapholunate advanced collapse pattern of degenerative arthritis. J Hand Surg. 1984;9(3):358–65.

13. Luchetti R, Corella F. The "4R" Algorithm of Treatment. In: Corella F, Heras-Palou C, Luchetti R, editors. Carpal ligament injuries and instability. First. Stuttgart, Germany: Thieme; 2023. p. 97–102.
14. Corella F, Ocampos M, Del CM. Arthroscopic Scaphoid 3D Test for Scapholunate Instability. J Wrist Surg. 2017;1(212):2–5.
15. Wang P, Stepan JG, An T, Osei DA. Equivalent Clinical Outcomes Following Favored Treatments of Chronic Scapholunate Ligament Tear. HSS J. 2017;13(2):186–93.
16. Brunelli GA, Brunelli GR. A new technique to correct carpal instability with scaphoid rotary subluxation: A preliminary report. J Hand Surg. 1995;20(3 PART 2):S82–5.
17. Van Den Abbeele KLS, Loh YC, Stanley JK, Trail IA. Early results of a modified Brunelli procedure for scapholunate instability. J Hand Surg. 1998;23(2):258–61.
18. Bain GI, Watts AC, McLean J, Lee YC, Eng K. Cable-augmented, quad ligament tenodesis scapholunate reconstruction: Rationale, surgical technique, and preliminary results. Tech Hand Up Extrem Surg. 2013;17(1):13–9.
19. Garcia-Elias M, Lluch AL, Stanley JK. Three-ligament tenodesis for the treatment of scapholunate dissociation: Indications and surgical technique. J Hand Surg. 2006;31(1):125–34.
20. Ross M, Loveridge J, Cutbush K, Couzens G. Scapholunate Ligament Reconstruction. J Wrist Surg. 2013;02(02):110–5.
21. Chee KG, Chin AYH, Chew EM, Garcia-Elias M. Antipronation spiral tenodesis—a surgical technique for the treatment of perilunate instability. J Hand Surg Am. 2012;37(12):2611–8. http://www.ncbi.nlm.nih.gov/pubmed/23174077.
22. Berger RA. The gross and histologic anatomy of the scapholunate interosseous ligament. J Hand Surg Am. 1996;21(2):170–8.
23. Berger RA, Imeada T, Berglund L, An KN. Constraint and material properties of the subregions of the scapholunate interosseous ligament. J Hand Surg Am. 1999;24(5):953–62.
24. Corella F, Del Cerro M, Ocampos M, Larrainzar-Garijo R. Arthroscopic ligamentoplasty of the dorsal and volar portions of the scapholunate ligament. J Hand Surg. 2013;38(12):2466–77. https://doi.org/10.1016/j.jhsa.2013.09.021.
25. Corella F, Del Cerro M, Ocampos M, Simon de Blas C, Larrainzar-Garijo R. Arthroscopic Scapholunate Ligament Reconstruction, Volar and Dorsal Reconstruction. Hand Clin. 2017;33(4):687–707.
26. Henry M. Reconstruction of both volar and dorsal limbs of the scapholunate interosseous ligament. J Hand Surg. 2013;38(8):1625–34.
27. Ho P, Wong C, Tse W. Arthroscopic-Assisted combined dorsal and volar scapholunate ligament reconstruction with tendon graft for chronic SL instability. J Wrist Surg. 2015;04(04):252–63.
28. Kakar S, Greene R. Scapholunate Ligament Internal Brace 360-Degree Tenodesis (SLITT) Procedure. J Wrist Surg. 2018;07(04):336–40.
29. Kakar S, Greene RM, Garcia-Elias M. Carpal Realignment Using a Strip of Extensor Carpi Radialis Longus Tendon. J Hand Surg. 2017;42(8):667.e1–8.
30. Sandow M, Fisher T. Anatomical anterior and posterior reconstruction for scapholunate dissociation: preliminary outcome in ten patients. J Hand Surg. 2020;45(4):389–95.
31. Carratalá V, Lucas FJ, Alepuz ES, Guisasola E, Calero R. Arthroscopically Assisted Ligamentoplasty for Axial and Dorsal Reconstruction of the Scapholunate Ligament. Arthrosc Tech. 2016;5(2):e353–9.
32. Short WH, Werner FW, Fortino MD, Palmer AK, Mann KA. A dynamic biomechanical study of scapholunate ligament sectioning. J Hand Surg. 1995;20(6):986–99.
33. Short WH, Werner FW, Green JK, Sutton LG, Brutus JP. Biomechanical Evaluation of the Ligamentous Stabilizers of the Scaphoid and Lunate: Part III. J Hand Surg Am. 2007;32(3):297–309.
34. Salva-Coll G, Garcia-Elias M, Hagert E. Scapholunate Instability: Proprioception and Neuromuscular Control. J Wrist Surg. 2013;02(02):136–40.

35. Mitsuyasu H, Patterson RM, Shah MA, Buford WL, Iwamoto Y, Viegas SF. The Role the Dorsal Intercarpal Ligament in Dynamic and Static Scapholunate Instability. J Hand Surg. 2004;29(2):279–88.
36. Hagert E. Proprioception of the Wrist Joint: A Review of Current Concepts and Possible Implications on the Rehabilitation of the Wrist. J Hand Surg. 2010;23(1):2–17.
37. Hagert E, Ljung BO, Forsgren S. General innervation pattern and sensory corpuscles in the scapholunate interosseous ligament. Cells Tissues Organs. 2004;177(1):47–54.
38. Hagert E, Persson JKE, Werner M, Ljung BO. Evidence of Wrist Proprioceptive Reflexes Elicited After Stimulation of the Scapholunate Interosseous Ligament. J Hand Surg. 2009;34(4):642–51.

Chapter 16
Chronic Scapholunate Instability: The Role of the Three-Ligament Tenodesis

Shruti Raut and Sumedh C. Talwalkar

Case

A 29-year-old, fit and well construction worker was referred to our institution with a 1-year history of dorso-radial wrist pain after a fall from scaffolding. X-rays at his local Emergency Department were normal (Fig. 16.1), and he was discharged with a diagnosis of a wrist sprain. He had ongoing dorso-radial wrist pain and a sensation of clicking, so was subsequently referred to our unit. Examination revealed tenderness in the dorsal scapholunate interval with a positive Kirk Watson test. X-rays were within normal limits. MRI showed increased signal in the region of the scapholunate ligament but normal carpal alignment and preserved articular cartilage.

He underwent fluoroscopic evaluation (Fig. 16.2) and although static images were normal, when asked to replicate the click and upon making a tight fist, there was notable scapholunate diastasis. Subsequent wrist arthroscopy showed a Geissler grade 2 scapholunate injury and dorsal synovitis but normal cartilage.

Considering the ongoing symptoms and clinical findings, he was counselled for surgery and subsequently underwent three-ligament tenodesis.

The normal scapholunate articulation is maintained by the C-shaped scapholunate interosseous ligament (SLIL), composed of dorsal, membranous and palmar portions. The dorsal component is a true ligament, the strongest of the three, and the most critical in stability of the scapholunate joint [1, 2] as the primary restraint to distraction, translation and rotation. The palmar portion is thinner but provides additional stability in rotation. Scapholunate dissociation is the most common type of carpal instability [3]. The typical mechanism of injury is a fall onto the outstretched hand with forced dorsiflexion and ulnar deviation of the wrist and intercarpal supination, resulting in failure, first of the palmar and finally the dorsal SLIL. This gives

S. Raut (✉) · S. C. Talwalkar
Wrightington Hospital, Wigan, UK
e-mail: Shruti.raut2@nhs.net

J. Yao (ed.), *Carpal Instability*, https://doi.org/10.1007/978-3-031-55869-6_16

S. Raut and S. C. Talwalkar

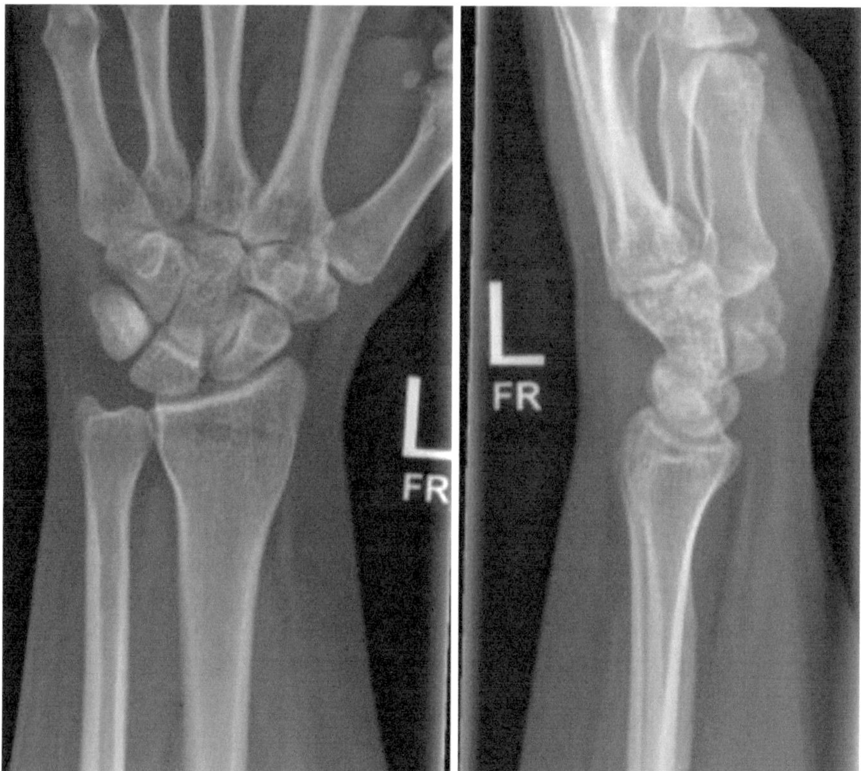

Fig. 16.1 Preoperative radiographs show normal carpal alignment

a spectrum of injury, as described by Mayfield, from SLIL sprains to frank lunate dislocation [4, 5]. If only the palmar component is injured, this is likely a stable injury with no scapholunate diastasis [6, 7]. If there is complete division of the SLIL, there is more substantial disruption to carpal kinematics but usually no immediate diastasis or malalignment unless there is associated disruption to the critical secondary stabilisers of the proximal carpal row, namely the scapho-trapezio-trapezoid, long radiolunate and dorsal intercarpal (DIC) ligaments. The DIC is now recognised as having equal importance to the SLIL in scapholunate stability [8–11]. Disruption to the secondary stabilisers may not occur at the time of injury but may be chronic attenuation due to loss of a primary stabilising SLIL.

Chronic SLIL injuries are generally considered those beyond 6 weeks from the time of injury, especially with injuries involving the mid-substance of the ligament with poor healing potential. Bony avulsions may still maintain some healing capacity for up to 12 weeks. Several options for the management of chronic SLIL injury have been proposed over the years. Treatment should consider the age, comorbidities and professional and recreational demands of the patient. In addition to these patient factors, Garcia-Elias proposed considering the following five injury factors

Fig. 16.2 Fluoroscopy demonstrating scapholunate diastasis

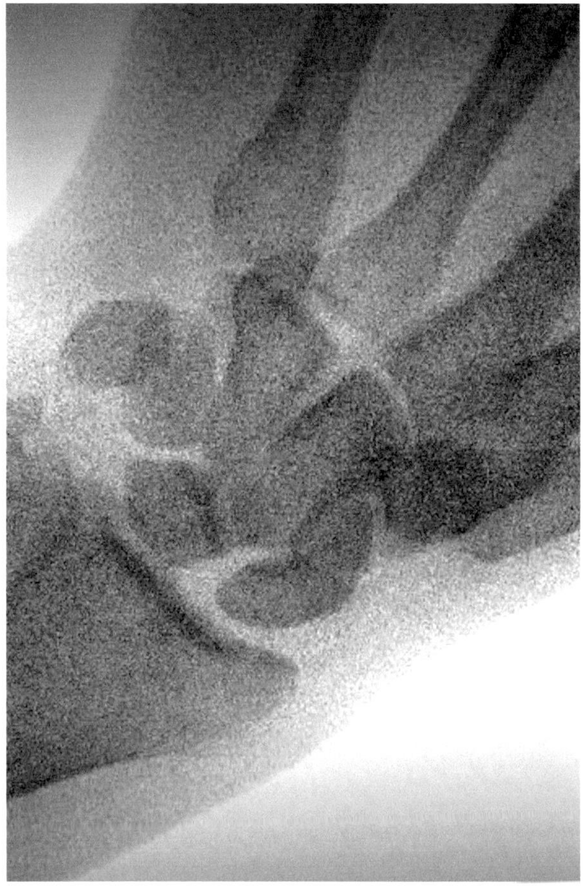

Table 16.1 Modified from Garcia-Elias, M., Lluch, A. L. & Stanley, J. K. Three-ligament tenodesis for the treatment of scapholunate dissociation: indications and surgical technique. *J Hand Surg Am* 31, 125–34 (2006)

	Stage-1	Stage-2	Stage-3	Stage-4	Stage-5	Stage-6
Dorsal SLIL intact?	Yes	No	No	No	No	No
Repairable?	Yes	Yes	No	No	No	No
Normal scaphoid alignment?	Yes	Yes	Yes	No	No	No
Reducible?	Yes	Yes	Yes	Yes	No	No
Articular cartilage intact?	Yes	Yes	Yes	Yes	Yes	No

when planning treatment, thus stratifying chronic SLIL injuries into six stages (Table 16.1) and providing an algorithm for management [12]:

1. Is the dorsal SLIL intact?
2. If it is a complete lesion, is it repairable with good healing potential?
3. Is scaphoid alignment normal? i.e. are the secondary stabilisers intact?

4. Is the carpal malalignment easily reducible?
5. Is the radiocarpal and midcarpal articular cartilage intact?

The above questions can be answered through a combination of clinical, radiographic and arthroscopic assessment.

Diagnosis

History

Most wrist problems, and in particular carpal instability, can be diagnosed based on history and examination [13, 14].

It is important to elicit a history of trauma, particularly of axial load to the wrist. There may have been other wrist injuries, for example, a distal radius fracture, which were treated while the SLIL injury remained undiagnosed. There may be a history of a rotational injury of the carpus about a fixed radius, such as a twist while hanging from a bar, which can result in rupture of the dorsal portion of the SLIL first.

Pain is typically dorso-radial, at the scapholunate interval and there may be a history of "clunking", weak grip or orthosis use.

Examination

Tenderness over the dorsal scapholunate interval or occasionally the volar distal pole of the scaphoid may be elicited.

The scaphoid shift test described by Watson [15] can aid in diagnosis of subacute injuries. This may cause pain over the dorsal scapholunate interval, due to associated synovitis, or a "clunk" once the volar pressure is released, allowing the subluxed scaphoid to reduce back into the scaphoid fossa of the distal radius. A normal scaphoid shift test does not, however, exclude scapholunate ligament injury.

Wrist range of motion should be routinely assessed as those with underlying degenerative change and restricted range of motion will be poor candidates for reconstruction.

Investigations

Radiographs

Features of SLIL injury include:

- Scapholunate interval >3 mm—the "Terry Thomas sign [16]"
- Flexed scaphoid ("signet ring sign")
- Dorsal tilt of the lunate and increased scapholunate angle (normal = 30–60°)
- Dorsal translation of the scaphoid [17] on lateral radiographs, indicating loss of the secondary scaphoid stabilisers

Radiographs should ideally be compared to the uninjured side and interpreted with caution if there is a history of hyperlaxity or inflammatory arthropathy, especially in the absence of trauma.

Stress radiographs can be useful to demonstrate dynamic SLIL instability, including:

- Clenched fist view: clenching the fist applies an axial load to the carpus making dynamic scapholunate diastasis more apparent.
- Bilateral ulnar deviation and supination view [18].

At our unit, we perform a "6-shot series" of radiographs for suspected scapholunate injuries which includes the standard 4 projections of a scaphoid series plus clenched-fist and loaded clenched-fist views.

Fluoroscopy

Fluoroscopy can highlight dynamic instability and demonstrate reducibility of carpal malalignment.

Magnetic Resonance Imaging

MRI aids in assessing the integrity of the SLIL, the secondary stabilisers and the state of the articular cartilage. MR arthrography is an extremely sensitive diagnostic tool, but may reveal asymptomatic pathologies, potentially leading to overtreatment. A normal MRI, however, does not exclude scapholunate ligament injury, reiterating the importance of a thorough history and examination.

Arthroscopy

Considered the diagnostic gold standard. It allows grading of the SLIL injury as per the Geissler grade [19] and direct visualisation of the articular cartilage. The author's preference is to perform diagnostic arthroscopy first, progressing to reconstruction as a second stage, if appropriate.

Management

Reconstruction should be reserved for patients with chronic SLIL injuries who meet specific criteria- a symptomatic patient with a complete SLIL tear not amenable to direct repair, provided the carpal malalignment remains reducible and there is no carpal collapse or degenerative change, i.e. Garcia-Elias stage 3 or 4.

It is important to recognise the three distinct deformities occurring in chronic SLIL injury and attenuation of the secondary stabilisers (scapholunate diastasis, scaphoid flexion-pronation, dorsal subluxation of the scaphoid). Any successful reconstruction should aim to correct all three (Fig. 16.3). Recently, however, it has been found that correction of the dorsal scaphoid translation is a more sensitive predictor of post-operative pain relief compared to all other commonly used radiological parameters, including scapholunate angle, radiolunate angle and scapholunate gap [20].

Reconstructive procedures fall into three broad categories:

1. Dorsal weaves
2. Axis methods
3. Box methods

The three ligament tenodesis (3LT) [12] is an example of a dorsal weave technique and an evolution of that initially described by Brunelli and Brunelli [21].

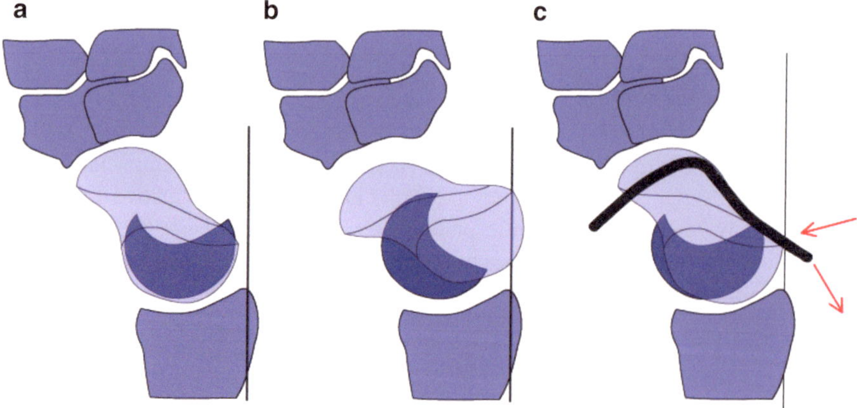

Fig. 16.3 Lateral view of the wrist showing **a)** normal alignment, **b)** DISI with dorsal scaphoid translation, **c)** 3LT depressing the scaphoid

Surgical Technique

A longitudinal dorsal incision is performed centred over Lister's tubercle and full-thickness flaps elevated, with care to protect dorsal sensory branches of the radial and ulnar nerves. The third extensor compartment is opened with an oblique incision and EPL taken radially. The septum between the third and fourth compartment is divided and the fourth compartment taken ulnarwards (Fig. 16.4). A dorsal ligament-sparing capsulotomy [22] is performed and once again, the articular cartilage and reducibility of the carpus are evaluated using K-wires as joysticks. It is important to counsel the patient that occasionally it may become necessary to change to a salvage strategy on table.

We utilise a two-incision volar technique to harvest the flexor carpi radialis (FCR) graft, via an extended FCR approach at the wrist, exposing the scaphoid tubercle and FCR and a 2 cm transverse skin incision over the FCR tendon, 8 cm proximal to the wrist. The FCR tendon is sectioned, taking approximately 3 mm width and harvested using a curved tendon passer. The fibres of the FCR tendon rotate ulnar to radial as they pass proximal to distal and one must untwist the fibres prior to passing the graft. "TROTTUR- Tendon Rotates Over The Top from Ulnar to Radial" serves as a useful aide memoire, as described by Professor John Stanley (Fig. 16.5). The distal attachment of FCR is maintained.

A 1.1 mm K-wire is passed from the scaphoid waist dorsally to the volar scaphoid tuberosity under fluoroscopic guidance (Fig. 16.6). The K-wire is then drilled over with a 2.5 mm cannulated drill. This is a more distal wire placement [23] than described by Garcia-Elias et al., but in our experience, serves to extend the scaphoid and successfully allows the FCR to reduce the dorsal subluxation.

The harvested FCR tendon is passed volar to dorsal through the scaphoid, brought to lie dorsally over the lunate and passed around the dorsal radio-luno-triquetral ligament (Fig. 16.7). The carpus is held reduced, and the graft is tensioned and tenodesed to itself using a 4-0 PDS suture, bedding down the proximal pole of

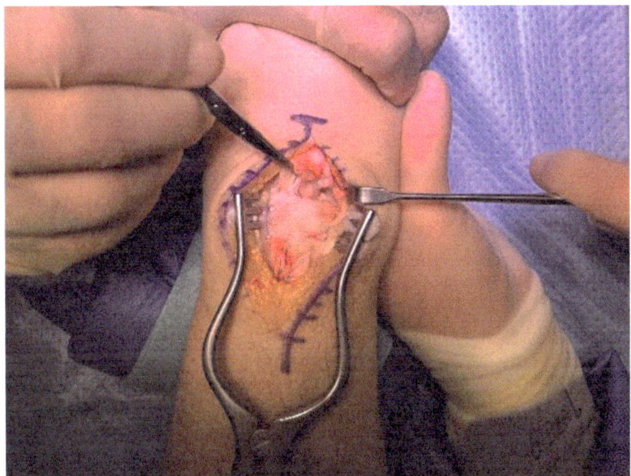

Fig. 16.4 Dorsal approach with a radially-based, ligament-sparing capsular flap

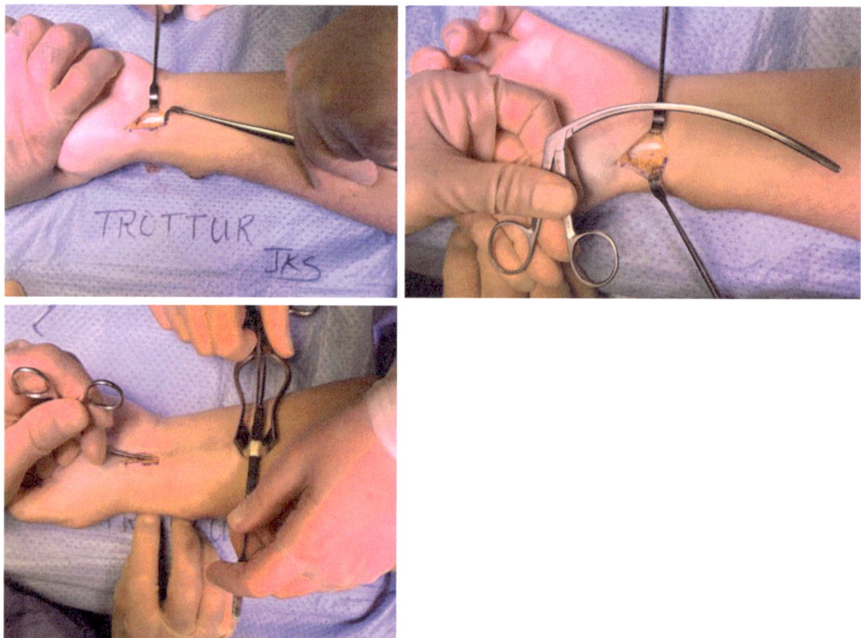

Fig. 16.5 Dual-incision technique for FCR tendon harvest

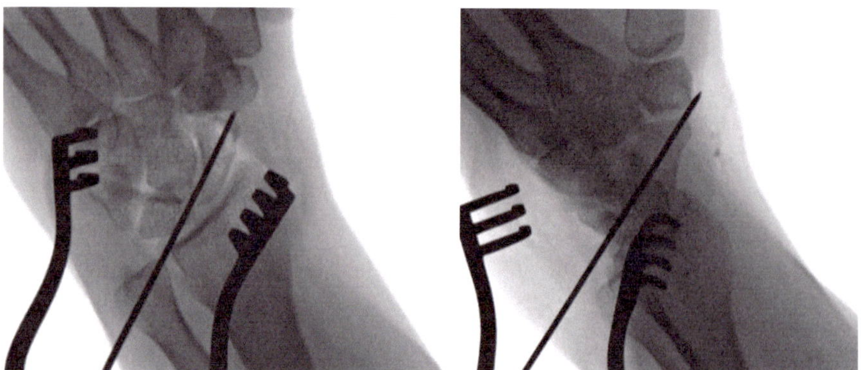

Fig. 16.6 Fluoroscopically-guided guidewire placement from dorsal to volar, along the long axis of the scaphoid

the scaphoid. Satisfactory reduction is confirmed on fluoroscopy (Fig. 16.8) and closure is performed in layers, exteriorising the EPL tendon when repairing the retinaculum.

Post-operatively, the patient is immobilised in a below-elbow plaster for 6 weeks, changed at 10–14 days for a wound check. Rehabilitation is commenced from 6 weeks post-operatively under the guidance of a hand therapist, with advice to

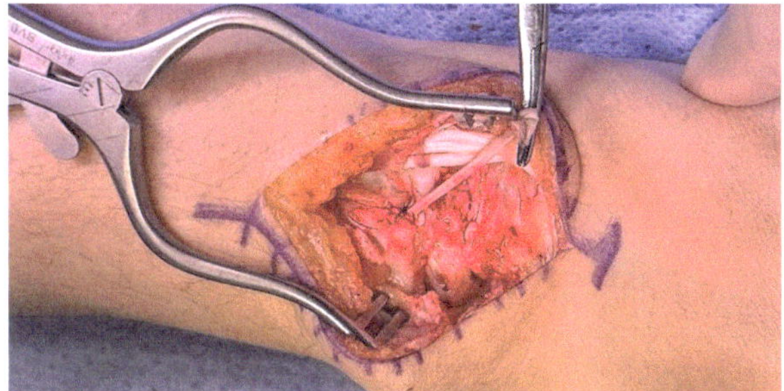

Fig. 16.7 FCR tendon passed volar to dorsal and around the dorsal radio-luno-triquetral ligament

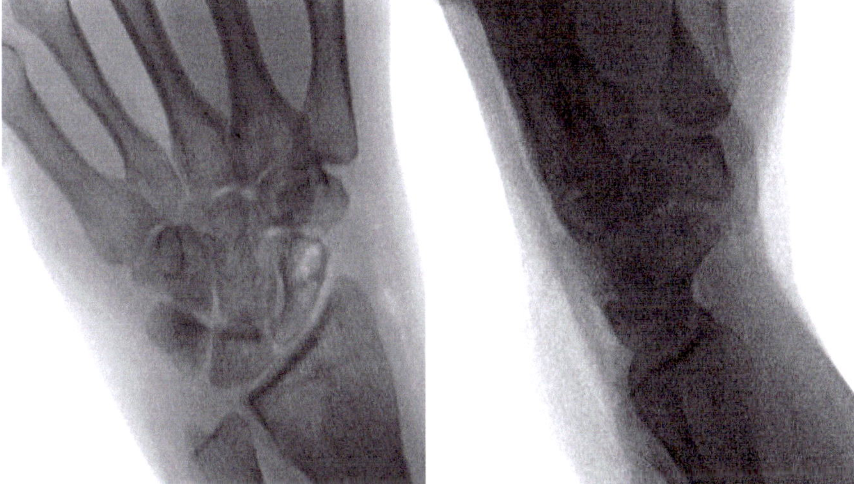

Fig. 16.8 Final carpal alignment

avoid heavy lifting for a minimum of 3 months and patients are provided with a removable splint for this duration.

We have previously reported the outcomes of 162 patients undergoing the 3LT and found that 62% of patients had no/mild pain with a VAS of 3.67. 79% of patients were satisfied with the results of the surgery and 88% felt they would undergo the surgery again [24].

Discussion

The ideal treatment for chronic SLIL injury remains an unsolved problem. While several surgical techniques have been described ([25–28]), results can be inconsistent and long-term outcomes are currently lacking. Compared with many newer reconstructive techniques, long-term results of the 3LT have been published [24,

29]. There are concerns regarding ligament reconstructions using tendon graft resulting in creep, especially when there is increased distance between the two fixation points of the graft [28] as in box reconstructive methods. Other potential complications with techniques using transosseous tunnels include carpal fracture, avascular necrosis and poor healing of the graft to endosteal bone [30]. We believe the 3LT is a successful procedure in the treatment of chronic scapholunate dissociation provided there is appropriate patient selection, early diagnosis to ensure reducibility of the carpus and the absence of degeneration. This technique is successful in reducing dorsal subluxation of the proximal scaphoid and is therefore of particular benefit where this deformity is present. While the 3LT certainly remains the workhorse of our practice, there are occasions, particularly with drive-through lesions or more advanced Geissler grade 3 or 4 lesions, where other reconstructive techniques, such as the Corella [31], may be more suitable.

References

1. Berger RA. The gross and histologic anatomy of the scapholunate interosseous ligament. J Hand Surg Am. 1996;21(2):170–8. https://doi.org/10.1016/S0363-5023(96)80096-7.
2. Berger RA, et al. Constraint and material properties of the subregions of the scapholunate interosseous ligament. J Hand Surg Am. 1999;24(5):953–62. https://doi.org/10.1053/jhsu.1999.0953.
3. Kitay A, Wolfe SW. Scapholunate instability: current concepts in diagnosis and management. J Hand Surg Am. 2012;37(10):2175–96. https://doi.org/10.1016/j.jhsa.2012.07.035.
4. Mayfield JK. Mechanism of carpal injuries. Clin Orthop Relat Res. 1980;(149):45–54.
5. Mayfield JK, Johnson RP, Kilcoyne RK. Carpal dislocations: pathomechanics and progressive perilunar instability. J Hand Surg Am. 1980;5(3):226–41. https://doi.org/10.1016/S0363-5023(80)80007-4.
6. Rohman EM, et al. Scapholunate interosseous ligament injuries: a retrospective review of treatment and outcomes in 82 wrists. J Hand Surg Am. 2014;39(10):2020–6. https://doi.org/10.1016/j.jhsa.2014.06.139.
7. Waters MS, et al. Biomechanical evaluation of scaphoid and lunate kinematics following selective sectioning of portions of the scapholunate interosseous ligament. J Hand Surg Am. 2016;41(2):208–13. https://doi.org/10.1016/j.jhsa.2015.11.009.
8. Badida R, et al. The role of scapholunate interosseous, dorsal intercarpal, and radiolunate ligaments in wrist biomechanics. J Biomech. 2021;125:110567. https://doi.org/10.1016/j.jbiomech.2021.110567.
9. Pérez AJ, et al. Role of ligament stabilizers of the proximal carpal row in preventing dorsal intercalated segment instability. J Bone Joint Surg. 2019;101(15):1388–96. https://doi.org/10.2106/JBJS.18.01419.
10. Raja S, et al. New concepts in carpal instability. In: Geissler WB, editor. Wrist and elbow arthroscopy with selected open procedures. 3rd ed. Cham: Springer International Publishing; 2022. p. 173–85. https://doi.org/10.1007/978-3-030-78881-0.
11. Short WH, et al. Biomechanical evaluation of ligamentous stabilizers of the scaphoid and lunate. J Hand Surg Am. 2002;27(6):991–1002. https://doi.org/10.1053/jhsu.2002.35878.
12. Garcia-Elias M, Lluch AL, Stanley JK. Three-ligament tenodesis for the treatment of scapholunate dissociation: indications and surgical technique. J Hand Surg Am. 2006;31(1):125–34. https://doi.org/10.1016/j.jhsa.2005.10.011.

13. Rhee PC, et al. Examination of the wrist: ulnar-sided wrist pain due to ligamentous injury. J Hand Surg Am. 2014;39(9):1859–62. https://doi.org/10.1016/J.JHSA.2014.07.004.
14. Sauvé PS, et al. Examination of the wrist: radial-sided wrist pain. J Hand Surg Am. 2014;39(10):2089–92. https://doi.org/10.1016/J.JHSA.2014.07.036.
15. Kirk Watson H, Ashmead D, Vincent Makhlouf M. Examination of the scaphoid. J Hand Surg Am. 1988;13(5):657–60. https://doi.org/10.1016/S0363-5023(88)80118-7.
16. Frankel VH. The Terry-Thomas sign. Clin Orthop Relat Res. 1978;(135):311–312.
17. Chan K, et al. Radiographs detect dorsal scaphoid translation in scapholunate dissociation. J Wrist Surg. 2019;8(3):186–91. https://doi.org/10.1055/S-0038-1677536.
18. Puig de la Bellacasa I, et al. Bilateral ulnar deviation supination stress test to assess dynamic scapholunate instability. J Hand Surg Am. 2022;47(7):639–44. https://doi.org/10.1016/j.jhsa.2022.02.021.
19. Geissler WB, et al. Intracarpal soft-tissue lesions associated with an intra-articular fracture of the distal end of the radius. J Bone Joint Surg Am. 1996;78(3):357–65. https://doi.org/10.2106/00004623-199603000-00006.
20. Vutescu ES, et al. Postoperative pain is correlated with scaphoid dorsal translation following scapholunate interosseous ligament reconstruction. J Wrist Surg. 2020;9(6):487–92. https://doi.org/10.1055/s-0040-1713656.
21. Brunelli GA, Brunelli GR. A new technique to correct carpal instability with scaphoid rotary subluxation: a preliminary report. J Hand Surg Am. 1995;20(3 Pt 2):S82–5. https://doi.org/10.1016/s0363-5023(95)80175-8.
22. Berger RA, Bishop AT, Bettinger PC. New dorsal capsulotomy for the surgical exposure of the wrist. Ann Plast Surg. 1995;35(1):54–9. https://doi.org/10.1097/00000637-199507000-00011.
23. Howlett JPC, et al. Distal tunnel placement improves scaphoid flexion with the Brunelli tenodesis procedure for scapholunate dissociation. J Hand Surg Am. 2008;33(10):1756–64. https://doi.org/10.1016/J.JHSA.2008.08.022.
24. Talwalkar SC, et al. Results of tri-ligament tenodesis: a modified Brunelli procedure in the management of scapholunate instability. J Hand Surg Br. 2006;31(1):110–7. https://doi.org/10.1016/j.jhsb.2005.09.016.
25. Ho P, Wong C, Tse W. Arthroscopic-assisted combined dorsal and volar scapholunate ligament reconstruction with tendon graft for chronic SL instability. J Wrist Surg. 2015;4(4):252–63. https://doi.org/10.1055/s-0035-1565927.
26. Kakar S, Greene R. Scapholunate ligament internal brace 360-degree tenodesis (SLITT) procedure. J Wrist Surg. 2018;7(4):336–40 https://doi.org/10.1055/s-0038-1625954.
27. Ross M, et al. Scapholunate ligament reconstruction. J Wrist Surg. 2013;2(2):110–5. https://doi.org/10.1055/s-0033-1341962.
28. Yao J, Zlotolow D, Lee S. Scapholunate axis method. J Wrist Surg. 2016;5(1):59–66. https://doi.org/10.1055/s-0035-1570744.
29. Goeminne S, et al. Long-term follow-up of the three-ligament tenodesis for scapholunate ligament lesions: 9-year results. Hand Surg Rehabil. 2021;40(4):448–52. https://doi.org/10.1016/j.hansur.2021.03.020.
30. Bain GI, Amarasooriya M. Scapholunate instability: why are the surgical outcomes still so far from ideal? J Hand Surg Eur. 2023;48(3):257–68. https://doi.org/10.1177/17531934221148009.
31. Corella F, et al. Arthroscopic ligamentoplasty of the dorsal and volar portions of the scapholunate ligament. J Hand Surg Am. 2013;38(12):2466–77. https://doi.org/10.1016/j.jhsa.2013.09.021.

Chapter 17
Antipronation Spiral Tenodesis for the Treatment of Chronic Reducible Scapholunate Instability with Associated Radiolunate or Perilunate Instability

Ana Scott-Tennent, Mireia Esplugas, Alex Lluch, and Marc García-Elías

Case Presentation

A 39-year-old male with no relevant medical history presented with wrist pain and impairment 6 months after a motorcycle accident. He had been immobilized for 3 weeks after trauma, but no other treatment since.

Diagnosis

- Physical examination: Dorsoradial tenderness and limited range of active motion (ROM). Finger extension test with pain around the dorsal scapholunate joint (SLj). Asymmetric Watson test with clunk and pain in dorsal SLj. Beighton's criteria ruled out hyperlaxity.
- PA radiographic view (bilateral): Widened SL space and decreased radiolunate contact area compared to the contralateral wrist. (Fig. 17.1a)
- Lateral radiographic view (bilateral): Increased SL angle compared with the contralateral side (DISI). (Fig. 17.1b)
- Fluoroscopy (bilateral): Widening of SL space and ulnar displacement of the lunate compared to contralateral wrist. Asymmetry became more evident with

A. Scott-Tennent
Hospital Arnau de Vilanova, Lleida, Spain

M. Esplugas · M. García-Elías
Institut Kaplan, Barcelona, Spain

A. Lluch (✉)
Institut Kaplan, Barcelona, Spain

Hand and Wrist Unit, Hospital Vall d'Hebron, Barcelona, Spain

© The Author(s), under exclusive license to Springer Nature Switzerland AG 2024
J. Yao (ed.), *Carpal Instability*, https://doi.org/10.1007/978-3-031-55869-6_17

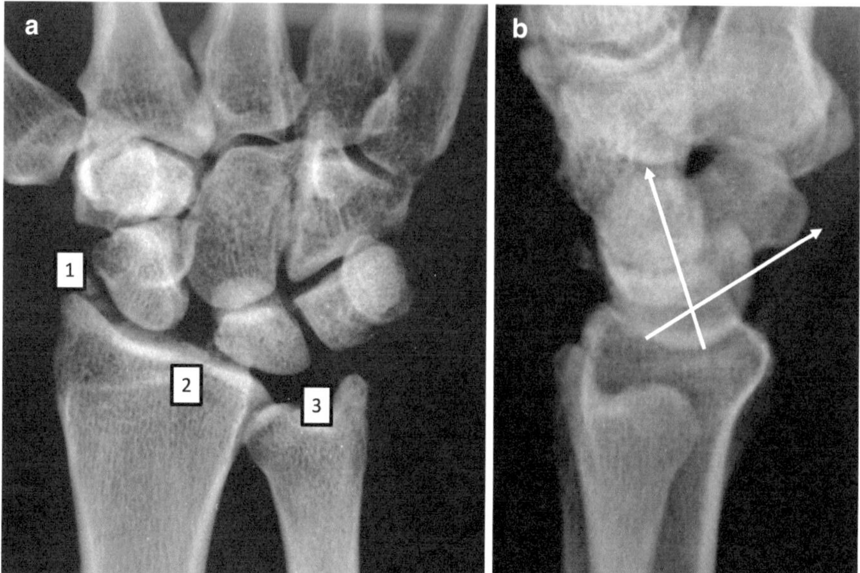

Fig. 17.1 (**a**) Wrist PA X-ray showing classical signs of stage 5 SL dysfunction: Rotatory subluxation of scaphoid (1), widened SL space (2), possible ulnar translocation of the lunate when compared to contralateral side (3). (**b**) Wrist lateral X-ray showing increased SL angle

ulnar inclination and supination against resistance (BUDS test [1]) and with axial compression. Axial traction of the wrist and gentle manipulation allowed for improvement of wrist alignment.

- Magnetic resonance imaging: Direct or indirect signs of complete scapholunate ligament (SLL) rupture, and insufficiency of the dorsal radiocarpal ligament (DCR), dorsal intracarpal ligament (DIC) and volar radiocarpal ligament, dorsal and volar radiocarpal synovitis. No signs suggesting bony or cartilage damage.

Management

Treatment Plan (Indication)

Planification is crucial in scapholunate dysfunction (SLD) management [2].

- *First step: Recognition of the stage of SL injury*
- After the diagnostic workup, the patient was suspected to suffer from a Stage 5 SLD: Complete SL and radiolunate ligament injury, non-repairable, with reducible rotatory subluxation of the scaphoid and *ulnar translocation of the lunate* [2] (Fig. 17.2).
- *Second step: Treatment decision*

Fig. 17.2 Recognition of SLD stage by answering 6 Yes/No questions. Patient's suspected Stage was 5

	I	II	III	IV	V	VI	VII
Partial injury	Yes	No	No	No	No	No	No
Repairable	Yes	Yes	No	No	No	No	No
Normal RS angle	Yes	Yes	Yes	No	No	No	No
Stable lunate	Yes	Yes	Yes	Yes	No	No	No
Reducible	Yes	Yes	Yes	Yes	Yes	No	No
Normal cartilage	Yes	Yes	Yes	Yes	Yes	Yes	No

Complete rupture, carpal collapse, ulnar translocation lunate, reducible

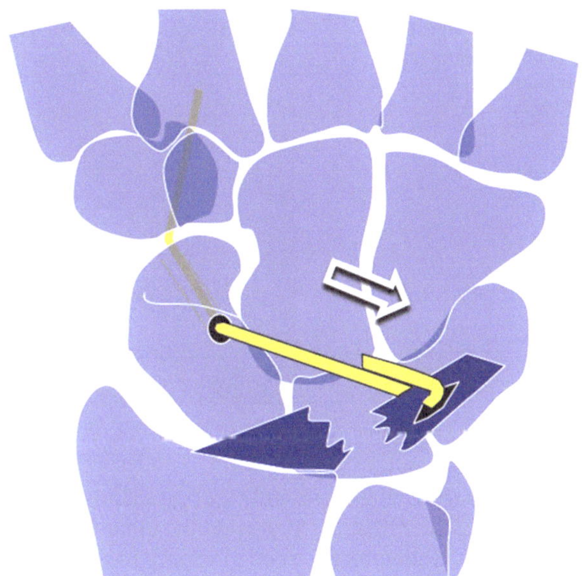

Fig. 17.3 Schematic representation showing the reason why isolated SL reconstruction techniques such as 3LT are prone to fail if there is radiolunate instability. Dorsal radiocarpal ligament is not strong enough to support the reconstruction to maintain the scapholunate complex in place

- *Surgical treatment* is indicated in cases of symptomatic SLD in active individuals. An initial period of conservative treatment, even as a preparation for the protocol after ligament reconstruction, is highly recommended [3].
- *Third step: Type of surgery needed according to SLD stage and patient's requirements.*
- Healthy active patients with suspicion of SLD Stage 5 may be treated by *tendon reconstruction*. Hyperlaxity is a specific condition to take into account when deciding the type of ligament reconstruction for any stage.
- In cases where the radiolunate joint is unstable (Stage 5), tendon reconstruction of the SLj alone, such as a three-ligament tenodesis (3LT), are prone to fail [4] (Fig. 17.3).

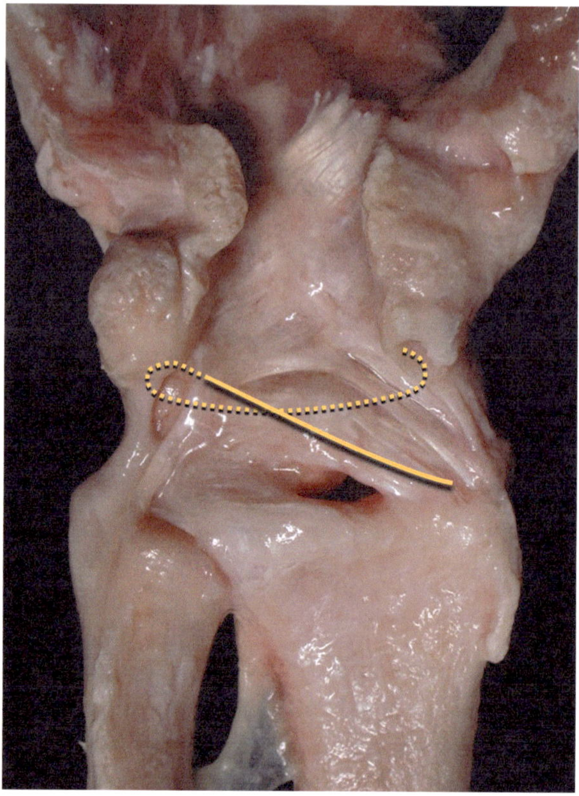

Fig. 17.4 Cadaveric dissection of a carpus showing the direction of the so-called antipronation isodynamic ligaments, from distal to proximal: Palmar SC ligament, Dorsal SL ligament, Dorsal Intercarpal ligament (dotted yellow line), Palmar LTq ligament, Long RL ligament (continuous yellow line). Note the spiral conformation that gives name to the surgical tendon reconstruction technique

- Instead, the Antipronation Spiral Tenodesis (AST) has been designed to reconstruct a complex of ligaments (antipronation isodynamic ligaments) (Fig. 17.4) including those that try to prevent the ulnar translocation of the lunate [5].
- However, tendon reconstruction is only recommended if:

  1. The malalignment is easily reducible (either preoperatively by gentle manipulation under fluoroscopy or intraoperatively under anesthesia to avoid muscle contraction)
  2. The cartilages are not injured.

- The previous requisites can be suspected by the diagnosis workout, but SLD stage needs to be confirmed intraoperatively before the definitive treatment is applied [2, 4, 5].

Surgical Treatment

- *First step: Intraoperative confirmation of the stage of SL injury*

- The extent of injury and ligaments involved, the cartilage status and reducibility of SLj need to be confirmed intraoperatively. This can be done using:

    (a) **Wrist Arthroscopy**

    Standard radiocarpal (3–4 and 6R) and midcarpal dorsal (MCR, MCU) portals for *Confirmation of SLD Stage 5:*

    1. Checking extent of injury and *ligaments involved:* in this case, complete SLL rupture and extrinsic ligaments (DIC, RSC, LRL, SRL) (EWAS IV) was found [6]
    2. Thorough assessment of the articular *cartilage status* of both the radio-carpal and midcarpal joints: Cartilage was preserved in this patient.
    3. *Reducibility*: Releasing tower traction and confirming that malalignment is easily reducible with a probe through midcarpal portals or under fluoroscopy.

    In this case, SLj was reduced without struggle using the probe through MCR, while MCU was used as a viewing portal. For ulnar translocation reduction, the wrist had to be withdrawn from traction and gentle axial traction had to be applied. Correction of the alignment was checked under fluoroscopy.

    (b) **Open Approach**

    – Standard dorsal wrist approach. Wide exposure from E2 to E5.
    – Visual assessment of the PIN:

    If thickened, irregular or suspicion of neuroma → denervation of the terminal PIN and Berger et al. capsulotomy [7]
    If found normal → preservation of PIN and nerve-sparing dorsal cap-sulotomy as described by Hagert et al. [8]

    – At this moment, if not done previously by scoping the wrist, *Confirmation of SLD Stage 5* need to be done:

    Checking extent of injury and *ligaments involved.*
    Thorough assessment of the articular *cartilage status* of both the radiocarpal and midcarpal joints (Fig. 17.5)
    Reducibility: If reduction of the carpal malalignment is not easy by slight traction or gentle manual manipulation, pure soft tissue techniques are likely to fail and palliative techniques may be considered.

- *Second step: After Confirmation of stage 5: tendon reconstruction using Antipronation Spiral Tenodesis (AST)* (Fig. 17.6a, b) [5, 9]

    1. Scaphoid tunnel: An oblique transscaphoid Kirschner wire (KW) is preset under fluoroscopy, from dorsal to palmar, entering at the level of the original insertion of the dorsal SL ligament, aiming at the palmar tuberosity. A 2.7 mm cannulated drill is then passed to create the transscaphoid tunnel. The tunnel is then widened with a 3.0 mm drill and the strip of tendon graft is passed through the tunnel using a wire loop or a tendon passer (Fig. 17.7).

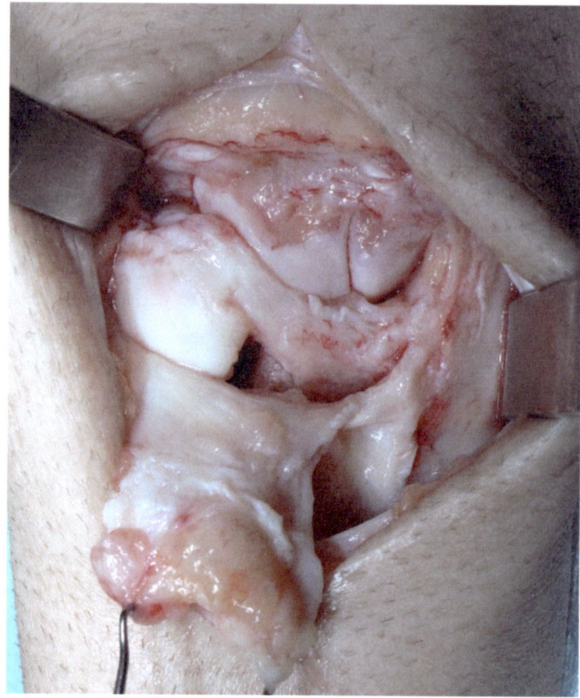

Fig. 17.5 Intraoperative confirmation of Stage 5 SLD through dorsal nerve-sparing capsulotomy from a dorsal standard wrist approach

2. Anterolateral incision: 2-cm skin over the volar radial aspect of the wrist from the scaphoid tuberosity to the direction of the radial styloid is done.

3. Tendon strip: As a preference, an Extensor Carpi Radialis Longus (ECRL) tendon strip is obtained. It has to be long enough to ensure the complete reconstruction (around 15 cm). Maintaining its distal insertion, the tendon strip is passed from dorsal to volar through the STT capsule. Although the ECRL seems to be better in counteracting the flexion and pronation deformity of the scaphoid [10], a Flexor Carpi Radialis (FCR) tendon strip may be used alternatively.

4. SLj reduction: Classically, under fluoroscopic guidance, the SL joint is reduced and stabilized using two 1.5 mm KW. We now prefer the use of inter-ferential screws and augmentation with internal bracing that helps to maintain reduction. That may prevent any chondral damage created by the KW and allow for earlier motion. The first interferential screw is placed in the distal scaphoid in a retrograde manner.

5. Fixing the tendon to the dorsum of the lunate: A transverse trough is then made over the dorsum of the lunate with a rongeur, exposing cancellous bone from the dorsum of the lunate. To obtain intimate contact between the tendon strip and the lunate cancellous bone, an optional small anchor suture may be placed into the floor of the lunate (Fig. 17.8).

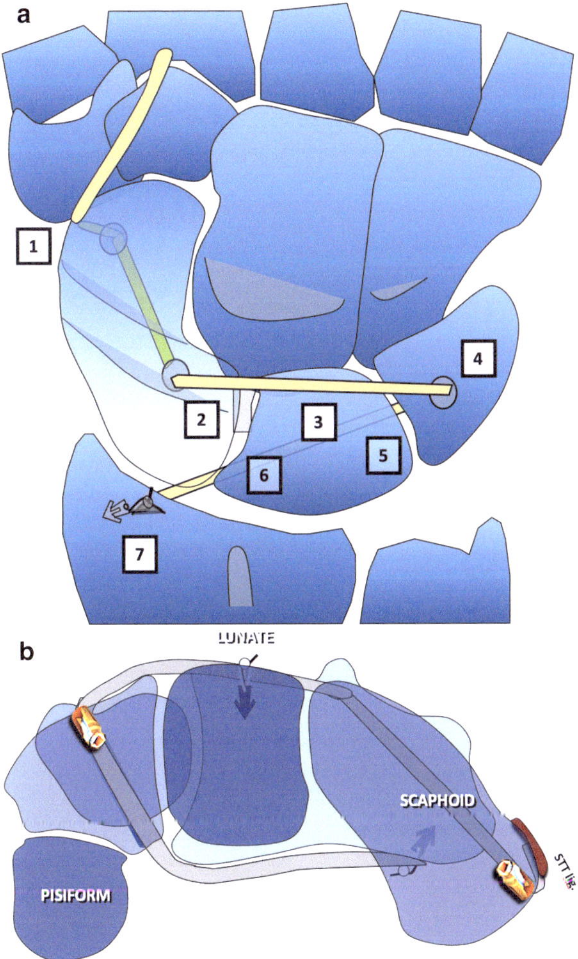

Fig. 17.6 Schematic representation and description of the Antipronation Spiral Tenodesis (AST), (**a**) (coronal view), (**b**) (axial view): (1) The strip of extensor carpi radialis longus tendon is passed across the scaphoid bone. It may be fixed with an interferential screw at the entrance of the tunnel. (2) The tendon emerges at the insertion site of the dorsal scapholunate ligament. (3) From the insertion site of the dorsal scapholunate ligament, the tendon takes a transverse course toward the dorsal ridge of the triquetrum bone. At this point, an anchor suture may be used to fix the tendon to the lunate. (4) The tendon enters a tunnel across the triquetrum bone and may be fixed with an interferential screw. (5) After passing through the tunnel, the tendon exits on the floor of the carpal tunnel. The exit point of the tendon is medial to the pisotriquetral joint. (6) Once inside the carpal tunnel, the strip of tendon is passed deep to the Flexor Digitorum Profundus tendon and Flexor Pollicis Longus tendon. (7) Finally, the strip of tendon is inserted onto the volar (palm-side) aspect of the radial styloid. An anchor suture is used to secure the tendon in place

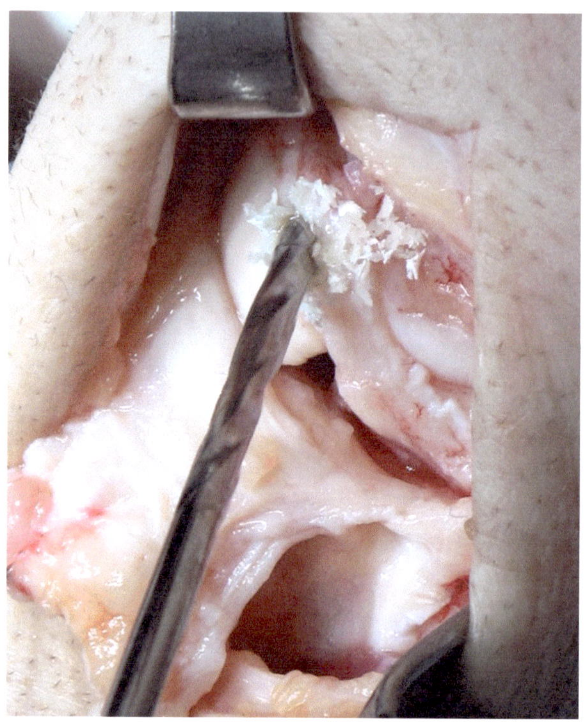

Fig. 17.7 Intraoperative image showing how the scaphoid tunnel is made with a cannulated drill

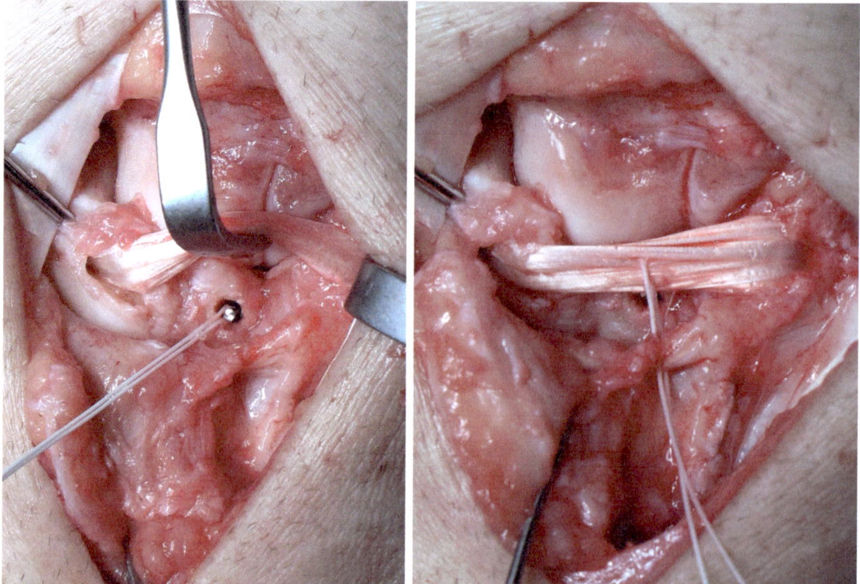

Fig. 17.8 Intraoperative image showing fixation of the tendon to the lunate

6. Carpal tunnel incision (Fig. 17.9) to expose the radial and volar part of the triquetrum, close to the pisotriquetral joint.
7. Triquetrum tunnel: The tendon graft has been brought to the dorsum of the triquetrum. An anteroposterior KW along the radial margin of the pisiform is passed. A cannulated 2.7 mm drill from palmar to dorsal through the carpal tunnel incision is made (Fig. 17.10). The tunnel is then widened with a 3.0 mm drill and the tendon graft is passed from dorsal to volar. An interferential screw is placed through the dorsal part of this second tunnel while the graft is tensioned from volar.
8. Passing the tendon to the volar radial edge of the wrist: The tendon is grasped and pulled radially by a curved mosquito through the anterolateral incision, under the carpal tunnel contents. It is important to protect the radial artery.
9. Securing the tendon to the volar radial styloid: The tendon graft is brought to the volar aspect of the radial styloid and secured by means of either a bone anchor or threaded through another drill hole across the radial styloid, directed at the floor of the second compartment where it can be attached to Lister's tubercle with transosseous sutures or using a third interferential screw (Fig. 17.11).

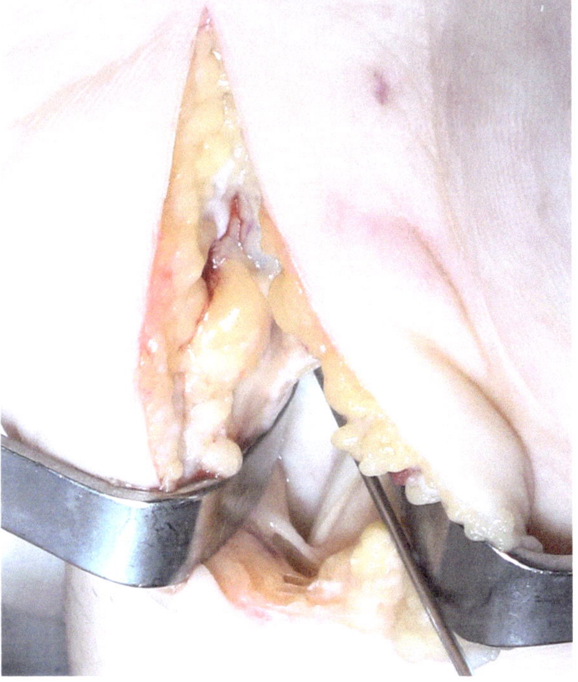

Fig. 17.9 Intraoperative image showing carpal tunnel incision. The incision can be shortened and centered at the level of the radial margin of the triquetrum

Fig. 17.10 Intraoperative image showing a dorsal view of the carpus after SL reduction. In this case, temporary fixation with a KW and tendon graft has passed through the triquetrum from dorsal to volar

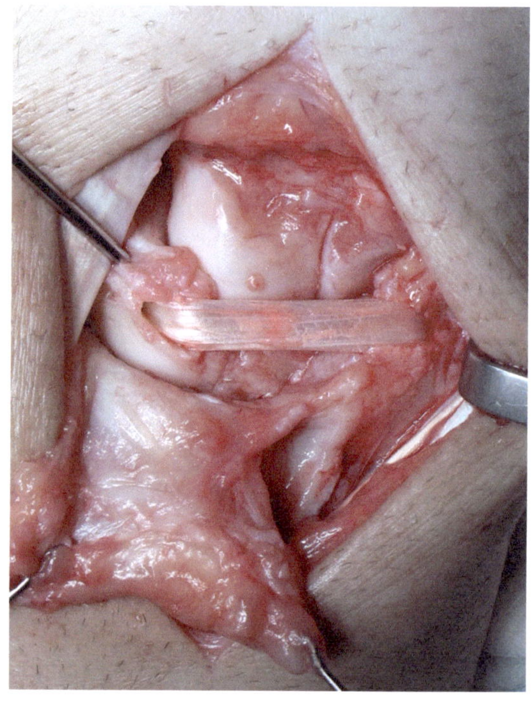

Fig. 17.11 Intraoperative image showing how the tendon graft is brought to the volar aspect of the radial styloid before being secured to the radial styloid

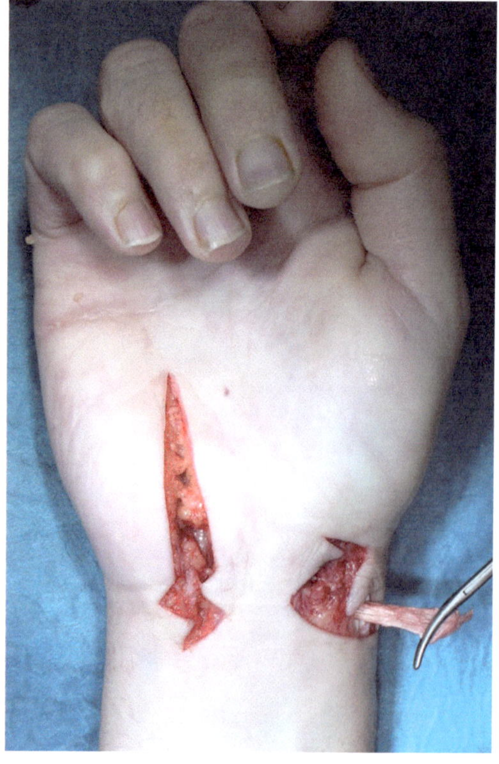

Postoperative Care

If carpal reduction is maintained with KW:

- Immobilization for 4–6 weeks
- Protective removable splint for 4 weeks more, allowing rest between supervised physiotherapy sessions. Start with midcarpal motion, followed by flexion/extension and radial/ulnar deviations.
- Intracarpal supinator muscle strengthening exercises starting 10 weeks after surgery. Avoid loading in forearm supination [3]
- Contact sports should be avoided for 4 months.

If tendon augmentation and interferential screws are used:

- Immobilization for 2 weeks.
- Protective removable splint. 2–4 weeks allowing midcarpal motion. 4–6 weeks flexion/extension and radial/ulnar deviations.
- Intracarpal supinator muscle strengthening exercises starting 6–12 weeks. Avoid loading in forearm supination [3]
- Contact sports should be avoided for 4 months.

Outcomes

At 39-month follow-up, the patient sustained 85% of contralateral grip strength and functional wrist mobility (Fig. 17.12). X-ray showed maintenance of alignment (Fig. 17.13).

Pearls and Pitfalls

- Staging is the first step in SLD management. Failure to recognize SLD stage is related to treatment failure.
- Intraoperative confirmation of suspected SLD stage needs to be done. Wrist arthroscopy is less harmful and allows the surgeon to replan the treatment strategy "in situ," or simply back down and redesign the plan with the patient before any definitive treatment.
- No soft tissue reconstruction can achieve effective stability if the malalignment cannot be reduced with minimal force.
- If the lunate is unstable, an Antipronation Spiral Tenodesis should be chosen instead of isolated SLL reconstruction procedures.

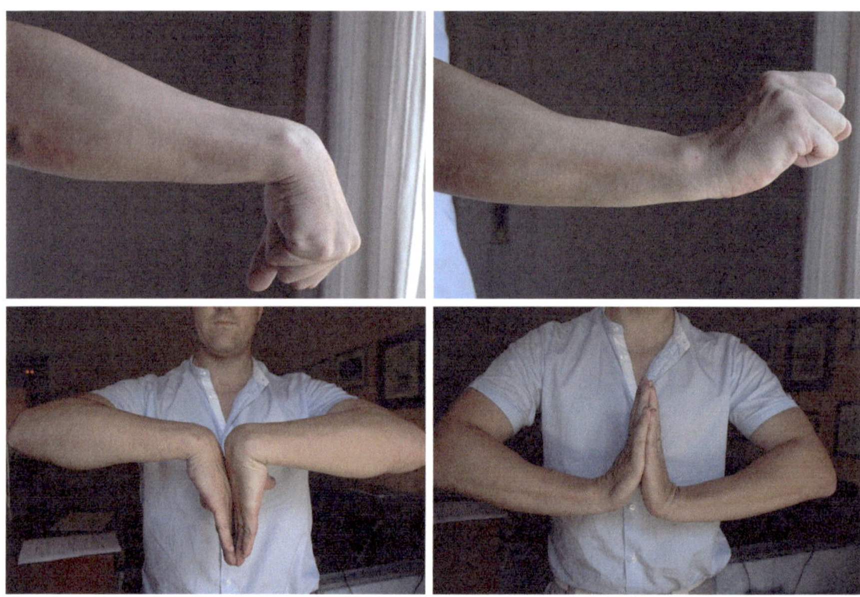

Fig. 17.12 Patient ROM after 39 follow-up

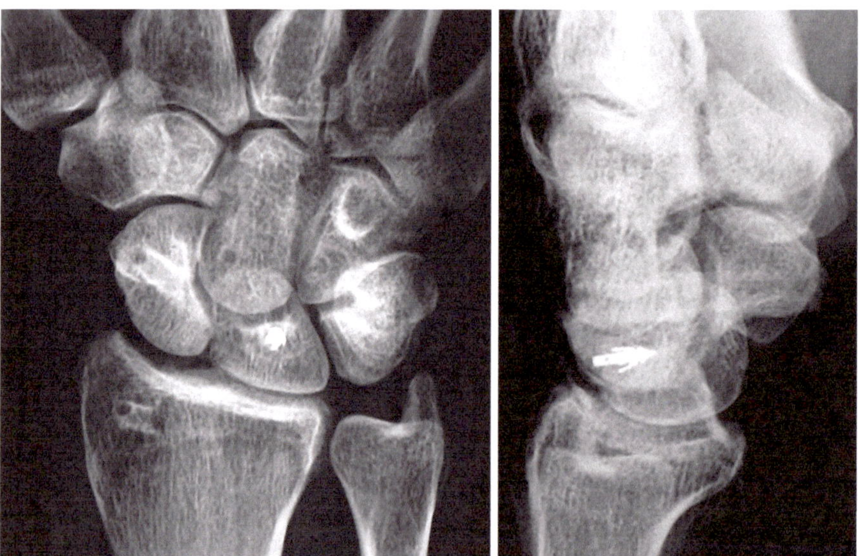

Fig. 17.13 Postoperative X-ray after 39 follow-up

Literature Review

The antipronation spiral tenodesis has also been described to solve perilunate instabilities involving SL and LT ligament ruptures [5, 9]. However, this technique does not provide an anatomic reconstruction of the volar LT ligament, but rather the volar extrinsic ligaments. Also, other ligament reconstruction techniques aiming to provide a more anatomical LT ligament reconstruction have been designed for this purpose [11].

In cases of SLD with rotatory subluxation of the scaphoid, the lunate and triquetrum rotate abnormally into extension, creating a dorsal intercalated segment instability (DISI). If, in these circumstances, the short radiolunate ligament is also torn or insufficient, the lunate will follow its natural tendency of sliding down the ulnarly inclined distal radial surface and will appear translocated ulnarly and palmarly. This situation corresponds to Stage 5 of SLD, before any cartilage degeneration appears.

The authors of this chapter consider that the AST provides a more suitable reconstruction in these cases, by providing a reconstruction of the so-called isodynamic antipronation ligament complex that includes not only the interosseous ligaments but also extrinsic ligaments. As experience accumulates, the AST is being chosen more frequently over the 3LT, as the radiocarpal instability component of most SL deficient wrists is often underestimated.

References

1. Puig de la Bellacasa I, Salva-Coll G, Esplugas M, Quintas S, Lluch A, Garcia Elias M. Bilateral ulnar deviation supination stress test to assess dynamic scapholunate instability. J Hand Surg Am. 2022;47(7):639–44.
2. Garcia-Elias M, Lluch AL, Stanley JK. Three-ligament tenodesis for the treatment of scapholunate dissociation: indications and surgical technique. J Hand Surg Am. 2006;31A:125–34.
3. Salva-Coll G, Garcia-Elias M, Hagert E. Scapholunate instability: proprioception and neuromuscular control. J Wrist Surg. 2013;2(2):136–40.
4. Ananos D, García-Elias M. Open surgery for chronic scapholunate injury. In: del Piñal F, et al., editors. Distal radius fractures and carpal instabilities. New York: Thieme; 2019. p. 220–3.
5. Chee KG, Chin AY, Chew EM, Garcia-Elias M. Antipronation spiral tenodesis—a surgical technique for the treatment of perilunate instability. J Hand Surg Am. 2012;37(12):2611–8.
6. Messina JC, Van Overstraeten L, Luchetti R, Fairplay T, Mathoulin CL. The EWAS classification of scapholunate tears: an anatomical arthroscopic study. J Wrist Surg. 2013;2(2):105–9.
7. Berger RA, Bishop AT, Bettinger PC. New dorsal capsulotomy for the surgical exposure of the wrist. Ann Plast Surg. 1995;35:54–9.
8. Hagert E, Ferreres A, Garcia-Elias M. Nerve-sparing dorsal and volar approaches to the radiocarpal joint. J Hand Surg Am. 2010;35A:1070–4.
9. Chin AYH. Scapholunate reconstruction 3LT and spiral tenodesis. In: Geissler WB, editor. Wrist and elbow arthroscopy with selected open procedures. Cham: Springer; 2022.
10. Kakar S, Green RM, Garcia-Elias M. Carpal realignment using a strip of extensor carpi radialis longus tendon. J Hand Surg Am. 2017;42(8):667.e1–8.
11. Corella F, Ocampos M, Laredo R, Tabuenca J, Corella MA, Larrainzar-Garijo R. Arthroscopic "S"-shaped ligamentoplasty for floating lunate. Tech Hand Up Extrem Surg. 2020;24(4):194–206.

Chapter 18
Reduction and Association of the Scaphoid and Lunate (RASL) Reconstruction for Chronic Static Scapholunate Instability

Melvin P. Rosenwasser

Introduction

The reduction and association of the scaphoid and lunate (RASL) procedure can provide a predictable and satisfactory means to treat irreparable, symptomatic scapholunate (SL) ligament tears [1–3]. SL, ligament tears can occur as an isolated injury due to a fall on the extended wrist involving axial load, wrist extension, intercarpal supination, and ulnar deviation or in conjunction with associated injuries such as distal radius fractures, which may lead to a missed or delayed diagnosis [4]. Carpal ligament injuries represent a spectrum from isolated and partial SL ligament tears involving only the thin central membranous portion to perilunate or lunate dislocations with involvement of both intrinsic and extrinsic carpal ligaments. Ascertainment of the severity of injury can be difficult and a "wrist sprain" may not recover with benign neglect. Fifty-five percent of patients with chronic tears develop a predictable pattern of arthritis called scapholunate advanced collapse (SLAC) [5]. Thus, a timely diagnosis and effective treatment are crucial for an optimal long-term outcome.

Wrist motion in one plane is due to the composite effects of individual carpal bones that undergo unique multiplanar and often reciprocal motions. Radial and ulnar deviation occurs in the coronal plane, with the proximal capitate serving as the center of rotation. Additionally, during ulnar deviation, the scaphoid and lunate extend and during radial deviation they flex [6, 7]. Finally, the proximal row pronates and the distal row supinates during radial deviation, with the opposite occurring during ulnar deviation [8]. Thus, out of plane motion of the scaphoid and lunate

M. P. Rosenwasser (✉)
Department of Orthopedic Surgery, Columbia University Medical Center, New York, NY, USA
e-mail: mpr2@cumc.columbia.edu

255

J. Yao (ed.), *Carpal Instability*, https://doi.org/10.1007/978-3-031-55869-6_18

is more apparent during wrist radial-ulnar deviation than during wrist flexion and extension [9]. Furthermore, within the proximal carpal row, there is disproportionate flexion and extension between the scaphoid and lunate, with the scaphoid rotating fastest and to a larger degree (approximately 20°). It is this obligatory rotation that produces the most stress on SL reconstructions.

SL ligament injury can be categorized based on radiographic patterns of instability. *Static* instability occurs when abnormal scaphoid and lunate alignment is present on routine posteroanterior (PA) and lateral radiographs (Fig. 18.1). *Dynamic* instability occurs when abnormalities occur only during stress radiographs (e.g., pronated grip or ulnar deviation PA views). *Pre-dynamic* instability consists of a history and physical examination suggestive of SL injury, with SL interval pain on palpation, a negative Watson's maneuver, and no radiographic changes on any views. Dorsal intercalated segment instability (DISI) refers to the position of the lunate, with its distal articular surface facing dorsally (Fig. 18.2), as measured by an abnormal increase in the radiographic carpal angles (Table 18.1).

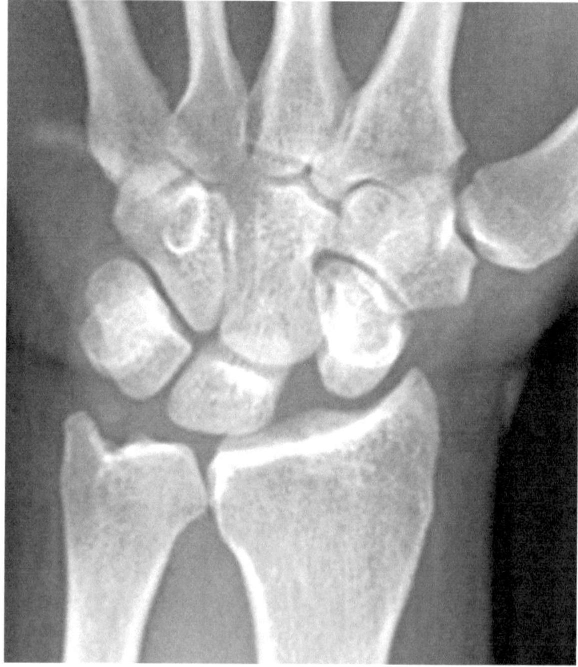

Fig. 18.1 Posteroanterior radiograph of a 53-year-old man with 2 months of wrist pain that began while moving large fertilizer bags by hand. The radiographs demonstrate significant scapholunate diastasis and static instability. The distal scaphoid appears as a circle highlighting the cortical ring sign caused by the flexed scaphoid. The scaphoid appears shortened and the capitate descends proximally

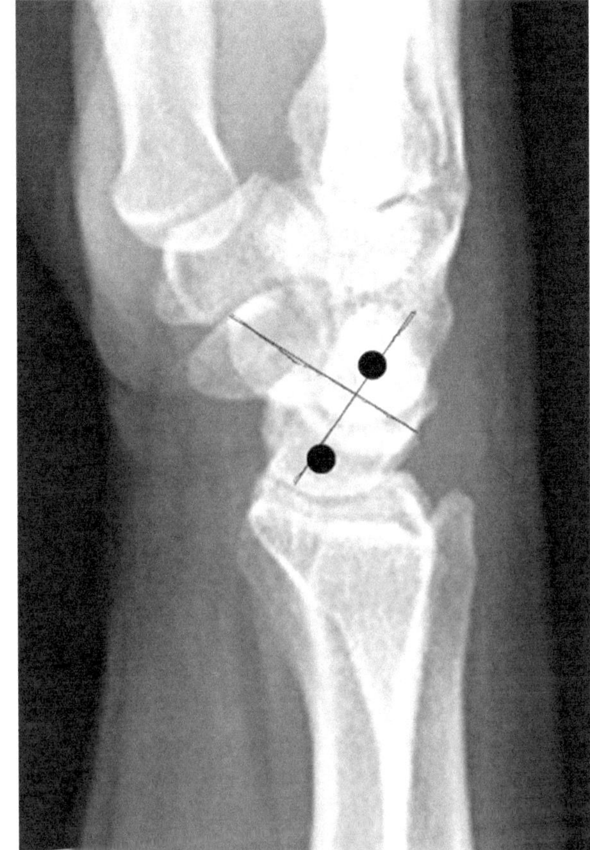

Fig. 18.2 Lateral radiograph of the same patient (Fig. 18.1). Note, the dorsal intercalated segment instability pattern with lunate extension, an increased capitolunate angle (35°, an increased scapholunate angle (90°), and dorsal translation of the capitate indicated by the offset position of the center of rotation of the lunate and capitate (black circles)

Table 18.1 Normal lateral radiographic angles

Angle	Average (degrees)	Range (degrees)
Scapholunate [10]	47	35–70
Radiolunate (61)	7	−9 to 12
Capitolunate [10]	0	−20 to 15

Contraindications for the RASL Procedure

We would like to emphasize that the RASL procedure is contraindicated in the presence of a repairable SL ligament. The authors strongly believe that a primary repair should be attempted in all patients with an SL ligament that has sufficient tissue quality and quantity to withstand suture placement and healing. When the ligament is avulsed from bone, typically off the lunate, suture anchors can be used to reattach the ligament. Supplemental SL and scapho-capitate trans-articular pinning with Kirschner (K) wires and external immobilization should be employed to protect the repair during healing for 8 weeks, particularly when carpal derotation is performed. Repairable ligaments are typically found in the acute setting, arbitrarily defined as less than 6 weeks. However, we recommend examination of the ligament at surgery in all cases as some may be repairable despite being chronic. The RASL procedure is also contraindicated in the presence of significant capitolunate arthritis. Focal arthritis between the radial styloid and scaphoid is not a contraindication because radial styloidectomy is part of the procedure and will adequately decompress this contact region.

Indications for the RASL Procedure

The degree of instability and the chronicity of the injury can guide surgical decision-making. Partial ligament injuries which are stable may be treated with arthroscopic debridement alone [11] or arthroscopic debridement and thermal shrinkage [12, 13]. Complete ligament tears with static instability may be treated with arthroscopic debridement alone [14], reduction and temporary SL trans-articular pinning [15], ligament repair with or without dorsal capsulodesis [16–21], dorsal capsulodesis alone [22], ligament reconstruction using various tendon weaves or bone-soft tissue-bone constructs [23], tenodeses with various wrist tendons [10, 24–26], limited intercarpal fusions [27–32], or the RASL [1–3]. Each of these procedures has different strategies to reduce and control carpal instability. Some disrupt the normal carpal kinematics more than others, but none completely restore motion and stability.

In the author's opinion, the RASL procedure is indicated in a symptomatic patient without a repairable SL ligament and without significant pan-carpal arthritis. A patient may present with chronic dorsal wrist pain after having received a report of normal initial radiographs (pre-dynamic instability) and then over time may develop additional cumulative minor injuries which progresses to a readily apparent dynamic or static instability on subsequent radiographs. Alternatively, initial symptoms may have been mild or resolved shortly after injury and the patient presents for evaluation for the first time with an acute on chronic unrecognized and asymptomatic injury. In these cases, the SL ligament is often attenuated, fibrotic, with limited vascularity and capacity to hold a suture. Additionally, the repetitive loading on an incompetent SL ligament often leads to secondary intercarpal ligamentous stretching and attenuation in the dorsal intercarpal ligament and leads to wide diastasis and maximal rotatory instability precluding capsulodesis procedures alone. Patients who present after a failed primary surgical reconstruction such as SL ligament repair, SL pinning, or a dorsal capsulodesis, but who have not yet developed arthritis are also candidates for the RASL procedure.

Considerations for Preoperative Planning

Confirmation of an SL tear is based upon a history with an appropriate mechanism of injury, correlative physical examination signs, and findings on imaging studies. Physical examination consists of observation, palpation, range of motion, and provocative maneuvers on both wrists to elicit asymmetry. The SL ligament can be palpated with deep pressure applied in the interval just distal and ulnar to Lister's tubercle which is the location of the 3–4 portal for wrist arthroscopy. Watson's scaphoid shift test is a provocative maneuver to assess for SL injury [33]. The scapho-trapezial joint and the radiocarpal joints are palpated to assess the possibility of associated distal and volar ligamentous injuries.

Complete sectioning of all three regions of the SL ligament in cadavers does not create static SL diastasis as viewed on a standard PA radiograph or DISI deformity on a lateral radiograph, or dynamic changes produced by stress views [7]. Associated ligamentous injury is required to produce abnormal carpal relationships such as the volar extrinsic (radiolunate, radio-scapho-capitate) [6, 34], the distal intrinsic (scapho-trapezial) [6, 35], or the dorsal intercarpal ligaments [36]. However, these ligament injuries may be in evolution and are not apparent on routine or stress radiographs until the carpus has experienced sufficient load and time from the injury to produce these classic findings.

Plain radiographs are critical and should be obtained as the first imaging study in every patient. The following radiographs should be obtained: PA in neutral rotation, PA in ulnar and radial deviation, clenched fist PA in pronation, a true lateral in neutral rotation, and two 45° oblique views. Comparison views of the contralateral normal wrist should be obtained as here is a wide range of normal angles. These radiographs may document the instability pattern that confirms the SL injury and grades the extent of arthritis.

On the PA radiograph, several radiographic changes may be noted. A widening of the SL joint space (SL dissociation) that is asymmetric with respect to the contralateral normal wrist is suggestive of an SL ligament injury. The SL distance has been measured at the proximal or mid aspect of the joint space and ranged from 2.5 to 5.0 mm in normal wrist radiographs [37, 38].

The scaphoid cortical ring sign occurs when excessive palmar flexion of the scaphoid causes the radiographic beam to be parallel with rather than perpendicular to the distal scaphoid [39]. Rotation of the scaphoid shortens the distance between its proximal and distal ends. Additionally, with progressive lunate extension, the lunate shape changes from trapezoidal to triangular. The clenched fist and ulnar deviation PA views load the SL joint and may increase the gap. Gilula defined three arciform lines drawn along the proximal surface of the proximal carpal row, the distal surface of the proximal carpal row, and the proximal surface of the distal carpal row [40]. A step off in any of these arcs suggests a carpal ligamentous injury, which may be enhanced by applying longitudinal traction to the wrist.

In SL ligament injuries, the scaphoid flexes and the lunate extends leading to abnormal SL angles on the lateral radiograph should be compared to the normal opposite wrist (Table 18.1). In the normal wrist, the central axis of the distal radius, lunate, and capitate should be aligned. In SL dissociation, these three bones become malaligned as the capitate collapses proximally and translates dorsally, forcing the lunate to rotate into extension (dorsal tilt) which increases the radiolunate [41] and capitolunate angles, decreases carpal height, and creates a DISI pattern.

Other imaging modalities have limited usefulness in current management of suspected SL tears. Since abnormal arthrographic findings have been found in 74% of asymptomatic patients, wrist arthrography is seldom used [42]. Magnetic resonance imaging (MRI) is commonly employed, but its accuracy is dependent on observer experience, signal sequences, strength of magnet, and use of dedicated wrist coils resulting in variable sensitivities, specificities, and accuracies. In a prospective study of arthroscopically confirmed SL tears, MRI was only able to correctly diagnose acute and chronic SL tears in 75% of cases, with no added benefit to employing intravenous contrast [43]. The sensitivity was 63% and specificity was 86%. However, in another study using MRI arthrography with a 1.5 T magnet, MRI was able to detect complete tears of the SL ligament with an improved sensitivity of 92%, specificity of 100%, and accuracy of 99% [44]. Detection of partial tears had a lower sensitivity of 63%, but specificity and accuracy were still high at 100% and 95%, respectively.

Surgical Technique for the RASL Procedure

The first step in the RASL procedure is to confirm via wrist arthroscopy the integrity of the capitolunate articular cartilage. Any significant damage to that articulation contraindicates the RASL procedure. Either regional or general anesthesia can be used, with administration of preoperative prophylactic intravenous antibiotics. The patient is placed supine on the operating room table with the arm on an arm board and a sterile tourniquet is applied and elevated to 250 mmHg after extremity exsanguination. The hand is suspended from a traction tower device and radiocarpal and midcarpal arthroscopy is performed to assess the carpal ligaments, articular cartilage, and degree of instability. If an SL tear is confirmed, no repairable dorsal ligament is observed, and no significant arthritis is present, an arthroscopic or open RASL procedure can be performed. It is recommended that arthroscopic RASL be attempted only after considerable experience with the open procedure. The arthrotomy respects and preserves the dorsal intercarpal ligament by transverse windows proximal and distal to its course.

The hand is removed from the traction tower and a 6 cm midline, longitudinal incision is made on the dorsal wrist just ulnar to Lister's tubercle centered over the radiocarpal joint.

The retinaculum is incised through the fourth dorsal compartment. The extensor pollicis longus is gently retracted radially and the extensor digitorum communis tendons are retracted ulnarly to permit transverse capsular incision to be made over the SL joint between the dorsal intercarpal and dorsal radio-triquetral ligaments. A second longitudinal incision is made centered over the radial styloid. Branches of the dorsal sensory radial nerve and the dorsal radial artery are protected. The first dorsal compartment is incised, the tendons gently retracted, and the capsule is incised. The radial styloid is exposed subperiosteally and a limited styloidectomy is performed, preserving the scaphoid fossa and extrinsic ligaments. Styloidectomy provides access to the radial proximal scaphoid for screw placement in the lunate center axis and at the same time eliminates radioscaphoid impingement and early radioscaphoid arthritis (SLAC 1).

A 0.062 in. K-wire is placed into the most proximal dorsal surface of the extended lunate angled from proximal to distal (Fig. 18.3). It is important to place the wire proximal to the lunate center on the lateral fluoroscopic image to prevent interference with the insertion of the headless screw. The wire is pushed distally, causing the wire to become perpendicular to the dorsal surface of the wrist which causes palmar flexion of the lunate. If this wire is maximally flexed, but the lunate is still not anatomically reduced, it may be necessary to place a second wire into the newly exposed dorsal and proximal part of the lunate, remove the first wire, and then translate the second wire distally until the lunate is fully reduced. When the proximal uncovered capitate articular surface is fully covered by the lunate, reduction of the

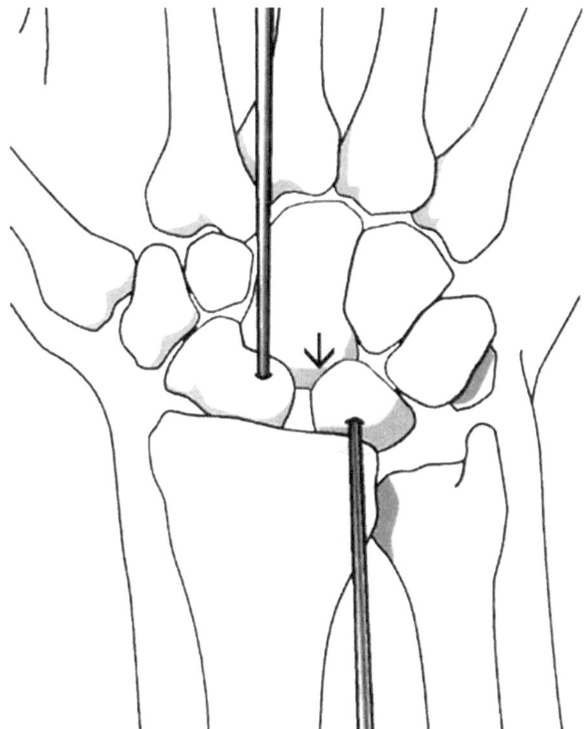

Fig. 18.3 Coronal view of the carpus illustrating the orientation of the scaphoid Kirschner (K) wire in a distal to proximal oblique direction and of the lunate K-wire orientation in a proximal to distal oblique direction. Lunate extension causes the capitate head to be abnormally uncovered (arrow). Proximal lunate descent causes loss of carpal height and increases scapholunate diastasis. (Source: Adapted from [2])

lunate is anatomic. This can be confirmed fluoroscopically by observing a capitolunate angle of 0° with both bones collinear on the lateral view. A K-wire is also placed into the dorsal scaphoid distal pole at an oblique angle from distal to proximal so that when wire is pulled proximally to extend the palmar flexed scaphoid, the wire becomes perpendicular to the dorsal surface of the wrist (Fig. 18.4). This is a reduction by derotation of the scaphoid and lunate.

With the wires reducing the scaphoid and lunate, the articular cartilage is carefully removed from the opposing scaphoid and lunate surfaces with a mechanical bur or for more safety curettes, until punctuate subchondral bleeding is observed (Fig. 18.5). This facilitates ingrowth of fibrous connective tissue. If a remnant of the SL ligament is present, it is not debrided but left to add to the fibrous connective tissue at the interface. A Kocher clamp is placed across the joystick K-wires after reduction is confirmed (Fig. 18.6). A guide wire for a cannulated dumbbell-shaped headless bone screw is placed into the radial mid waist of the scaphoid exiting the scaphoid at the mid-point of its articular surface opposite the lunate, across the joint, and then into the center of the lunate pointing towards the medial vertex on the coronal image and the middle of the lunate on the lateral image (Figs. 18.7 and 18.8). This starting point is critical and should be at or just proximal to the dorsolateral ridge of the scaphoid. Getting this starting point is greatly facilitated by the radial styloidectomy as previously described. The cannulated drill is placed over the guide wire and the hole is drilled. Then, the screw length is measured with a cannulated guide and the screw is advanced over the guide wire. The length should be slightly less than the length measured from the guide wire to allow countersinking of the screw beneath the scaphoid surface. When the K-wires are unclamped, they should not move as the screw is maintaining reduction. The K-wires are then removed.

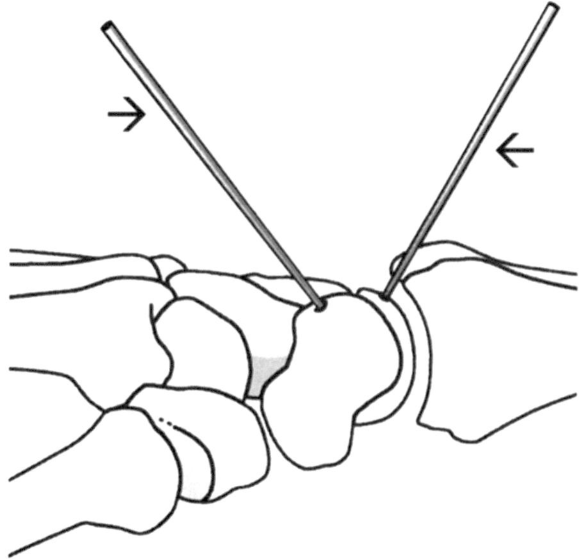

Fig. 18.4 Sagittal view of carpal Kirschner-wire orientation. The scaphoid wire is pushed toward the radius (arrow to right) to derotate the scaphoid out of palmarflexion and the lunate wire is pushed towards the hand (arrow to left to derotate the lunate out of extension. After reduction, the wires should be roughly parallel rather than divergent. (Source: Adapted from [2])

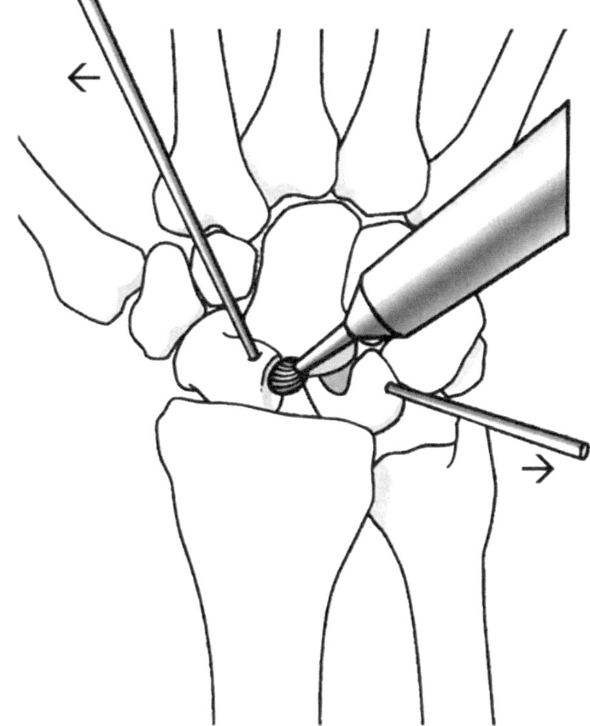

Fig. 18.5 Wires can be used to slightly increase scapholunate (SL) diastasis to facilitate insertion of a burr that is used to carefully remove cartilage in the SL interval until punctate bleeding is observed. This stimulates formation of a fibrous neoligament. *SL* scapholunate. (Source: Adapted from [2])

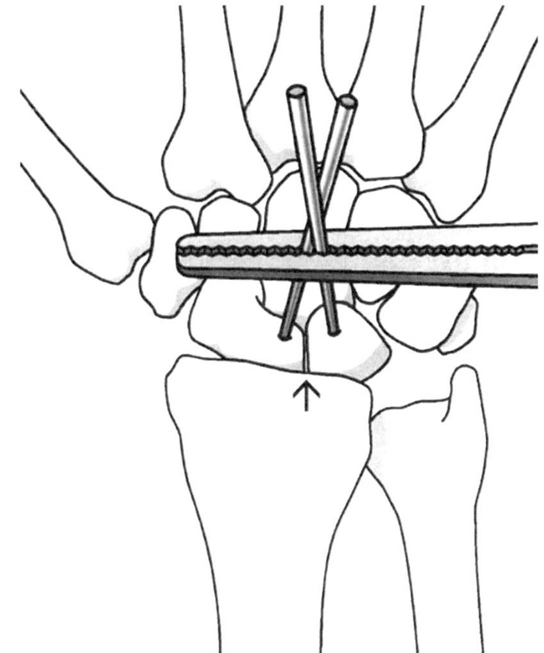

Fig. 18.6 A Kocher clamp is used to hold the joysticks that have been used to derotate the scaphoid and lunate into their reduced position. Note, scapholunate diastasis is also corrected (arrow). (Source: Adapted from [2])

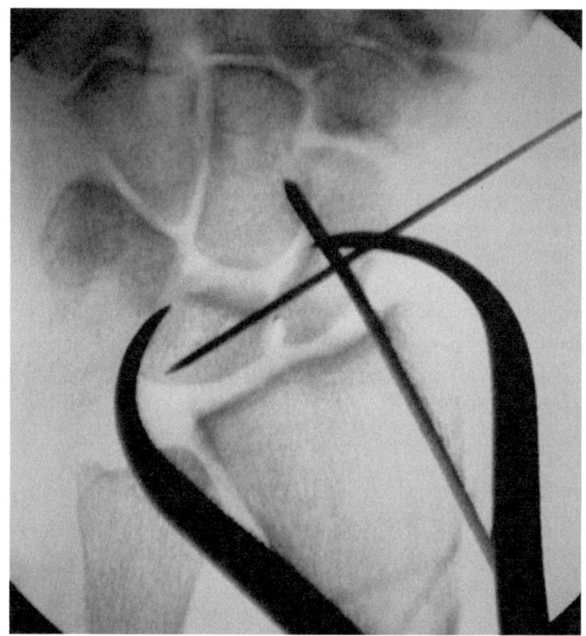

Fig. 18.7 Intra-operative fluoroscopic posteroanterior image of guidance wire placement prior to cannulated screw placement. The wire is placed into the midwaist of the scaphoid exiting the scaphoid at the midpoint of its articular surface opposite the lunate, and then into the center of the lunate at the medial vertex on the coronal image

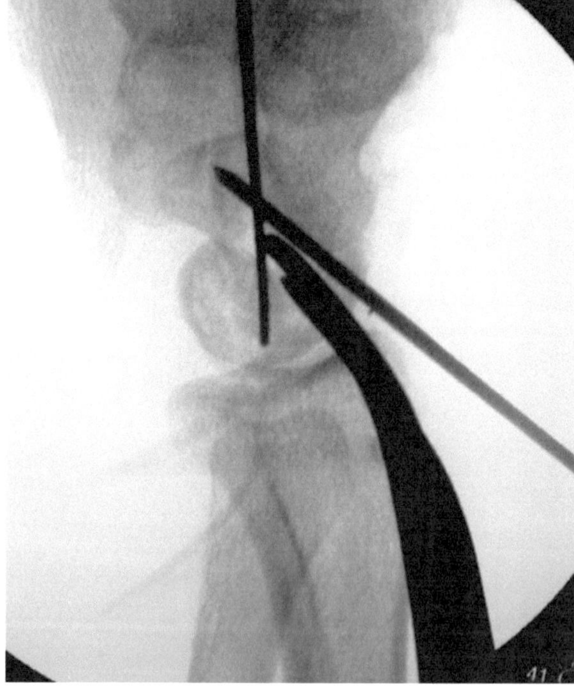

Fig. 18.8 Intra-operative fluoroscopic lateral image of wire placement prior to cannulated screw. The wire is appropriately positioned through the scaphoid and into the middle of the lunate on the lateral image

The radial capsule and periosteal sleeve are closed with interrupted absorbable sutures. The first dorsal retinaculum is transposed and cover the area of the radial styloidectomy. The dorsal wrist capsule is left unsutured to prevent loss of motion postoperatively. The EPL is left within its sheath. The wrist is immobilized in a volar splint for 2–3 weeks to allow for capsular healing; then early motion in a supervised occupational therapy program is begun. At 6 weeks, gradual strengthening is begun with unrestricted activity permitted at 4–6 months.

The arthroscopic RASL procedure is essentially the same as described above without the use of the dorsal and radial incisions. The radial styloidectomy and decortication of the opposing scaphoid and lunate articular surfaces are performed with an arthroscopic bur through standard portals. The K-wires for scaphoid and lunate derotation and for headless bone screw guidance are placed percutaneously by manually pushing the wires down to bone and then advancing them with a wire driver to minimize wrapping up of soft tissues. To drill, measure, and place the headless bone screw, a small incision is made radially.

Complications

There have been no occurrences of major intraoperative or postoperative complications consisting of infection, nerve injury, or screw breakage. Accurate measurement of screw length is important with placement of a screw slightly shorter than the measured length of the guide wire so that adequate countersinking below the surface of the radial aspect of the scaphoid can be performed. No headless bone screw threads should cross the SL interval to allow intercarpal rotation of the scaphoid and lunate around the smooth central axis. Furthermore, it is critical that the screw entry site be at the dorsal lateral ridge of the scaphoid and the axis of the guide wire be central or slightly palmar to central on the sagittal view to allow for the obligatory SL intercarpal rotation of 25°. Increasing screw obliquity or deviation from the lunate center may create asymmetric oscillation of the bones rather than axis rotation. Despite ideal positioning one can expect some non-progressive lucency around the leading threads of the lunate end of the screw.

Reduction of DISI deformity is important to preserve wrist motion and longevity. Incomplete SL reduction may predispose to abnormal carpal loading and kinematics that cause excessive screw loosening and progressive arthritis. This may partially explain why 3 of 24 patients who underwent the RASL procedure needed a subsequent surgical treatment with a proximal row carpectomy or arthrodesis procedure due to recurrent instability and symptoms.

The radial styloidectomy must be performed to obtain the best screw axis but the amount of bone that is removed is small which insures preservation of the origins of the radioscaphocapitate, dorsal radiocarpal, and long radiolunate ligaments.

Summary

From cadaver studies, we know that normal wrist ligaments maintain the carpal height and alignment through balanced tension that results in stored potential energy. When one or more ligaments is compromised, the potential energy is released as kinetic energy, as the carpal bones rotate, translate, and collapse into a more stable configuration [45].

The first part of the RASL procedure is reduction of the scaphoid and lunate back to stable alignment with the lunate colinear with the radius and capitate and the scaphoid in a mid-flexed posture with respect to the radius. Simultaneously, the critical midcarpal capitolunate relationship is restored when the proximal pole of the capitate is captured by the concave distal articular surface of the lunate and the ulnar aspect of the scaphoid.

The second part of the procedure is the association of the scaphoid and lunate with a headless bone screw while a fibrous neo-ligament forms, both of which establish long-term carpal stability. Permanent, planned retention of the screw distinguishes this technique from the one described by Herbert [46]. This is critical to allow for sufficient remodeling and strengthening of the fibrous neo-ligament. The prevention of carpal collapse may prevent or slow progression to SLAC arthritis. The RASL technique prevents dorsal subluxation of the proximal pole of the scaphoid in its facet. The RASL procedure allows radiocarpal and intercarpal motion. It does not link the rows via arthrodesis.

Results

This procedure has been used over the last 30 years and has been a reliable treatment for chronic static SL instability without advanced SLAC arthritis. The average follow-up of the initial series of 35 consecutive patients is 12 years with high patient satisfaction and excellent function and a low revision rate of 11%. These included conversion to total wrist fusion, proximal row carpectomy, and hardware removal.

SL ligament tears are common causes of chronic wrist pain and can lead to progressive patterns of arthritis. A thorough understanding of wrist anatomy and kinematics is necessary to select the appropriate treatment. The RASL procedure is an effective technique to restore carpal alignment, preserve motion, and improve symptoms without limiting future surgical treatments including intercarpal fusions, proximal row carpectomy, or wrist arthrodesis, should fixation fail or arthritis progress.

Summation Points

Indications

Initial treatment or after a failed alternative surgical treatment for an irreparable, symptomatic SL ligament tear with any degree of instability.

Contraindications

Progressive SLAC arthritis > Stage 1.

Outcomes

Excellent pain relief, improved function, maintenance of functional wrist motion, and maintenance of carpal alignment at average of 12 years.

References

1. Lipton CB, Ugwonali OF, Sarwahi V, et al. Reduction and association of the scaphoid and lunate for scapholunate ligament injuries (RASL). Atlas Hand Clin. 2003,8(2):249–60.
2. Rosenwasser MP, Miyasaka KC, Strauch RJ. The RASL procedure: reduction and association of the scaphoid and lunate using the Herbert screw. Tech Hand Up Extrem Surg. 1997;1(4):263–72.
3. Lipton C, Ugwonali O, Sarwahi V, et al. The treatment of chronic scapholunate dissociation with reduction and association of the scaphoid and lunate (RASL). Atlas Hand Clin. 2003;8(1):95–105.
4. Lindau T, Arner M, Hagberg L. Intraarticular lesions in distal fractures of the radius in young adults. A descriptive arthroscopic study in 50 patients. J Hand Surg Br. 1997;22(5):638–43.
5. Watson HK, Weinzweig J, Zeppieri J. The natural progression of scaphoid instability. Hand Clin. 1997;13(1):39–49.
6. Short WH, Werner FW, Green JK, et al. Biomechanical evaluation of ligamentous stabilizers of the scaphoid and lunate. J Hand Surg Am. 2002;27(6):991–1002.
7. Hurkmans HL, Kooloos JG, Meijer RS. Scapho-lunate dissociation and arthrodesis. An experimental study with lesions of the interosseous ligament and fusions with -wires. Clin Biomech (Bristol, Avon). 1996;11(4):220–6.
8. Linscheid RL, Dobyns JH. Dynamic carpal stability. Keio J Med. 2002;51(3):140–7.
9. Short WH, Werner FW, Fortino MD, et al. Analysis of the kinematics of the scaphoid and lunate in the intact wrist joint. Hand Clin. 1997;13(1):93–108.

10. Talwalkar SC, Edwards AT, Hayton MJ, et al. Results of tri-ligament tenodesis: a modified Brunelli procedure in the management of scapholunate instability. J Hand Surg Br. 2006;31(1):110–7.
11. Ruch DS, Smith BP. Arthroscopic and open management of dynamic scaphoid instability. Orthop Clin North Am. 2001;32(2):233–40; see also vii.
12. Darlis NA, Weiser RW, Sotereanos DG. Partial scapholunate ligament injuries treated with arthroscopic debridement and thermal shrinkage. J Hand Surg Am. 2005;30(5):908–14.
13. Hirsh L, Sodha S, Bozentka D, et al. Arthroscopic electrothermal collagen shrinkage for symptomatic laxity of the scapholunate interosseous ligament. J Hand Surg Br. 2005;30(6):643–7.
14. Weiss AP, Sachar K, Glowacki KA. Arthroscopic debridement alone for intercarpal ligament tears. J Hand Surg Am. 1997;22(2):344–9.
15. Whipple TL. The role of arthroscopy in the treatment of scapholunate instability. Hand Clin. 1995;11(1):37–40.
16. Bickert B, Sauerbier M, Germann G. Scapholunate ligament repair using the Mitek bone anchor. J Hand Surg Br. 2000;25(2):188–92.
17. Bloom HT, Freeland AE, Bowen V, et al. The treatment of chronic scapholunate dissociation: an evidence-based assessment of the literature. Orthopedics. 2003;26(2):195–203; quiz 204–5.
18. Lavernia CJ, Cohen MS, Taleisnik J. Treatment of scapholunate dissociation by ligamentous repair and capsulodesis. J Hand Surg Am. 1992;17(2):354–9.
19. Uhl RL, Williamson SC, Bowman MW, et al. Dorsal capsulodesis using suture anchors. Am J Orthop. 1997;26(8):547–8.
20. Szabo RM, Slater RR Jr, Palumbo CF, et al. Dorsal intercarpal ligament capsulodesis for chronic, static scapholunate dissociation: clinical results. J Hand Surg Am. 2002;27(6):978–84.
21. Wyrick JD, Youse BD, Kiefhaber TR. Scapholunate ligament repair and capsulodesis for the treatment of static scapholunate dissociation. J Hand Surg Br. 1998;23(6):776–80.
22. Wintman BI, Gelberman RH, Katz JN. Dynamic scapholunate instability: results of operative treatment with dorsal capsulodesis. J Hand Surg Am. 1995;20(6):971–9.
23. Almquist EE, Bach AW, Sack IT, et al. Four-bone ligament reconstruction for treatment of chronic complete scapholunate separation. J Hand Surg Am. 1991;16(2):322–7.
24. Glickel SZ, Millender LH. Ligamentous reconstruction for chronic intercarpal instability. J Hand Surg Am. 1984;9(4):514–27.
25. Brunelli GA, Brunelli GR. A new surgical technique for carpal instability with scapho-lunar dislocation. (Eleven cases). Ann Chi Main Memb Super 1995; 14(4–5):207–213.
26. Van Den Abbeele KL, Loh YC, Stanley JK, et al. Early results of a modified Brunelli procedure for scapholunate instability. J Hand Surg Br. 1998;23(2):258–61.
27. Watson HK, Belniak R, Garcia-Elias M. Treatment of scapholunate dissociation: preferred treatment-STT fusion vs. other methods. Orthopedics. 1991;14(3):365–8; discussion 368–70.
28. Watson HK, Weinzweig J, Guidera PM, et al. One thousand intercarpal arthrodeses. J Hand Surg Br. 1999;24(3):307–15.
29. Roman MB, Manske PR, Pruitt DL, et al. Scaphocapitolunate arthrodesis. J Hand Surg Am. 1993;18(1):26–33.
30. Hom S, Ruby LK. Attempted scapholunate arthrodesis for chronic scapholunate dissociation. J Hand Surg Am. 1991;16(2):334–9.
31. Kleinman WB. Management of chronic rotary subluxation of the scaphoid by scapho-trapezio-trapezoid arthrodesis. Rationale for the technique, postoperative changes in biomechanics, and results. Hand Clin. 1987;3(1):113–33.
32. Hastings DE, Silver RL. Intercarpal arthrodesis in the management of chronic carpal instability after trauma. J Hand Surg Am. 1984;9(6):834–40.
33. Watson HK, Ashmead D, Makhlouf MV. Examination of the scaphoid. J Hand Surg Am. 1988;13(5):657–60.
34. Ruby LK, An KN, Linscheid RL, et al. The effect of scapholunate ligament section on scapholunate motion. J Hand Surg Am. 1987;12(5 Pt 1):767–71.

35. Boabighi A, Kuhlmann IN, Kenesi C. The distal ligamentous complex of the scaphoid and the scapho-lunate ligament. An anatomic, histological and biomechanical study. J Hand Surg Br. 1993;18(1):65–9.
36. Mitsuyasu H, Patterson RM, Shah MA, et al. The role of the dorsa intercarpal ligament in dynamic and statie scapholunate instability. J Hand Surg Am. 2004;29(2):279–88.
37. Meade TD, Schneider LH, Cherry K. Radiographic analysis of selective ligament sectioning at the carpal scaphoid: a cadaver study. J Hand Surg Am. 1990;15(6):855–62.
38. Baratz ME, Dunn MJ. Ligament injuries and instability of the carpus: scapholunate joint. In: Berger RA, Weiss AP, editors. Hand surgery. Philadelphia: Lippincott Williams and Wilkins; 2004. p. 481–94.
39. Cautilli GP, Wehbe MA. Scapho-lunate distance and cortical ring sign. J Hand Surg Am. 1991;16(3):501–3.
40. Gilula LA. Carpal injuries: analytic approach and case exercises. AJR Am J Roentgenol. 1979;133(3):503–17.
41. Mack GR, Bosse MJ, Gelberman RH, et al. The natural history of scaphoid non-union. J Bone Joint Surg Am. 1984;66(4):504–9.
42. Herbert TJ, Faithfull RG, McCann DJ, et al. Bilateral arthrography of the wrist. J Hand Surg Br. 1990;15(2):233–5.
43. Schadel-Hopfner M, Iwinska-Zelder J, Braus T, et al. MRI versus arthroscopy in the diagnosis of scapholunate ligament injury. J Hand Surg Br. 2001;26(1):17–21.
44. Schmitt R, Christopoulos G, Meier R, et al. Direct MR arthrography of the wrist in comparison with arthroscopy: a prospective study on 125 patients. Rofo. 2003;175(7):911–9.
45. Cohen MS. Ligamentous injuries of the wrist in the athlete. Clin Sports Med. 1998;17(3):533–52.
46. Herbert TJ. Acute rotary dislocation of the scaphoid: a new technique of repair using Herbert screw fixation across the scapho-lunate joint. World J Surg. 1991;15(4):463–9.

Chapter 19
Chronic, Reducible Scapholunate Ligament Injury: Scapholunate Axis Method (SLAM)

Arin E. Kim and Steve K. Lee

Case Presentation

The patient is a 44-year-old right-hand dominant man who presented 6 months after injuring his left wrist while sailing. He continued to sail with a wrist splint, and while the pain improved from the initial injury, he remained debilitated by his wrist pain which was symptomatic at work, with activities of daily living, and while sailing.

On physical examination, he was tender to palpation over the scapholunate (SL) interval with a positive Watson scaphoid shift test. He had full range of motion of his wrist. He had a palmaris tendon. He was distally neurovascularly intact.

Radiographs demonstrated 5.7 mm gap of the left SL interval and dorsal intercalated segmental instability (DISI). The radiolunate angle was 30° and SL angle was 85° (Fig. 19.1a, b). MRI showed a complete SLIL tear with dorsal scaphoid translation and SL gap, positive DISI deformity, intact radiocarpal, and midcarpal cartilage (Fig. 19.2a–c).

A. E. Kim
Montefiore Medical Center, Bronx, NY, USA
e-mail: arkim@montefiore.org

S. K. Lee (✉)
Hospital for Special Surgery, New York, NY, USA
e-mail: lees@hss.edu

J. Yao (ed.), *Carpal Instability*, https://doi.org/10.1007/978-3-031-55869-6_19

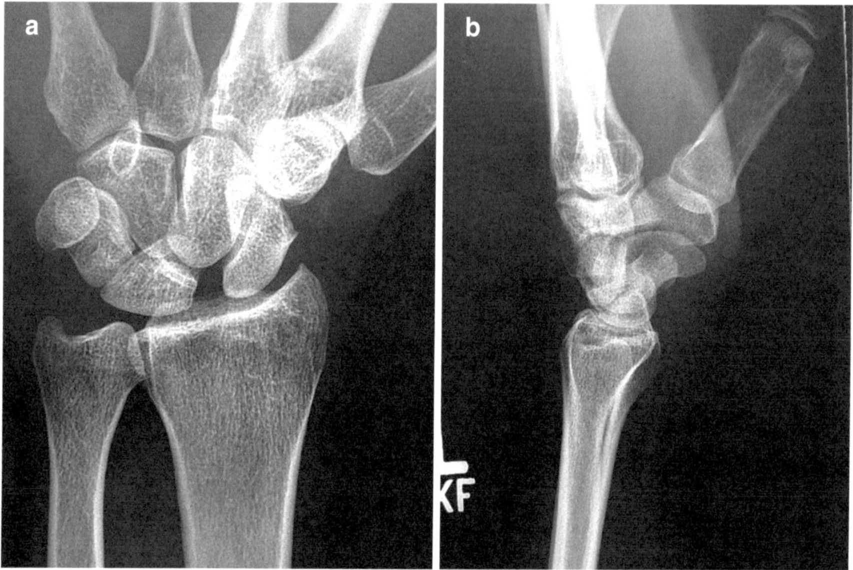

Fig. 19.1 (**a**) PA view of the left wrist demonstrates widening of the scapholunate interval. (**b**) Lateral view of the left wrist demonstrates DISI deformity

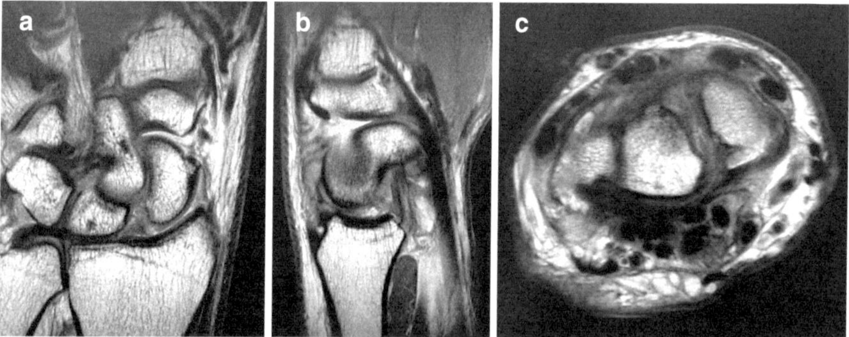

Fig. 19.2 (**a**) Coronal T1-weighted MRI of the wrist demonstrates intact radioscapholunate and midcarpal cartilage and SL widening. (**b**) Sagittal T1-weighted MRI of wrist demonstrates dorsal subluxation of the scaphoid. (**c**) Axial T1-weighted MRI of the wrist shows widening of the SL interval due to chronic SLIL tear

Management Options

A wide array of treatment options has been proposed for scapholunate ligament injuries. Although the debate continues, consideration for treatment options should be based on the patient age and activity demands, symptoms, dynamic instability, reducibility, chronicity, and the presence of arthritic changes [1]. SLIL injuries are truly on a spectrum from mild ligamentous sprains to severe degenerative changes due to loss of normal carpal kinematics and stability. In a partial SLIL injury, pinning, capsulodesis, and arthroscopic debridement or thermal shrinkage have been described to be sufficient in restoring stability to the SL interval [2–4]. In patients with dynamic instability or complete dissociation with repairable tissue and reducible injury, scapholunate repair and dorsal capsulodesis are recommended. Repair is best performed in patients with acute or subacute injuries in which there is sufficient tissue for repair and no degenerative changes [5, 6]. In contrast, on the other end of the spectrum are patients with scapholunate advance collapse (SLAC) requiring salvage or fusion options such as proximal row carpectomy and partial or complete wrist fusions.

Chronic SLIL injuries without degenerative changes land in the middle of this spectrum and are perhaps the most vexing challenge for surgeons. These injuries warrant reconstructive methods to restore carpal kinematics to prevent the natural history of progression to SLAC wrist. The current patient fits the picture of symptomatic chronic scapholunate dissociation without a repairable SLIL in the absence of degenerative changes. Several options have been proposed for this problem.

Early options included scapholunate fusion, but this has since been abandoned as it does not preserve the natural kinematics of the wrist and isolated fusion is difficult to achieve [7]. The Reduction Association Scaphoid and Lunate (RASL) procedure creates a tether by placing a screw as close as possible the axis of rotation [8]. While this links the scapholunate articulation near its axis of rotation, a stiff screw cannot mimic the fluid motion of normal carpal kinematics. Flexor carpi radialis (FCR) tendon for tenodesis and reconstruction has been described and modified as well as use of the extensor carpi radialis brevis tendon (ECRB) [9, 10]. The three ligament tenodesis (3LT) technique also uses the FCR tendon to reconstruct the dorsal SLIL, augment palmar tissues, and prevent ulnar translation of the lunate as a modification of previously described techniques [11]. While this technique corrects the flexion and dissociation of the scaphoid, it is a tendon reconstruction with expected creep along the length of the tendon. Lastly, dorsal capsulodesis has been shown to have similar results to 3LT [12]. However, capsulodesis only limits scaphoid flexion and does not address the extension of the lunate or SL widening.

Management Chosen for this Case with Rationale

The patient is a young, active who leads a demanding lifestyle. He has no arthritic changes as confirmed by radiographs and advanced imaging. The goals of the surgery were to improve the relationship, stability, and motion of the carpus in a sustainable way for an active patient. The rationale for the SLAM technique is to use a flexible, biological graft to reconstruct the SLIL in the central axis of rotation. Fixation close to the scapholunate joint minimizes creep to provide long-term approximation of normal carpal alignment and kinematics. Furthermore, the second limb of autograft is passed dorsally to the lunate to reconstruct the dorsal SLIL, which is the critical stabilizing portion [13].

Clinical Course and Outcome

At 9 months from date of injury, the patient underwent SLAM procedure as follows.

Surgical Technique: An incision is made over the dorsal wrist, in line with the third ray. Skin flaps are raised, careful to avoid injury to the cutaneous nerves. The third compartment is opened and extensor pollicis longus (EPL) is transposed radially and the second and fourth compartments are opened. A posterior interosseous nerve neurectomy is performed at the floor of the fourth compartment. An inverted T-capsulotomy is performed to reveal a full tear of the scapholunate ligament with a flexed scaphoid, wide SL gap, and dorsally subluxated scaphoid in DISI. A radial sided incision is made and careful dissection past critical structures to approach the scaphoid. A palmaris longus tendon graft is harvested and debulked to approximately 2 mm to easily pass through the 3.5 mm × 7 mm tendon anchor (Arthrex, Naples, FL).

The deformity is reduced by manual palmar pressure on the capitate to reduce the lunate out of DISI into the neutral position. Next, scapholunate compression is applied, followed by a 0.045-inch K-wire in the scaphoid and lunate to hold the reduction. The c-shaped reduction guide can also be used for the reduction and as a drill guide (Fig. 19.3). The K-wire in the mid axis of the scaphoid and lunate is confirmed on fluoroscopy (Fig. 19.4). It is critical that this is correctly placed in the coronal and sagittal planes. An additional scaphocapitate wire can be placed for stability. The K-wire is overdrilled (Arthrex, Naples, FL) (Fig. 19.5). The palmaris

Fig. 19.3 The C-ring guide can be used to insert the K-wire in the central axis. (Photo courtesy of Dan Zlotolow MD)

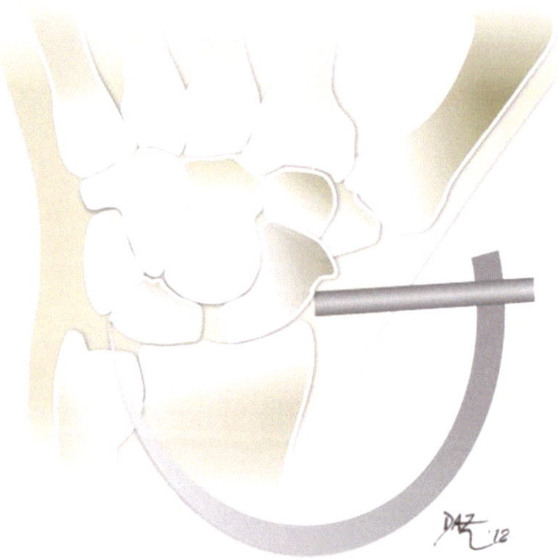

Fig. 19.4 The wire is placed in the center-center position across the scaphoid and lunate and a secondary stabilization wire can be used (Courtesy of Dan Zlotolow MD)

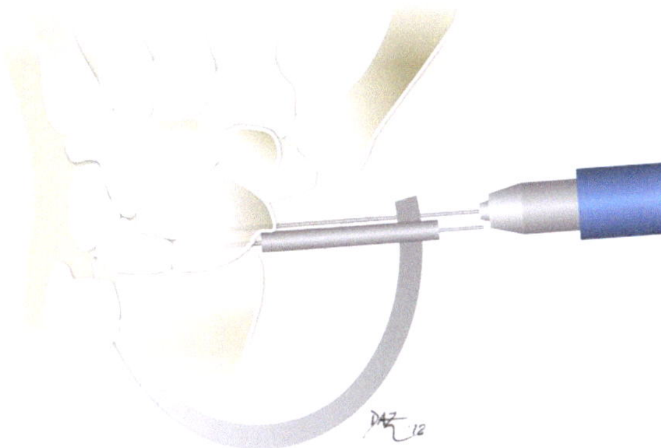

Fig. 19.5 The K-wire is overdrilled (Courtesy of Dan Zlotolow MD)

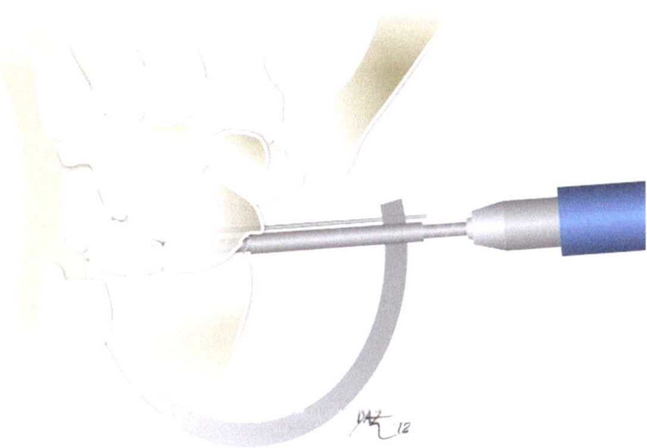

longus graft is threaded through the tendon anchor (Arthrex, Naples, FL). The drill hole is irrigated with saline through a spinal needle to remove any debris that may block easy passage of the tendon graft. The graft is placed into the drill hole and tamped into place with a mallet (Fig. 19.6). Fluoroscopic imaging should be taken to assess excellent position on the anchor which is within the lunate and near the proximal ulnar corner. The tendon is tensioned tightly and a 4 mm × 10 mm interference screw (Arthrex, Naples, FL) is placed into the scaphoid (Fig. 19.7). The excess tendon graft is passed radially and dorsally over the carpus and fixed to the dorsal aspect of the lunate by suturing to any remnant dorsal SLIL or dorsal radiocarpal ligament (Fig. 19.8). The dorsal aspect of the lunate and scaphoid is decorticated under where the tendon graft lies to provide a healing bony bed. The wound is irrigated and the capsule and retinaculum are closed with the EPL transposed. If used, the scaphocapitate K-wire is cut and buried under the skin. After closing the skin, a sterile dressing is placed followed by a volar and dorsal wrist splint in neutral.

Fig. 19.6 The anchor and graft is inserted and impacted (Courtesy of Dan Zlotolow MD)

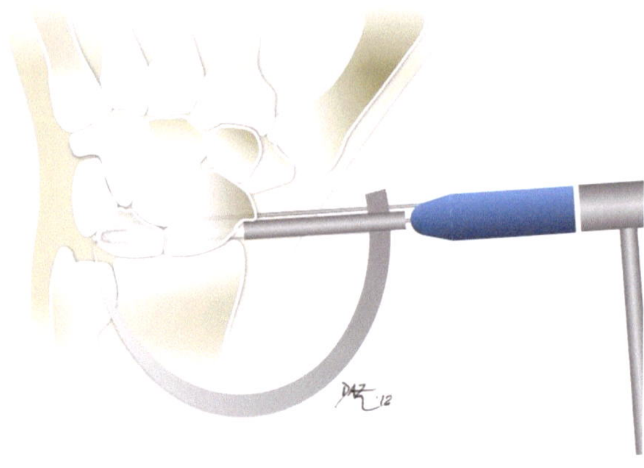

Fig. 19.7 An interference screw is placed into the scaphoid with the graft in tension (Courtesy of Dan Zlotolow MD)

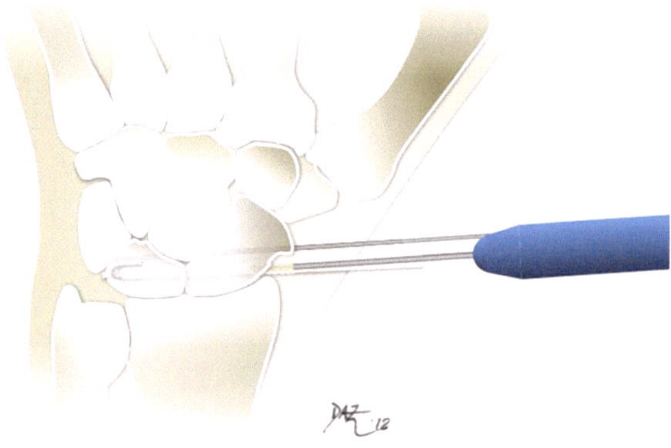

Fig. 19.8 Dorsal stabilization is performed with the remainder of the graft laid across the dorsal scaphoid and lunate (Courtesy of Dan Zlotolow MD)

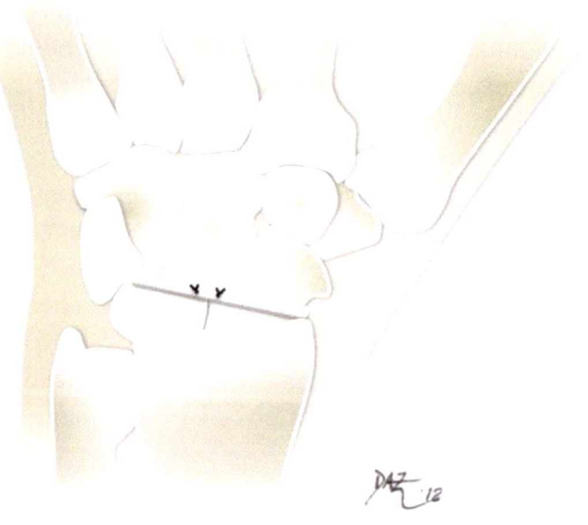

Clinical Course

The patient was seen 2 weeks after surgery. His sutures were removed and he was transitioned from the splint to a short arm cast for 4 weeks. At 6 weeks, he was transitioned to a thermoplastic splint. He remained nonweightbearing without range of motion of the wrist. Pin was removed at 9 weeks from date of initial surgery in the operating room under local anesthesia. The patient started hand therapy for gentle wrist range of motion.

Postoperative radiographs demonstrated central position of the anchor and reduced SL interval (Fig. 19.9a, b).

The patient was seen in clinic at 2-month intervals. He was pain free and continued to improve his range of motion. He began sailing again 5 months postoperatively. At 1 year postop, he had 0 out of 10 pain and returned to competitive sailing and weight training without pain. His range of motion showed 60 degrees of flexion, 50° extension, 20 degrees of radial deviation, 33 degrees of ulnar deviation, and 80 degrees of symmetric pronation and supination (Fig. 19.10a–d). His tip to palm distance was 0 cm and grip strength 60 lbs. in the third position. Pinch strength was 16 lbs. Radiographs continued to show improved carpal position (Fig. 19.11a, b).

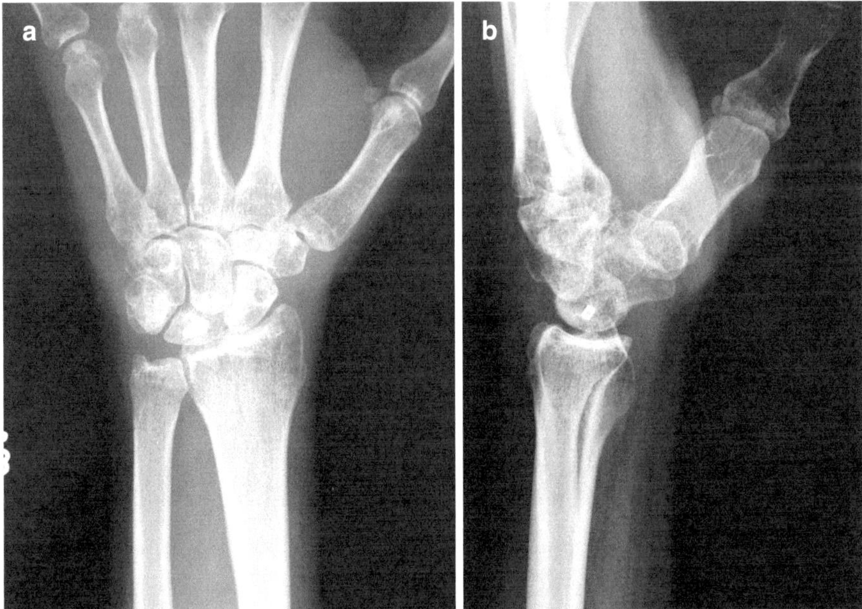

Fig. 19.9 (a) PA view of the postoperative wrist demonstrates reduction of SL interval now at 2.5 mm. (b) Lateral view of the postoperative wrist demonstrates centrally placed anchor in the lunate with improvement of DISI deformity

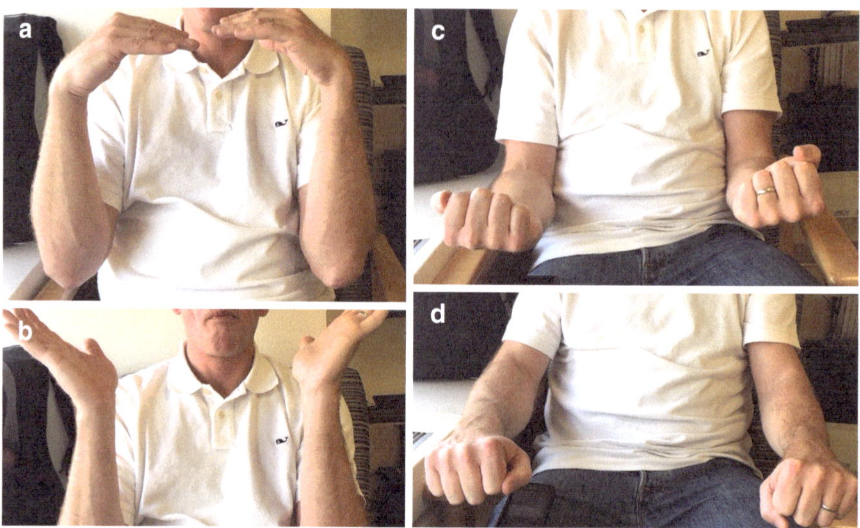

Fig. 19.10 Range of motion at 1 year from surgery with (**a**) flexion, (**b**) extension, (**c**) supination, (**d**) pronation now nearly symmetric to the contralateral side

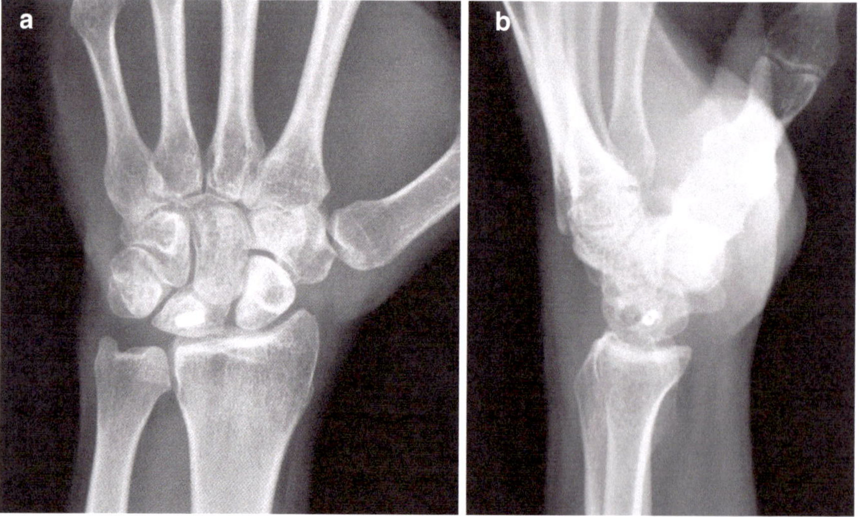

Fig. 19.11 Radiographs at 1 year demonstrate (**a**) PA and (**b**) lateral views showing maintained reduction of the SL interval and improvement of DISI deformity

Clinical Pearls and Pitfalls

- The guidewire must be in the central axis of the scaphoid and lunate in the sagittal plane and aiming to the proximal ulnar corner of the lunate in the coronal plane.
- Eccentric placement of the bone tunnel can lead to vascular compromise or unreliable fixation or fracture [14, 15].
- To pass the tendon graft easily, irrigate the drill hole with saline using a spinal needle and trim the tendon graft as needed.
- Instead of using the step drill, a double drilling separately of the scaphoid and lunate are possible through the scapholunate interval (Fig. 19.12a–d).

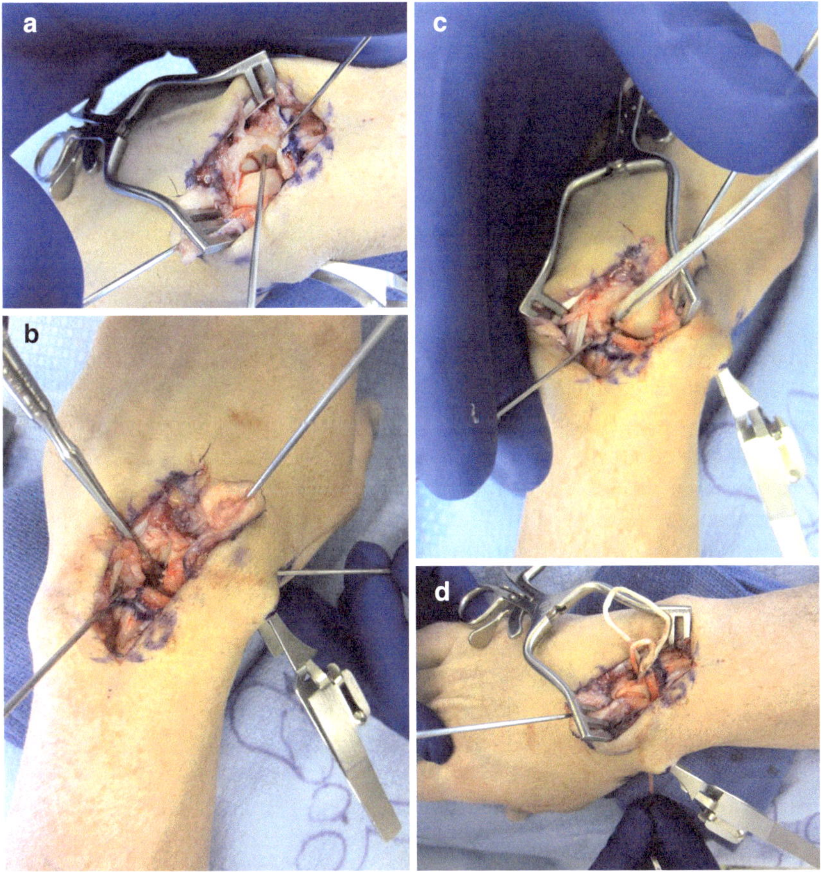

Fig. 19.12 (**a**) Using the scapholunate interval, the first guidewire is placed in the center of the articular surface of the lunate toward the proximal ulnar corner. Once the position is confirmed on fluoroscopy it is drilled and the guidewire removed. (**b**) Another guidewire is placed at the ulnar aspect of the scaphoid and drilled radially and drilled after confirming position on fluoroscopy. (**c**) The graft and anchor are first impacted into the lunate. (**d**) The tails of the graft are passed through the scaphoid from the ulnar to radial aspect

Literature Review and Discussion

Scapholunate ligament injuries are the most frequently injured ligament in the wrist and cause symptoms of pain, clicking, and decreased grip strength [1]. The natural history of SLIL deficiency is progression to SLAC wrist [16, 17]. This is a challenge in young, active patients who do not have a repairable ligament. The goal of surgery is to improve carpal kinematics.

SLAM is a technique that aims to reconstruct the central and dorsal SLIL with biologic tissue and place fixation points close to the scapholunate joint to minimize creep. Preliminary results have been excellent. In the preliminary review of 13 patients, the mean preoperative scapholunate gap was 5.4 mm compared to 2.1 mm postop. The mean preoperative scapholunate angle of 70° was improved to 59° post-operatively. The mean postoperative wrist flexion and extension were 45 and 56°, respectively. The mean grip strength was 62% of the contralateral side and the mean visual analog scale for pain postoperatively was 1.7 [28].

In this same cohort, there was one failure. The oldest patient in the cohort was 65 years old and had postoperative widening of the gap with pain and was ultimately treated with proximal row carpectomy. For older patients, salvage procedures should be considered. One published complication of this technique was avascular necrosis of the lunate [14]. In this case, there was eccentric placement of the anchor that likely violated the volar cortex of the lunate compromising its blood supply [15]. Thus, it is critical that the transosseous tunnel be placed in the central axis position for the best fixation and to prevent vascular compromise.

In the absence of degenerative changes, other soft tissue procedures that are used are dorsal capsulodesis and tenodesis procedures. Dorsal capsulodesis can be used alone or in conjunction with SLIL repair in cases when the ligament is repairable [5, 18]. Dorsal capsulodesis prevents scaphoid flexion but does not prevent SL gapping. In a retrospective series of 17 patients, flexion and extension loss averaged 11° each [19]. Grip strength improved by 11.2 kg and average pain and activity score was good (60.8/80). Another retrospective analysis examined 31 patients who underwent dorsal capsulodesis procedures [20]. They found a 20% decrease in wrist motion and no improvement in grip strength after surgery. While most patients had improvement in pain, only two had complete relief and there was loss of radiographic maintenance of carpal alignment at final follow-up. Later studies showed that dorsal capsulodesis does not prevent radiographic deterioration and degenerative changes in the long term, but may still improve functional outcomes [21, 22].

Tendon graft reconstruction has been attempted with FCR, ECRB, and extensor carpi radialis longus (ECRL) [9, 10, 23]. The original Brunelli tenodesis involves a strip of FCR tendon passed through the scaphoid and anchored to the distal radius [10]. This was modified by anchoring the tendon to the dorsum of the lunate [24]. The 3LT technique combines these earlier versions by replicating the scaphotrapeziotrapezoid, dorsal SLIL, and dorsal radiotriquetral ligaments [11]. The authors report range of motion approximately 25% less than the contralateral side, grip strength 65% of the contralateral side, and pain relief in 74% of patients. Short-term outcomes show improvement in patient function, satisfaction, and pain relief in 80% of patients [25]. The 3LT technique did show improvement in pain compared to previous tenodesis techniques [26].

Comparison of tenodesis and capsulodesis showed that both groups had decreased motion postoperatively, and similar grip strength and Mayo wrist scores between groups [12]. Biomechanical studies of SLAM, modified Brunelli tenodesis, Blatt capsulodesis showed that SLAM and Brunelli tenodesis did better than capsulodesis at recreating the SL interval and SLAM trended toward better correction of the SL angle [27]. SLAM creates a double tether in the central and dorsal planes and theoretically has biomechanical advantage over isolated capsulodesis and decreased creep compared to 3LT.

Conclusion

The SLAM technique is for a static reducible scapholunate dissociation without cartilage degeneration. It is technically demanding but can lead to satisfactory clinical outcomes for the well-selected patient.

References

1. Kuo CE, Wolfe SW. Scapholunate instability: current concepts in diagnosis and management. J Hand Surg Am. 2008;33(6):998–1013. https://doi.org/10.1016/j.jhsa.2008.04.027. PMID: 18656780.
2. Darlis NA, Weiser RW, Sotereanos DG. Partial scapholunate ligament injuries treated with arthroscopic debridement and thermal shrinkage. J Hand Surg Am. 2005;30(5):908–14. https://doi.org/10.1016/j.jhsa.2005.05.013. PMID: 16182044.
3. Rosa ND, Sapino G, Vita F, di Summa PG, Adani R. Modified Viegas dorsal capsuloplasty for chronic partial injury of the scapholunate ligament in young athletes: outcomes at 24 months. J Hand Surg Eur Vol. 2020;45(9):945–51. https://doi.org/10.1177/1753193420939490. Epub 2020 Jul 12. PMID: 32659131.
4. Weiss AP, Sachar K, Glowacki KA. Arthroscopic debridement alone for intercarpal ligament tears. J Hand Surg Am. 1997;22(2):344–9. https://doi.org/10.1016/S0363-5023(97)80176-1. PMID: 9195439.
5. Lavernia CJ, Cohen MS, Taleisnik J. Treatment of scapholunate dissociation by ligamentous repair and capsulodesis. J Hand Surg Am. 1992;17(2):354–9. https://doi.org/10.1016/0363-5023(92)90419-p. PMID: 1564287.
6. Pomerance J. Outcome after repair of the scapholunate interosseous ligament and dorsal capsulodesis for dynamic scapholunate instability due to trauma. J Hand Surg Am. 2006;31(8):1380–6. https://doi.org/10.1016/j.jhsa.2006.07.005. PMID: 17027803.
7. Hom S, Ruby LK. Attempted scapholunate arthrodesis for chronic scapholunate dissociation. J Hand Surg Am. 1991;16(2):334–9. https://doi.org/10.1016/s0363-5023(10)80122-4. PMID: 2022849.
8. Rosenwasser MP, Miyasajsa KC, Strauch RJ. The RASL procedure: reduction and association of the scaphoid and lunate using the Herbert screw. Tech Hand Up Extrem Surg. 1997;1(4):263–72. PMID: 16609495.

9. Almquist EE, Bach AW, Sack JT, Fuhs SE, Newman DM. Four-bone ligament reconstruction for treatment of chronic complete scapholunate separation. J Hand Surg Am. 1991;16(2):322–7. https://doi.org/10.1016/s0363-5023(10)80120-0. PMID: 2022847.

10. Brunelli GA, Brunelli GR. Une nouvelle intervention pour la dissociation scapho-lunaire. Proposition d'une nouvelle technique chirurgicale pour l'instabilité carpienne avec dissociation scapho-lunaire (11 cas) [A new surgical technique for carpal instability with scapho-lunar dislocation. (Eleven cases)]. Ann Chir Main Memb Super. 1995;14(4–5):207–13. French. https://doi.org/10.1016/s0753-9053(05)80415-6. PMID: 8519586.

11. Garcia-Elias M, Lluch AL, Stanley JK. Three-ligament tenodesis for the treatment of scapholunate dissociation: indications and surgical technique. J Hand Surg Am. 2006;31(1):125–34. https://doi.org/10.1016/j.jhsa.2005.10.011. PMID: 16443117.

12. Moran SL, Ford KS, Wulf CA, Cooney WP. Outcomes of dorsal capsulodesis and tenodesis for treatment of scapholunate instability. J Hand Surg Am. 2006;31(9):1438–46. https://doi.org/10.1016/j.jhsa.2006.08.002. PMID: 17095371.

13. Berger RA. The gross and histologic anatomy of the scapholunate interosseous ligament. J Hand Surg Am. 1996;21(2):170–8. https://doi.org/10.1016/S0363-5023(96)80096-7. PMID: 8683042.

14. Chan K, Engasser W, Jebson PJL. Avascular necrosis of the lunate following reconstruction of the scapholunate ligament using the scapholunate axis method (SLAM). J Hand Surg Am. 2019;44(10):904.e1–4. https://doi.org/10.1016/j.jhsa.2018.10.028. Epub 2018 Dec 20. PMID: 30579687.

15. Zlotolow DA, Lee SK, Yao J. Technical errors in the implantation of the scapholunate axis method (SLAM) resulting in avascular necrosis of the lunate. J Hand Surg Am. 2020;45(7):e1. https://doi.org/10.1016/j.jhsa.2020.03.012. Epub 2020 Apr 20. PMID: 32327335.

16. Watson HK, Ballet FL. The SLAC wrist: scapholunate advanced collapse pattern of degenerative arthritis. J Hand Surg Am. 1984;9(3):358–65. https://doi.org/10.1016/s0363-5023(84)80223-3. PMID: 6725894.

17. Watson HK, Weinzweig J, Zeppieri J. The natural progression of scaphoid instability. Hand Clin. 1997;13(1):39–49. PMID: 9048182.

18. Blatt G. Capsulodesis in reconstructive hand surgery. Dorsal capsulodesis for the unstable scaphoid and volar capsulodesis following excision of the distal ulna. Hand Clin. 1987;3(1):81–102. PMID: 3818814.

19. Muermans S, De Smet L, Van Ransbeeck H. Blatt dorsal capsulodesis for scapholunate instability. Acta Orthop Belg. 1999;65(4):434–9. PMID: 10675938.

20. Moran SL, Cooney WP, Berger RA, Strickland J. Capsulodesis for the treatment of chronic scapholunate instability. J Hand Surg Am. 2005;30(1):16–23. https://doi.org/10.1016/j.jhsa.2004.07.021. PMID: 15680551.

21. Gajendran VK, Peterson B, Slater RR Jr, Szabo RM. Long-term outcomes of dorsal intercarpal ligament capsulodesis for chronic scapholunate dissociation. J Hand Surg Am. 2007;32(9):1323–33. https://doi.org/10.1016/j.jhsa.2007.07.016. PMID: 17996765.

22. Megerle K, Bertel D, Germann G, Lehnhardt M, Hellmich S. Long-term results of dorsal intercarpal ligament capsulodesis for the treatment of chronic scapholunate instability. J Bone Joint Surg Br. 2012;94(12):1660–5. https://doi.org/10.1302/0301-620X.94B12.30007. PMID: 23188908.

23. Linscheid RL, Dobyns JH. Treatment of scapholunate dissociation. Rotatory subluxation of the scaphoid. Hand Clin. 1992;8(4):645–52. PMID: 1460063.

24. Van Den Abbeele KL, Loh YC, Stanley JK, Trail IA. Early results of a modified Brunelli procedure for scapholunate instability. J Hand Surg Br. 1998;23(2):258–61. https://doi.org/10.1016/s0266-7681(98)80191-5. PMID: 9607676.

25. Blackburn J, van der Oest MJW, Poelstra R, Selles RW, Chen NC, Feitz R, Hand-Wrist Study Group. Three-ligament tenodesis for chronic scapholunate injuries: short-term outcomes in 203 patients. J Hand Surg Eur Vol. 2020;45(4):383–8. https://doi.org/10.1177/1753193419885063. Epub 2019 Nov 11. PMID: 31711344.

26. Wagner JM, Stammler A, Harenberg P, Reinkemeier F, Lehnhardt M, Behr B. Did implementation of three ligament tenodesis improve patient outcome after chronic scapholunate instability? A retrospective study. Arch Orthop Trauma Surg. 2022;142(9):2397–403. https://doi.org/10.1007/s00402-022-04435-z. Epub 2022 Apr 11. PMID: 35411494.
27. Lee SK, Zlotolow DA, Sapienza A, Karia R, Yao J. Biomechanical comparison of 3 methods of scapholunate ligament reconstruction. J Hand Surg Am. 2014;39(4):643–50. https://doi.org/10.1016/j.jhsa.2013.12.033. Epub 2014 Feb 20. PMID: 24559758.
28. Yao J, Zlotolow DA, Lee SK. Scapholunate axis method. J Wrist Surg. 2016;5(1):59–66. https://doi.org/10.1055/s-0035-1570744. Epub 2016 Jan 6. Erratum in: J Wrist Surg. 2016 May;5(2):169. PMID: 26855838; PMCID: PMC4742262.

Further Reading

Kitay A, Wolfe SW. Scapholunate instability: current concepts in diagnosis and management. J Hand Surg Am. 2012;37(10):2175–96. https://doi.org/10.1016/j.jhsa.2012.07.035. PMID: 23021178.
Lee SK, Zlotolow DA, Sapienza A, Karia R, Yao J. Biomechanical comparison of 3 methods of scapholunate ligament reconstruction. J Hand Surg Am. 2014;39(4):643–50. https://doi.org/10.1016/j.jhsa.2013.12.033. Epub 2014 Feb 20. PMID: 24559758.
Yao J, Zlotolow DA, Lee SK. Scapholunate axis method. J Wrist Surg. 2016;5(1):59–66. https://doi.org/10.1055/s-0035-1570744. Epub 2016 Jan 6. Erratum in: J Wrist Surg. 2016 May;5(2):169. PMID: 26855838; PMCID: PMC4742262.
Zlotolow DA, Lee SK, Yao J. Technical errors in the implantation of the scapholunate axis method (SLAM) resulting in avascular necrosis of the lunate. J Hand Surg Am. 2020;45(7):e1. https://doi.org/10.1016/j.jhsa.2020.03.012. Epub 2020 Apr 20. PMID: 32327335.

Chapter 20
Chronic, Reducible Scapholunate Ligament Injury: Scapho-Luno-Triquetral Tenodesis (SLT)

Mark Ross and Greg Couzens

Case Presentation

A 34-year-old male police officer fell 3 m off a wall sustaining multiple injuries including facial injuries and a serious wrist injury which initially went untreated. He was referred 5 months later when fully recovered from his other injuries with a weak painful wrist which had a trial of strengthening and other exercises. He complained of severe weakness and pain under load. He was unable to pass any of his return-to-work tests for active-duty policing.

Diagnosis

Physical Examination

There was marked swelling and tenderness over the dorsal central carpus. Wrist flexion was 40° and extension 30° and Grip Strength was 6 kg compared to 45 kg on the opposite side. His scaphoid shift test was painful, and there was a dorsal lump but no dynamic shift of the scaphoid. Luno-triquetral ballottement demonstrated increased translation.

M. Ross (✉)
Brisbane Hand and Upper Limb Research Institute, University of Queensland, Brisbane, QLD, Australia
e-mail: markross@upperlimb.com

G. Couzens
Brisbane Hand and Upper Limb Research Institute, Queensland University of Technology, Brisbane, QLD, Australia
e-mail: greg.couzens@upperlimb.com

J. Yao (ed.), *Carpal Instability*, https://doi.org/10.1007/978-3-031-55869-6_20

Imaging

Plain radiographs demonstrated a static scapholunate interval of 11 mm and a scapholunate angle of 80° with some ulnar translation of both scaphoid and lunate (Fig. 20.1).

MRI demonstrated dorsal subluxation of the proximal scaphoid and capsular stripping from the dorsal lunate. The long radiolunate ligament had some high signal but was intact (Fig. 20.2).

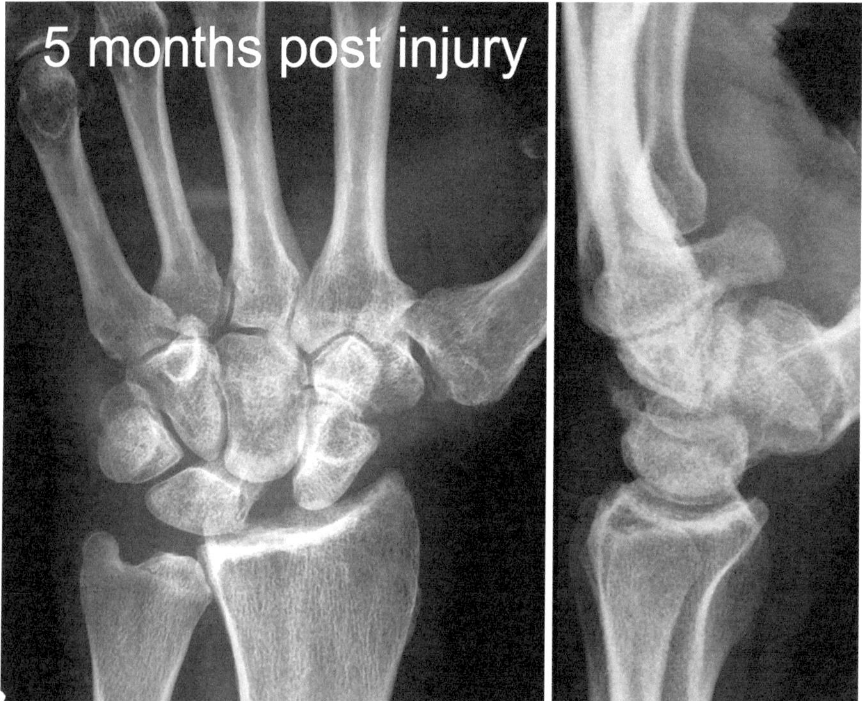

Fig. 20.1 Preoperative radiographs 5 months post injury

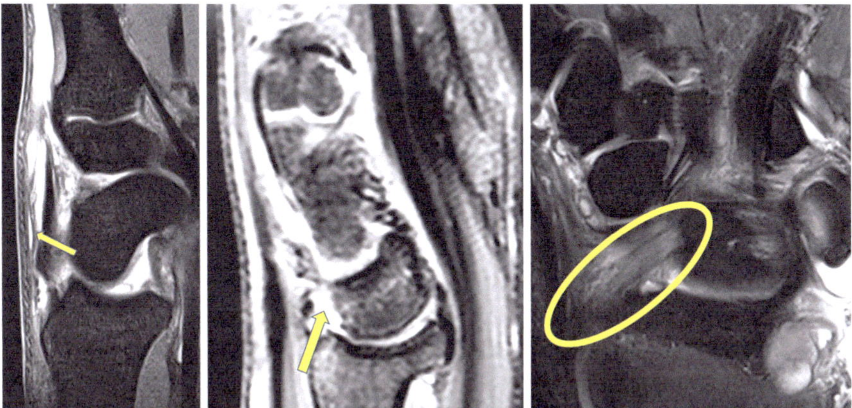

Fig. 20.2 MRI demonstrating dorsal translation of the scaphoid, lunate bare area, and intact LRL

Management

Management Options

The patient had a severe incapacity with inability to return to work and very concerning imaging findings. The uncertainties of controlling this degree of carpal malalignment even with a tendon weave procedure were discussed; however, the patient had concerns about his ability to return to active policing with a partial fusion procedure. It was decided to perform an SLT reconstruction [1].

Operative Management

Initial arthroscopic assessment demonstrated an 8 × 10 mm area of cartilage loss on the proximal pole of the scaphoid (Fig. 20.3) and confirmed the ligamentous disruption noted on imaging. An open dorsal exposure was performed utilizing a "window" approach which we initially described in 2014 [2] (Fig. 20.4) and was further defined by Wolfe et al. in 2021 [3], rather than the Mayo ligament splitting capsulotomy [4]. This approach avoids further stripping of the dorsal capsular ligaments from the proximal row [3, 5]. It also allows preservation of the posterior interosseous nerve which plays a role in proprioception [6] (Fig. 20.5).

A small volar incision was made over the scaphoid tubercle and 40% of the FCR (approximately 3 mm diameter) was harvested. A guide wire was passed from the dorsal scaphoid proximal pole towards the tubercle. The starting point is just dorsal

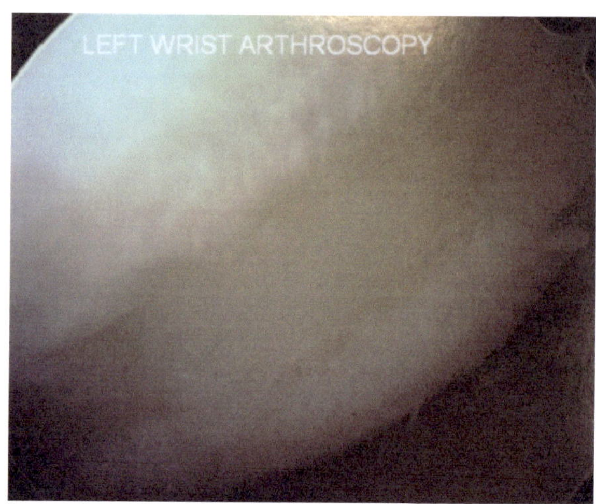

Fig. 20.3 Arthroscopy demonstrated 10 × 8 mm cartilage loss on proximal scaphoid

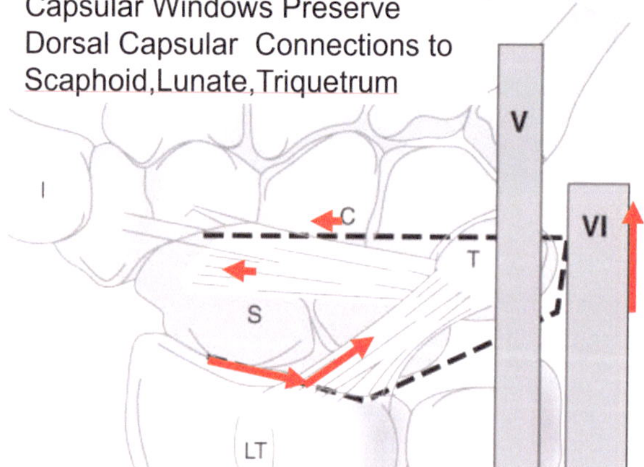

Fig. 20.4 The window approach is designed to minimize dorsal capsular damage—the red arrows indicate the lesser capsular incisions compared to the original capsulotomy described in our first publication [1]

Fig. 20.5 Window approach: The blue arrow indicates the avulsion of the dorsal capsule from the lunate. The posterior interosseous nerve is preserved. With preservation of the residual DICL and DRCL connections to the proximal row there is adequate exposure for SLIL surgery

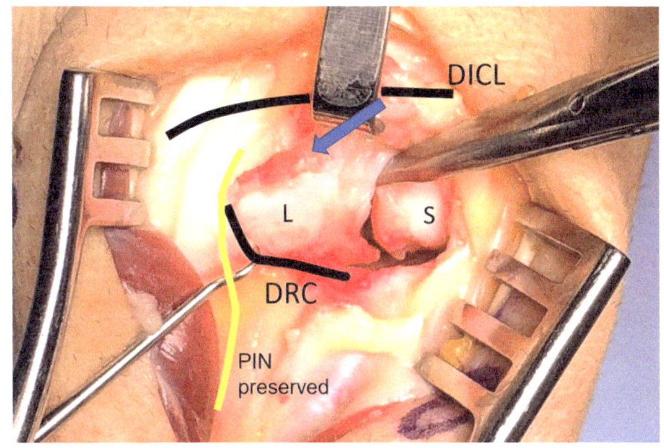

to the center of the articular facet for the lunate, and the exit is as close as possible to ulnar half of the scaphoid tubercle while remaining fully inside the scaphoid and not perforating the midcarpal joint. A 3 mm cannulated drill was used to create the tunnel. A disposable tendon passer was used to pass the tendon from volar to dorsal through the scaphoid. At this point, the graft was checked to ensure no laxity prior to entering the volar scaphoid. A 3 × 8 mm biocomposite interference screw was inserted into the volar tunnel on the scaphoid tubercle with the graft tensioned and the scaphoid held in extension.

Attention was then turned to the luno-triquetral (LT) tunnel. The original description for the SLT made the LT tunnel with a single pass [1]. The starting point on the lunate is just volar to the center point of the facet for the scaphoid. This offset with the scaphoid tunnel maximizes correction of dorsal scaphoid subluxation when the graft is tensioned. Drilling the LT tunnel in one pass can make it difficult to start the tunnel in the ideal location on the lunate and still exit in the center of the triquetrum without perforating the midcarpal joint. This is even more pronounced in smaller individuals. In addition, if the LT tunnel is drilled in one pass a temporary wire must be placed across the LT joint to ensure that the two tunnels do not offset making it impossible to pass the tendon. In this case, we chose to drill the tunnel from the lunate starting point to exit the lunate dorsally just at the dorsal aspect of the LT joint, and then drill a second tunnel from the dorsal corner of the triquetrum adjacent to the LT joint where the lunate tunnel exited, back to the ulnar border of the triquetrum. This also allows a second anchoring point for the dorsal pass of the graft to emulate/reconstruct the deep proximal limb of the DICL, the Dorsal Scapho-Luno-Triquetral ligament (DSLT) [7]. The graft that has exited the lunate facet of the proximal scaphoid was then passed sequentially through the lunate tunnel and the triquetral tunnel. The graft was again tensioned by pulling it ulnarwards from the triquetrum back across the carpus to pronate the LT segment towards the scaphoid with the wrist in neutral to slight ulnar deviation, closing the SL interval. With tension maintained, another 3 × 8 mm interference screw was inserted into the triquetral tunnel from the ulnar side, volar to the tendon graft.

Fig. 20.6 The tendon graft is passed through separate tunnels in the lunate and triquetrum then sutured back to the graft at the LT interval and the lunate bare area and the dorsal scaphoid to reconstruct the DSLT. The pull of the graft pronates the LT segment towards the scaphoid to close the dorsal SL gap

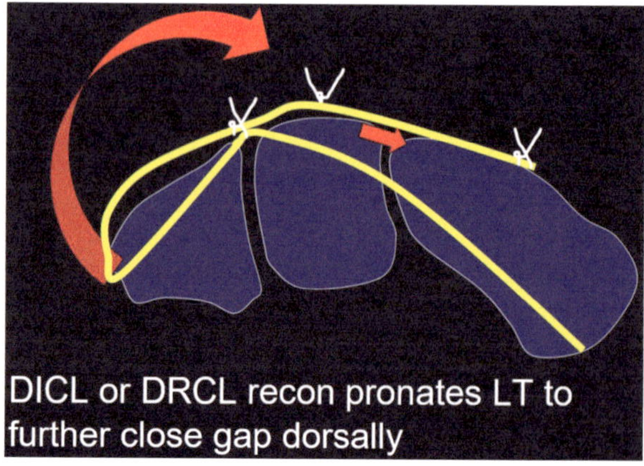

Supplementary sutures were placed between the graft and the periosteum/soft tissue on the ulnar border of the triquetrum to improve security in addition to the interference screw. The graft was then passed from its exit on the ulnar border of the triquetrum, deep to the ECU and EDM back below the fourth compartment over the dorsum of the LT interval using a straight artery forceps.

The graft was then sutured to itself at the point where it had previously exited the LT interval. An all-suture anchor was placed in the bare area of the lunate which was passed through the DICL and DRC and then the extracapsular portion of the graft. This creates an open RADiCL repair (See Chap. 10) [8] to deal with the dorsal capsular avulsion and also reconstructs/reinforces the DSLT with a well-anchored graft. Finally, the graft was secured to the dorsal scaphoid using an anchor placed in the dorsal ridge (Fig. 20.6).

One of the key principles of the SLT reconstruction is that graft tensioning reduces the scaphoid subluxation and gapping, and the SL interval should not be pinned prior to reduction with the graft. It is the correct placement and tensioning of the graft that achieves the reduction and confirms its efficacy. However, in cases as severe as this with such a severe static dissociation, we chose to insert a temporary k-wire between the scaphoid and the lunate for 6 weeks after graft tensioning. Assessing the severity of the static deformity is quite subjective, but in general terms a static situation with an SL gap greater than 5 mm combined with a radiolunate angle greater than 20° and SL angle greater than 80° may push the surgeon to consider a temporary pin. Another factor would be the amount of tension required on the graft to reduce the scaphoid dorsal subluxation. We have found that the correctly placed graft can almost always reduce the dorsal subluxation of the proximal scaphoid; however, the amount of tenson required is subjectively variable. We have not quantified the required tension.

Postoperative Management

The patient was immobilized in a volar plaster slab which was changed to a removable thermoplastic splint the following day at hand therapy. Therapy focused on digital motion and forearm rotation and the splint was removed for gentle dart throwing motion and flexion/extension of 20° in each direction.

At 6 weeks post-surgery, the temporary k-wire was removed and the splint was discontinued at 8 weeks. Orthogonal and dart throwing motion was increased at that point. Strengthening and increased activities and a return to light duties commenced at 12 weeks.

Outcomes

The patient completed firearms recertification at 18 weeks post-surgery and returned to active duties. He has continued to function at a high level with excellent clinical (Table 20.1) and radiographic outcomes at 2 years post-surgery (Fig. 20.7).

Table 20.1 Pre-op and 2-year post-op scores

	Pre-op	2 years
Pain with normal activities	70	5
Satisfaction	5	96
GRC symptoms (± 7point scale)		+7
GRC function (± 7point scale)		+7
PRWE	87	10
QuickDASH	80	6
Flexion—Right wrist	40	50
Extension—Right wrist	30	60
Grip strength	6 kg	42 kg

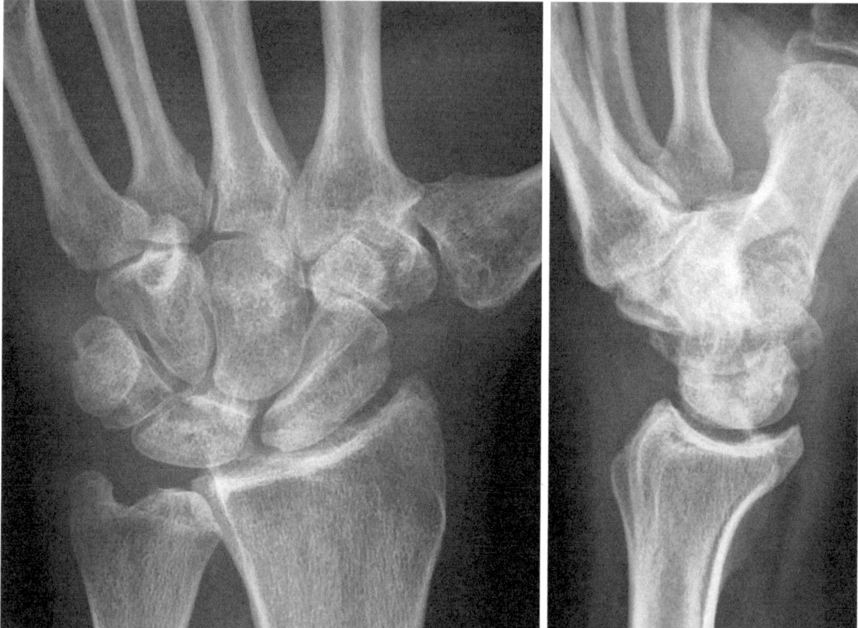

Fig. 20.7 A 2-year follow-up radiographs demonstrate good maintenance of improved carpal alignment

Pearls and Pitfalls

- There is no clear literature on how much articular cartilage loss on the proximal pole of the scaphoid is compatible with reconstruction versus salvage (such as partial fusion). However, in our experience we have consistently achieved good outcomes with up to 10 mm^2 of full-thickness cartilage loss.
- Avoid further iatrogenic compromise of dorsal capsular attachments by utilizing a window approach rather than a Mayo ligament splitting capsulotomy [2, 3, 5].
- Exercise extreme care when drilling tunnels through carpal bones—use the smallest possible diameter and irrigate extensively while drilling to diminish thermal injury.
- In cases with such severe chronic separation of the SL interval, we prefer to remove the cartilage from between the scaphoid and lunate to increase biological activity for healing between the bones. In some ways, this could be considered a "biological RASL." [9]
- Careful imaging is needed to ensure the scaphoid tunnel does not perforate the scapho-capitate joint and the L-T tunnel does not perforate the capito-lunate joint.
- The anchors in the dorsal scaphoid and lunate should be placed while the cannulated drill for the tunnels is in the bone to ensure the anchors do not conflict

with tunnels. Similarly, if a temporary k-wire is going to be used it should be passed through the scaphoid while the drill is in place.

- Extra care should be taken to ensure that the graft does not catch the ECU or EDM tendons when passing it deep to those tendons from the 6U interval to the 3–4 interval.

References

1. Ross M, Loveridge J, Cutbush K, Couzens G. Scapholunate ligament reconstruction. J Wrist Surg. 2013;2(2):110–5. https://doi.org/10.1055/s-0033-1341962.
2. Ross M, Peters SE, Couzens GB. Scapho-luno-triquetral tenodesis. In: Shin A, editor. Advances in scapholunate ligament treatment. American Society for Surgery of the Hand; 2014.
3. Loisel F, Wessel LE, Morse KW, Victoria C, Meyers KN, Wolfe SW. Is the dorsal fiber splitting approach to the wrist safe? A kinematic analysis and introduction of the "Window" approach. J Hand Surg Am. 2021;46(12):1079–87.
4. Berger RA, Bishop AT, Bettinger PC. New dorsal capsulotomy for the surgical exposure of the wrist. Ann Plast Surg. 1995;35:54–9.
5. Raja S, Williams D, Wolfe S, Couzens G, Ross M. New concepts in carpal instability. In: Geissler WB, editor. Wrist and elbow arthroscopy with selected open procedures; 2022.
6. Salva-Coll G, Garcia-Elias M, Hagert E. Scapholunate instability: proprioception and neuromuscular control. J Wrist Surg. 2013;2:136–40. https://doi.org/10.1055/s-0033-1341960.
7. Wessel LE, Kim J, Morse KW, Loisel F, Koff MF, Breighner R, Doty S, Wolfe SW. The dorsal ligament complex: a cadaveric, histology and imaging study. J Hand Surg Am. 2022;47(5):480.e1–9.
8. Williams D, Raja S, Ross M. The RADiCL procedure: repair/augmentation of dorsal intercarpal ligament. In: Geissler WB, editor. Wrist and elbow arthroscopy with selected open procedures; 2022.
9. Rosenwasser M, Miyasajsa K, Strauch R. The RASL procedure: reduction and association of the scaphoid and lunate using the Herbert screw. Tech Hand Up Extrem Surg. 1997;1(4):263–72.

Chapter 21
Chronic, Reducible Scapholunate Ligament Injury: ANAFAB

Michael Sandow and Zheng Xu Cheng

Case Presentation

A 36-year-old Electrician presented following a fall onto his non-dominant outstretched right hand 2 months previously. He experienced sudden pain and a tearing sensation at the time of the fall and had difficulty using his hand.

The pain settled partly with rest and he was more comfortable in a splint, he failed to regain function to allow him to continue his normal duties. He continued to perform lighter work.

Initially, his injury was thought to be a minor strain so he kept working, but his wrist was becoming progressively more painful. He presented to his family physician who arranged plain radiology, which suggested possible ligament injury and he was referred for consultation.

Diagnosis

Physical examination revealed tenderness dorsally on the wrist but with an almost normal range of motion. He reported pain at the extremes of motion. There was pain and a subluxation sensation on performing the scaphoid shift test. His grip strength was approximately 75% of the contralateral normal wrist.

Plain radiographs demonstrated widening of the scapholunate interval which was exacerbated with stressed ulnar deviation (Fig. 21.1), demonstrating extension of the lunate and flexion of the scaphoid (Fig. 21.2).

M. Sandow (✉) · Z. X. Cheng
Wakefield Orthopaedic Clinic, and Centre of Orthopaedic and Trauma Research, University of Adelaide, Adelaide, SA, Australia
e-mail: msandow@woc.com.au

J. Yao (ed.), *Carpal Instability*, https://doi.org/10.1007/978-3-031-55869-6_21

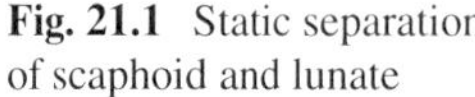

Fig. 21.1 Static separation of scaphoid and lunate

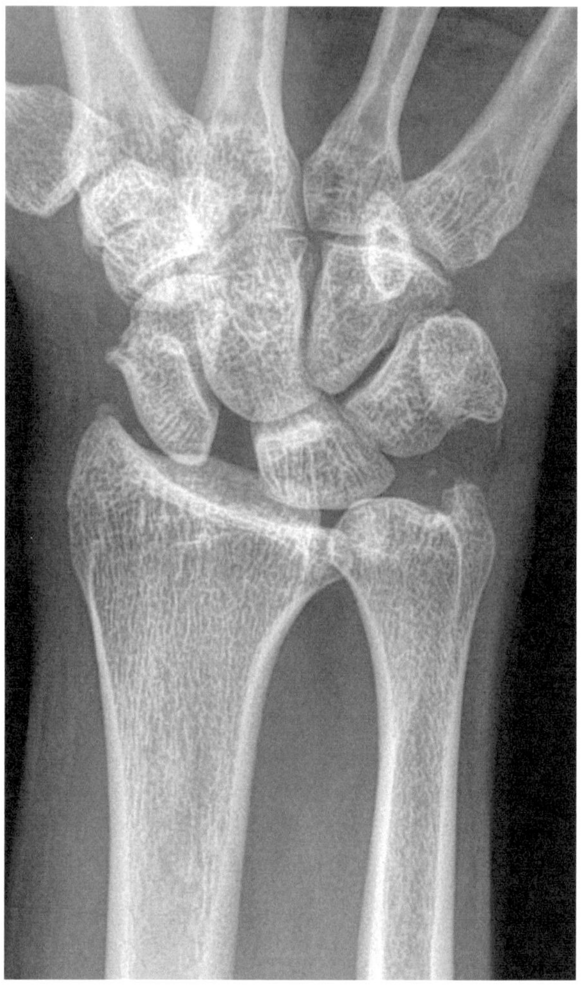

CT scanning was performed and a 3D model was created from the scan data (Fig. 21.3). This confirmed diastasis of the normal scapholunate attachments, flexion, and dorsal translation of the proximal pole of the scaphoid and lunate extension.

The diagnosis of scapholunate dissociation with carpal instability was made. This was deemed a static scapholunate diastasis and constituted reducible carpal instability. Where wrist motion is largely retained, and X-rays show minimal degenerative changes, anatomical reduction of the scaphoid and lunate malalignment is usually possible although may require a variable extent of soft tissue release and scar clearance.

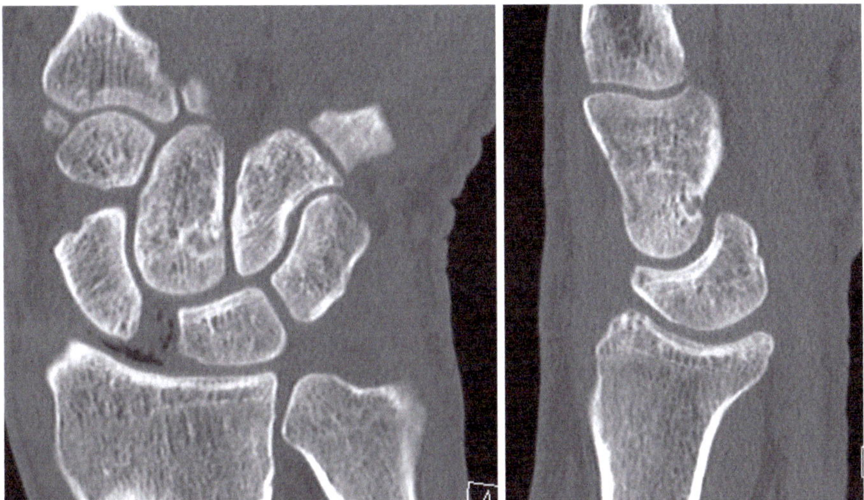

Fig. 21.2 Scapholunate diastasis confirmed on CT scan, with dorsal angulation of lunate

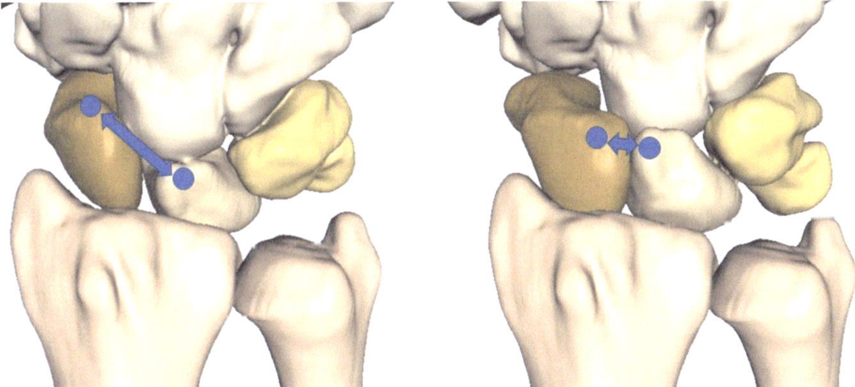

Fig. 21.3 3D model of scapholunate disruption showing extent of separation of scapholunate ligament attachments and planned virtual reduction of proximal row (www.truelifeanatomy.com)

Management Options

In the consideration of what management was indicated, the assertion of carpal instability implies a departure from carpal stability—and an understanding of what comprises stability is the key to what constitutes the contrary. The prehensile wrist has the very specific purpose of placing the central axis of the wrist and hand into a functional arc of motion which has only two degrees of freedom (pitch and yaw). The key functional element of the upper limb is the second and third metacarpals which are rigidly attached to the distal carpal row—around which the more mobile thenar and hypothenar elements move [1–3].

Multiple reconstructive solutions proposed to restore wrist function following injury. Carpal research has been largely empirical and not based on an understanding of the holistic nature of carpal stability, and surgical solutions are often the result of opportunistic utilization of locally available tendons or synthetic materials to replace observed, and thus presumed critical ligament deficits.

The Stable Central Column Theory (SCCT) of Carpal mechanics [4] provides a theoretical basis on which the biomechanics of the wrist can be explained. The presence of isometric connections between the various carpal bones and the radius provides an explanation for the dynamic stability of the wrist, and in particular the proximal row. The motion of the distal row is dependent on the stable connections to the radius via the proximal carpal row, and wrist instability is most commonly due to a loss of dynamic control of the motion of the proximal carpal row, and in particular the lunate.

The lunate is stabilized by balanced ligamentous restraints on the volar and dorsal aspects and is able to rotate into flexion and extension by a complex interaction of coronal translation on the radial articular surface and the obliquity of the volar and dorsal ligament restraints.

Lunate motion is thus controlled and stability maintained by a combination volar and dorsal restraints. Extension is controlled or restrained on the dorsal aspect by the dorsal scapholunate interosseous ligament, and the connections to the dorsal extrinsic ligament—DIC (dorsal intercarpal ligament) and DRC (dorsal radiocarpal ligament) as part of the DCSS (dorsal capsuloligamentous scapholunate septum), and on the volar side, primarily by the long radiolunate ligament. Flexion of the lunate is controlled on the dorsal side, again by connections to the scaphoid and dorsal extrinsic ligament complex, and on the volar side by the lunato-triquetral ligament.

The scaphoid and triquetrum are similarly controlled by volar and dorsal ligaments.

The stability of the proximal row can be anatomically aligned at rest but may fail under load or may adopt a collapse pattern even at rest. Patients may present with variable extent between these extremes, and it can be surmised that the extend of static or dynamic carpal instability will be the result of a variable extent of ligamentous disruption on both the dorsal and volar aspects.

The notion of ligament-specific reconstruction [5–7] should provide an explanation for the variation in surgical approaches. The appropriate reconstructive choice should be linked to the identified ligamentous disruption.

The long radiolunate ligament is a critical static restraint to lunate extension [4–6, 8, 9]. However, it is clear the lunate alignment is also governed by dorsal constraints in the form of the scapholunate interosseous ligament and the DCSS. While mild lunate extension may occur with an intact LRL ligament, a high frequency of disruption of that ligament has been noted in S-L dissociation.

The choice of reconstruction for this patient was based on the presumed ligamentous disruption and using an interactive 3D analytical imagery, disruption to the

SLIL, LRL, and STT was proposed. A reconstructive technique that addressed all these damaged tissues was regarded as a logical therapeutic approach.

The ANAFAB procedure is a theory driven, defect correction-based reconstruction that aims to restore the anatomical mechanical constraints on both volar and dorsal aspects of the carpus—where they are likely to have been involved. It is based on the SCCT and has achieved a consistent recovery of carpal stability and grip strength, without significant loss of motion.

In lower grades of scapholunate disruption, (EWAS grade 3a, 3b, and 3c), where the extent of injury is less extensive, alternate reconstruction would more appropriate [10]. These would include arthroscopic dorsal scapholunate ligament repair, and reattachment of the DCSS to the dorsal lunate. In this case, it was deemed that there has been a dorsal and volar disruption, causing a static, but reducible deformity and thus a volar and dorsal reconstruction was required.

Management Chosen for this Case with Rationale

Based on the diagnosis of longitudinal instability of the carpus with likely loss of dorsal and volar constraints, a reconstructive approach was selected that addresses both the dorsal and volar structures.

Anatomical Front and Back (ANAFAB) Repair

Surgical Technique

The reconstruction was performed through a volar and dorsal approach.

The first incision was dorsal along the line of the extensor carpi radialis brevis tendon, taking care to protect and mobilize the extensor pollicis longus tendon. A window was developed between the distal and proximal limbs of the DIC ligament and carefully extended to gain access to the dorsal scapholunate region. Once the extent of ligamentous disruption was confirmed, the bones were mobilized as well as scar released to allow anatomical reduction of the scaphoid proximal pole into the radial articular surface fossa and approximation of the scaphoid and lunate.

The origins of the dorsal scapholunate ligament were identified on the scaphoid and lunate and a 2 mm drill hole created to mark the location, and define a target for subsequent bone tunnel placement.

Through a volar approach, the antero-lateral facet of the trapezium was exposed. An anchor attached to a synthetic tape was inserted into the central portion of the antero-lateral facet of the trapezium and a distally based strip of flexor carpi radialis tendon, 3 mm wide and 15 cm long was raised. The tape plus the, distally based strip of FCR tendon was passed from the volar trapezium to the scaphoid tuberosity, and then trans-osseously to the dorsal scaphoid at the location of the dorsal S/L attachment. Care is taken to maintain an adequate bony bridge to the medial scaphoid. The tape/tendon hybrid was then passed trans-osseously from dorsal to volar through the lunate and then volarly to the radial styloid where it was tensioned as tight as possible and secured with an interference screw (Fig. 21.4). A second reinforcement screw was inserted to secure the end of the tape/tendon.

A further 3 mm (or smaller) interference screw is inserted into the dorsal lunate drill hole to secure the tape/tendon hybrid along its path. Prior to inserting the interference screw, a multiple throw knot is placed about halfway along a No. 1 braided polyester suture and the created knot inserted into the dorsal lunate tunnel. This was secured into the hole by the interference screw and was used to reattach the dorsal capsule and DCSS. No stabilizing wires were used.

The wounds (volar and dorsal) were closed and the wrist placed in a splint. At 5 days, the wrist was placed in a cast for 6 weeks.

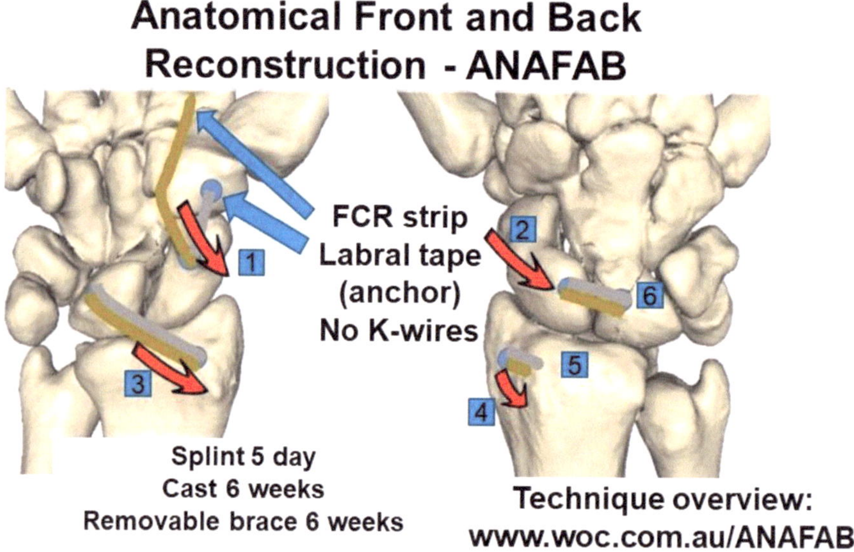

Fig. 21.4 ANAFAB reconstruction. Hybrid tape and tendon strip secured to trapezium and passed into scaphoid tuberosity drill hole (1), tape/tendon passed through scaphoid and across to lunate (2), tape/tendon passed dorsal to volar through lunate and across to volar radial styloid (3), tape/tendon passed through distal radius and secured dorsally (4), plus an additional anchor fixation (5), and finally an interference screw with non-absorbable suture inserted into dorsal lunate (6)

Clinical Course and Outcome

The patients were reviewed at 5 days postoperatively and a cast applied. This is left on for 6 weeks.

Radiographs were obtained at 1 week, and then at 6 weeks (on cast removal), and at 3 months prior to full mobilization. Final radiographs are taken at 12 months (Fig. 21.5).

At 6 months postoperatively the patient had regained 90% grip strength, and 110° arc of wrist motion, with a negative scaphoid shift sign. He returned to full-time duties on a graduated basis from 2 month postoperatively, and on to normal duties at 6 months. His wrist function continued to improve out to the final review at 2 years.

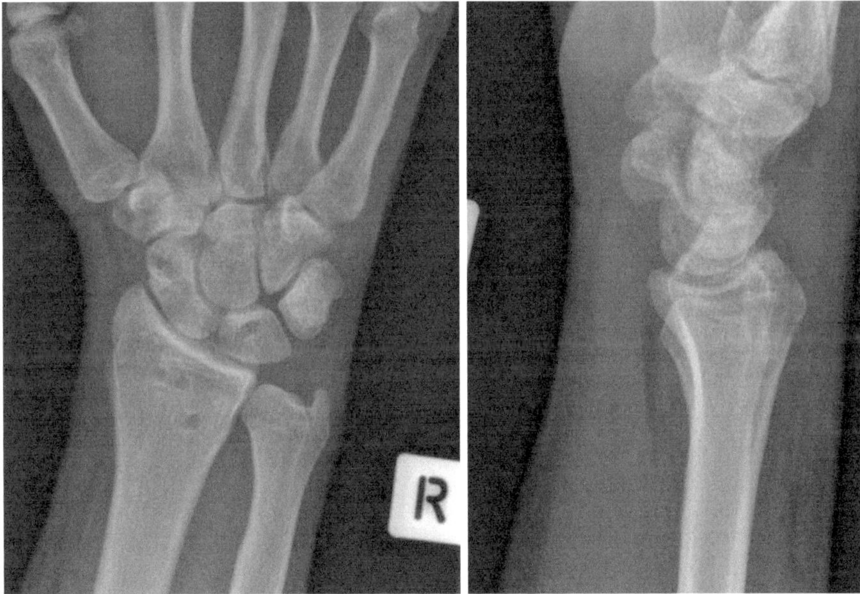

Fig. 21.5 Final result at 12 months. Some tunnel enlargement is evident

Pearls and Pitfalls

- Fixed scapholunate dissociation with scaphoid subluxation and lunate extension likely due to indicate volar and dorsal ligamentous disruption. The key is to restore anatomical alignment using volar and dorsal stabilization and avoid rigid non-physiological intercarpal fixation.
- Bony fixation requires either anchors or drill holes—using tendon strips alone or combined with tape/suture. Tendon repairs are unlikely to retain adequate strength through the healing period to maintain reduction. Tape or suture fixation only has been less reported, and is now preferred. Using only tape and no tendon weave, the drill hole size can be reduced. Tendon may not be critical to the reconstruction, but there is inadequate long term follow-up to indicate that a tape only repair is appropriate.
- Bone tunnel enlargement remains a major concern and the cause and sequelae are unclear. Many current fixation compound sutures and tapes are composed of polyethylene which can potentially produce wear particles that have been implicated in osteolysis [11]. Concentric bone tunnel enlargement suggests that the cause is not pure mechanical wearing. The fixation material is at the surgeon's choosing; however, due to uncertainty about the viability and contribution of the tendon strip, the current preference is a tape only repair using a woven polyester rather than polyethylene tape - to avoid possible adverse bone effects of polyethylene wear particles. Braided polyester suture does not have adequate abrasion resistance properties and is not favored over tape.
- Where there is dorsal disruption only, a dorsal only approach, arthroscopic or open is appropriate. However, where there is volar and dorsal disruption, as indicated by wide scapholunate diastasis and lunate extension, a dorsal and volar reconstruction is needed.
- The repair performed for this patient restored the volar and dorsal restraints of the proximal row and allowed incorporation with DIC by securing the dorsal scapholunate reconstruction to the transverse mobile component of the DRC and DIC.

References

1. Sandow M. The why, what, how and where of 3D imaging. J Hand Surg Eur Vol. 2014;39(4):343–5.
2. Sandow M, Fisher T. Anatomical anterior and posterior reconstruction for scapholunate dissociation: preliminary outcome in ten patients. J Hand Surg Eur Vol. 2020;45(4):389–95. PMID: 31718405. https://doi.org/10.1177/1753193419886536.
3. Sandow MJ. Can the wrist be explained? Macropace products. Adelaide; 2020. www.woc.com.au/wrist.pdf.
4. Sandow MJ, Fisher TJ, Howard CQ, Papas S. Unifying model of carpal mechanics based on computationally derived isometric constraints and rules-based motion: the stable central column theory. J Hand Surg Eur Vol. 2014;39:353–63.

5. Badida R, Akhbari B, Vutescu E, Moore DC, Wolfe SW, Crisco JJ. The role of scapholunate interosseous, dorsal intercarpal, and radiolunate ligaments in wrist biomechanics. J Biomech. 2021;125:110567. https://doi.org/10.1016/j.jbiomech.2021.110567. Epub 2021 Jun 12. PMID: 34246909.
6. Pérez AJ, Jethanandani RG, Vutescu ES, Meyers KN, Lee SK, Wolfe SW. Role of ligament stabilizers of the proximal carpal row in preventing dorsal intercalated segment instability: a cadaveric study. J Bone Joint Surg Am. 2019;101(15):1388–96. https://doi.org/10.2106/JBJS.18.01419.
7. Rainbow MJ, Wolff AL, Crisco JJ, Wolfe SW. Functional kinematics of the wrist. J Hand Surg Eur Vol. 2016;41(1):7–21.
8. Sandow MJ. 3D dynamic analysis of the wrist. Hand Surg. 2015;20(3):366–8.
9. Sandow M. The application of computer-based quantitative analysis to explain carpal biomechanics. J Hand Surg Eur Vol. 2021;46(1):97–102. https://doi.org/10.1177/1753193420970449. Epub 2020 Nov 12. PMID: 33183145.
10. Mathoulin CL. Indications, techniques, and outcomes of arthroscopic repair of scapholunate ligament and triangular fibrocartilage complex. J Hand Surg Eur. 2017;42:551–66.
11. Lovric V, Goldberg MJ, Heuberer PR, Oliver RA, Stone D, Laky B, Page RS, Walsh WR. Suture wear particles cause a significant inflammatory response in a murine synovial airpouch model. J Orthop Surg Res. 2018;13(1):311. https://doi.org/10.1186/s13018-018-1026-4. PMID: 30522505.

Chapter 22
Chronic, Reducible Scapholunate Ligament Injury: 360 Reconstruction

John R. Fowler

Case Presentation

A 51-year-old F, active in CrossFit, presented to the office with about 4 weeks of left dorsal wrist pain and "clunking." She said that she was throwing a 75-lb medicine ball over her shoulder and felt a pop in the left wrist. She reported pain with wrist extension and inability to perform pushups or plank type activities with the left wrist. Handstand walks and other CrossFit activities were painful and nearly impossible to perform.

Diagnosis

- Physical Assessment/Relevant Maneuvers
  There was mild dorsal wrist swelling. Wrist range of motion was grossly maintained. Wrist flexion was 70° (compared to 80° on the contralateral wrist) and wrist extension was 75° (compared to 75° on the contralateral wrist). She was mildly tender to palpation over the scapholunate interval. There was a positive scaphoid shift test.
- Diagnostic Studies
  Radiographs (Fig. 22.1a–c) demonstrated static scapholunate widening and a DISI deformity. Based on the static widening, I did not feel the need to obtain additional imaging.

J. R. Fowler (✉)
Department of Orthopedics, University of Pittsburgh Medical Center, Pittsburgh, PA, USA

© The Author(s), under exclusive license to Springer Nature Switzerland AG 2024
J. Yao (ed.), *Carpal Instability*, https://doi.org/10.1007/978-3-031-55869-6_22

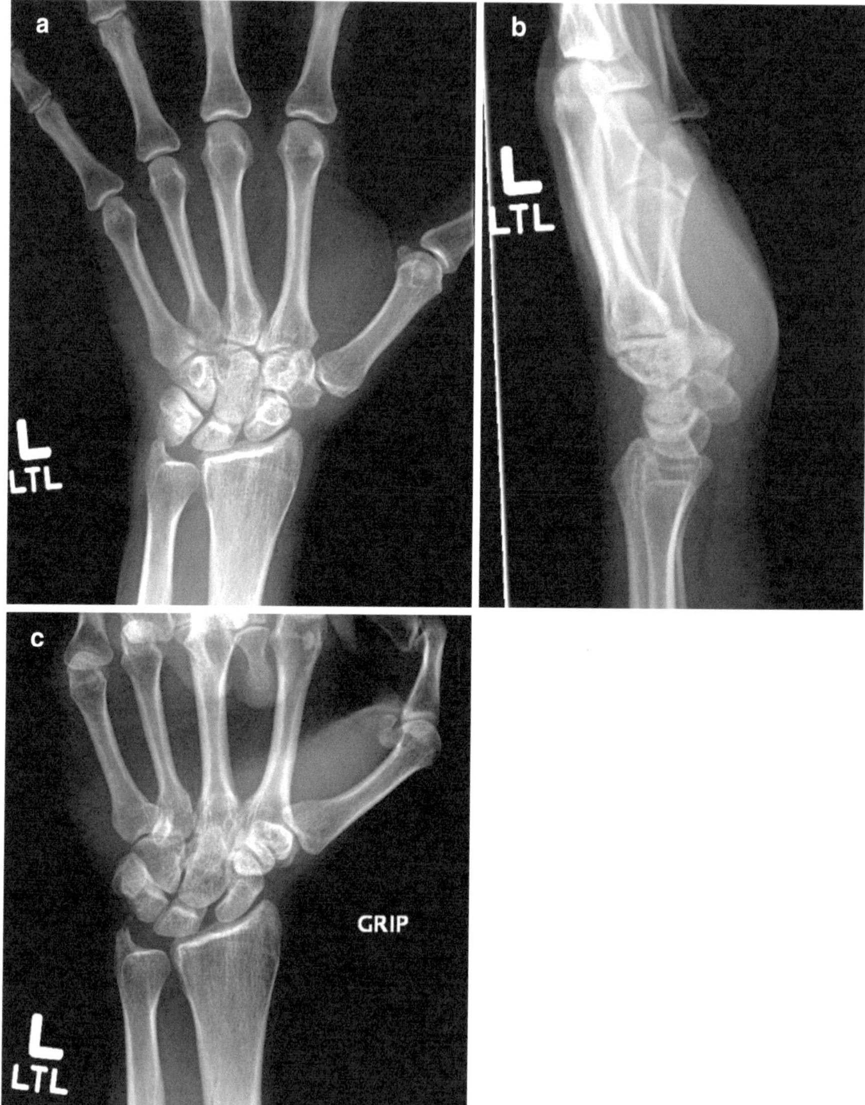

Fig. 22.1 (**a**) Posteroanterior (PA) radiograph, (**b**) lateral radiograph, and (**c**) grip view demonstrating widening of the scapholunate interval and dorsal intercalated segment instability (DISI)

Management Options

Management of an acute scapholunate ligament tear is a challenging problem, particularly in a 51-year-old active female. One could advocate for doing nothing acutely and allowing the patient to develop arthritis 10–15 years down the road. Consideration could be given to proximal row carpectomy or scaphoid excision intercarpal fusion at that point. The downside to this approach is that the patient would be unlikely to participate fully in CrossFit, something she very much enjoys, and is almost certainly committing to a salvage procedure in the future. Given that she has static widening despite only 4 weeks of symptoms, it is likely that this current episode is an acute exacerbation of a chronic injury. Acute repair of the scapholunate ligament will not be possible. One could consider a procedure such as Reduction and Association of the Scaphoid and Lunate (RASL). However, I would be concerned that once the screw is removed, without reconstruction of the ligaments, a CrossFit enthusiast would be likely to widen again in the future. In cases with static widening, it is clear that both the volar and dorsal scapholunate ligaments are disrupted. The majority of current reconstruction techniques only reconstruct the dorsal ligaments. For young, active patients, procedures that reconstruct both of these dorsal and volar ligaments would theoretically be preferred. Based on all of these factors and in discussion with the patient, a 360-degree reconstruction was chosen.

Given the increased exposure required for the 360-degree reconstruction, in particular the added potential morbidity with the volar approach, I reserve it for high-demand patients with evidence of both volar and dorsal ligament full-thickness tears. In patients with dorsal only scapholunate ligament tears, I typically perform a dorsal only repair using suture anchors with or without suture augmentation. In lower demand patients, I have also performed a dorsal capsulodesis using the proximal half of the dorsal intercarpal ligament. I have found this procedure to result in widening of the scapholunate ligament at long-term follow-up, but it appears to prevent or at least delay development of scapholunate advanced collapse.

Management Chosen for this Case with Rationale

A longitudinal incision is made on the dorsum of the wrist in line with Lister's tubercle and the third metacarpal (Fig. 22.2). The extensor pollicis longus (EPL) is identified and protected. The interval between the second and fourth dorsal compartment tendons is developed. While protecting the EPL, the distal one-third of the extensor retinaculum is "vented" to gain more exposure. This author does not routinely transpose EPL or perform a posterior interosseous nerve neurectomy (Fig. 22.3). An "inverted T" is made in the dorsal wrist capsule and the scapholunate dissociation identified (Fig. 22.4).

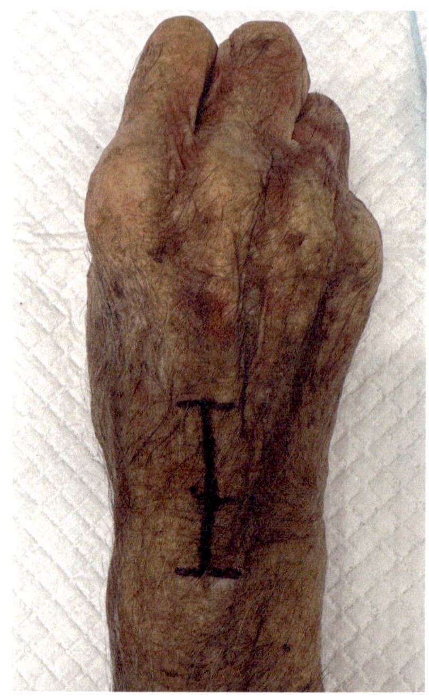

Fig. 22.2 Planned dorsal incision in line with Lister's tubercle and the third metacarpal

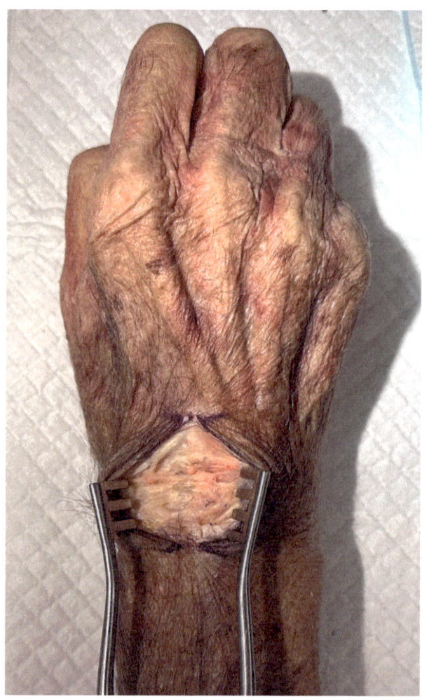

Fig. 22.3 The dorsal capsule is exposed by developing the interval between the second and fourth compartments

Fig. 22.4 An inverted "T" is made in the capsule to expose the carpus and the scapholunate interval

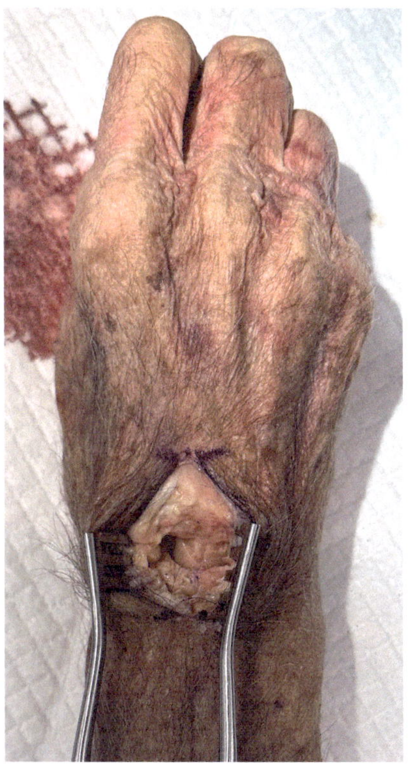

Attention is then turned volarly and an extended carpal tunnel release is performed to gain exposure to the volar wrist capsule (Fig. 22.5a). Once the flexor tendons and median nerve have been safely retracted (Fig. 22.5b), a 1.1 mm k-wire is placed from dorsal to volar in the scaphoid (Fig. 22.6a, b). As the scaphoid is typically in flexion, the k-wire is directed from dorsal distal to proximal volar. Next attention is turned to the lunate. A 1.1 mm k-wire is placed from dorsal proximal to volar distal to correct the lunate extension (Fig. 22.6c). Care is taken to remain central in the lunate to prevent fracture. Radiographs are obtained to ensure appropriate k-wire placement (Fig. 22.7a, b). The scaphoid k-wire is then overdrilled with a cannulated 2.5 mm drill. The lunate k-wire is then overdrilled with a cannulated 3.0 mm drill. A suture passer is used to pass a 1 mm palmaris graft (either autograft or allograft) dorsal to volar through the lunate (Fig. 22.8a), volar to dorsal through the scaphoid (Fig. 22.8b, c), and dorsal to volar back through the lunate again (Fig. 22.8d). The graft is tensioned and reduction of the scapholunate interval and the DISI is confirmed. A 3 × 8 mm biotenodesis screw (Arthrex, Naples, FL) is then placed from dorsal to volar in the scaphoid (Fig. 22.9a) and lunate (Fig. 22.9b) to hold the graft and tension. Next, a non-absorbable braided suture tape (FiberTape,

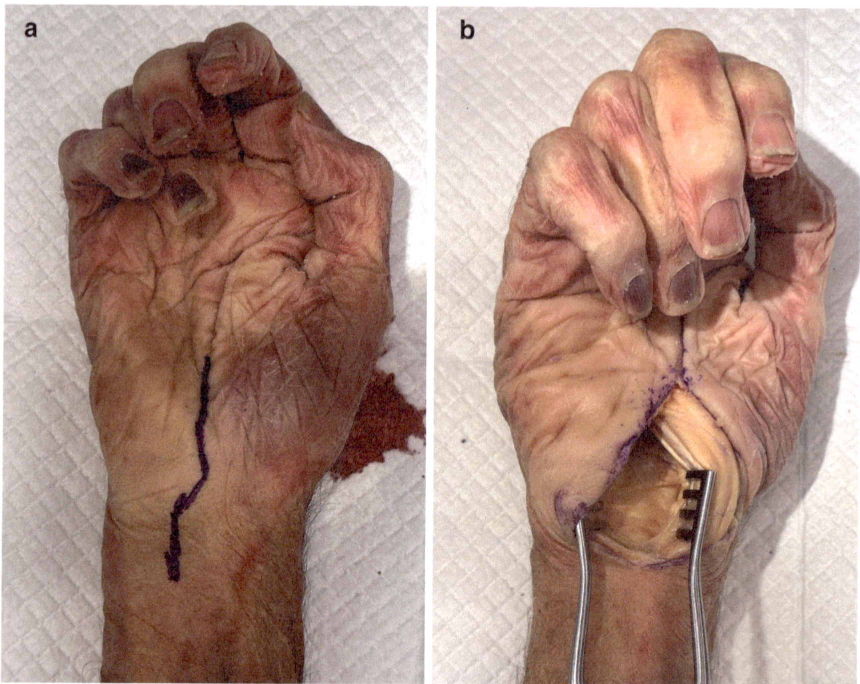

Fig. 22.5 (**a**) Planned volar incision as an extended carpal tunnel release; (**b**) the flexor tendons and median nerve are retracted to expose the volar capsule

Arthrex Naples, FL, Fig. 22.10) is passed from dorsal to volar through the scaphoid biotenodesis screw and the lunate biotenodesis screw and tied volarly (Fig. 22.11). The scapholunate interval is examined dorsally to ensure closure (Fig. 22.12).

The capsule is closed with non-absorbable sutures and skin closed with 4-0 nylon. The patient is placed into a volar splint. The splint is maintained for 2 weeks and then transitioned to a removable volar splint for another 4 weeks.

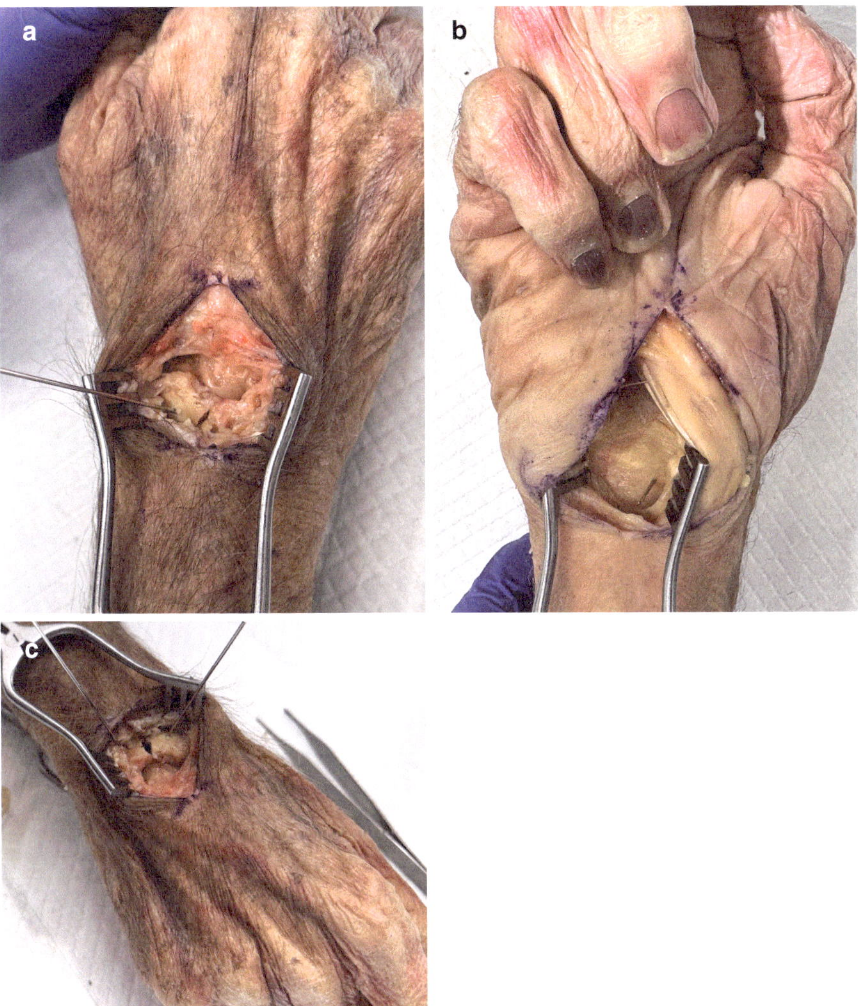

Fig. 22.6 (**a**) A 1.1 mm k-wire is placed in the scaphoid from dorsal distal to volar proximal to correct the scaphoid flexion; (**b**) the flexor tendons and median nerve are protected and the k-wire is brought out through the volar capsule; (**c**) a 1.1 mm k-wire is placed in the scaphoid from dorsal proximal to volar distal to correct the lunate extension

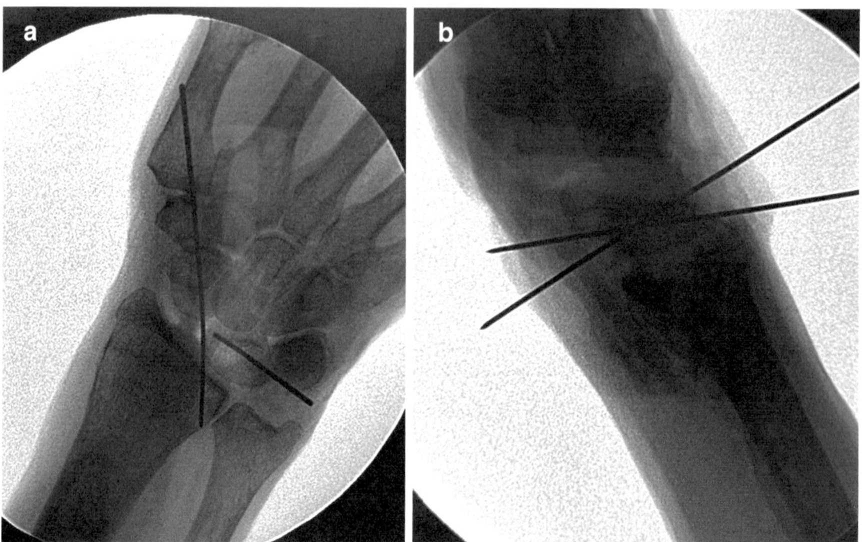

Fig. 22.7 (**a**) PA radiograph and (**b**) lateral radiograph demonstrating appropriate placement of the k-wires in the scaphoid and lunate

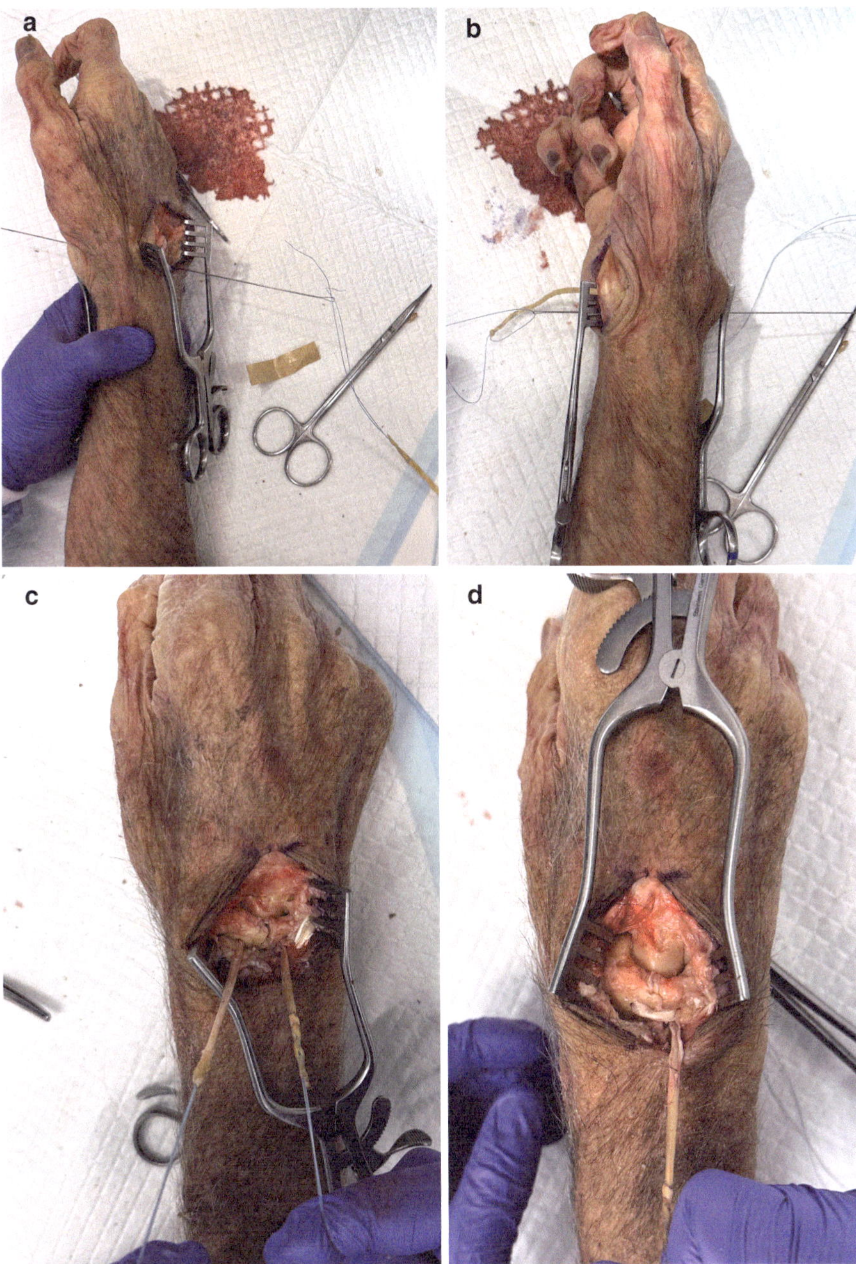

Fig. 22.8 (**a**) The palmaris graft is passed from dorsal to volar through the lunate; (**b**) the graft is then passed from volar to dorsal through scaphoid; (**c**) both ends of the graft are now coming out dorsally; (**d**) the scaphoid end of the graft is then passed again through the lunate from dorsal to volar

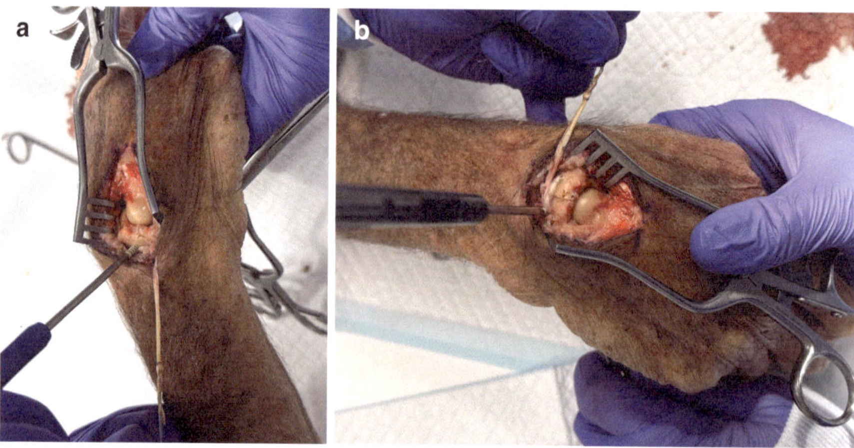

Fig. 22.9 While holding tension on both limbs of the graft, a 3 × 8 mm interference screw is placed into the scaphoid (**a**) and lunate (**b**)

Fig. 22.10 A suture tape is passed through the interference screws from dorsal to volar in the scaphoid and the other end is passed from dorsal to volar in the lunate

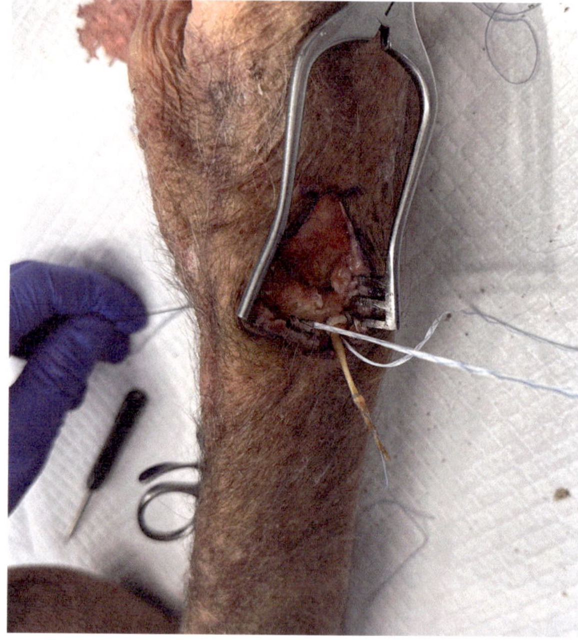

Fig. 22.11 The suture tape is tied volarly over the capsule

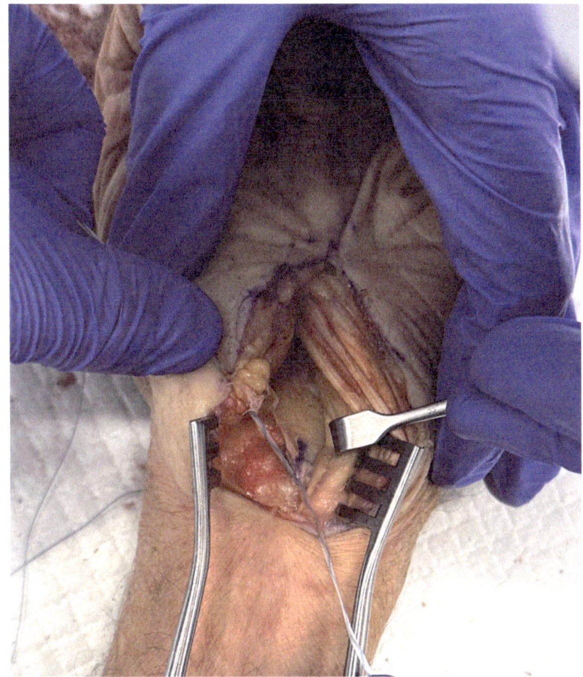

Fig. 22.12 The reconstruction is examined dorsally to ensure closure of the scapholunate interval

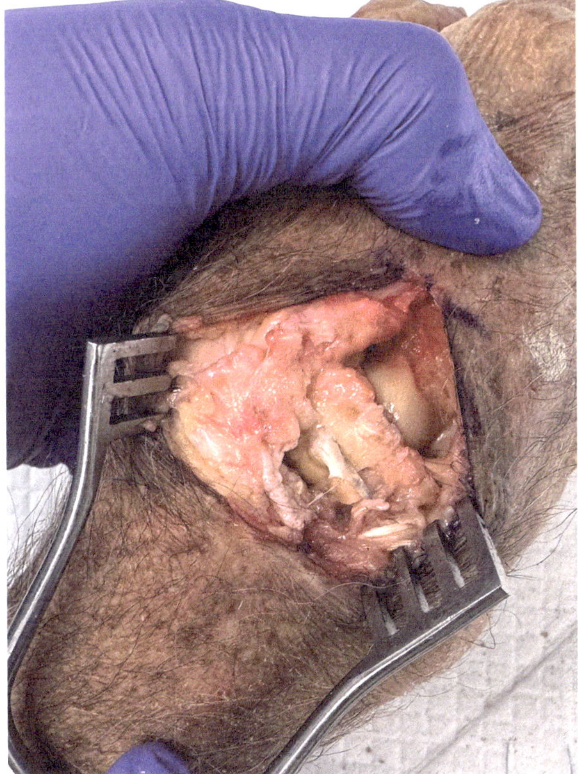

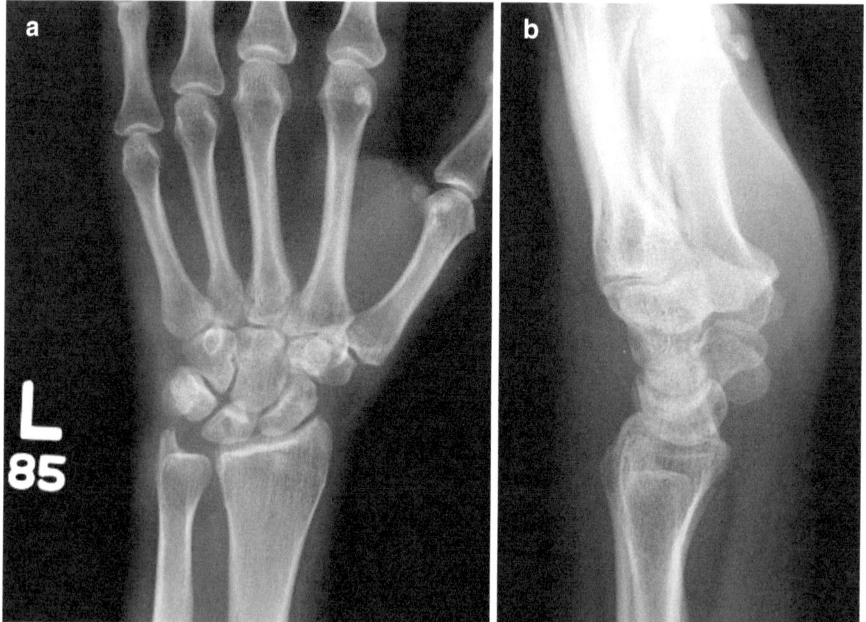

Fig. 22.13 PA (**a**) and lateral (**b**) radiographs are obtained to ensure resolution of the DISI alignment

Clinical Course and Outcome

The patient did well after surgery and returned to all CrossFit activities without restrictions. Her wrist extension returned to 80°, but her wrist flexion remained decreased at 45° at final follow-up (2.5 years). Her grip strength was equivalent to the contralateral side (115-lbs on Jamar 2). Her radiographs at 2-year follow-up show maintenance of the scapholunate interval with slight DISI (Fig. 22.13a, b).

Clinical Pears/Pitfalls

- It is imperative to have a 1-mm graft as anything larger than this will not fit well through the holes.
- It is essential to stay central in the lunate as the 3 mm drill and interference screw can cause a lunate fracture if you are eccentric.
- Lubricate the graft with mineral oil to help with graft passage.

Literature Review and Discussion

There is minimal literature using the 360 reconstruction. Two biomechanical studies support the benefits of the 360 reconstruction over other techniques. Chae and colleagues performed a cadaver study to determine how well three different SL reconstruction techniques closed the SL interval both dorsally and volarly [1]. The authors compared the 360 reconstruction, modified Brunelli reconstruction, and a dorsal only reconstruction. The 360 reconstruction was the only method that effectively closed and maintained the volar SL gap/interval. Kakar et al. performed a biomechanical study to determine if adding the suture tape to the construct improved stiffness and load to failure of the reconstruction [2]. The authors found that the mean load to failure nearly doubled and the stiffness was greater in the group with the suture augmentation.

From a clinical outcome standpoint, only one case series describes the 360 reconstruction technique. Logli and colleagues reported on 9 patients who underwent the 360° SL reconstruction [3]. At mean follow-up of 34 months, mean SL gap improved from 5.1 mm pre-operatively to 2.8 mm post-operatively. Mean SL angle improved from 71° pre-operatively to 57° post-operatively. VAS pain scores at final follow-up were 0 in 6 of 9 patients.

References

1. Chae S, Nam J, Park IJ, Shin SS, McGarry MH, Lee TQ. Biomechanical analysis of three different reconstruction techniques for scapholunate instability: a cadaveric study. Clin Orthop Surg. 2022;14(4):613–21.
2. Kakar S, Greene RM, Denbeigh J, Van Wijnen A. Scapholunate ligament internal brace 360 tenodesis (SLITT) procedure: a biomechanical study. J Wrist Surg. 2019;8(3):250–4.
3. Kakar S, Logli AL, Ramazanian T, Gaston RG, Fowler JR. Scapholunate ligament 360° procedure: a preliminary outcome report. Bone Joint J. 2021;103(5):939–45.

Further Reading

Kakar S, Greene RM. Scapholunate ligament internal brace 360-degree tenodesis (SLITT) procedure. J Wrist Surg. 2018;7(4):336–40.

Kakar S, Greene RM, Denbeigh J, Van Wijnen A. Scapholunate ligament internal brace 360 tenodesis (SLITT) procedure: a biomechanical study. J Wrist Surg. 2019;8(3):250–4.

Kakar S, Logli AL, Ramazanian T, Gaston RG, Fowler JR. Scapholunate ligament 360° procedure: a preliminary outcome report. Bone Joint J. 2021;103(5):939–45.

Chapter 23
Chronic, Reducible Scapholunate Ligament Injury: Bone-Ligament-Bone (BLB) Reconstruction

Jack C. Casey and Arnold-Peter C. Weiss

Case Presentation

An active, 48-year-old right hand dominant man presented to our orthopedic clinic unable to undertake load activities with his right wrist. The injury occurred 3 months prior when the patient fell onto an outstretched hand. The patient had been evaluated by an orthopedic hand surgeon out of state prior with a radiographic SL gap of 3.5 mm on the static PA view, 1 cm gap on the power grip view and an SL angle of 65° on the lateral view. A scaphoid shift test was positive with a clunk and pain. These physical exam and radiographic findings were consistent with a dynamic scapholunate ligament tear. The patient was referred to our clinic for reconstruction.

Diagnosis

In a patient who presents with pain poorly localized to the peri-scaphoid region, injury to the scapholunate ligament should be considered. These patients often have a history of a fall that involved force to the hypothenar area and may present with wrist effusion or diffuse swelling. In a swollen wrist with normal appearing X-rays, arthrocentesis can be performed to assess for hemarthrosis which may be indicative of ligamentous injury [1]. In the setting of a subacute scapholunate ligament injury, patients may also have decreased grip strength and complain of painful popping or clicking with activities.

J. C. Casey · A.-P. C. Weiss (✉)
Department of Orthopaedics, Alpert Medical School of Brown University & Medical University of South Carolina, Providence & Charleston, RI & SC, USA
e-mail: Jack_casey@brown.edu; apcweiss@brown.edu; weissar@musc.edu

J. Yao (ed.), *Carpal Instability*, https://doi.org/10.1007/978-3-031-55869-6_23

The scaphoid shift test is a helpful provocative test in which the clinician applies pressure with their thumb to the scaphoid tubercle while moving the patient's wrist from ulnar deviation and partial extension into radial deviation and partial flexion. In a patient with a structurally intact wrist, the scaphoid will flex and pronate. In a patient with scaphoid instability, the proximal scaphoid will subluxate from the scaphoid fossa onto the dorsal articular lip of the radius due to pressure from the thumb. The patient will likely report pain during this maneuver, and removing thumb pressure will enable the proximal scaphoid to reduce which is often palpated and audible as a clunk [2]. It is worth noting that just over a third of people with structurally intact wrists will have false positive scaphoid shift tests, likely due to ligamentous hyperlaxity and capitate dorsal subluxation from the capitolunate joint. Therefore, fluoroscopic confirmation of positive scaphoid shift tests can be valuable [3].

For patients with a suggestive history and clinical exam, as well as a positive scaphoid shift test, the clinician should obtain posteroanterior, lateral, navicular, and anteroposterior grip radiographs of both wrists for comparison. If static radiographs appear normal, stress radiographs or motion studies are indicated to assess for dynamic scaphoid instability [1]. The diagnosis can be confirmed via advanced imaging or arthroscopy.

Scapholunate ligament tears were historically assessed with triple-injection wrist cinearthrogram or wrist arthroscopy [4, 5] although arthroscopy is more accurate and normal arthrographic findings should not necessarily rule out a scapholunate ligament tear [6]. Cineradiography and arthroscopy, in addition to fluoroscopy, enable kinematic assessment of the ligaments which can be useful to assess structural damage. Computed tomography scanning along the axis of the scaphoid is helpful in determining carpal bone geometric relationships and the presence of fractures. High-resolution magnetic resonance imaging with a 3-T MRI is another accurate choice for confirmation of the diagnosis [7].

Management Options

Scapholunate ligament disruption ultimately causes degenerative joint disease, pain, and morbidity [8]. Surgery is therefore often indicated to prevent secondary joint collapse and the resultant degenerative arthrosis. Non-surgical treatment should be considered and involves symptom management via splint immobilization, NSAIDs, and intraarticular steroid injections [9]. There are a variety of surgical options, and they can be organized into four categories. These include capsulodesis, tenodesis, bone-tissue-bone procedures, and scapholunate joint debridement and stabilization with temporary or dynamic fixation [10].

Management Chosen for this Case with Rationale

A scapholunate reconstruction was performed using the bone-retinaculum-bone autograft technique stabilized by single mini-screws in each bone plug and multiple Kirschner wires [11]. This procedure began with an 8 cm longitudinal dorsal wrist incision centered over Lister's tubercle. The autogenous graft was taken from Lister's tubercle, composed of a 20 × 8 × 8 mm bone block that included the overlying periosteum and retinaculum. This bone block was shaped using a fine rongeur. A bridge-like structure was created by removing a 2–3 mm wide section of bone from the middle, leaving the overlying periosteum and retinaculum intact. The final construct consists of a block of bone with a short intervening segment of retinaculum/periosteum connected to another block of bone.

The capsule between the second and fourth compartments was then longitudinally incised to expose the scapholunate interval (Fig. 23.1). With the wrist flexed to 45°–60°, Kirschner wires (K-wires) were drilled into the scaphoid and lunate to use as joysticks. The scaphoid and lunate were aligned and checked fluoroscopically. Two slightly crossed 0.045-inch smooth K-wires were drilled from the anatomic snuffbox through the scaphoid and lunate to maintain the alignment. The joysticks were removed once alignment was established, and the scaphoid and lunate were prepared for implantation of the graft. A small osteotome was used to create a trough in both bones, directly adjacent to the scapholunate joint (Fig. 23.2). A benefit of the bone-retinaculum-bone procedure is the bone-to-bone healing, as opposed to bone-tendon healing which can be less predictable. It is therefore important to create steep trough walls to promote an interdigitated autograft fit. The graft was then placed into the troughs and pressed down using digital pressure. A single

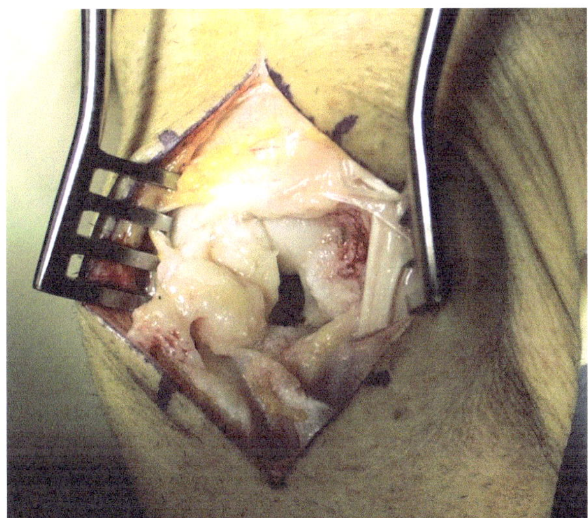

Fig. 23.1 Left: intraoperative photo showing troughs carved out of the scaphoid and lunate to prepare for autograft placement. Right: intraoperative photo showing the autograft in place, bridging the scaphoid and lunate. A single mini screw stabilizes each bone plug

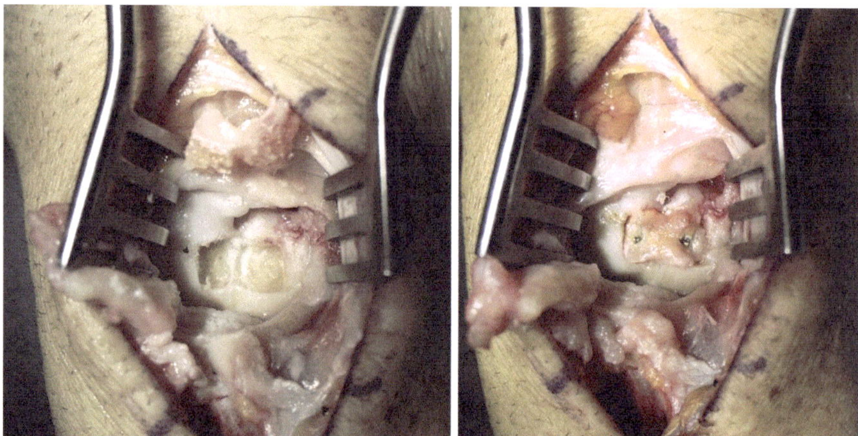

Fig. 23.2 Intraoperative photo of the dorsal wrist showing scapholunate widening and a high-grade tear of the scapholunate ligament

Fig. 23.3 Posteroanterior radiograph showing anatomic alignment of the scaphoid and lunate. Four K-wires are in place holding the fixation, and single mini-screws can be seen in each bone plug

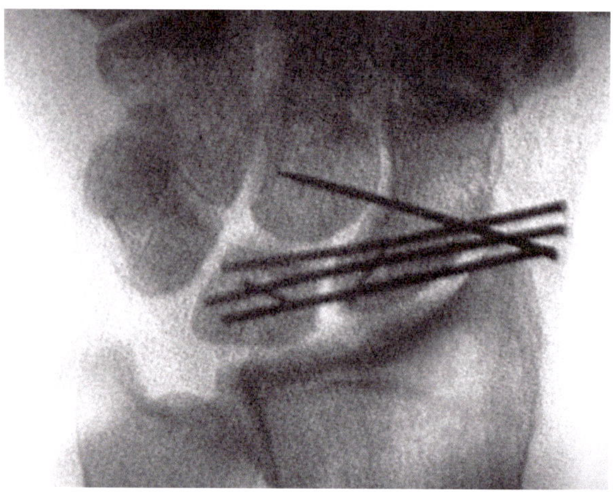

mini screw was placed in each bone plug to hold the construct in place (Fig. 23.2). The dorsal lip of the distal radius was used to further lock the autograft by slightly distracting the wrist and putting it into 30° of extension. The capsule is closed primarily; however, this technique does not preclude augmenting the repair with a capsulodesis incorporating a portion of the intrinsic ligaments either in forward or reverse manner.

Posteroanterior radiographs were obtained to check for anatomical alignment of the scaphoid and lunate (Fig. 23.3).

Clinical Course and Outcome

The patient was immobilized in a cast postoperatively for 8 weeks, with subsequent removal of all K-wires. This was followed by 3 months of hand therapy. The patient regained wrist extension of 45°, wrist flexion of 55°, radial deviation of 10°, and ulnar deviation of 25° at 6-month follow-up examination. Radiographs 5-years post-op demonstrated maintenance of the scapholunate interval with no evidence of radiocarpal arthritis (Fig. 23.4) or an increased scapholunate angle on lateral radiographs (Fig. 23.5). The patient was able to return to playing tennis with the reconstructed wrist at 8 months and has remained relatively symptom-free playing sports for nearly two decades following the procedure. Overall wrist range of motion has not increased with further time.

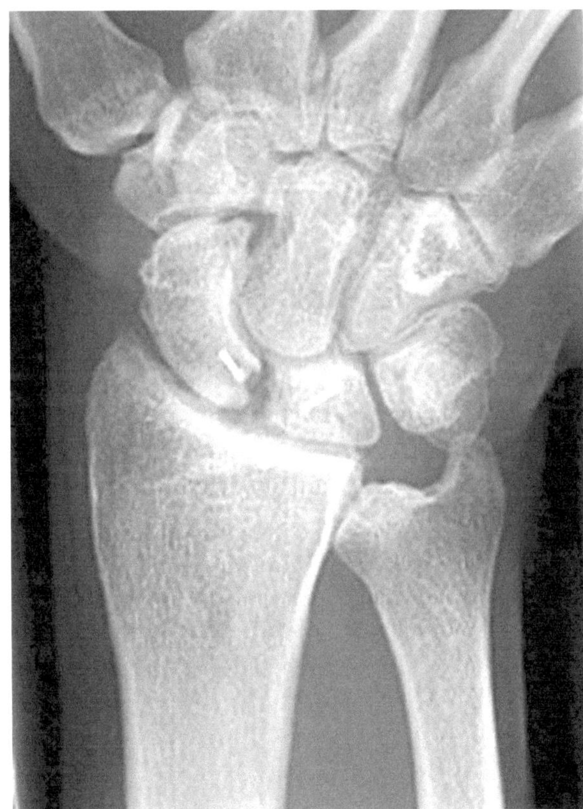

Fig. 23.4 Five-year postoperative anteroposterior radiograph showing maintenance of the scapholunate interval with no evidence of radiocarpal arthritis

Fig. 23.5 Five-year postoperative lateral radiograph showing restoration of the scapholunate angle

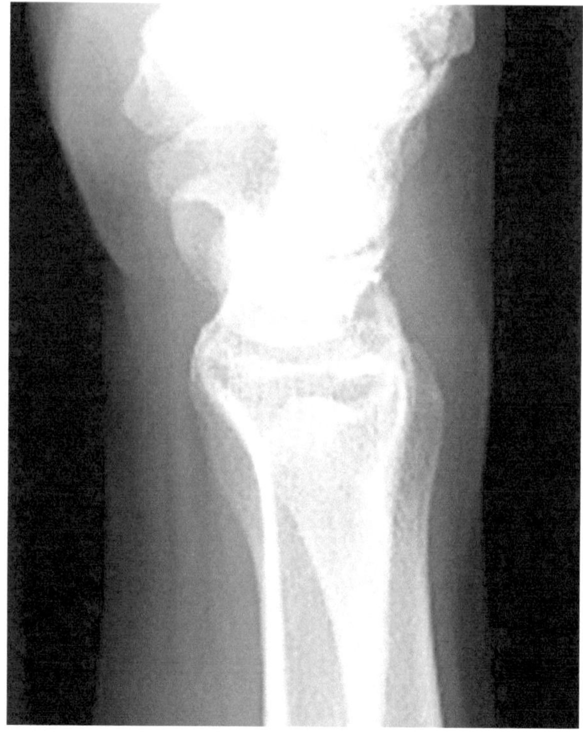

Bulleted Clinical Pearls/Pitfalls

- Do not use this technique for fixed SL gap patients; a reduction intra-op with K-wires should be able to be accomplished without struggle. Dynamic instability or early, non-fixed SL gap patients are ideal.
- Do not take too small a graft to start with; one can always trim the size down with a rongeur.
- Do not make the recipient scaphoid and lunate bone troughs too large; a trough approximately 8 mm (high) × 7 mm (wide) × 6 mm (deep) is adequate.
- Keep the K-wires in the volar half of the carpal bones otherwise they may interfere with the trough opening.
- Cut K-wires below the skin then check via the still open dorsal wrist incision using a dissecting scissor that the sensory branch of the radial nerve fibers are free of the K-wire ends by blunt dissection radially.

Literature Review and Discussion

The scaphoid and lunate carpal bones are connected by the scapholunate ligament, an intrinsic structure composed of dorsal and palmar ligaments and a proximal fibrocartilaginous membrane [12]. The dorsal aspect of the scapholunate ligament is the strongest, made up of transversely oriented collagen fibers that support against distraction as well as torsional and translational forces. The palmar component contributes rotational stability to the scapholunate joint, while the proximal region provides little support [1]. Scapholunate ligament injuries that result in scapholunate dissociation are most often caused by a fall onto an extended and ulnarly deviated wrist. Scapholunate dissociation is the most common carpal instability and is found in 13.4% of patients with a distal radius fracture [1, 13]. Scapholunate ligament damage leads to abnormal cartilage wear, and ultimately a form of wrist arthritis termed scapholunate advanced collapse (SLAC) [8]. The differential diagnosis in patients with carpal instability should include causes of wrist arthritis that require significantly different treatment like pseudogout, inflammatory arthritis, and Kienböcks disease [14].

Many surgical options for scapholunate ligament disruption have been proposed. While this chapter highlights the bone-retinaculum-bone reconstruction, one may also consider a primary repair in dynamic instability if a stout SL ligament remains for primary repair. In addition, one might consider other non-biologic suture tapes for strength if some ligament tissue is present. The bone-retinaculum-bone autograft is ideal if no stout SL ligament exists for repair. Cadaver studies comparing bone-retinaculum-bone tissue to the native dorsal scapholunate ligament show that autograft tissue is equally strong per unit area relative to native tissue, but overall weaker as there is less tissue present [15].

References

1. Kitay A, Wolfe SW. Scapholunate instability: current concepts in diagnosis and management. J Hand Surg Am. 2012;37(10):2175–96.
2. Watson HK, Ashmead D 4th, Makhlouf MV. Examination of the scaphoid. J Hand Surg Am. 1988;13:657–60.
3. Wolfe SW, Gupta A, Crisco JJ 3rd. Kinematics of the scaphoid shift test. J Hand Surg Am. 1997;22:801–6.
4. Ruch DS, Bowling J. Arthroscopic assessment of carpal instability. Arthroscopy. 1998;14(7):675–81.
5. Weiss AP, Akelman E. Diagnostic imaging and arthroscopy for chronic wrist pain. Orthop Clin North Am. 1995;26(4):759–67.
6. Weiss AP, Akelman E, Lambiase R. Comparison of the findings of triple-injection cinearthrography of the wrist with those of arthroscopy. J Bone Joint Surg Am. 1996;78(3):348–56.

7. Magee T. Comparison of 3-T MRI and arthroscopy of intrinsic wrist ligament and TFCC tears. AJR Am J Roentgenol. 2009;192(1):80–5.
8. Watson HK, Ballet FL. The SLAC wrist: scapholunate advanced collapse pattern of degenerative arthritis. J Hand Surg Am. 1984;9(3):358–65.
9. Wahed K, Deore S, Bhan K, Vinay S, Jayasinghe G, Dutta A, Singh B. Management of chronic scapholunate ligament injury. J Clin Orthop Trauma. 2020;11(4):529–36.
10. Montgomery SJ, Rollick NJ, Kubik JF, Meldrum AR, White NJ. Surgical outcomes of chronic isolated scapholunate interosseous ligament injuries: a systematic review of 805 wrists. Can J Surg. 2019;62(3):1–12.
11. Weiss AP. Scapholunate ligament reconstruction using a bone-retinaculum-bone autograft. J Hand Surg Am. 1998;23(2):205–15.
12. Konopka G, Chim H. Optimal management of scapholunate ligament injuries. Orthop Res Rev. 2018;10:41–54.
13. Gunal I, Ozaksoy D, Altay T, Satoglu IS, Kazimoglu C, Sener M. Scapholunate dissociation associated with distal radius fractures. Eur J Orthop Surg Traumatol. 2013;23(8):877–81.
14. Trehan SK, Lee SK, Wolfe SW. Scapholunate advanced collapse: nomenclature and differential diagnosis. J Hand Surg Am. 2015;40(10):2085–9.
15. Shin SS, Moore DC, McGovern RD, Weiss AP. Scapholunate ligament reconstruction using a bone-retinaculum-bone autograft: a biomechanic and histologic study. J Hand Surg Am. 1998;23(2):216–21.

Further Reading

Shin SS, Moore DC, McGovern RD, Weiss AP. Scapholunate ligament reconstruction using a bone-retinaculum-bone autograft: a biomechanic and histologic study. J Hand Surg Am. 1998;23(2):216–21.
Weiss AP. Scapholunate ligament reconstruction using a bone-retinaculum-bone autograft. J Hand Surg Am. 1998;23(2):205–15.

Chapter 24
Volar Capsulodesis in the Management of Dynamic Scapholunate Instability

Steven L. Moran

Case Presentation

A 22-year-old collegiate offensive lineman presented with left nondominant wrist pain. The wrist pain developed following a block of an opposing defensive player. The patient reports that the injury occurred over a month prior and has continued to get worse despite splinting and taping. On physical exam, the patient was noted to have weak grip but good wrist range of motion, with mild decrease of flexion and extension. Pain was localized dorsally over the scapholunate interval, and provocative maneuvers showed a painful Watson's maneuver and tenderness to palpation over the ulnar aspect of the wrist, at the ulnar fovea. The patient wished to return to football for his final season and hoped to rehabilitate during the off-season.

Diagnosis

Physical Assessment/Relevant Maneuvers

There was mild dorsal wrist swelling. Wrist range of motion was grossly maintained. Wrist flexion was 60° (compared to 70° on the contralateral wrist), and wrist extension was 70° (compared to 75° on the contralateral wrist). The patient was

Supplementary Information The online version contains supplementary material available at https://doi.org/10.1007/978-3-031-55869-6_24.

S. L. Moran (✉)
Division of Plastic Surgery, Department of Orthopedics, Mayo Clinic, Rochester, MN, USA
e-mail: Moran.steven@mayo.edu

J. Yao (ed.), *Carpal Instability*, https://doi.org/10.1007/978-3-031-55869-6_24

tender to palpation over the scapholunate interval with the wrist in flexion. There was a positive scaphoid shift test.

Diagnostic Studies

Radiographs (Fig. 24.1) demonstrated no significant abnormalities, with no evidence of scapholunate widening and no DISI deformity. In the absence of abnormalities on plain radiographs, but pain on exam, a 3 T MRI of the wrist was ordered using dedicated wrist coils. MRI imaging showed evidence of a scapholunate ligament injury with evidence for membranous and volar tearing of the SL ligament (Fig. 24.2a). The lateral views showed evidence of a dorsal capsular avulsion of the dorsal radiocarpal (DRC) ligament off the dorsal horn of the lunate. The short radiolunate ligament remained intact. The MRI also noted evidence of a peripheral TFCC tear.

Arthroscopy was used to verify the MRI findings on the day of the surgery (Fig. 24.3). The arthroscopy revealed a membranous and volar tear of the SL ligament. The dorsal portion remained intact. Arthroscopy also identified evidence of a TFCC injury with foveal disruption.

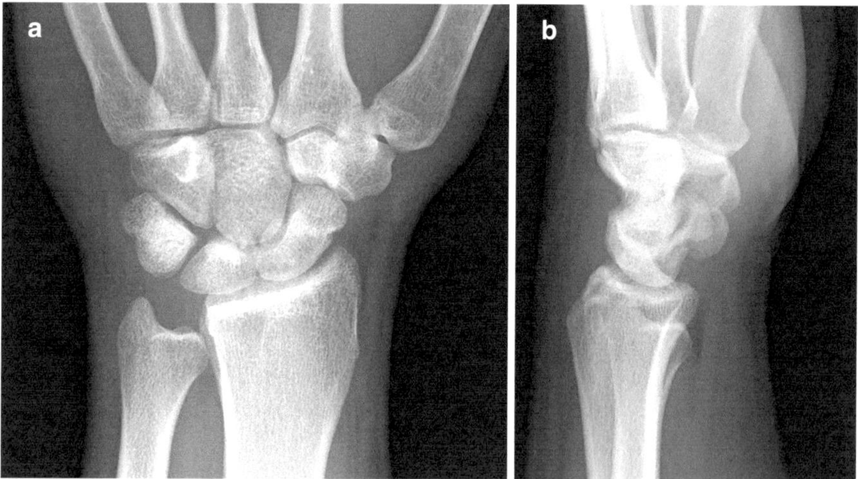

Fig. 24.1 (**a**) Posteroanterior (PA) radiograph, (**b**) lateral radiographs demonstrating no significant abnormalities

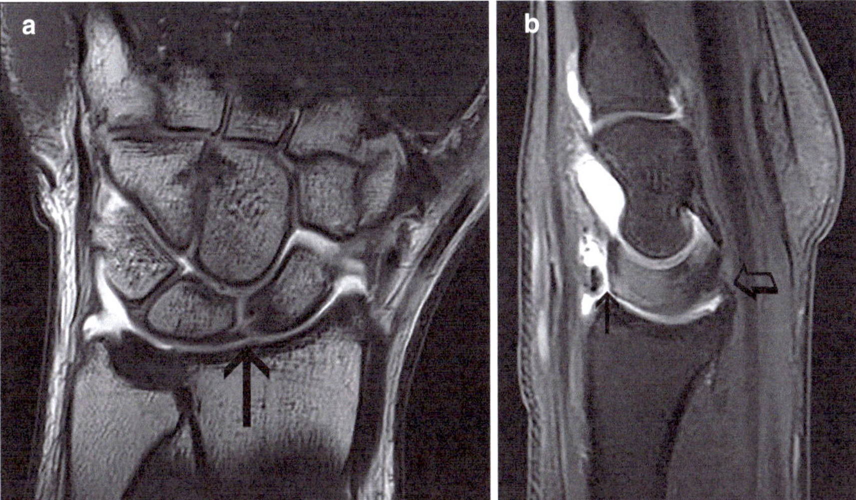

Fig. 24.2 (**a** and **b**) 3T MRI of wrist with representative coronal and lateral views. The coronal view shows tearing of the volar and membranous portions of the SL ligament (arrow), with ongoing edema in the proximal pole of the scaphoid. In this image, one can also appreciate avulsion of TFCC deep insertion. Lateral view (**b**) shows avulsion of the DRC from the lunate dorsal horn (arrow), and broad arrow points to intact short radiolunate ligament

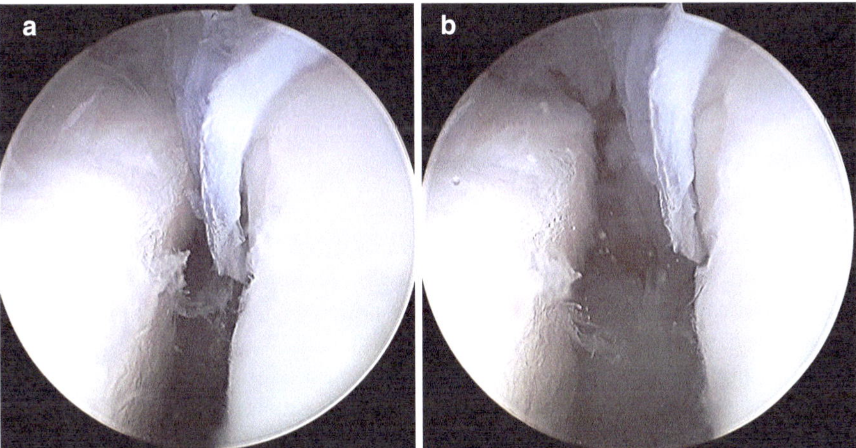

Fig. 24.3 (**a** and **b**) Arthroscopic view of the SL interval through the radial midcarpal portal. View (**a**) shows the palmar aspect of the scapholunate interval as seen from the radial midcarpal portal. Image **b** shows gapping of volar portion of scapholunate interval. If you look beyond the bones, you can identify the SL injury in background

Management Options

The patient has findings suggestive of a partial SL ligament tear. Based on the patient's exam and radiographic imaging, this patient presents with symptomatic dynamic scapholunate instability. Dynamic instability refers to an early injury within the spectrum of scapholunate instability, where plain radiographs fail to show any significant abnormalities, specifically with regard to scapholunate angle, radiolunate angle, or scapholunate diastasis. Dynamic stress radiographic views and MRI imaging should show evidence of SL injury.

It is thought that SL tears begin volarly and propagate dorsally. The thickness of the volar SL ligament is less than the dorsal component of the SL ligament, thus predisposing the volar limb of the ligament to rupture first [1, 2]. This is a mild injury to the SL ligament, with the majority of the secondary volar and dorsal stabilizers remaining intact. Secondary constraints to carpal motion include the long and short radiolunate ligaments, the radioscaphocapitate ligament, and the dorsal capsule [1]. In this patient, the MRI shows evidence of an avulsion of the DRC from the lunate. If injuries to the SL and secondary stabilizers are left unrepaired, attritional changes will develop and predispose the patient to subsequent injury, particularly with his desire to return to playing football [1].

Because of this patient's young age, desire to return to collegiate-level sports, and relatively early stage of injury, options for reconstruction could include primary scapholunate ligament reconstruction, arthroscopic stabilization procedures, capsulodesis, or tenodesis-based reconstruction. Based on the chronicity of the injury, the need for return to sports, *and the fact that the dorsal SL ligament is intact*, we opted for a *volar capsulodesis*. In this patient, the primary problem is the tear to the volar SL ligament injury. Options such as *dorsal capsulodesis* fail to address the injury directly and result in a limitation of wrist motion [3]. Tenodesis or "360" repairs with bone tunnels risk compromising postoperative motion and may injure the blood supply to the carpal bones [4, 5]. Minimally invasive repair techniques in this young individual are a more appealing option.

Capsulodesis is a term describing the use of a portion of either the volar or the dorsal wrist capsule to tether and control the motion of the carpal bones. This procedure was originally popularized by Blatt in the 1980s. Dr. Blatt originally described a dorsal capsulodesis using a proximally based strip of the dorsal capsule attached to the scaphoid. This capsular strip helped to maintain scaphoid extension despite scapholunate injury [6]. Since the description of the Blatt capsulodesis, multiple other capsulodesis procedures have been described, most notably by groups of researchers led by Viegas, Szabo, and Berger [3, 6–8]. All of these capsulodeses are dorsally based, utilizing the attachments of the dorsal radiocarpal and dorsal intercarpal ligaments to the scaphoid and lunate to tether the carpal bones in an attempt to prevent carpal collapse. Unfortunately, dorsal capsulodesis is primarily designed to prevent scaphoid flexion, and this is only one component of carpal instability following scapholunate injury. Most dorsal capsulodesis procedures have little ability to control lunate extension, scapholunate diastasis, and ulnar translation of the lunate.

While being an extremely popular option for the management of SL instability by hand surgeons for decades, dorsal capsulodesis produces inconsistent and at times poor results [3, 9]. Studies by Moran and others have shown that dorsal capsulodesis fails to restore normal carpal kinematics and does not prevent recurrence of diastasis or the long-term development of SLAC arthritis [3, 10, 11].

More recent attempts at arthroscopic based capsulodesis as described by Mathoulin utilize the attachment of the scapholunate ligament to portions of the dorsal capsule [12]. By placing a horizontal mattress suture through the dorsal capsule and through the dorsal remnants of the scapholunate ligament, Mathoulin and colleagues have shown that pain from scapholunate instability can be decreased [13, 14].

Newer options have focused on the use of an open volar capsulodesis for the treatment of scapholunate instability, particularly for isolated volar tears. The use of a volar capsulodesis attempts to tether the proximal pole of the scaphoid within the radial fossa [15, 16]. Work by Lee and colleagues has shown that dorsal translation of the scaphoid can be a major pain generator for patients with SL instability. Control of proximal pole migration may explain why the volar capsulodesis works well at resolving dynamic SL instability symptoms and pain [17].

Management Chosen: Volar Capsulodesis (Figs. 24.4 and 24.5)

Given the dynamic nature of the injury, we always proceed with wrist arthroscopy at the start of surgery. Arthroscopic findings guide our treatment course. Preoperatively, the patient is counseled on all possible treatment options to allow for flexibility when interpreting the intraoperative findings.

The findings in this case showed a volar SLIL tear. Figure 24.3 shows the volar SL widening as the scope is passed into the volar aspect of the SL interval. The patient was also noted to have an avulsion of the dorsal portion of the capsule from the lunate, as seen from the radiocarpal 3–4 portal. Finally, the patient also had a foveal TFCC injury.

The dorsal capsule avulsion was repaired with a suture anchor placed through the 4–5 portal as described by Mathoulin [13]. The TFCC foveal avulsion was repaired using standard technique through a limited open ulnar approach with a suture anchor. These two procedures were performed first prior to addressing the volar SL tear.

For repair of the volar SL injury, we chose to perform a limited open volar SL capsulodesis. The hand was taken out of the arthroscopy tower and placed on the operating room table. The volar capsulodesis can be performed through a proximal radial volar incision. This surgical approach is similar to the approach used for the treatment of a scaphoid fracture (Figs. 24.4 and 24.5). Once the volar capsule is

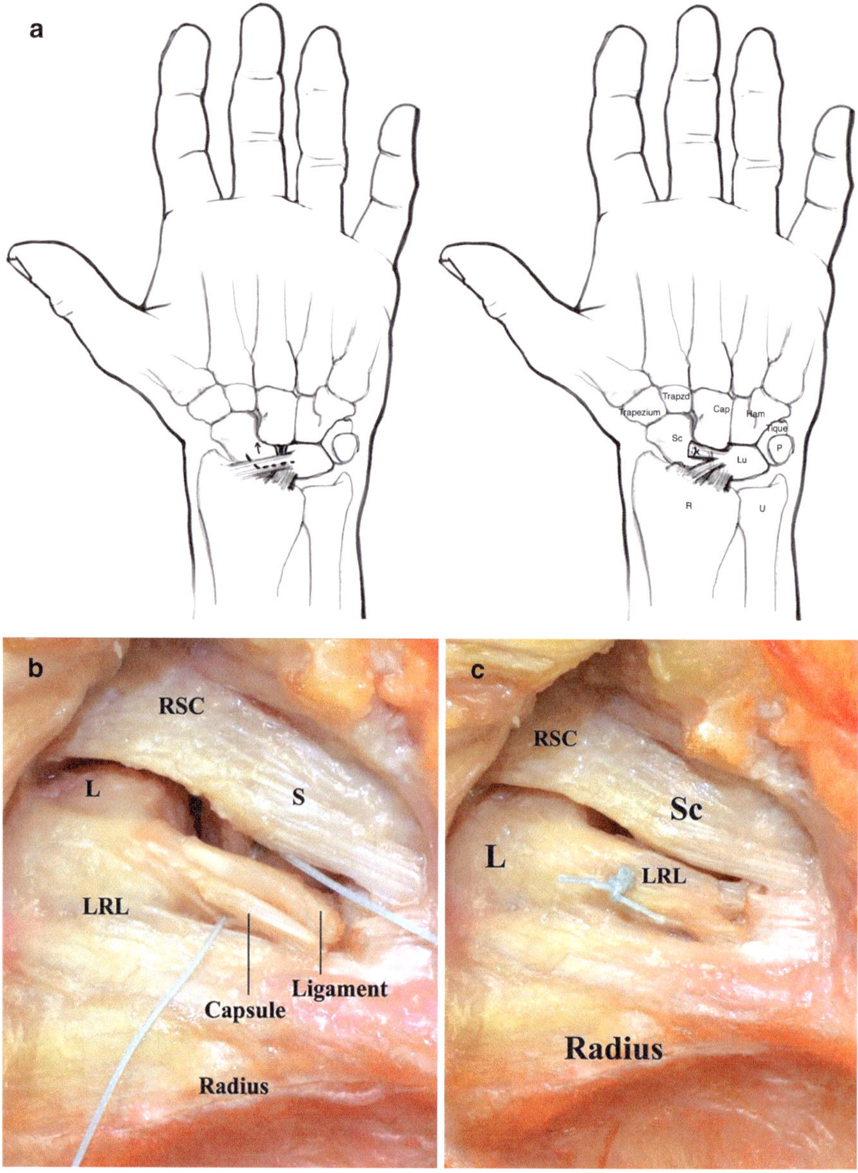

Fig. 24.4 (**a–c**) Schematic of technique for volar capsulodesis. A small strip of the volar capsule, which includes a portion of the long radiolunate ligament that is divided proximally off the radius and transferred to the waist of the scaphoid. The same procedure demonstrated on a cadaveric specimen is shown in images **b** and **c**. (**b**) The capsular strip is seen harvested and prepared for transfer. The suture anchor has been placed in the proximal pole of the scaphoid. (**c**) The capsulodesis has been completed, and the capsular strip has been transferred to the scaphoid. The capsulodesis tethers the scaphoid and lunate together palmarly and also prevents the proximal pole of the scaphoid from translating dorsally during gripping and wrist extension

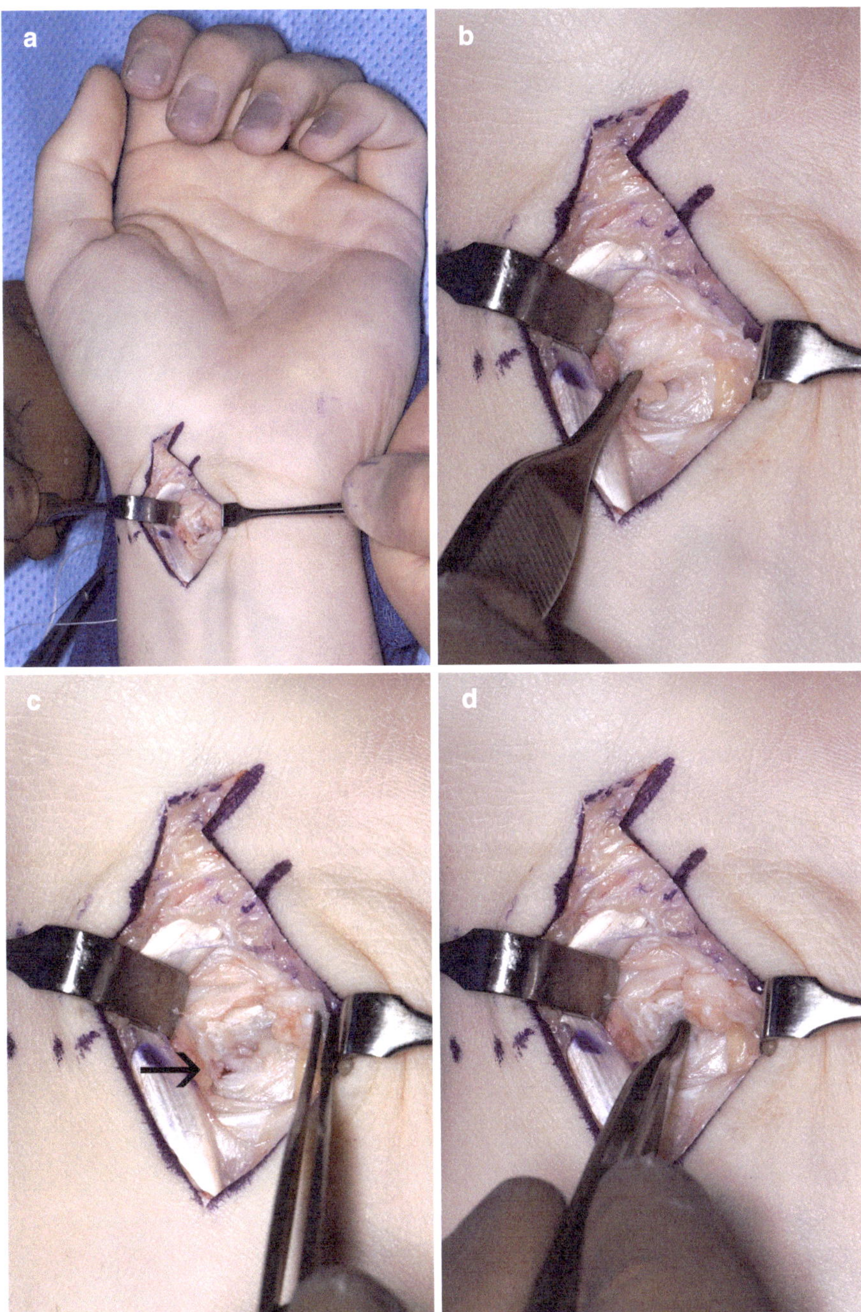

Fig. 24.5 (**a–d**) The surgical approach on our patient is performed through 4–5 cm incision localized just medial to the FCR. The FCR is mobilized radially, and the subsheath of the FCR is opened. This is similar to the volar approach for open treatment of scaphoid fractures. The wrist is brought into extension, and a K-wire is used to identify the SL interval. The volar ligaments and fibers can be seen at the base of the wound. (**b**) The forceps holding the flap after elevation, and (**c**) the capsular flap redirected toward the lunate. The arrow points to the tear in the volar SL ligament. (**d**) The forceps being placed into the SL interval through the rent in the ligament

reached, a K-wire is used to identify the SL interval. The outlines of the lunate and scaphoid are traced onto the volar capsule. A 2–3 mm strip of volar capsule, in line with the long radiolunate ligament, is harvested off the radius and left attached to the lunate. Elevation of this strip allows one to visualize the volar SL interval, which was torn in this patient (Fig. 24.5d). A suture anchor is then placed into the proximal pole of the scaphoid (Fig. 24.4). The wrist is brought into mild radial deviation, and the sutures are placed through the capsular strip and tied under mild tension. If the capsular strip is frayed, a modified Krakauer suture may be used to grasp the capsular flap more firmly. The tails of the suture anchors are then used to imprecate the capsular strip to both the radioscaphocapitate and long radiolunate ligaments. K-wires used for stabilization of the scaphoid and lunate are not routinely used but can be considered if there is concern for noncompliance with postoperative immobilization.

Postoperative therapy consists of 6–8 weeks of immobilization. This is followed by graded range of motion and strengthening therapy. Patients are allowed to return to weight training at 10 weeks once they have recovered wrist range of motion. Weight training is usually restricted to 25 lbs. within the operative hand for 3 months after surgery; after this period of time, patients may return to regular activities.

Clinical Course and Outcome (Figs. 24.6 and 24.7)

The patient was immobilized for 6 weeks and then started graded ROM exercises. He regained symmetric wrist motion as seen in Fig. 24.7 by 4 months. He was able to return to collegiate football for his senior year on the starting offensive line, and

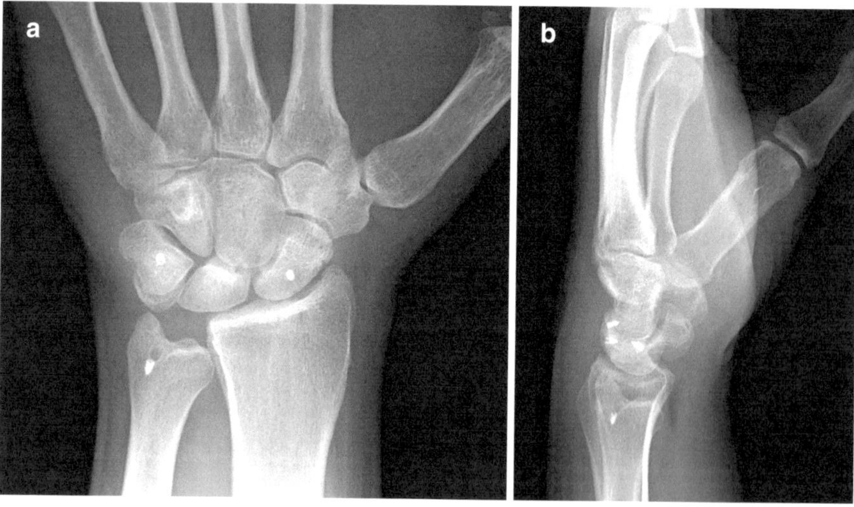

Fig. 24.6 Two-year postoperative radiographs showing stable carpal position with no signs of progressive midcarpal instability or arthritis

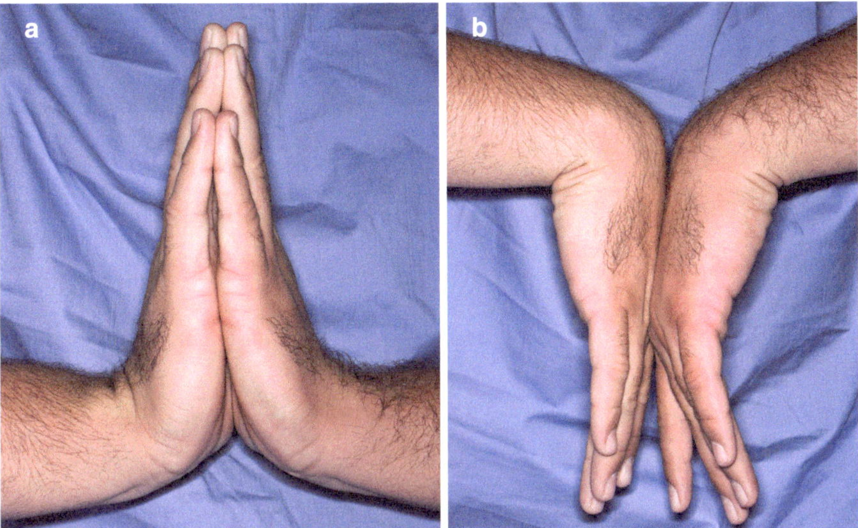

Fig. 24.7 Postoperative flexion and extension views showing preservation of excellent motion

he was capable of bench pressing close to 400 lbs. His grip strength was equivalent to the contralateral side. His radiographs have remained stable over his 5-year follow-up (Fig. 24.6).

Bullet Clinical Pears/Pitfalls (Fig. 24.8)

- Wrist arthroscopy is important to verify the diagnosis of a volar tear.
- Confirm with preoperative MRI or arthroscopy that the short and long lunate ligaments are intact prior to performing this technique.
- To identify the location of the long radiolunate ligament, follow the articular branch of the radial artery to the wrist capsule as seen in Fig. 24.8a. This artery usually passes below the long radiolunate ligament and distal to the rim of the volar radius. A K-wire is then placed into the wrist at this level and position confirmed with the fluoro-scanner (Fig. 24.8b and c).
- Bring the wrist into extension to stretch the volar capsule, which will better define the volar ligaments.
- Use the remaining tails of the suture anchor to imbricate the radioscaphocapitate and long radiolunate ligament during closure. This further reinforces the repair.

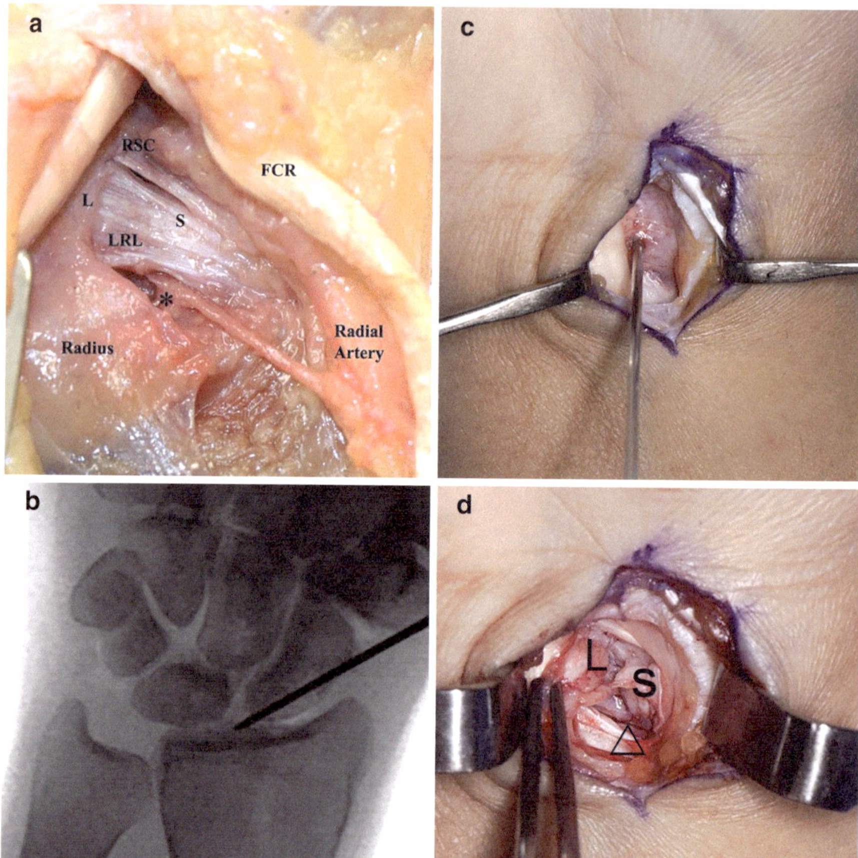

Fig. 24.8 (**a–d**): *Pearls for success*. (**a**) The location of the articular branch of the radial artery that consistently runs proximal to the long radiolunate ligament. This arterial branch can guide you toward the location of the SL interval. (**b** and **c**) The location of the SL interval with the aid of intraoperative radiography. A K-wire is used to mark the location of the SL interval on the capsule. Once the surgeon has become familiar with this technique, it can be performed through a 3–4 cm incision over the volar wrist with good exposure of the volar SL tear. (**d**) A complete volar SLIL tear with the capsular flap elevated off the lunate (L). The arrow points to the torn SLIL ligament (S = scaphoid)

Literature Review and Discussion

As the use of volar capsulodesis is a newer technique, long-term outcome studies are limited. Recent reports have described performing this procedure arthroscopically, making the technique more attractive when combined with other arthroscopic techniques [18–20]. Most recently, the long-term outcomes with volar repair have been reported by Sarcon and colleagues in a retrospective study of 28 patients followed for over 64 months [21]. Final wrist motion was flexion of 57°, extension of

61°, ulnar deviation of 29°, and radial deviation (RD) of 19°. Mean postoperative grip strength was 80% of the contralateral normal side. One patient required a revision (3.5%) for persistent pain over the 5-year follow-up period. Final patient-reported outcome scores were very good with an average DASH of 16.4 and PRWE of 24.6.

References

1. Chim H, Moran SL. Wrist essentials: the diagnosis and management of scapholunate ligament injuries. Plast Reconstr Surg. 2014;134(2):312e–22e.
2. Berger RA. The gross and histologic anatomy of the scapholunate interosseous ligament. J Hand Surg Am. 1996;21(2):170–8.
3. Moran SL, Cooney WP, Berger RA, Strickland J. Capsulodesis for the treatment of chronic scapholunate instability. J Hand Surg Am. 2005;30(1):16–23.
4. Chan K, Engasser W, Jebson PJL. Avascular necrosis of the lunate following reconstruction of the scapholunate ligament using the scapholunate axis method (SLAM). J Hand Surg Am. 2019;44(10):904.e1–4.
5. De Smet L, Sciot R, Degreef I. Avascular necrosis of the scaphoid after three-ligament tenodesis for scapholunate dissociation: case report. J Hand Surg Am. 2011;36(4):587–90.
6. Blatt G. Capsulodesis in reconstructive hand surgery. Dorsal capsulodesis for the unstable scaphoid and volar capsulodesis following excision of the distal ulna. Hand Clin. 1987;3:81–102.
7. Mitsuyasu H, Patterson RM, Shah MA, Buford WL, Iwamoto Y, Viegas SF. The role of the dorsal intercarpal ligament in dynamic and static scapholunate instability. J Hand Surg Am. 2004;29:279–88.
8. Gajendran VK, Peterson B, Slater RR, Szabo RM. Long-term outcomes of dorsal intercarpal ligament capsulodesis for chronic scapholunate dissociation. J Hand Surg Am. 2007;32:1323–33.
9. Zarkadas PC, Gropper PT, White NJ, Perey BH. A survey of the surgical management of acute and chronic scapholunate instability. J Hand Surg Am. 2004;29:848–57.
10. Deshmukh SC, Givissis P, Belluso D, Stanley JK, Trail IA. Blatt's capsulodesis for chronic scapholunate dissociation. J Hand Surg Br. 1999;24:215–20.
11. Moran SL, Ford KS, Wulf CA, Cooney WP. Outcomes of dorsal capsulodesis and tenodesis for treatment of scapholunate instability. J Hand Surg Am. 2006;31(9):1438–46.
12. de Villeneuve Bargemon JB, Mathoulin C, Jaloux C, Levadoux M, Gras M, Merlini L. Wide arthroscopic dorsal capsuloligamentous repair in patients with severe scapholunate instability. Bone Joint J. 2023;105-B(3):307–14.
13. Binder AC, Kerfant N, Wahegaonkar AL, Tandara AA, Mathoulin CL. Dorsal wrist capsular tears in association with scapholunate instability: results of an arthroscopic dorsal capsuloplasty. J Wrist Surg. 2013;2(2):160–7.
14. Mathoulin CL, Dauphin N, Wahegaonkar AL. Arthroscopic dorsal capsuloligamentous repair in chronic scapholunate ligament tears. Hand Clin. 2011;27(4):563–72.
15. van Kampen RJ, Bayne CO, Moran SL. A new technique for volar capsulodesis for isolated palmar scapholunate interosseous ligament injuries: a cadaveric study and case report. J Wrist Surg. 2015;4(4):239–45.
16. Trentadue TP, Lopez C, Breighner RE, Fautsch K, Leng S, Holmes Iii DR, Moran SL, Thoreson AR, Kakar S, Zhao KD. Evaluation of Scapholunate injury and repair with dynamic (4D) CT: a preliminary report of two cases. J Wrist Surg. 2023;12(3):248–60.

17. Vutescu ES, Wolfe SW, Sung K, Jethanandani R, Lee SK. Postoperative pain is correlated with scaphoid dorsal translation following scapholunate interosseous ligament reconstruction. J Wrist Surg. 2020;9(6):487–92.
18. Pérez AJ, Jethanandani RG, Vutescu ES, Meyers KN, Lee SK, Wolfe SW. Role of ligament stabilizers of the proximal carpal row in preventing dorsal intercalated segment instability: a cadaveric study. J Bone Joint Surg Am. 2019;101(15):1388–96.
19. Lui H, Kakar S. Arthroscopic-assisted volar scapholunate capsulodesis: a new technique. J Hand Surg Am. 2022;47(11):1124.e1–6.
20. Del Piñal F. Arthroscopic volar capsuloligamentous repair. J Wrist Surg. 2013;2(2):126–8.
21. Sarcon AK, Cantwell S, Pino PA, Selem O, Moran SL. Long-term functional outcomes of volar capsulodesis for treatment of scapholunate interosseus ligament injury: a case series. Presented at ASSH Annual meeting, 2023.

Further Reading

Moran SL, Cooney WP, Berger RA, Strickland J. Capsulodesis for the treatment of chronic scapholunate instability. J Hand Surg Am. 2005;30(1):16–23.
Trentadue TP, Lopez C, Breighner RE, Fautsch K, Leng S, Holmes Iii DR, Moran SL, Thoreson AR, Kakar S, Zhao KD. Evaluation of scapholunate injury and repair with dynamic (4D) CT: a preliminary report of two cases. J Wrist Surg. 2023;12(3):248–60.
van Kampen RJ, Bayne CO, Moran SL. A new technique for volar capsulodesis for isolated palmar scapholunate interosseous ligament injuries: a cadaveric study and case report. J Wrist Surg. 2015;4(4):239–45.

Chapter 25
Chronic Scapholunate Dissociation Reconstruction with Internal Brace

Steven J. Lee, Devin W. Collins, Justin Luis, and Michael J. Garcia

Case Presentation

A 49-year-old right-hand-dominant previously healthy male presented 6 weeks status post a fall on an outstretched right hand. He was initially seen at an urgent care center; X-rays were told to be negative for fracture; he was told that he had a sprain, placed in a splint, and told to follow up with an orthopedist. The patient complained of mostly dorsal wrist pain, but especially with dorsiflexion of the wrist.

The pertinent positive findings on exam included tenderness overlying the dorsal scapholunate ligament. Active range of motion was limited to 20% of extension of the contralateral side secondary to pain; passive volar flexion, pronation, supination, and radial and ulnar deviation were symmetric to the unaffected left side. A Watson's maneuver did not produce an obvious clunk but did elicit pain in the dorsal wrist as well as a "mushiness" to the scaphoid tubercle.

Plain radiographs revealed a mildly widened scapholunate interspace that increased to 3 mm with a pencil grip AP stress view. No gapping was noted on the opposite side. Scapholunate angle measured 72° compared to 50° on the opposite side. No arthritic changes were noted. MRI findings were consistent with a complete disruption of the scapholunate ligament (Figs. 25.1 and 25.2).

An extensive discussion of the management options concluded that no one definitive option could be unanimously determined and that the literature was highly controversial. One option included continued splinting followed by hand therapy

S. J. Lee (✉)
Hand and Upper Extremity, Lenox Hill Hospital, New York, NY, USA

D. W. Collins · M. J. Garcia
Florida Orthopedic Institute, Temple Terrace, FL, USA

J. Luis
Lenox Hill Hospital, New York, NY, USA
e-mail: jluis@northwell.edu

J. Yao (ed.), *Carpal Instability*, https://doi.org/10.1007/978-3-031-55869-6_25

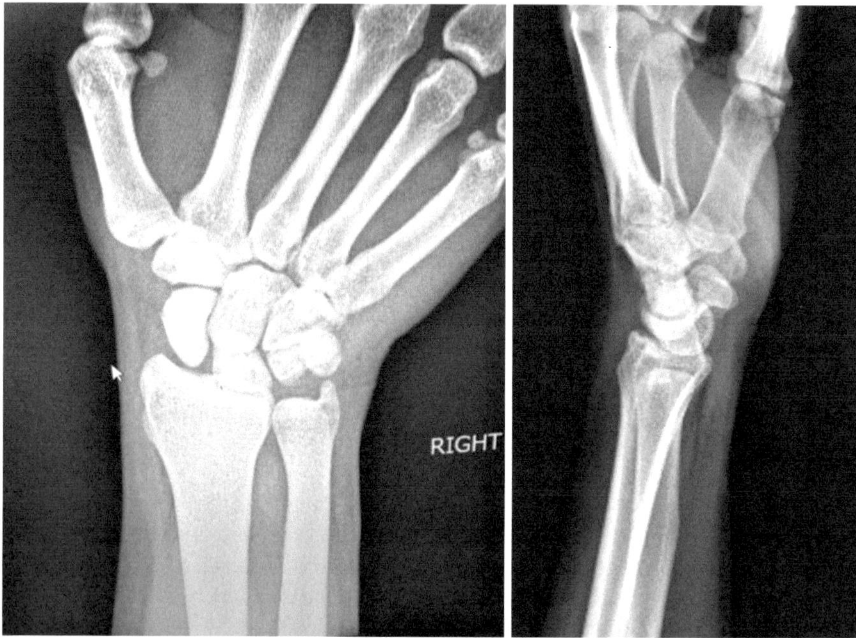

Figs. 25.1 and 25.2 Pre-op AP and Lat wrist X-rays

with the expectation that if pain persisted in the future, salvage options could be performed. Another option of denervation of the wrist was discussed. A number of repair options were presented, including a repair with suture anchors and pinning or repair with suture augmentation. Finally, various tendon graft reconstruction techniques were discussed.

The procedure that was performed for this patient was a scapholunate repair with suture augmentation, along with an anterior and posterior interosseous neurectomy. The rationale for this procedure included the fact that a repair could still produce relatively normal function and pain relief. It was discussed that suture augmentation, which has been used successfully in many other parts of the body (Lee), could help to protect the repair while avoiding the need for pins that could be potentially painful, a nidus for infection, or hardware removal. The addition of a neurectomy would potentially provide the patient with improved pain relief versus ligament repair alone [1].

The surgical technique involved a dorsal longitudinal approach, cauterizing and ligating the posterior interosseous nerve at the radial base of the fourth compartment. This was followed by incising a portion of the interosseous membrane to access and perform a neurectomy of the anterior interosseous nerve. A ligament-sparing dorsal capsulotomy was performed, and joysticks were placed into the scaphoid and lunate bones in such a manner that connecting them will simultaneously close the widened gap and also correct the DISI deformity. A forked anchor (3.5 DX SwiveLock SL, Arthrex, Naples, FL) that was simultaneously holding sutures (2-0 FiberLoop, Arthrex, Naples, FL) as well as the internal brace (Collagen Coated FiberTape, Arthrex, Naples, FL) was placed into the proximal pole of the scaphoid. The suture was used to repair the torn remnant of the scapholunate ligament (Fig. 25.3), and the FiberTape was used as a suture augmentation and secured onto the dorsal lunate with another SwiveLock anchor. Finally, the FiberTape was then secured into the distal pole of the scaphoid with a third SwiveLock anchor (Fig. 25.4). The sutures used for the repair were not cut after the knot was tied but used to secure the capsule down onto the dorsal aspect of the scaphoid and lunate (Fig. 25.5). The patient was then splinted for 6 weeks followed by hand therapy for 6 weeks. Progressive resistance exercises were begun with therapy for range of motion at 6 weeks postoperatively. Return to normal activities and sports was allowed at 3 months postoperatively. Light use of the hand was begun at the initiation of therapy.

One-year follow-up later, the patient's pre-op DASH score went from 67 preoperatively to 8. Grip strength decreased 20%, pinch strength decreased 5% from preoperatively, range of motion in dorsiflexion and palmar flexion decreased from 80/65 to 70/42 compared to the opposite side, and pronosupination was unchanged from the opposite side. Radiographs showed minimal S-L diastasis and improved

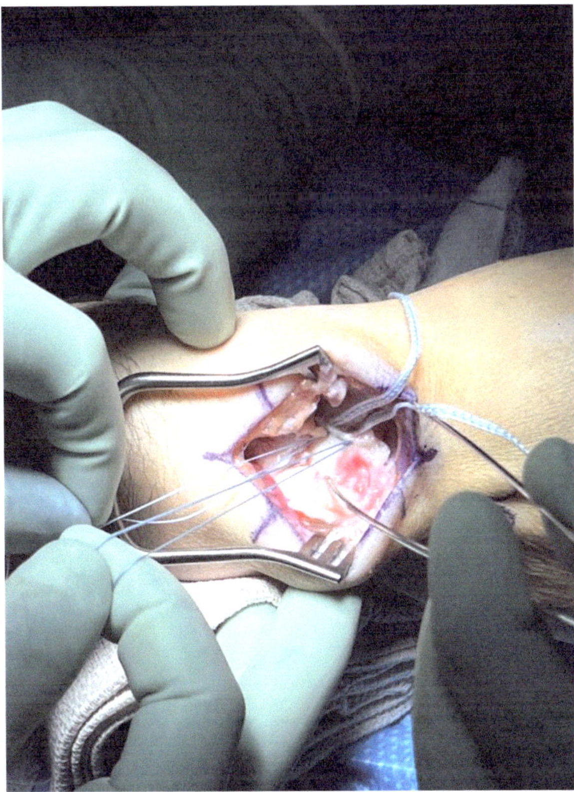

Fig. 25.3 S-L ligament repaired

Fig. 25.4 Internal brace secured

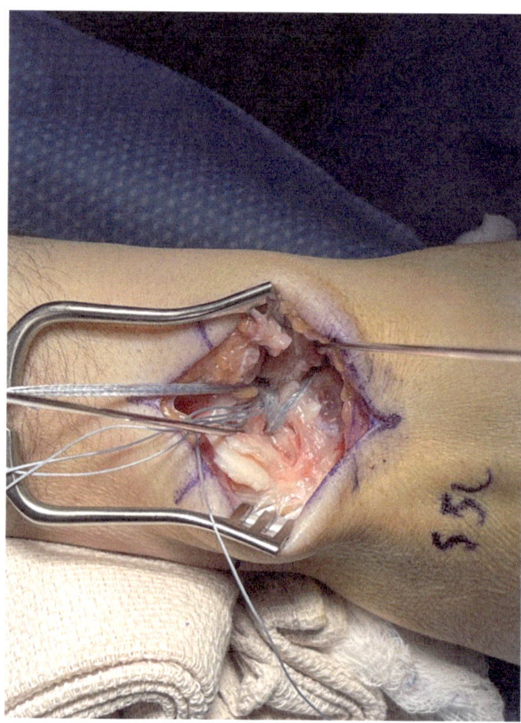

Fig. 25.5 Secure capsular closure tied to the lunate from sutures used to repair the S-L

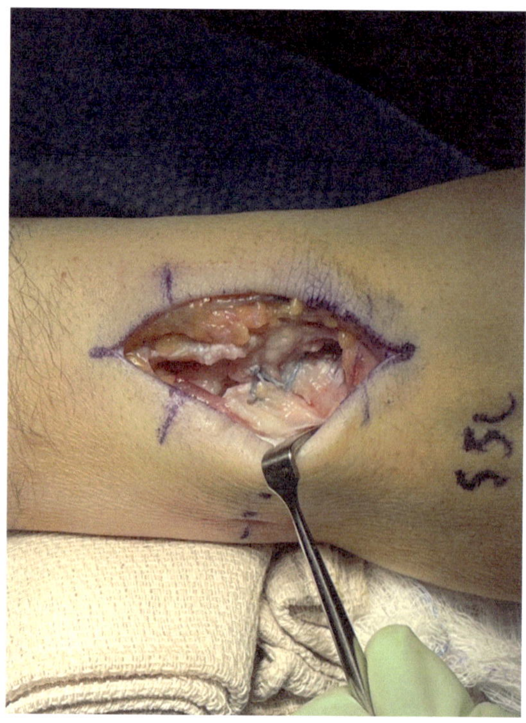

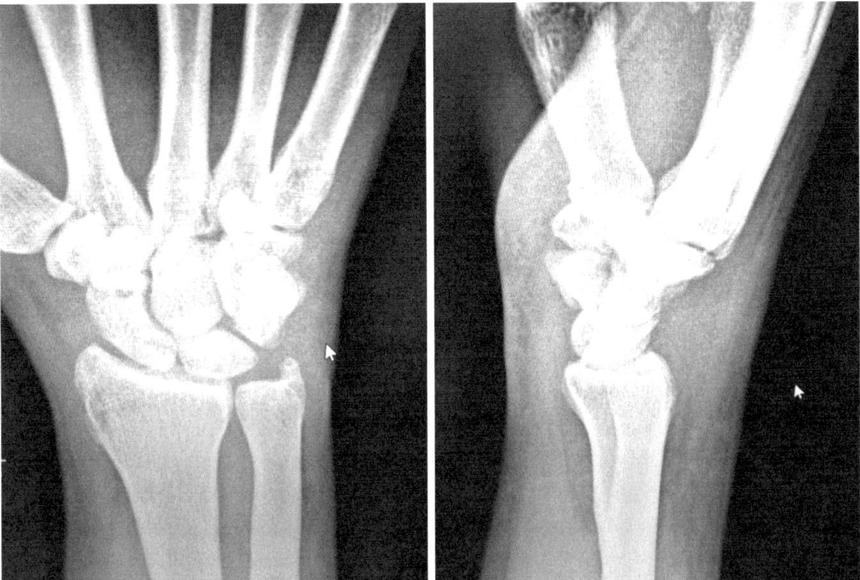

Figs. 25.6 and 25.7 Post-op AP and Lat X-rays

S-L angle (Figs. 25.6 and 25.7). He still complained of mild pain when attempting to perform push-ups, but otherwise was unhampered with his activities of daily living and his job as a wilderness guide, which entailed a fair amount of physical lifting activities.

Clinical Pearls/Pitfalls

- Many treatment options exist, and the optimal treatment is controversial.
- Best results occur when treatment is initiated in the acute/subacute phase.
- Internal bracing increases the repair strength and/or prevents tendon elongation.
- Despite this, some widening of the scapholunate space can be expected.

Literature Review and Discussion

Scapholunate ligament injuries are commonly caused by traumatic injuries to the surrounding soft tissue and osseous structures of the wrist by a fall onto an outstretched hand but can also be encountered in the nontraumatic setting. It is paramount to understand the normal anatomy and biomechanics of the wrist to understand the intricacies of instability, as they come in varying patterns and degrees of severity [2–5]. Frequently, these injuries can be missed in the acute setting and become chronic, debilitating conditions. A thorough history should be performed to elicit any acute or remote trauma. In addition, relevant past surgical procedures and medical and social history should be obtained.

Physical exam should include any tenderness to palpation about the radiocarpal, ulnocarpal, and midcarpal joints. Notable tenderness may be found over the scapholunate interval dorsally and volarly. There may be crepitance as the wrist is brought through range of motion. Flexion, extension, and radial and ulnar deviation of the wrist should be compared to the contralateral limb. A neurovascular assessment of digital perfusion, palpable pulses, sensation, and motor function should be performed on every patient.

Many dynamic tests have been described for carpal instability. Common tests include the Watson scaphoid shift, scapholunate ballottement, midcarpal shift, and shuck test. It is important to assess the contralateral limb when performing provocative maneuvers. The scaphoid shift test results in a palpable, sometimes audible "clunk" that can be painful or painless and assesses scapholunate ligament instability. The shuck and the ballottement tests are utilized to assess lunotriquetral ligament integrity. Instability and pain may be elicited upon palpation over the triquetrum with radially based pressure. The midcarpal shift test will cause a clunk and pain and is a standard diagnostic tool for midcarpal instability.

Radiographic series of the wrist may allow clinicians to evaluate carpal arcs, osseous structure, and abnormalities. Violation of the carpal arcs can be indicative of carpal injury and ultimately instability. Scapholunate widening can also be evaluated and compared to the contralateral side with a clenched fist view with widening of greater than 2 mm compared to the contralateral side being diagnostic for injury. It is important to note that instability has a wide spectrum, and not one specific test or study will elicit if a patient has injury to the scapholunate ligament complex; instead, it is the collective of the whole patient's history, their clinical picture, and subsequent diagnostic tests.

CT and MRI are also widely used to aid in cases of acute and chronic injuries. CT can aid in identifying osseous abnormalities not appreciated on normal radiographic series and can also aid in assessing other potential causes for pain. MRI allows the visualization of soft tissue-supporting structures of the radiocarpal, ulnocarpal, and midcarpal regions [6]. MRA has been shown to be superior to MRI in some studies [7]. Each patient's injury pattern is unique and may have varying levels of osseous and soft tissue injury. Ultrasound has become a new way to test dynamic instability and can be performed in real time and in the office setting. This has gained popularity in its ease of use and in office application. Additional diagnostic studies include intra-articular injections into the midcarpal joint or radiocarpal joint. Pain reduction after these injections may aid in diagnosing subtle injury or instability.

Management of scapholunate ligament complex injuries depends on the severity and chronicity. There have been many proposed treatment algorithms and techniques. Arthroscopic debridement and electrothermal shrinkage have been the proposed treatments in partial scapholunate ligament tears. There have been studies in adult and pediatric patients demonstrating efficacy for partial tears without mechanical instability in pain relief for patients [8–11]. Acute complete disruption of the scapholunate ligament complex is amenable to direct repair. Many techniques have been described with trans-osseous tunnels, bone anchors, periosteal local tissue repair, augmentation with braided wire or tape, and capsulodesis procedures, among others [12–14]. All of these techniques have shown variable results, but overall good outcomes. Recently, arthroscopic ligament repairs have been described with a variety of techniques, all showing positive outcomes [15]. The use of augmented suture tape in repairs of the scapholunate ligament complex has been compared to repair with suture anchors alone. They found in their biomechanical study that suture tape augmentation yielded higher load to failure rates compared to repair with anchors alone and concluded that augmentation may be beneficial to higher demand patients. Despite adequate reduction of the scapholunate interval at the time of surgery, diastasis of the interval does occur postoperatively as compared to the uninjured side, but this has not been shown to affect clinical outcomes.

Patients that have chronic scapholunate ligament complex disruptions often require reconstructive or salvage procedures. An in-depth review on the variety of techniques is out of the scope of this topic. In general, described techniques for irreparable ligaments with reducible carpal alignment include the Blatt capsulodesis, Brunelli tenodesis, Garcia-Elias tenodesis, scapholunate arthrodesis, Mayo capsulodesis, RASL procedures, and others [16–20]. When the ligament is irreparable and with non-reducible carpal alignment or there are arthritic changes noted, salvage procedures include wrist denervations, proximal row carpectomy, partial or total wrist fusions, and wrist arthroplasty [21, 22].

In conclusion, chronic scapholunate ligament disruption can be a debilitating injury. It is important to perform an in-depth history, physical exam, and appropriate diagnostic imaging. There must be a high index of suspicion for injuries, as acute/subacute treatment leads to the best clinical outcomes. Many surgical techniques for chronic scapholunate ligament injuries have been described including arthroscopic and open repair, trans-osseous bone tunnels, suture tape augmentation, tendon transfers, and others. Despite early treatment, diastasis of the scapholunate interval may always remain on imaging, but this has not been shown to affect clinical outcomes. In this chapter, we describe our technique for SL reconstruction in the chronic setting. Salvage options for chronic dissociation with arthritic changes include partial or total wrist fusion, proximal row carpectomy, and wrist arthroplasty.

References

1. Hofmeister EP, Moran SL, Shin AY. Anterior and posterior interosseous neurectomy for the treatment of chronic dynamic instability of the wrist. Hand (N Y). 2006;1(2):63–70.
2. Sokolow C, Saffar P. Anatomy and histology of the scapholunate ligament. Hand Clin. 2001;17:77–81.
3. Short WH, Werner FW, Green JK, et al. Biomechanical evaluation of ligamentous stabilizers of the scaphoid and lunate. J Hand Surg Am. 2002;27:991–1002.
4. Short WH, Werner FW, Green JK, et al. Biomechanical evaluation of the ligamentous stabilizers of the scaphoid and lunate: part II. J Hand Surg Am. 2005;30:24–34.
5. Short WH, Werner FW, Green JK, et al. Biomechanical evaluation of the ligamentous stabilizers of the scaphoid and lunate: part III. J Hand Surg Am. 2007;32:297–309.
6. Magee T. Comparison of 3-T MRI and arthroscopy of intrinsic wrist ligament and TFCC tears. AJR Am J Roentgenol. 2009;192:80–5.
7. Moser T, Dosch JC, Moussaoui A, et al. Wrist ligament tears: evaluation of MRI and combined MDCT and MR arthrography. AJR Am J Roentgenol. 2007;188:1278–86.
8. Darlis NA, Weiser RW, Sotereanos DG. Partial scapholunate ligament injuries treated with arthroscopic debridement and thermal shrinkage. J Hand Surg Am. 2005;30:908–14.
9. Earp BE, Waters PM, Wyzykowski RJ. Arthroscopic treatment of partial scapholunate ligament tears in children with chronic wrist pain. J Bone Joint Surg Am. 2006;88:2448–55.
10. Ruch DS, Poehling GG. Arthroscopic management of partial scapholunate and lunotriquetral injuries of the wrist. J Hand Surg Am. 1996;21:412–7.
11. Weiss AP, Sachar K, Glowacki KA. Arthroscopic debridement alone for intercarpal ligament tears. J Hand Surg Am. 1997;22:344–9.
12. Bickert B, Sauerbier M, Germann G. Scapholunate ligament repair using the Mitek bone anchor. J Hand Surg Br. 2000;25:188–92.
13. Minami A, Kaneda K. Repair and/or reconstruction of scapholunate interosseous ligament in lunate and perilunate dislocations. J Hand Surg Am. 1993;18:1099–106.
14. Yao J, Zlotolow DA, Lee SK. Scapholunate axis method. J Wrist Surg. 2016;5(1):169.
15. Del Piñal F, Studer A, Thams C, et al. An all-inside technique for arthroscopic suturing of the volar scapholunate ligament. J Hand Surg Am. 2011;36:2044–6.
16. Blatt G. Capsulodesis in reconstructive hand surgery. Dorsal capsulodesis for the unstable scaphoid and volar capsulodesis following the excision of the distal ulna. Hand Clin. 1987;3:81–102.
17. Brunelli GA, Brunelli GR. A new technique to correct carpal instability with scaphoid rotatory subluxation: a preliminary report. J Hand Surg Am. 1995;20(3 Pt 2):S82–5.
18. Garcia-Elias M, Lluch AL, Stanley JK. Three-ligament tenodesis for the treatment of scapholunate dissociation: indications and surgical technique. J Hand Surg Am. 2006;31(1):125–34. https://doi.org/10.1016/j.jhsa.2005.10.011.
19. Berger RA, Bishop AT, Bettinger PC. New dorsal capsulotomy for the surgical exposure of the wrist. Ann Plast Surg. 1995;35(1):54–9.
20. Rosenwasser MP, Miyasajsa KC, Strauch RJ. The RASL procedure: reduction and association of the scaphoid and lunate using the Herbert screw. Tech Hand Up Extrem Surg. 1997;1(4):263–72.
21. Lee SJ, Rabinovich RV, Kim A. Proximal row carpectomy using decellularized dermal allograft: preliminary results. J Wrist Surg. 2021;10(2):116–22.
22. Wolf AL, Garg R, Kraszewski AP, Hillstron HJ, Hafer JF, Backus SI, Lenhoff ML, Wolf SW. Surgical treatments for Scapholunate advanced collapse wrist: kinematics and functional performance. J Hand Surg. 2015;40(8):1547–53.

Chapter 26
Subacute Lunotriquetral Ligament Injury: Reconstruction

Lauren E. Dittman and Alexander Y. Shin

Case Presentation

A 30-year-old, right-hand-dominant male presented to the emergency department with right-hand pain and swelling after punching a punching bag. He states that he hit the punching bag with the dorsoradial aspect of his hand. Radiographs were obtained, which did not show any acute findings aside from soft tissue swelling (Fig. 26.1). He was placed into a splint for comfort. He was discharged home with pain control. He returned approximately 1 week later with continued pain, swelling, and ecchymosis. He had tenderness over the lunotriquetral (LT) interval dorsally on examination. He was noted to have LT instability with positive shear and Kleinman tests. Repeat radiographs remained negative, and there was no evidence of volar intercalated segment instability (VISI) deformity. An MRI was obtained, which showed that the dorsal LT ligament was not clearly visualized and was suspected to be at least partially torn (Fig. 26.2). The articular cartilage otherwise appeared healthy and intact. A trial of nonoperative treatment was attempted, and he was immobilized in a short arm cast for approximately 6 weeks. At his return visit, he continued to have ulnar-sided wrist pain and positive LT shear and Kleinman tests. A diagnostic injection was then pursued, which gave him complete, albeit temporary, relief of pain. The decision was made to proceed with diagnostic arthroscopy for the presumed diagnosis of LT injury.

L. E. Dittman · A. Y. Shin (✉)
Mayo Clinic, Rochester, MN, USA
e-mail: Dittman.lauren@mayo.edu; shin.alexander@mayo.edu

J. Yao (ed.), *Carpal Instability*, https://doi.org/10.1007/978-3-031-55869-6_26

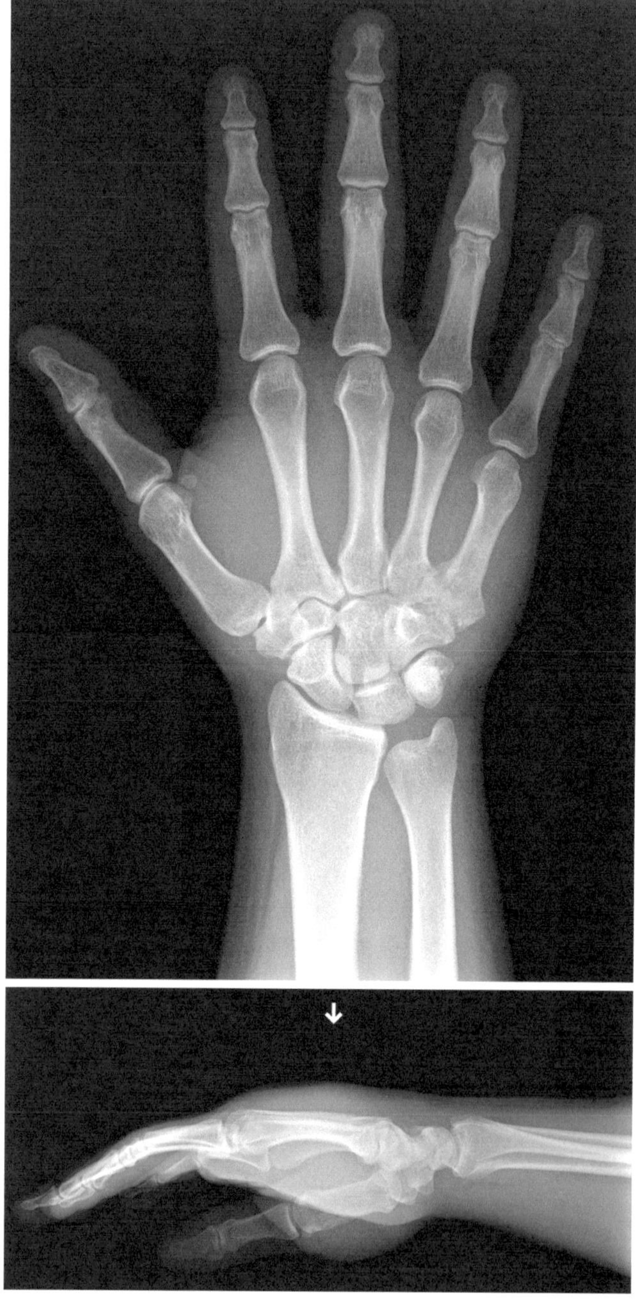

Fig. 26.1 PA and lateral radiographs at time of injury

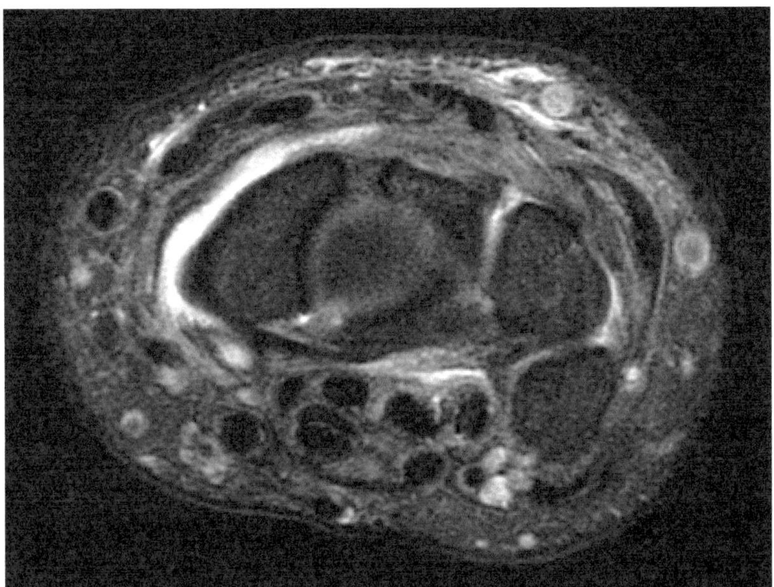

Fig. 26.2 Absence of the dorsal LT ligament on MRI

Diagnosis

Physical Exam

Patients with LT injuries typically present with ulnar-sided wrist pain and decreased grip strength after an acute injury. They will also have tenderness to palpation directly over the LT interval dorsally. Provocative exam maneuvers, including LT shear, lateral compression, and Kleinman tests, can help differentiate LT injury from other causes of ulnar-sided wrist pain [1]. These LT-specific exam findings were positive in the patient presented here, suggestive of LT injury.

Radiographs

Radiographs should always be obtained at the time of injury. However, unless there is acute dislocation due to significant ligamentous injury, radiographs are typically negative in the acute and subacute settings. Radiographs should also be scrutinized for VISI deformity or arthritic changes. As expected, the patient in this study had normal radiographs, aside from soft tissue swelling. With acute LT dislocation, the radiographs are often misinterpreted as a scapholunate dissociation. Careful evaluation of Gilula's arcs is necessary to fully understand the injury pattern.

MRI

MRI or MR arthrography can be useful when radiographs are negative and soft tissue injury is suspected. It is important to note that MRI sensitivity is variable based on the extent of LT injury [2]. Additionally, MRI is most valuable in the subacute setting, after initial soft tissue and bony edema has had time to convalesce, allowing for less background noise. This patient underwent MRI at 1 week post-injury. The dorsal LT ligament was unable to be visualized, suggesting at least partial tear.

Arthroscopy

Wrist arthroscopy remains the gold standard for diagnosis and staging of carpal instability, including LT injury [3, 4]. Geissler et al. proposed an arthroscopic classification system based on intraoperative ligament stability [5]. Grade I and II tears are considered low-grade or partial tears and can be managed conservatively. Grades III and IV are considered high-grade or complete tears and require surgical intervention. This patient underwent diagnostic arthroscopy and was found to have a grade IV tear (Fig. 26.3), thus confirming the diagnosis of complete LT injury and necessitating further surgical treatment.

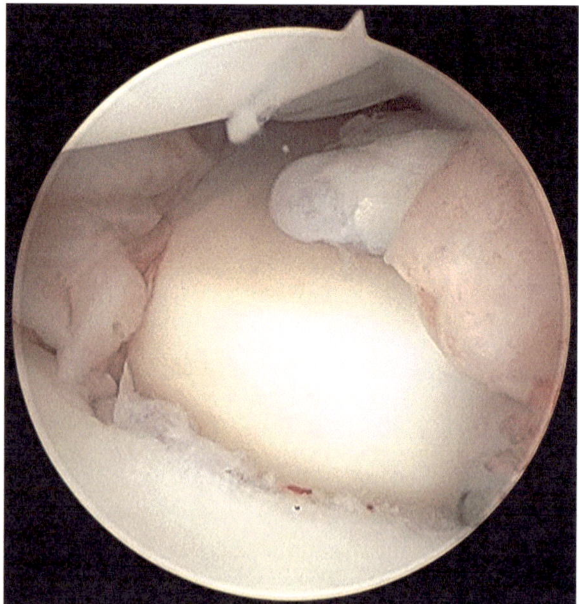

Fig. 26.3 Geissler Grade IV LT injury with associated LT step-off seen on diagnostic arthroscopy

Management

There are multiple considerations when determining appropriate treatment of LT ligament injuries. This includes both patient-specific factors, such as age and activity level, as well as the status of the wrist and extent of injury. Nonoperative treatment is typically reserved only for patients with acute, dynamic instability without associated VISI deformity [6–8]. A corticosteroid injection into the midcarpal joint can be helpful with both pain control and diagnostic confirmation.

When surgical intervention is pursued, there are multiple options, including debridement, direct ligament repair, ligament reconstruction, and arthrodesis. Direct ligament repair is indicated when adequate dorsal ligament is present and when the volar LT ligament remains intact. Reconstruction is the preferred technique if there is disruption of both the dorsal and volar LT ligaments. Generally speaking, LT ligament reconstruction should be considered in all patients in the acute and subacute settings, given its lower rate of re-rupture and decreased reoperation rate compared to direct repair [8]. Arthrodesis is indicated only in the setting of arthritic changes or irreducible VISI deformity. Arthroscopy is often useful for assessing the status of the LT ligament and articular cartilage. This can be done in isolation or can be at the time of planned definitive treatment, based on surgeon and patient preferences.

This patient underwent diagnostic arthroscopy followed by lunotriquetral ligament reconstruction using a distally based ECU tendon strip approximately 3 months after his initial injury. Of note, the patient was also found to have capitohamate instability intraoperatively and was treated with capitohamate arthrodesis using iliac crest autograft. We will focus on the author's preferred technique for LT ligament reconstruction using the ECU tendon.

After receiving general anesthesia, the patient is placed supine on the operating room table. The upper extremity is exsanguinated and a tourniquet inflated throughout the case. A standard arthroscopic setup is used, with the fingers hanging in 15 lbs. traction. The 3–4 portal is established first as the viewing portal, followed by an outflow portal at the ulnar sixth position. The 4–5 portal is also established, and a probe is used to explore the wrist. This patient has a Geissler IV abnormality with incongruity and step-off at the LT joint, confirming its instability (Fig. 26.3). Dynamic evaluation with arthroscopy demonstrated that the LT joint opened up abnormally both dorsally and volarly, consistent with an injury to both the volar and dorsal LT ligaments. Once diagnostic arthroscopy is complete, the arm is removed from the finger traps.

A dorsal, longitudinal incision is made, in line with the third metacarpal (Fig. 26.4). Dissection is carried down through subcutaneous tissue, until the extensor retinaculum is identified. The extensor pollicis longus tendon is identified, just ulnar to Lister's tubercle (Fig. 26.5). An incision is made over the tendon, and the third compartment is entered. An ulnarly based extensor retinacular flap is created and carried to expose the fourth and fifth compartments (Fig. 26.6). Care is taken to

Fig. 26.4 Dorsal midline incision in line with third metacarpal

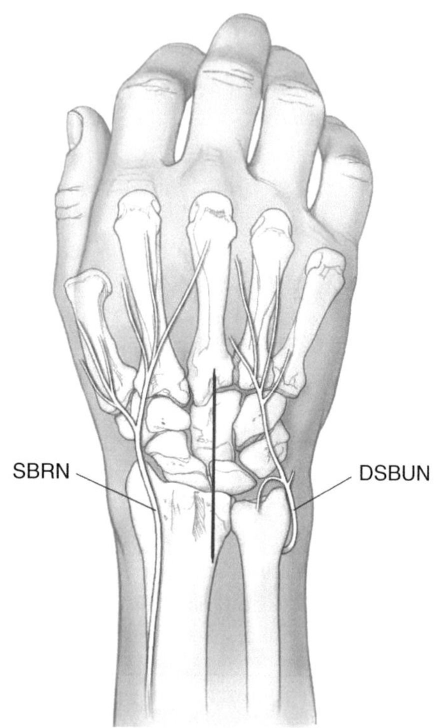

Fig. 26.5 Extensor retinaculum is exposed and EPL tendon is identified

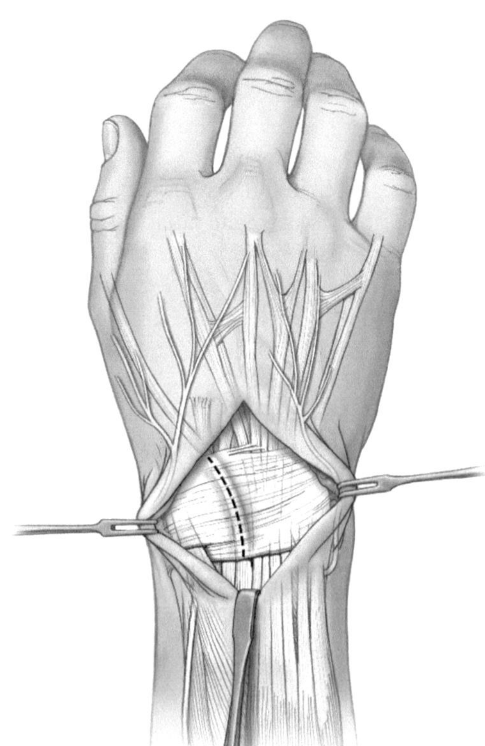

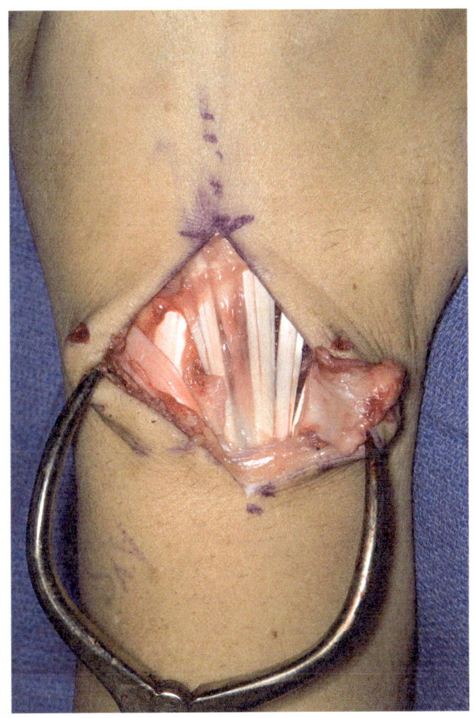

Fig. 26.6 The extensor tendons are exposed while preserving a flap of retinaculum for later repair

ensure the preservation of a thick extensor retinacular flap. Once fully exposed, the posterior interosseous nerve is identified on the floor of the first compartment, and a neurectomy can be performed.

The extensor tendons are retracted to visualize the dorsal wrist capsule. The dorsal radiocarpal and dorsal intercarpal ligaments are identified, and the midportion of the ligament is incised, creating a radially based ligament-sparing dorsal capsular flap (Fig. 26.7). This allows visualization into the radiocarpal joint. In this patient, this allowed confirmation of the LT ligament tear, as previously identified on arthroscopy (Fig. 26.8). The volar LT ligament competence is assessed with a Freer elevator. In this patient, both the dorsal and volar ligaments were incompetent. The distally based ECU reconstruction was next performed.

The ECU is identified at the level of the wrist, within the capsulotomy. Traction is placed on the tendon in order to identify its course proximally. Once identified, a 1 cm transverse incision is made over the proximal portion of the ECU tendon such that an 8–10 cm long graft can be harvested. Dissection is carried down through the subcutaneous tissue until the tendon can be isolated. A strip of the tendon, either 1/3 or 1/2 of its width, is cut proximally, and the free end is tied to a 28-gauge wire. An instrument such as a hemostat is placed through the ECU tendon sheath, moving from distal to proximal. The wire is then placed in the hemostat and pulled through, to allow passage of the cut strip of ECU tendon into the wound distally.

Fig. 26.7 Dorsal radiocarpal and dorsal intercarpal ligaments are incised, creating radiallybased capsular flap

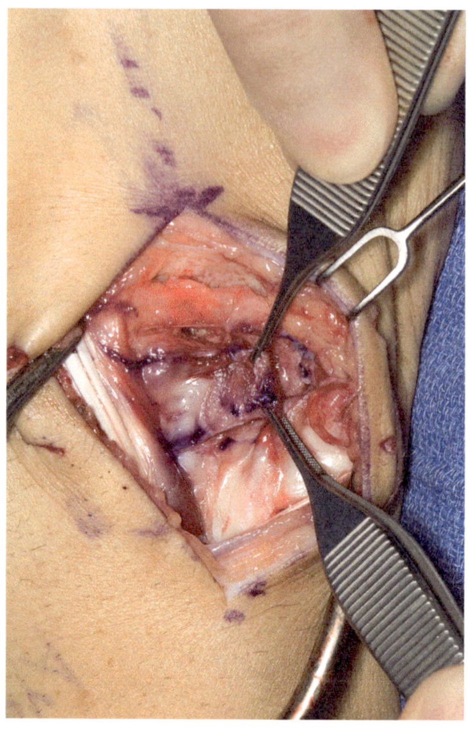

Fig. 26.8 Exposure of the LT interval and confirmation of LT ligament instability

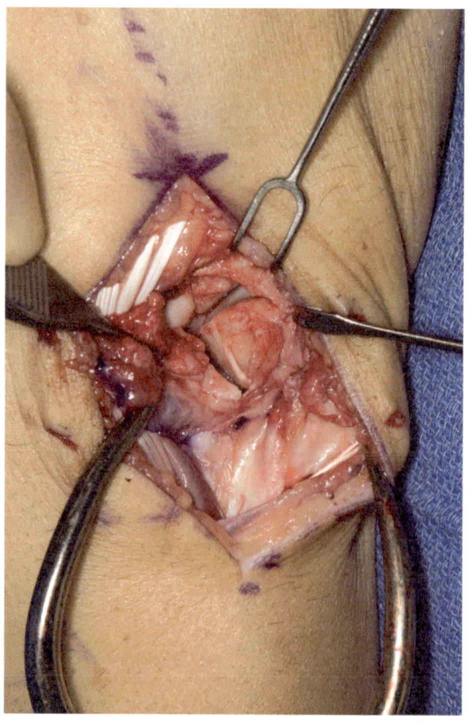

Two bone tunnels are then created using 0.045 K-wires. The K-wire is placed in a radial-dorsal to volar-ulnar direction in the lunate, and an ulnar-dorsal to volar-radial direction in the triquetrum (Fig. 26.9). The K-wires are overdrilled using cannulated drill bits to enlarge the tunnels. The wire with attached ECU tendon is then passed through the triquetrum and the lunate (Fig. 26.10). While holding the joint reduced and with tension on the ECU tendon strip, the LT joint is pinned with two 0.045" K-wires. The ECU tendon is folded back on itself and sutured into place using nonabsorbable sutures in multiple figure-of-eight fashion (Fig. 26.11). Fluoroscopy is used to ensure adequate reduction (Fig. 26.12).

The remnant native LT ligament can also be repaired to reinforce the construct. Two appropriate-sized suture anchors can be used, one in the lunate and one in the triquetrum, at the junction of the LT ligament. The remaining LT ligament is sutured down using these bone anchors. The repaired LT ligament is then sutured to the reconstructed ECU tendon using nonabsorbable sutures to reinforce the construct. Percutaneous K-wires are cut short under the skin, and removal is planned between 10 and 12 weeks post-surgery.

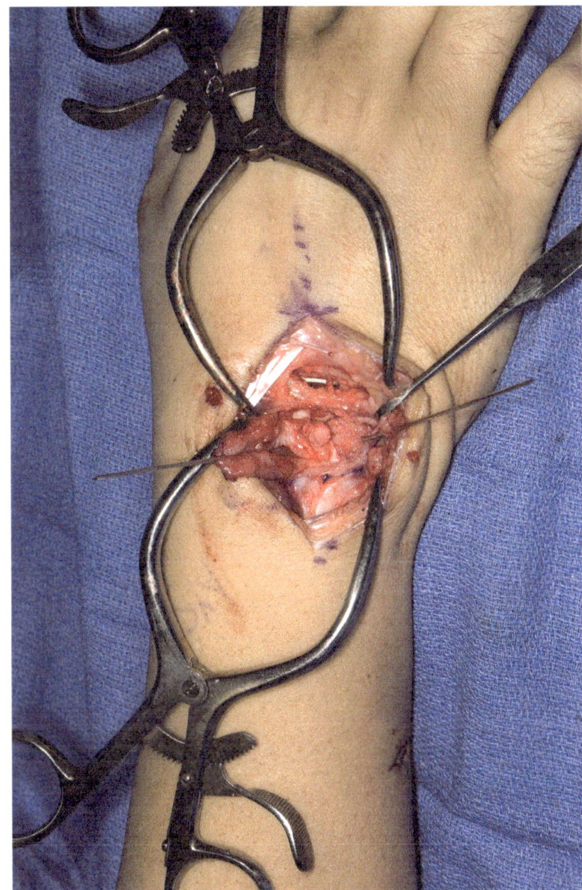

Fig. 26.9 K-wires placed in position of tunnels through lunate and triquetrum

Fig. 26.10 Use of wire to pass ECU tendon through bone tunnels

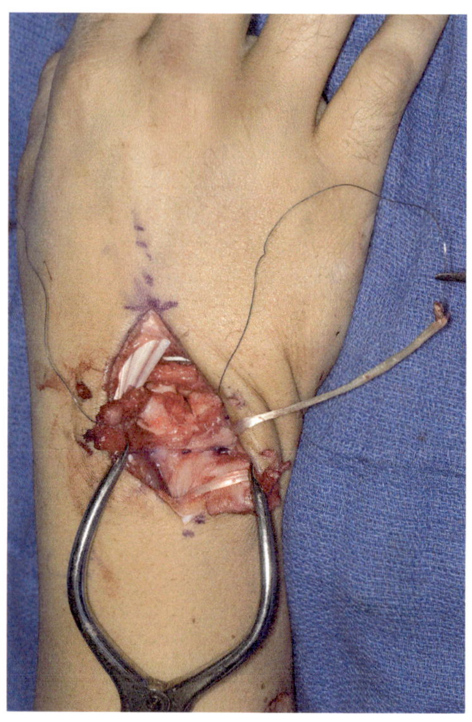

Fig. 26.11 After the ECU tendon is passed through the bone tunnels, it is sutured back on itself to secure

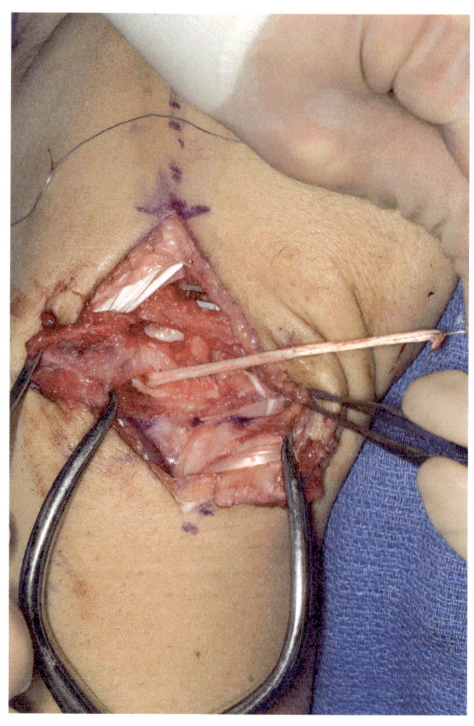

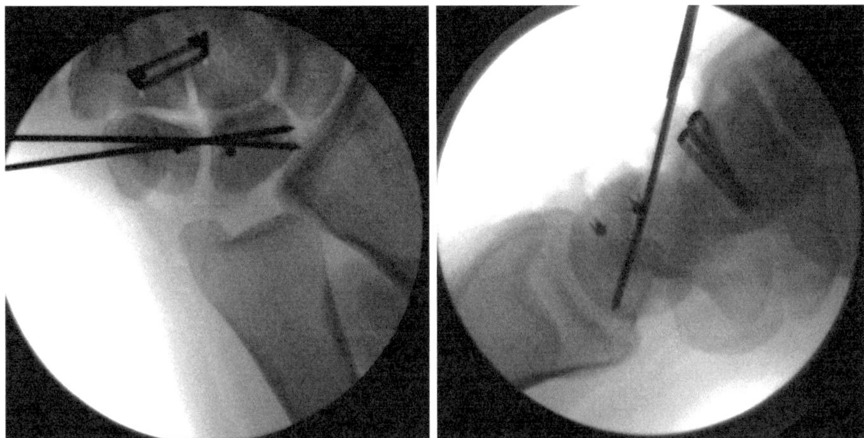

Fig. 26.12 Intraoperative PA and lateral radiographs after LT reconstruction

The capsule is closed, and the extensor retinaculum is repaired after transposing the EPL tendon. The wounds are thoroughly irrigated, and hemostasis is obtained. Skin is closed and sterile dressing placed. A sugar tong splint is applied for the first 2 weeks postoperatively. Sutures are removed at 2 weeks, and a Muenster-style cast is applied. This is worn until the 6-week postoperative mark, at which time a splint can be applied. The K-wires are removed at 10–12 weeks, the patient is transitioned to a removable splint, and therapy is begun.

Outcomes

The patient is now 13 years from his surgery and has returned to work as a laborer, without limitations. His most recent radiographs are shown in Fig. 26.13. Overall, LT ligament reconstruction has had favorable results. Reagan et al. were the first to publish the distally based ECU tendon reconstruction outcomes and reported satisfactory outcomes in all three patients included in this study [9]. A larger cohort study by Shahane et al. found that 40 out of 46 patients were satisfied with their outcome after LT reconstruction, with good or excellent Mayo Wrist Scores in 63% [10]. Another study by Pilny et al. reported good or excellent results in 90% of patients after LT reconstruction with ECU tendon in their cohort of 19 patients [11]. One comparative study by Shin et al. examined 57 patients with isolated LT injuries that were treated by arthrodesis, direct ligament repair, or reconstruction with ECU tendon. They found that reconstruction had the lowest rate of complications and need for revision surgery at 5 years [8]. Additionally, this study found that manual laborers and high-level athletes should undergo ligament reconstruction, when feasible, as they are at high risk for re-rupture and late failure of a direct ligament repair [8]. Given these results, the authors advocate for virtually all patients to undergo LT ligament reconstruction in both the acute and subacute settings.

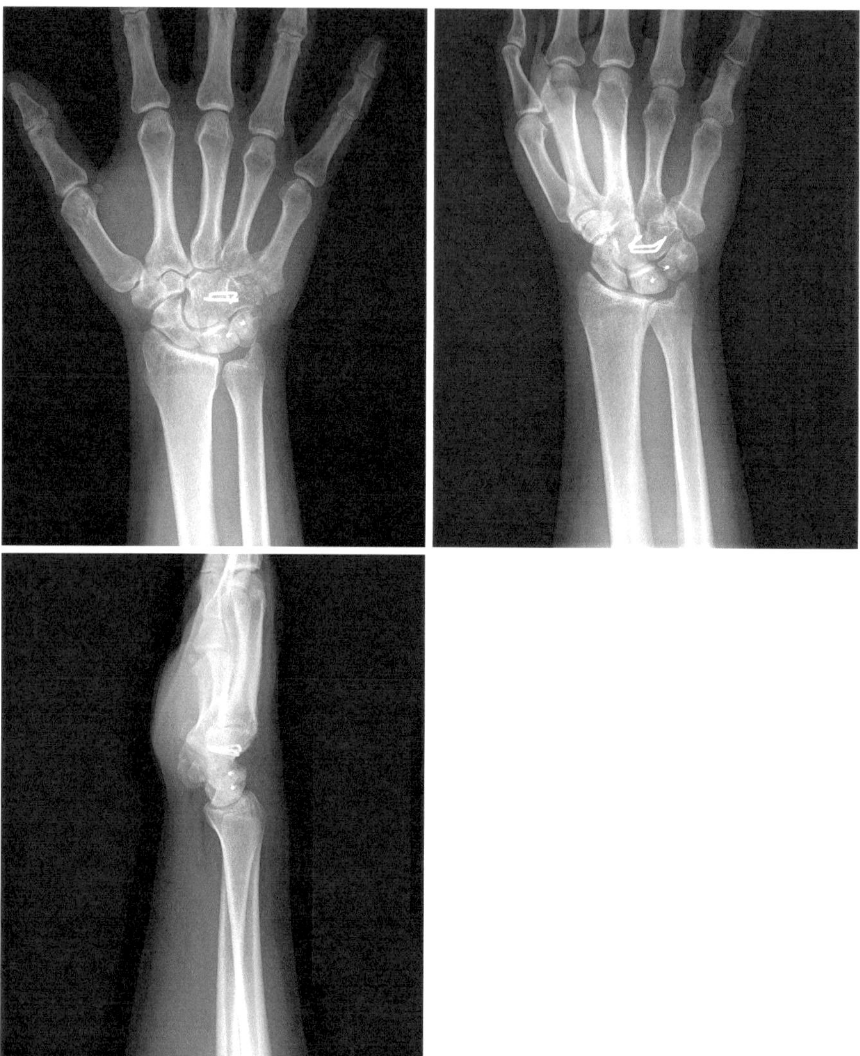

Fig. 26.13 Postoperative PA, lateral, and oblique radiographs

Pearls and Pitfalls

- Anatomic reduction is critical. A Freer elevator can be used to palpate the joint reduction. If you are able to visualize the entire LT joint easily, it is not reduced; the curvature of the joint should make it difficult to see when properly reduced.
- A 14-gauge angiocatheter needle can be used as a trochar for 0.045 inch or 1 mm K-wires. This allows better control during wire placement and protects soft tissues.

- Bone tunnels need to be carefully placed. Reduce the LT interval, estimate the placement of tunnels, and make sure that they are in the correct position to prevent distal/proximal translation when the ECU tendon is pulled taught.
- Create a loop on the 28-gauge wire prior to passing through the triquetral tunnel. A hook can then be created on the end of a 0.035 K-wire to hook the 28-gauge wire and allow easier passing through the tunnels.
- It is crucial to maintain adequate reduction of the LT joint while tensioning and securing the graft. A Kocher or Allis can be used to grasp the free edge of the tendon to allow better control while weaving and securing the tendon to itself.

Literature Review

There are several treatment options for patients with LT injury, including arthroscopic debridement/thermal shrinkage and capsulodesis, direct ligament repair, ligament reconstruction ulnar shortening osteotomy, and arthrodesis. Arthroscopic debridement is the most conservative option, allowing for a quicker recovery. After debridement, the LT joint is typically reduced and temporarily held with K-wires. A small dorsal incision can be used to aid in reduction. Weiss et al. reported good results with debridement alone followed by 2 weeks of immobilization. Seventy-eight percent of patients with complete LT tears and 100% of patients with partial tears reported symptomatic improvement [12]. While Ritt et al. reported similar successful results with debridement alone, not all studies echo these findings [13]. Westkaemper et al. reported the results of five patients who underwent isolated debridement for LT tears and found that only one of them had an acceptable outcome [14]. This difference is likely a factor of the extent of the tear and which portion of the ligament, dorsal or volar, was addressed.

Direct ligament repair is also an option for patients with LT ligament injury, which is typically utilized in the acute setting. Ligament repair can be done with either drill holes or suture anchors in either the lunate or the triquetrum, dependent upon from where the ligament avulsed. Percutaneous K-wires hold the joint reduced for 8–12 weeks after surgery to allow ligamentous healing. Previous studies have reported satisfactory outcomes after direct ligament repair alone. Reagan et al. reported an 85% satisfaction rate in their cohort of 7 patients, whereas Favero et al. reported a 90% satisfaction rate in their cohort of 21 patients [9, 15]. However, Shin et al. reviewed the largest cohort to date, including 27 patients with direct LT repair, and found that while they did have similar DASH scores compared to those who underwent LT reconstruction, they also had a 15% revision rate after direct LT repair [8]. Therefore, the authors prefer ligament reconstruction over direct LT repair alone.

Surgeons should also analyze preoperative radiographs to determine the patient's ulnar variance. Those with significant ulnar positivity and concomitant LT ligament injury may benefit from ulnar shortening osteotomy, alone or as an adjunct to LT ligament repair or reconstruction. Mirza et al. previously examined 53 patients with

LT ligament injury who were treated with isolated ulnar shortening osteotomy and found that 83% of patients reported good or excellent scores after surgery [16].

Arthrodesis is also an option after LT ligament injury; however, this is typically reserved for patients with static VISI deformity or arthritic changes in the carpus. Results of LT arthrodesis have been less than favorable thus far. In Reagan's study, all four patients who underwent arthrodesis continued to be symptomatic postoperatively [9]. Additionally, Shin et al. found that of the patients who underwent LT arthrodesis, 41% went on to nonunion and 78% required a second surgery [8]. Unfortunately, few other options remain in the setting of static deformity or concomitant arthritis.

LT ligament reconstruction remains the gold standard for treatment of acute and subacute LT injury. As previously mentioned, previous studies have shown to have good to excellent outcomes in these patients, with lower reoperation rates compared to other surgical techniques [8, 10, 11].

References

1. Kleinman WB. Physical examination of the wrist: useful provocative maneuvers. J Hand Surg Am. 2015;40(7):1486–500.
2. Yu J. MRI of the wrist. Orthopedics. 1994;17:1041–8.
3. Osterman AL, Seidman GD. The role of arthroscopy in the treatment of lunotriquetral ligament injuries. Hand Clin. 1995;11(1):41–50.
4. Weiss LE, Taras JS, Sweet S, Osterman AL. Lunotriquetral injuries in the athlete. Hand Clin. 2000;16(3):433–8.
5. Geissler WB, Freeland AE, Savoie FH, McIntyre LW, Whipple TL. Intracarpal soft-tissue lesions associated with an intra-articular fracture of the distal end of the radius. J Bone Joint Surg Am. 1996;78(3):357–65.
6. Beckenbaugh RD. Accurate evaluation and management of the painful wrist following injury. Orthop Clin N Am. 1984;15(2):289–306.
7. Nicoson MC, Moran SL. Diagnosis and treatment of acute lunotriquetral ligament injuries. Hand Clin. 2015;31(3):467–76.
8. Shin A, Weinstein L, Berger R, Bishop A. Treatment of isolated injuries of the lunotriquetral ligament: a comparison of arthrodesis, ligament reconstruction and ligament repair. J Bone Joint Surg Br. 2001;83(7):1023–8.
9. Reagan DS, Linscheid RL, Dobyns JH. Lunotriquetral sprains. J Hand Surg Am. 1984;9(4):502–14.
10. Shahane SA, Trail IA, Takwale VJ, Stilwell JH, Stanley JK. Tenodesis of the extensor carpi ulnaris for chronic, post-traumatic lunotriquetral instability. J Bone Joint Surg Br. 2005;87(11):1512–5.
11. Pilný J, Svarc A, Perina M, Siller J, Visna P. Chronic lunotriquetral instability of the wrist. Presentation of our method of treatment. Acta Chir Orthop Traumatol Cechoslov. 2009;76(3):208–11.
12. Weiss AP, Sachar K, Glowacki KA. Arthroscopic debridement alone for intercarpal ligament tears. J Hand Surg Am. 1997;22(2):344–9.
13. Ritt MJ, Linscheid RL, Cooney WP 3rd, Berger RA, An KN. The lunotriquetral joint: kinematic effects of sequential ligament sectioning, ligament repair, and arthrodesis. J Hand Surg Am. 1998;23(3):432–45.

14. Westkaemper JG, Mitsionis G, Giannakopoulos PN, Sotereanos DG. Wrist arthroscopy for the treatment of ligament and triangular fibrocartilage complex injuries. Arthroscopy. 1998;14(5):479–83.
15. Favero K, Bishop A, Linscheid R. Lunotriquetral ligament disruption: a comparative study of treatment methods. Procs 46th Annual Meeting American Society for Surgery of the Hand. 1991.
16. Mirza A, Mirza JB, Shin AY, Lorenzana DJ, Lee BK, Izzo B. Isolated lunotriquetral ligament tears treated with ulnar shortening osteotomy. J Hand Surg Am. 2013;38(8):1492–7.

Chapter 27
Subacute Lunotriquetral Ligament Injury: Arthrodesis

Maureen O'Shaughnessy and Marco Rizzo

Case Presentation

A 57-year-old male presented with chronic, dorso-ulnar wrist pain and complaints of diminished grip. Exam showed a midcarpal clunk and positive Kleinman shear test. Radiographs demonstrated chronic cystic change within the lunate (Fig. 27.1a, b). This confirmed chronic lunotriquetral pathology with end-stage degenerative changes, yet preserved radiocarpal and midcarpal joint spaces.

M. O'Shaughnessy (✉)
University of Kentucky, Lexington, KY, USA

M. Rizzo
Mayo Clinic, Rochester, MN, USA
e-mail: rizzo.marco@mayo.edu

J. Yao (ed.), *Carpal Instability*, https://doi.org/10.1007/978-3-031-55869-6_27

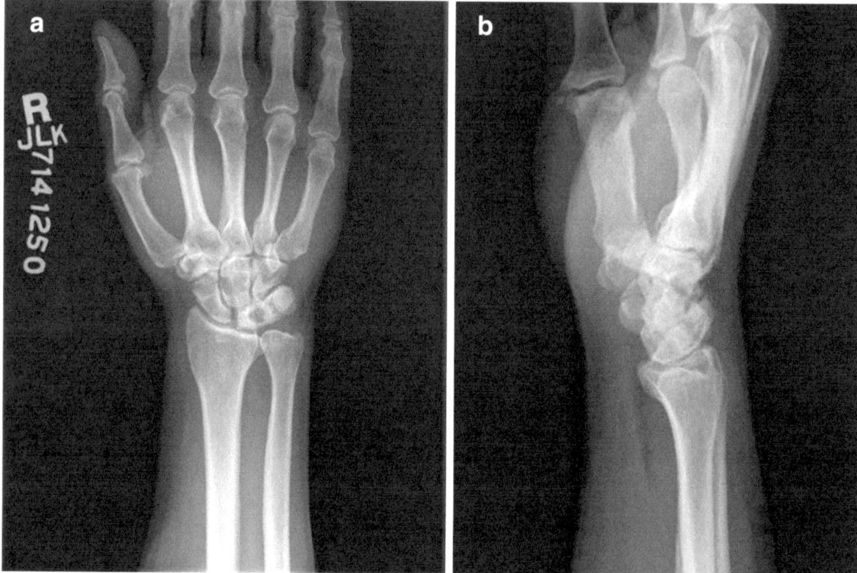

Fig. 27.1 Shows the PA (**a**) and lateral views (**b**) of patient with chronic dorso-ulnar wrist pain. Note the cystic, degenerative changes at the LT joint, with preserved LT angle and no evidence of VISI on the lateral

Diagnosis

Compared to SL injuries, LT injuries are less common and are often difficult to diagnose. Acute injury to the lunotriquetral interosseous ligament (LTIL) is often associated with injury to adjacent carpal ligaments and/or bones including a perilunate injury pattern. LT injury is also seen in ulnocarpal impaction syndrome and inflammatory disease.

Anatomic studies have shown that sectioning of the ligament leads to disruption of the intricate balance between the radiocarpal and midcarpal rows with a resultant extension of the lunate and flexion of the triquetrum, leading to VISI deformity [1]. When high-grade injury occurs, the lunate flexes palmarly leading to volar intercalated segmental instability (VISI) deformity of the wrist, leading to altered carpal kinematics. Anatomic studies have shown that the volar LTIL component is the primary stabilizer of the joint. Ritt et al. found that sectioning of the proximal and dorsal component of the LT ligament had little effect on carpal kinematics, but sectioning of the proximal and volar component of the LT ligament resulted in flexion of the lunate and triquetrum, producing a VISI pattern deformity [1].

The adjacent secondary stabilizers of the joint include the palmar radiotriquetral and dorsal radiocarpal ligaments. Over time, these secondary stabilizers also become incompetent leading to the resultant VISI deformity. However, even complete sectioning of the ligament typically does not lead to static divergence of the LT interval, making recognition on initial radiographs difficult and often leading to a delayed diagnosis [2].

Physical assessment should include a thorough history and physical. The clinical diagnosis of LT pathology is generally very subtle. Patients generally complain of ulnar sided wrist pain and reduced grip strength. In acute injuries, patients may report a fall onto a dorsiflexed wrist with the ulnar side being the primary site of impact. More chronic lesions endorse a vague generalized dorsal ulnar wrist pain without a concrete traumatic event.

Ulnar sided wrist pain has an extensive differential diagnosis that must be considered. In the acute setting, this includes TFCC injury, ECU pathology, extrinsic ligament injury, nerve entrapment, triquetral avulsion fractures, and pisotriquetral and distal radioulnar joint pathology. In the more chronic setting, additional factors to consider include all of the former in addition to ulnar impaction syndrome, congenital coalition, hamate arthrosis lunotriquetral ligament (HALT) lesion, and Kienbock's avascular necrosis.

In cases of LT injury or pathology, physical examination will often reveal pain with direct palpation and compression of the LT interval. There are several other described maneuvers. The triquetral compression test is performed by applying a radial directed force in the ulnar snuffbox and will elicit pain. The lunotriquetral shear (Kleinman shear) test is performed with the elbow flexed and the forearm in neutral position. The examiner stabilizes the radial carpus including the lunate in the nondominant hand and applies a shear to the triquetrum with the dominant hand in a palmar to dorsal direction. The force transmitted across the LT joint causes very precise pain. The Reagan shuck test is performed by stabilizing the radial wrist and carpus including the lunate in one hand, and the other hand supporting the pisiform and triquetrum. The two hands are shucked in opposite directions and elicit discomfort. The LT ballottement test includes stabilizing the lunate between the thumb and index of one hand while using the other hand to displace the triquetrum in a volar and dorsal direction. Comparison with the contralateral side is essential to differentiate congenital laxity from pathology.

Diagnostic studies include standard plain radiographs with true PA and lateral views; however, these are generally normal even in the case of a complete LTIL injury. Examination for subtle or dramatic disruption of Gilula's lines on the posterior-anterior wrist film can be helpful. The LT ligament may be widened on PA, although this is rarely seen. On the lateral view, VISI deformity can be seen with volar tilting of the lunate in relation to the capitolunate line, though this is more likely seen in chronic cases. The LT angle may be decreased on the lateral view.

Computed tomography (CT) scan can be considered, but not infrequently is nondiagnostic for ligament injury. In acute cases, fracture to the lunate and/or triquetrum may be identified that were missed on plain films. In more chronic cases, degenerative changes including cystic changes or cortical irregularity can be seen.

Magnetic resonance imaging (MRI) is particularly useful to evaluate the interosseous ligaments of the wrist. MRI may demonstrate changes in the LTIL; however, the frequency of missed injury is relatively high. Recent work by De Santis et al. compared MRI imaging with wrist arthroscopy for intrinsic wrist ligaments and TFCC injury detection and found that MRI failed to confirm LT ligament lesion in 70% of cases with positive arthroscopy [3]. Diagnostic wrist arthroscopy remains the gold standard for diagnosing and staging LT pathology and not only serves as a means of direct evaluation for making the diagnosis, but also provides an avenue for treatment [4].

Viegas et al. described a classification system for LT injury [5]. Grade I includes partial or incomplete tear without evidence of VISI deformity, grade II is complete tear with dynamic VISI, and grade III is complete tear with static VISI deformity. The Geissler classification system (I–IV) can also be applied to LT pathology based on findings at the time of arthroscopy [6].

Management Options

Initial management of the majority of LTIL lesions is nonoperative. Nonsurgical management including steroid injection, oral and topical nonsteroidal medications, bracing, casting, and hand therapy is attempted initially. When symptoms persist, surgical options may be considered. The choice of procedure is predicated on the degree of injury to the ligament, the chronicity of the injury, and the presence or absence of associated degenerative changes [4]. Goals of surgical repair or reconstruction focus on restoring equilibrium to the carpal kinematics.

Arthroscopy may be initially employed as the LT ligament and joint can be difficult to visualize and diagnose even with advanced MRI techniques, with false-negative rates approaching 70% [3]. Arthroscopy can help diagnose and stage the degree of tearing, as well as adjacent joint chondral changes, in addition to staging and possible treatment of other pathologies including ulnar impaction, proximal hamate arthrosis (HALT lesion), and TFCC injury. Diagnostic arthroscopy can answer questions regarding repairability of the ligament and quality of the cartilage before embarking upon a planned reconstruction or salvage procedure.

When a chronic, complete LT ligament injury is confirmed, surgical options considered include LT reconstruction, LT or other limited intercarpal fusion, arthroscopic debridement and/or temporary pinning, and more recently described ulnar shortening osteotomy. The intricacies of each technique and its unique risks and benefits are described in their respective chapters. The authors caution that in the case of any evidence of degenerative chondral changes noted within the ulnar midcarpal joint, a midcarpal fusion should be considered rather than limited LT fusion.

Management Chosen for This Case with Rationale

We discussed various surgical options including arthroscopy with debridement, ulnar shortening osteotomy, and limited arthrodesis procedures. After a thorough discussion, and given cystic changes noted in the lunate, this patient elected for an isolated LT fusion.

The theory behind LT fusion arises from the finding that patients with congenital coalition (fusion) of the joint have largely normal wrist motion and grip strength. The procedure was first described by Reagan and colleagues in 1984 [7]. The benefits of this technique include pain relief from fusion of a painful joint, in addition to the ability to control chronic instability and/or degenerative joint changes.

While reconstruction remains a viable option for joint salvage in cases of chronic LT pathology, fusion should also be considered. The authors find that the best indications for LT fusion are patients with chronic instability, joint space narrowing between the lunate and triquetrum, and/or cystic changes between the bones (as seen in this case).

Clinical Course and Outcome

The patient was taken to the operating room for planned LT arthrodesis. A dorsal longitudinal incision ulnar to Lister's tubercle was utilized. The retinaculum was elevated and capsule revealed. A ligament-sparing capsulotomy was performed to visualize the carpus.

Formal ligament-sparing capsulotomy was made, and the carpus was exposed. A critical step is to confirm suspected complete and chronic interosseous ligament tear, as well as evaluate the adjacent midcarpal and radiocarpal joint cartilage to ensure that no full-thickness chondral changes have developed that might lead to ongoing pain. The surgeon should discuss this with the patient preoperatively and have a shared plan in the event that intraoperative findings preclude planned limited LT fusion.

The LT interspace was carefully prepared, removing all remaining ligament and cartilage, followed by formal decortication and decompression of any cysts down to bleeding bone. Autograft may be harvested locally from the distal radius or at surgeon's preferred site. Allograft may also be considered. Careful attention to joint preparation and judicious selection and use of bone graft are keys to successful bony healing.

Any chronic VISI deformity is corrected using two K-wires as joysticks to reduce the LT interval. This is confirmed clinically and radiographically, ensuring that the lunate is in neutral flexion/extension. The preferred fixation construct is then used. The authors utilized Kirschner wires for this case as this was performed prior to the advent of more modern implants (Fig. 27.2a, b). However, other fixation techniques can be used including cannulated headless compression screws, staples, or plate fixation. The authors find that solid rigid internal fixation can allow earlier motion and potentially decrease risks of nonunion or malunion. One can consider using temporary stabilizing K-wires across the proximal and distal carpal rows to reduce strain across the fusing joint. These can be removed at 4–6 weeks postoperatively.

The patient is immobilized in a postoperative short arm splint for 2 weeks and then transitioned to a short arm cast or removable orthosis for an additional 4–8 weeks until evidence of clinical and/or radiographic healing, which is generally seen by the eighth week of postoperative visit. Strengthening commences when clinical and radiographic union of the arthrodesis is confirmed. This gentleman had the K-wires removed at 8 weeks after confirmation of appropriate healing, with final radiographs at 2.5 years post-surgery (Fig. 27.3a, b) showing a well-healed fusion.

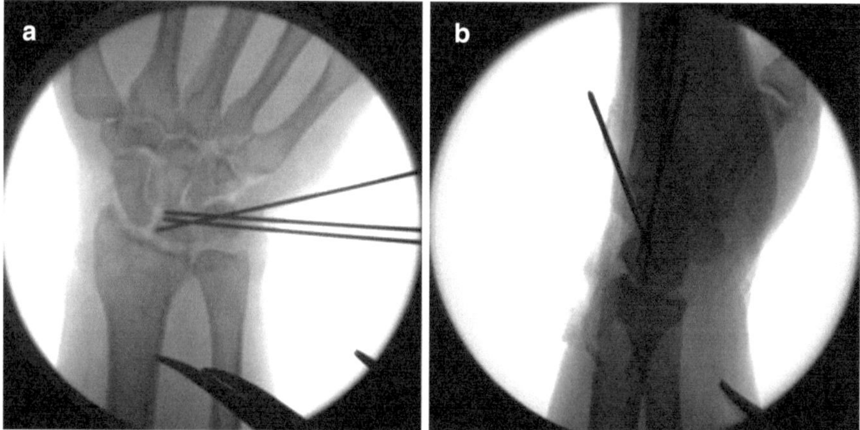

Fig. 27.2 Demonstrates the immediate postoperative PA (**a**) and lateral (**b**) showing pin fixation across prepared LT joint

Fig. 27.3 Shows the follow-up PA (**a**) and lateral (**b**) films of patient at the final follow-up showing successful consolidation of LT fusion, with maintained alignment of Gilula's arcs and no midcarpal or radiocarpal degenerative changes

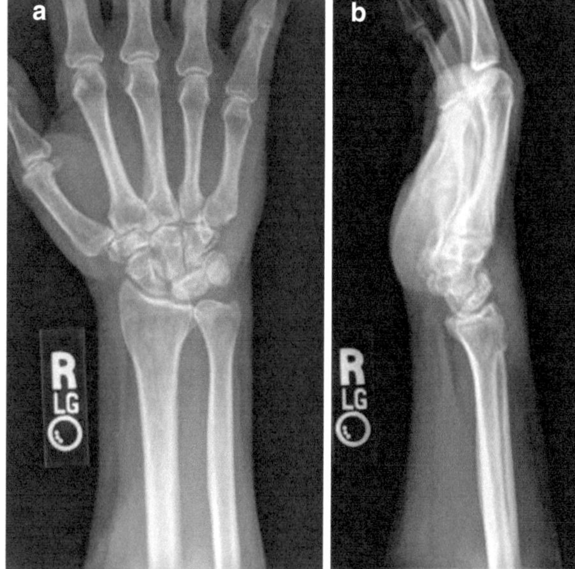

Bulleted Clinical Pearls/Pitfalls

- LTIL ligament injuries are less common, often hard to diagnose, and can lead to VISI deformity.
- Wrist arthroscopy can be considered to confirm a suspected diagnosis, as well as confirm staging of the tear with assessment of the degree of ligament injury and any associated chondral changes.

- LT fusion can be considered for patients with subacute to chronic, full-thickness tear who do not want to proceed with reconstruction attempt or with evidence of joint degeneration.
- In the presence of chondromalacia in the ulnar midcarpal joint, consideration should be given to four-corner fusion procedure.
- A paucity of literature exists regarding LTIL injuries, particularly in the chronic setting.
- Current limited evidence reports a comparatively higher rate of complications in the LT arthrodesis cohort; however, the authors feel that modern surgical techniques and implants may have more favorable outcomes than the historical reports.

Literature Review and Discussion

LT arthrodesis remains controversial with as many articles criticizing the technique [8–11] as favoring it [2, 12–15]. Critics cite relatively high nonunion rates, complication rates, and unreliable pain relief. In general, outcomes vary widely, and the reported outcomes and satisfaction are inconsistently measured. Heterogeneous surgical techniques, and fixation techniques, are reported. Nonunion after LT arthrodesis ranges from 0% [12, 14] to as high as 41% [9], 47%, [10], 50% [16], and 57% [8]. Complications are similarly heterogeneous and include symptomatic hardware, pin tract infection, nerve injury, nonunion, dorsal sensory nerve injury, and ulnocarpal impaction.

Shin et al. reported on a cohort study comparing outcomes of isolated LT injury with surgical management. The series included patients treated with repair ($n = 21$) or reconstruction of the ligament ($n = 8$), and arthrodesis ($n = 22$). Average follow-up was 9.5 years. The authors found a higher amount of complications and revision surgery in the fusion group. However, the cohort is heterogeneous, without controlling for age of patient and chronicity or severity of ligament injury, and the surgical management in the fusion cohort ranged from staples to screws to K-wires, making conclusions very limited.

Nickel et al. evaluated 28 patients over a 15-year period with distal radius autograft and single percutaneous headless compression screw fixation [2]. The series noted a union rate of 82% with average time to union of 8.8 weeks. Three patients (11%) developed radiographic nonunion but remained pain-free at the final follow-up. One patient (4%) with symptomatic nonunion was treated with four-corner fusion. No patients required removal of hardware. The senior author reports two key principles to the success of the operation:

1. Use of modern headless compression screws to provide strong compression.
2. Strong internal fixation and use of primary bone grafting using cancellous autograft at the time of fusion.

When successful, the benefits of LT fusion include pain relief and maintenance of carpal alignment. The authors find that the best indications for LT fusion are patients with chronic instability, joint space narrowing between the lunate and triquetrum, and/or cystic changes between the bones. Careful surgical precision is warranted to ensure appropriate joint preparation, judicious use of bone grafting, and, in the modern era, solid internal fixation.

Regarding the alternatives to LT fusion in the chronic setting, LT reconstruction can be considered when there is no evidence of degeneration or cystic changes in a patient desirous of attempt at reconstruction. Ulnar shortening osteotomy has emerged as an exciting alternative to fusion or reconstruction in cases of chronic LT pathology as it maintains motion and may potentially afford pain relief by unloading the pathologic joint.

In summary, LTIL injury remains a relatively infrequent injury, with a paucity of literature on the management and outcomes in these patients. The literature on LT fusion is limited to small case series given the rarity of the pathology, limiting any conclusions that can be made. Additionally, most of the articles report heterogeneous surgical methods including type of internal fixation and use of bone graft. The authors feel that the more modern series demonstrating relatively high union and satisfaction rate likely more accurately reflect our current understanding of surgical techniques and indications for LT fusion. Additional long-term outcome data is warranted to understand the appropriate surgical indications and expected outcomes of the various management techniques, including LT arthrodesis.

References

1. Ritt MJPF, et al. The lunotriquetral joint: kinematic effects of sequential ligament sectioning, ligament repair, and arthrodesis. J Hand Surg Am. 1998;23(3):432–45.
2. Nickel KJ, Curran MWT, Morhart M. Revisiting lunotriquetral arthrodesis in chronic lunotriquetral ligamentous injuries. J Wrist Surg. 2022;11(06):479–83. https://doi.org/10.1055/s-0041-1742205.
3. De Santis S, et al. Comparison between MRI and arthroscopy of the wrist for the assessment of posttraumatic lesions of intrinsic ligaments and the triangular fibrocartilage complex. J Wrist Surg. 2022;11(01):028–34. https://doi.org/10.1055/s-0041-1729757.
4. Wilson MS. Diagnosis and Management of Lunotriquetral Ligament Injuries. Curr Rev Musculoskelet Med. 2023;16(2):55–9. https://doi.org/10.1007/s12178-022-09819-7.
5. Viegas SF, et al. Ulnar-sided perilunate instability: an anatomic and biomechanic study. J Hand Surg Am. 1990;15(2):268–78. https://doi.org/10.1016/0363-5023(90)90107-3.
6. Geissler WB, et al. Intracarpal soft-tissue lesions associated with an intra-articular fracture of the distal end of the radius. J Bone Joint Surg. 1996;78(3):357–65. https://doi.org/10.2106/00004623-199603000-00006.
7. Reagan DS, Linscheid RL, Dobyns JH. Lunotriquetral sprains. J Hand Surg Am. 1984;9(4):502–14. https://doi.org/10.1016/S0363-5023(84)80101-X.
8. Sennwald GR, Fischer M, Mondi P. Lunotriquetral arthrodesis: a controversial procedure. J Hand Surg Br Eur. 1995;20(6):755–60.

9. Shin AY, et al. Treatment of isolated injuries of the lunotriquetral ligament. A comparison of arthrodesis, ligament reconstruction and ligament repair. J Bone Joint Surg (Br). 2001;83(7):1023–31.
10. De Smet L, Janssens I, Van De Sande W. Chronic lunotriquetral ligament injuries: arthrodesis or capsulodesis. Acta Chir Belg. 2005;105(1):79–81. https://doi.org/10.1080/00015458.2005.11679671.
11. Vandesande W, De Smet L, Van Ransbeeck H. Lunotriquetral arthrodesis, a procedure with a high failure rate. Acta Orthop Belg. 2001;67(4):361–7.
12. Guidera PM, et al. Lunotriquetral arthrodesis using cancellous bone graft. J Hand Surg. 2001;26(3):422–7. https://doi.org/10.1053/jhsu.2001.24969.
13. Nelson DL, et al. Lunotriquetral arthrodesis. J Hand Surg. 1993;18A:1113–20.
14. Pin PG, et al. Management of chronic lunotriquetral ligament tears. J Hand Surg. 1989;14(1):77–83. https://doi.org/10.1016/0363-5023(89)90062-2.
15. Wagner ER, Elhassan BT, Rizzo M. Diagnosis and treatment of chronic lunotriquetral ligament injuries. Hand Clin. 2015;31(3):477–86. https://doi.org/10.1016/j.hcl.2015.04.006.
16. McAuliffe JA, Dell PC, Jaffe R. Complications of intercarpal arthrodesis. J Hand Surg Am. 1993;18(6):1121–8. https://doi.org/10.1016/0363-5023(93)90413-W.

Further Reading

De Santis S, et al. Comparison between MRI and arthroscopy of the wrist for the assessment of posttraumatic lesions of intrinsic ligaments and the triangular fibrocartilage complex. J Wrist Surg. 2022;11(01):028–34. https://doi.org/10.1055/s-0041-1729757.
Nickel KJ, Curran MWT, Morhart M. Revisiting lunotriquetral arthrodesis in chronic lunotriquetral ligamentous injuries. J Wrist Surg. 2022;11(06):479–83. https://doi.org/10.1055/s-0041-1742205.
Wagner ER, Elhassan BT, Rizzo M. Diagnosis and treatment of chronic lunotriquetral ligament injuries. Hand Clin. 2015;31(3):477–86. https://doi.org/10.1016/j.hcl.2015.04.006.
Wilson MS. Diagnosis and management of lunotriquetral ligament injuries. Curr Rev Musculoskelet Med. 2023;16(2):55–9. https://doi.org/10.1007/s12178-022-09819-7.

Chapter 28
Management of Chronic Lunotriquetral Intercarpal Ligament Injuries

Spencer B. Chambers and Eric R. Wagner

Introduction

The lunotriquetral (LT) interosseous ligament creates an equilibrium of forces on the lunate with the scapholunate (SL) interosseous ligament, between the extension moment of the triquetrum (transmitted through the LT ligament) and the flexion moment of the scaphoid (transmitted through the SL ligament) [1]. The most critical aspect involves the volar LT ligament that is associated with the volar ulnocapitate and ulnolunate ligaments, transmitting the extension moment of the triquetrum when it engages the hamate [2, 3]. The secondary stabilizers of the LT ligament include the thinner dorsal LT ligament, as well as the radiotriquetral, radioscapholunate, and radiolunate ligaments [2, 4]. The pathologic process underlying LT injuries is not as well understood as the SL injuries, but thought to occur in the acute setting from a fall on a pronated and radially deviated wrist in flexion [5] or in the chronic setting from ulnocarpal impaction [6, 7]. Both of these processes place stress on the volar LT ligament, as well as the extrinsic ulnocapitate ligament. Therefore, although there are many treatment options for LT injuries, including LT arthrodesis [8–10], debridement [11, 12], capsulodesis [13], repair [8], and reconstruction [8, 14], the ulnar shortening osteotomy (USO) [3, 15] should be another consideration. We present a case in which a patient was successfully treated with an ulnar shortening osteotomy after prior attempts at arthroscopic debridement and open repair of the ligament.

S. B. Chambers
Department of Plastic and Reconstructive Surgery, St. Joseph's Hand and Upper Limb Clinic, Western University, London, ON, Canada

E. R. Wagner (✉)
Department of Orthopaedic Surgery, Emory University, Upper Extremity Center, Atlanta, GA, USA
e-mail: eric.r.wagner@emory.edu

J. Yao (ed.), *Carpal Instability*, https://doi.org/10.1007/978-3-031-55869-6_28

Case Presentation (Diagnosis and Evaluation)

A 42-year-old right-hand-dominant male presented with a 3-year history of bilateral ulnar sided wrist pain that radiates into the forearm, with the right side worse than the left. The pain is dull, constant, and exacerbated by activities such as playing tennis and golf, as well as typing on the computer. It improves with rest. There are no complaints of numbness, tingling, crepitus, or snapping with wrist motion. The patient is otherwise well, denies smoking, and works as an airline pilot.

The patient had previously trialed immobilization for over 6 months, including a 3-month protocol focused on stabilizing the LT through extensor carpi ulnaris (ECU) strengthening [16]. He also underwent injections with both corticosteroids and platelet-rich plasma at an outside institution without improvement. He previously underwent an LT arthroscopic debridement of the LT and repair of the triangular fibrocartilage complex (TFCC) repair 3 years prior, and then an open LT repair 18 months prior at outside institutions. Neither of these procedures were associated with any improvement in his wrist symptoms.

On examination, he had pain associated with the palpation of the dorsal LT ligament, with pain associated with the shear test. There was also pain localized to the LT interval in pronation and ulnar deviation. Plain radiographs did not demonstrate any LT widening or volar intercalated segment instability (VISI), with neutral ulnar variance (Fig. 28.1). MRI and CT images were carried out at another establishment

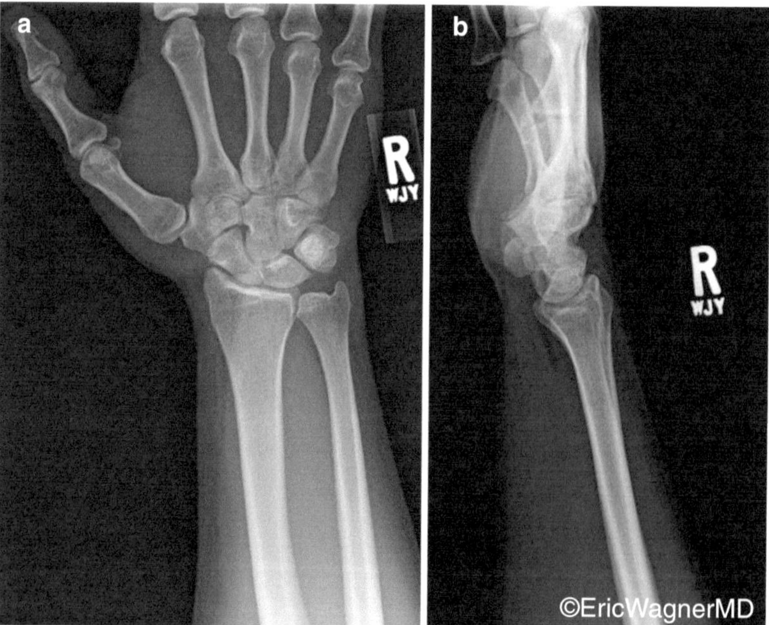

Fig. 28.1 Preoperative radiographs. Anterior-posterior (**a**) and lateral (**b**) radiographs demonstrating a neutral ulnar variance and no occult evidence of arthritic changes or malalignment within the carpus

and were not available, but reports noted that maintained carpal alignment increased signal at the ulnocarpal joint and LTIL. Nerve conductive studies had also been deemed normal. The patient also underwent an ultrasound-guided lidocaine injection to the LT articulation, which relieved 90% of his symptoms in clinic.

Diagnosis of LT Injuries

The differential diagnosis for chronic ulnar sided wrist pain is extensive (Table 28.1) [17]. There is considerable crossover in clinical examination of many causes, making accurate diagnosis challenging and requiring a high index of suspicion for the identification of lunotriquetral intercarpal ligament (LTIL) injuries.

Table 28.1 Various provocative tests for pathologies causing ulnar sided wrist pain. The differential diagnosis for ulnar sided wrist pain is broad, and accurate clinical exam and diagnostics tests are required to accurately assess for LTIL injury

Pathology	Provocative testing
Tendon and ligamentous	
Lunotriquetral ligament injury	• Tenderness to palpation over LT interval • Shuck test • Shear test • Pain with LT compression
Triangular fibrocartilage complex injury	• Foveal tenderness • Ballottement test • Piano key sign • Compression test
Extensor carpi ulnaris tendonitis	• Synergy test • Pain with resisted wrist extension • Pain with supination and ulnar deviation
Osseus	
Pisotriquetral arthritis	• PT Shuck test • Pisiform compression • Resisted wrist flexion
Distal radial ulnar joint arthritis	• Ballottement test • Piano key sign • Compression test • Grind test
Ulnar styloid fracture/malunion	• Foveal tenderness
Hamate fracture	• Ulnar nerve paresthesia • Pain on palpation
Neurovascular	
Ulnar nerve neuritis	• Sensory changes to fourth and fifth digits
Ulnar artery thrombosis	• Intrinsic hand weakness • Sensory changes to fourth and fifth digits • Pain over Guyon's canal
Ulnar artery aneurysm in Guyon's canal	• Intrinsic hand weakness • Sensory changes to fourth and fifth digits • Pain over Guyon's canal

Physical Assessment/Relevant Maneuvers

Assessment for LTIL injuries begins with a comprehensive evaluation of the total upper limb. Visual deformities, range of motion, strength, and neurovascular status are noted in a standard fashion. Specific provocative tests from the LTIL include dorsal LT tenderness through manual palpation, as well as a palpable clunk with ulnar deviation and pronation (ballottement test) [18]. The LT shear test can also be used to elicit pain through shucking the triquetrum and lunate separately [19].

Diagnostic Studies

Plain-film radiographs of both wrists are the preliminary investigation in all cases. In the case of LT disruptions, chronic injuries may demonstrate carpal malalignment with proximal and ulnar displacement of the triquetrum with associated extension of the lunate (VISI). However, often signs are more subtle, and these findings tend to manifest only in long-standing injuries after attenuation of the secondary stabilizers. To extenuate minor anomalies, grip views and dynamic radiographs during radial-ulnar deviation are helpful, but more advanced imaging is typically indicated.

Computed tomography or magnetic resonance imaging assists in revealing subtle carpal alignment changes, and MRI may demonstrate soft tissue edema without the ligament or LT articulation, and ligamentous discontinuity. If all diagnostic tests are negative but clinically the patient is symptomatic, diagnostic injections can help identify anatomic causes of pain. When all other tests have failed, arthroscopy remains the gold standard for assessment of ligamentous injury within the wrist including the LTIL (Fig. 28.2) and TFCC (Fig. 28.3).

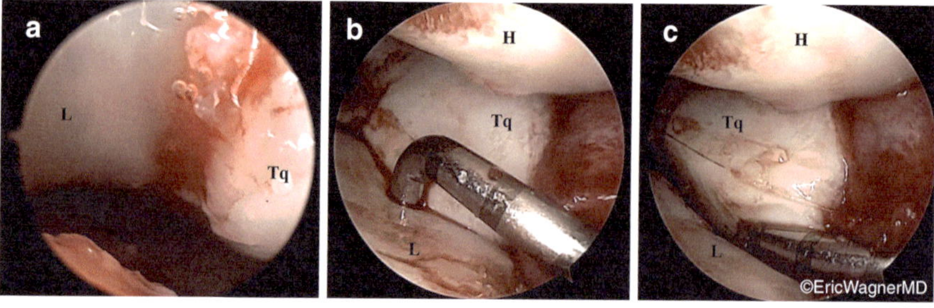

Fig. 28.2 Arthroscopic assessment of lunotriquetral intercarpal ligament stability. Assessing the lunotriquetral intercarpal ligament involves visual assessment in the radial-carpal joint (**a**) in addition to testing from the midcarpal joint (**a** and **b**). Viewing from the radial midcarpal portal the interval between the lunate (L) and triquetrum (Tq) is visualized (**a**) and an arthroscopic probe is inserted to assess gapping and stability (**b**). Hamate (H). The probe is able to be twisted (**c**)

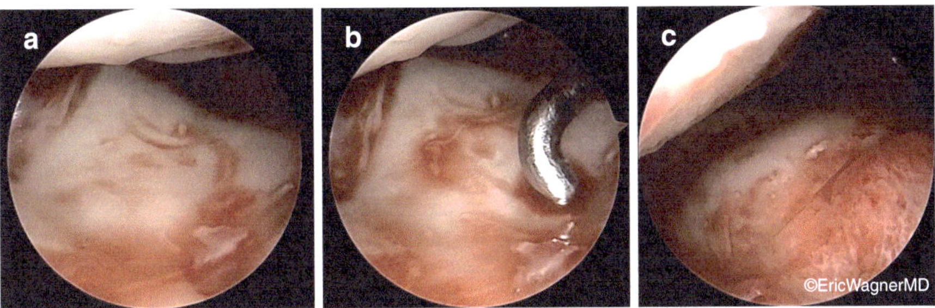

Fig. 28.3 Arthroscopic triangular-fibrocartilage complex assessment. Triangular fibrocartilage complex (TFCC) injuries can independently cause ulnar sided wrist pain and mimic lunotriquetral intercarpal ligament instability. TFCC assessment with MRI is sensitive but arthroscopic examination is specific (**a**). Viewing from a dorsal radial portal a trampoline test (**b**) is used to test the tightness of the ligament and a hook test (**c**) is performed by inserting an arthroscopic hook deep to the TFCC to assess foveal attachments

Case Presentation (Treatment and Outcome)

In the presented case, the patient had previously undergone arthroscopic TFCC debridement and attempted repair in addition to numerous injections without durable symptom relief. Diagnostic imaging was limited and nonspecific, given postsurgical changes and negative nerve studies and chronicity of pain pointed to ligamentous instability of the LTIL as a likely cause. The patient was offered arthroscopic evaluation of the joint in addition to an LTIL reconstruction versus an ulnar shortening osteotomy (USO) if the ligament was confirmed to be torn. Given the prior failures of arthroscopic interventions, the patient opted for an USO without arthroscopy. Although we generally recommend wrist arthroscopy in addition to USO as we do feel that a volar and/or dorsal capsulodesis can augment the benefits of the USO, in the setting of a prior failed repair, this is not always necessary. In the setting of chronic LTIL instability, USO is thought to restore stability to the triquetrum through tightening of ulnocapitate, ulnotriquetral, and ulnolunate ligaments that works in conjunction with the thick volar LT ligament [2, 3, 20], while also off-loading the ulnocarpal joint and pressure on the LT articulation [2, 3].

The USO was performed using a direct ulnar approach, placing the plate volarly on the ulna (Figs. 28.4 and 28.5). We prefer the volar to dorsal or lateral plate positioning as it allows the bulky flexor tendon muscles to pad the plate. However, in someone who is skinnier and types a lot on the computer, then a dorsal plate can be considered. We targeted 2–3 mm of shortening based on biomechanical studies suggesting that 2 mm is enough to tighten the extrinsic ulnar sided ligament stabilizers [20]. When dissecting around the osteotomy site, we prefer avoiding electrocautery, using a surgical knife to expose the site and to facilitate the removal of the sliver of bone. For a uniform cut, we use the cutting

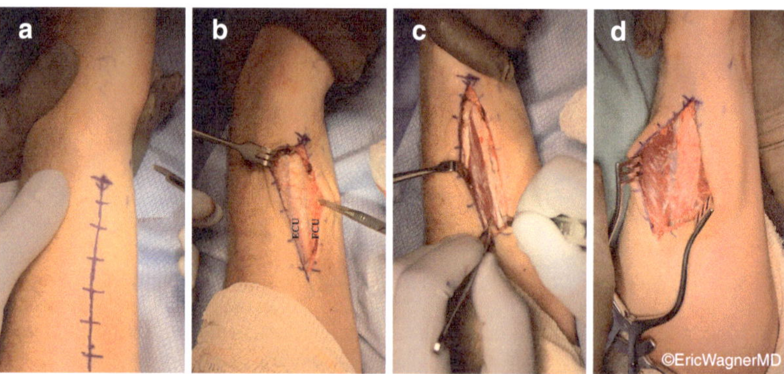

Fig. 28.4 Surgical approach and exposure of ulna for shortening osteotomy. Under tourniquet control the arm is positioned with the hand elevated and a 7–8 cm incision is marked over the border of the ulna (**a**). Subcutaneous dissection progresses, taking care to identify and protect any branches of the dorsal sensory branch (**b**). The extensor carpi ulnaris (ECU) and flexor carpi ulnaris (FCU) are identified and an interval between is developed (**b** and **c**) to approach the ulna (*) which is stripped of soft tissues (**d**)

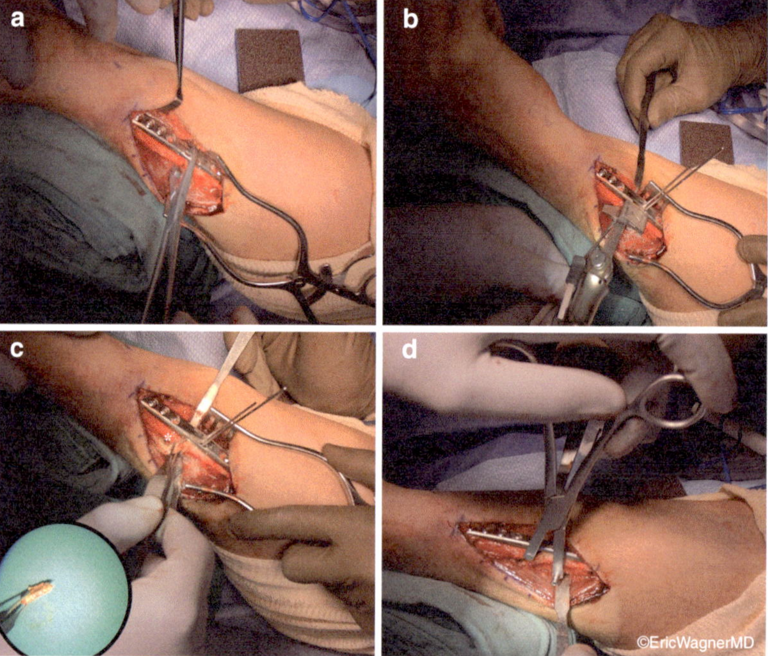

Fig. 28.5 Plate assisted ulnar shortening osteotomy. After exposure of the ulna is complete, the arm is positioned on an arm table and plate provisionally placed with the assistance of fluoroscopy (**a**). All distal screws are secured as well as a proximal screw in the gliding hole prior to securing the cutting jig with Kirshner wires. The osteotomy is carried out with a sagittal saw (**b**). A second osteotomy is created after adjusting the cutting jig before removing the wafer (*) and ensuring the osteotomy is complete (**c**). The ulna is shortened and compressed prior to securing the remaining proximal screws and ensuring reduction is maintained (**d**)

block and a sagittal saw. For maximal compression, when placing the lag screw, we clamp the bone to the plate to help improve the overall compression into the "axilla" formed by the bone and the plate.

Following USO, the patient's wrist was immobilized for 2 weeks in a sugar tong splint, and then another 4 weeks in a forearm Muenster cast while encouraging digital motion. Typical postoperative healing without complication ensued and at 6 weeks was transitioned to forearm-based splints for an additional 2 weeks (Fig. 28.6). At the completion of 2 months of immobilization, the patient began physical therapy focused on wrist mobilization and strengthening. By 12 weeks, the patient's pain and motion were significantly improved, and strengthening and range-of-motion exercises were initiated (Fig. 28.7). At 12 months postoperatively, the patient was extremely pleased with the outcome, with a VAS score of 0/10, wrist subjective value of 90%, and DASH score of 5. He ultimately requested a USO be carried out on the contralateral side for similar LT-related symptoms and pathology (Fig. 28.8). In this case, we elected to perform the osteotomy more proximally, as the patient felt the distal aspect of the prior plate.

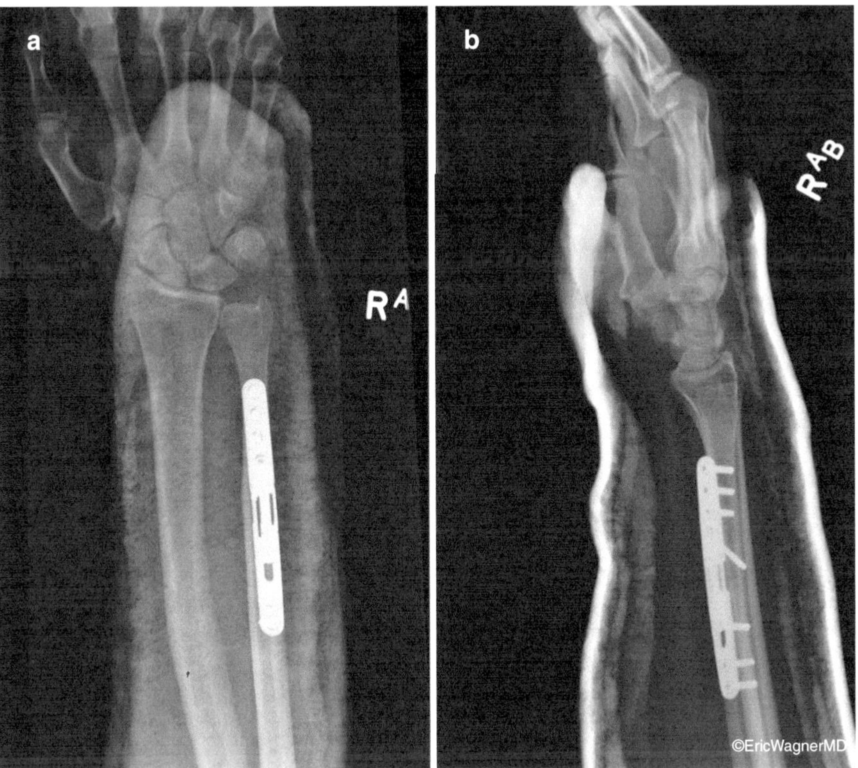

Fig. 28.6 Postoperative radiographs after ulnar shortening osteotomy. Anterior-posterior (**a**) and lateral (**b**) radiographs demonstrating a negative ulnar variance with volar plate in-situ

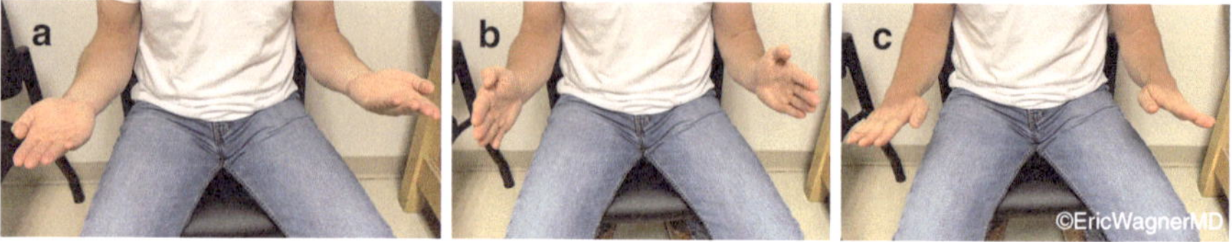

Fig. 28.7 Postoperative motion at 3 months. After 6 weeks of cast-immobilization range of motion rehabilitation with physiotherapy begins. This patient obtained full painless range of motion from supination (**a**), neutral (**b**), and pronation (**c**)

Fig. 28.8 Postoperative radiographs of bilateral ulnar shortening osteotomies. After significant symptom relief on the right side (**b**) the patient requested ulnar shortening on the left for similar pain and LT symptoms (**a**)

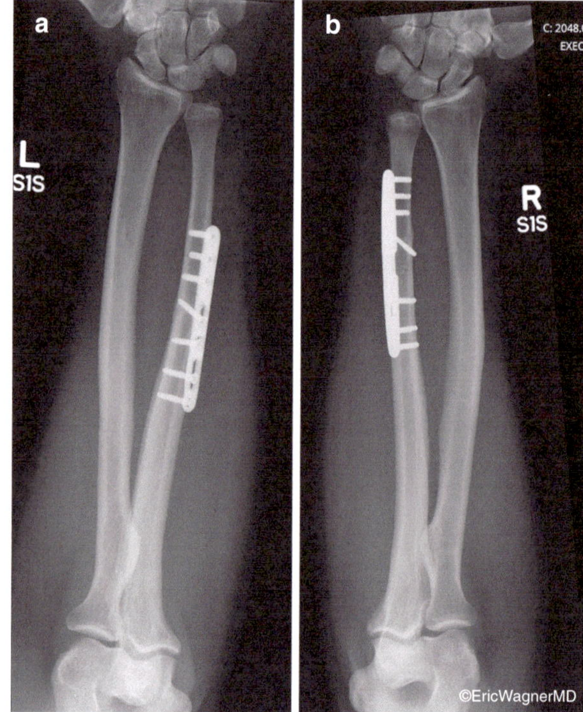

Review of LT Treatment Options

Management of chronic LTIL injuries includes various nonoperative and surgical interventions. Stepwise management is prudent with appropriate patient expectations as recovery and immobilization can be prolonged.

Conservative Management

Acute LT injuries can be treated with oral anti-inflammatories and wrist immobilization for 8–12 weeks [21]. The duration of immobilization and healing potential of chronic injuries are not known. Although this has shown promise in the acute setting, the outcomes of conservative management in the chronic setting are more guarded with successful outcomes as low as 25% [18]. In the chronic setting, we advocate trials of ultrasound-guided injections with corticosteroids, but the utility of this intervention is not well reported. Furthermore, physical therapy regimens focused on strengthening the extensor carpi ulnaris (ECU) with proprioception training have the potential to stabilize the LT joint and improve the patient's symptoms [16]. As demonstrated in the study by Leon-Lopez et al., sectioning of the LT ligament leads to flexion and supination of the triquetrum [16]. However, the ECU is able to reverse this process, exhibiting an extension and supination moment on the triquetrum. Thus, focusing on strengthening and retraining the ECU to fire during various wrist-loading activities has the potential to improve symptoms associated with LT insufficiency.

Operative Management

After failure of conservative measures, chronic LT injuries may be addressed with various surgical interventions including LT arthrodesis [8–10], debridement [11, 12], capsulodesis [13], repair [8], reconstruction [8, 14], and ulnar shortening osteotomy (USO) [3, 15]. The primary goal is to re-establish the balance of the proximal carpal row, stabilizing the lunate [17, 21]. Classic descriptions of these interventions involve an open approach, but more recently arthroscopic techniques have been described [22]. When restoring balance is not feasible by restoring the primary LT stabilizers, joint denervation, partial wrist arthrodesis, or proximal row carpectomy may be considered [15, 23].

LT Debridement, Repair, and/or Capsulodesis

The outcomes of LT pathologies are not as well studied as their SL counterparts. Arthroscopic debridement alone has variable outcomes, with some studies showing promise [11], while others showing poor outcomes [12]. Primary repair of the LT ligament is considered when there is no static VISI or LT widening. In the setting of dynamic instability with a structurally intact volar ligament, dorsal repair alone [7, 18, 24], or in combination with a dorsal capsulodesis [24], has shown promise. Dorsal capsulodesis alone has also shown promise in case series with a structurally intact volar ligament alone [10, 13, 25].

However, there remains a paucity of studies examining the long-term outcomes of dorsal repair or capsulodesis. In a comparison study to LT reconstruction and LT arthrodesis, LT repair had only a 23% survival free of reoperation rate at 5 years [8]. Thus, attempted treatment focusing only on the dorsal stabilizing structures will not be successful unless the volar structures remain intact, thus enabling an anatomic restoration of motion between the lunate and triquetrum.

LT Reconstruction and Arthrodesis

When there is a combined volar and dorsal LT pathology, or those with reducible VISI or LT interval gapping, LT reconstruction has shown promising potential [5, 8, 14, 18, 24, 25]. The two primary methods described involved either an LT tenodesis using ECU [14] or the extensor retinaculum [25]. However, both of these techniques are dependent on a reducible LT joint, ideally in an isolated LT pathologic state as confounding concomitant injuries lead to poor outcomes [14, 25].

LT arthrodesis is another option to treat LT pathologies, particularly if there is concern for the reducibility of the LT articulation. Although initial reports were promising [9, 26], subsequent studies showed high rates of nonunion, ulnocarpal impingement, and variable pain relief [8, 10, 18]. The ideal candidate for LT arthrodesis is still unknown and where it should fit in the therapeutic algorithm.

One study compared LT repair ($n = 27$), LT reconstruction with a distally based ECU tenodesis ($n = 8$), and LT arthrodesis ($n = 22$) [8]. At 5 years, the predicted probability of a complication for reconstructions, repairs, and arthrodesis was 31%, 86%, and 99%, respectively, while the probability of a required revision procedure was 31%, 77%, and 79%, respectively. Clinical outcomes were better for repairs or reconstructions than arthrodesis. Re-rupture rates after repair were the highest in high-demand laborers and athletes.

LT Arthroscopic Treatment

With advances in arthroscopic management of carpal injuries, chronic LTIL instability can also be addressed using minimally invasive techniques. Haugstvedt described an arthroscopic assisted version of the classic technique that limits disruption of capsular ligaments. Using intra-articular visualization of the lunate and triquetrum, bone tunnels can be accurately created [22]. A slip of extensor carpi ulnaris (ECU) is then harvested and passed through this tunnel before being secured with interference screws after ensuring reduction using fluoroscopic and arthroscopic guidance. Although novel, early outcomes are promising with symptomatic relief in two patients at almost 3 years described in this series. Alternatively, in partial injuries where a remnant of the LTIL is present, it is the practice of the senior author to carry out a suture-based capsuloligamentous repair arthroscopically. This involves standard dorsal arthroscopic portals in addition to exposure of the volar ulnar wrist capsule by developing an interval between the flexor carpi ulnaris (FCU) and carpal tunnel (Fig. 28.9). With complete exposure, shuttling sutures are passed from volar to dorsal beginning in the radiocarpal joint and through the LT ligament remnant before being retrieved from the midcarpal joint (Fig. 28.10). A nonabsorbable braided suture is then passed using these shuttling sutures while capturing dorsal capsule to create a ligament repair augmented by capsule for stability.

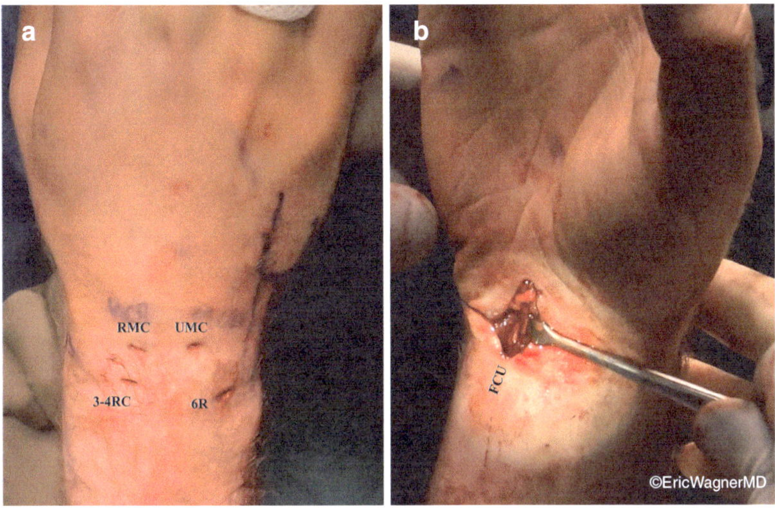

Fig. 28.9 Arthroscopic Assisted Lunotriquetral Intercarpal Ligament (LTIL) Repair Incisions. (**a**) Prior to repair the LTIL is assessed arthroscopically from the radiocarpal joint using the 3–4 radiocarpal (3–4RC) and 6 radial (6R) portals. The ligament is additionally tested using the radial and ulnar midcarpal portals (RMC, UMC). (**b**) If repair or reconstruction is needed, a volar incision over flexor carpi ulnaris (FCU) is made to expose the volar wrist capsule, protecting the neurovascular structures

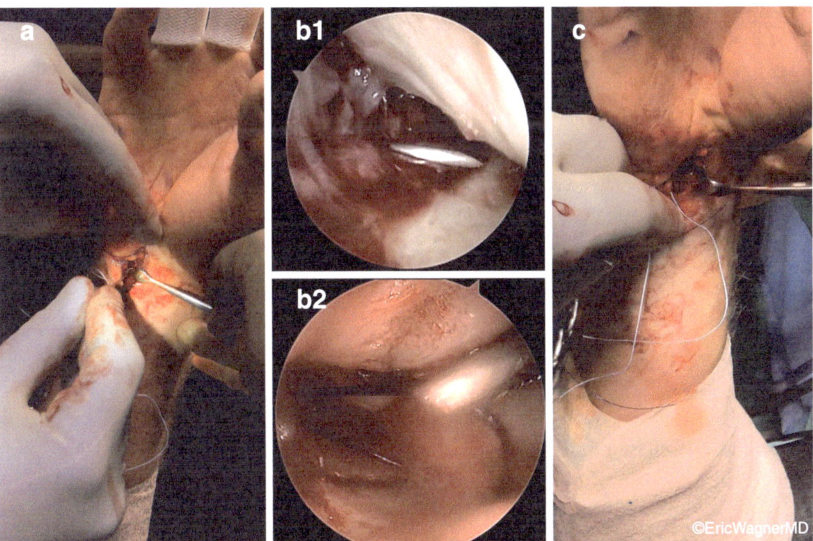

Fig. 28.10 Suture placement for LTIL repair. After assessment and exposure monofilament passing sutures can be introduced into the radiocarpal joint from the volar incision using 22-gauge needles under arthroscopic guidance (**a** and **b1**). This suture is then oriented distal into the midcarpal joint while capturing the ulnar aspect of the LTIL and is then retrieved with an arthroscopic grasper (**b2**). A second suture is placed in a similar fashion on the radial aspect of the LTIL and together these shuttling sutures are used to place a non-absorbable braided suture (**c**) that will be tied volarly, capturing the LTIL and dorsal capsule creating a capsuloligamentous repair

Ulnar Shortening Osteotomy

The ulnar shortening osteotomy remains a viable alternative for patients with chronic LT pathologies with a maintained LT articulation and no mechanical malalignment. There are two reasons why this treatment is effective:

1. Extrinsic and volar LT ligaments: Shortening the ulna tensions the critical volar extrinsic ligaments, the ulnocapitate, ulnolunate, and ulnotriquetral ligaments, that work in conjunction with the critical volar LT ligament. These act together to transmit the extension moment of the triquetrum on the lunate, after the triquetrum engages the hamate [2]. The USO reduces the strain of the LT ligament by tensioning the volar extrinsic ligaments and improving their ability to stabilize the LT biomechanics [3].
2. Off-loading the LT articulation: By reducing ulnar positive or even neutral variance, the forces transmitted through the triquetrum during ulnar deviation are reduced, thus off-loading the pressure on the LT ligament and secondary stabilizers [3].

The ulnar shortening osteotomy requires the LT articulation to be reduced without mechanical malalignment, given its dependence on the secondary extrinsic stabilizers. However, it is a powerful tool for treating LT injuries, particularly those not responsive to other procedures. In a study of 53 patients with post-traumatic LT pathologies, ulnar shortening osteotomy led to excellent or good outcomes in 83% of patients [15]. We ultimately decided against a revision LT repair given the prior failure of an open repair and concern for ligament tissue quality, and given that there was no static deformity we did not feel that a reconstruction or arthrodesis was necessary. Alternatively, the USO offered an option to augment the LT stability using the volar extrinsic ligaments, thus not having to rely on previously operated ligament tissue.

Bulleted Clinical Pearls/Pitfalls

Pearls

Ulnar Shortening Osteotomy

- Obtain neutral films of the wrist with the shoulder abducted to 90° and elbow flexed at 90° to ensure that a true ulnar variance is obtained.
- A reduced LT articulation is required without static LT widening or VISI.
- An ultrasound-guided injection of lidocaine into the LT articulation can be helpful to rule in or out LT pathologies at the location of the patient's ulnar sided wrist pain.
- A shortening of 2 mm is biomechanically sufficient to unload the ulnocarpal joint and tighten the extrinsic stabilizers [20].
- Placement of the plate on the volar surface of the ulna underneath the flexor muscles can minimize symptomatic hardware prominence. Low-BMI patients should be counselled preoperatively of the possibility of requiring hardware removed secondarily.

- Wrist arthroscopy can be combined with USO, particularly if there is a history of no prior surgical treatments, as a volar or dorsal LT repair and/or capsulodesis can be a helpful augmentation to stabilize the LT articulation.
- Prolonged immobilization may be required to ensure ulnar osteotomy healing, and the patient must be cooperative to avoid nonunion. If there is no clear radiographic healing by or before 3 months, we obtain a CT scan to evaluate the osteotomy healing potential. If there is <50% cortical healing, we continue lifting restrictions until the 4-month time point.

Pitfalls

Ulnar Shortening Osteotomy

- The dorsal sensory branch of the ulnar nerve may be encountered in the distal aspect of the incision and must be protected (Fig. 28.11).

Fig. 28.11 Ulnar dorsal sensory branch. In the distal extent of the incision of the subcutaneous approach to the ulna the crossing location of the dorsal sensory branch (white arrows) of the ulnar nerve is variable and care must be taken to identify and protect this structure

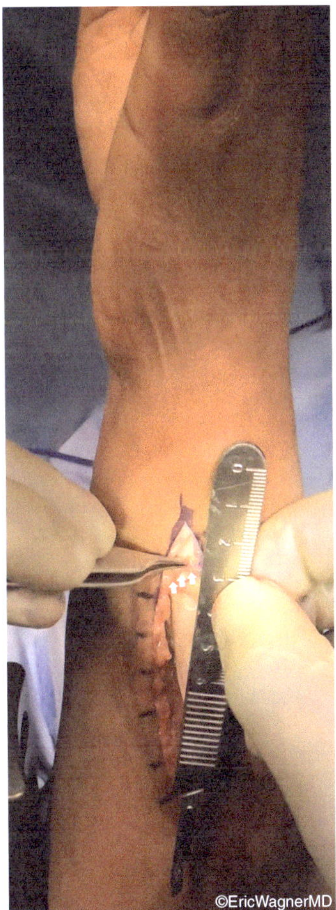

- Rotational control of the proximal and distal ulnar shaft must be maintained during the osteotomy. If not using a plate or jig when carrying out the osteotomy, a longitudinal line can be made on the diaphysis prior to the osteotomy. Preserved forearm rotation should be assessed during preliminary fixation if there are any concerns intraoperatively.

References

1. Kaufmann RA, Pfaeffle HJ, Blankenhorn BD, Stabile K, Robertson D, Goitz R. Kinematics of the midcarpal and radiocarpal joint in flexion and extension: an in vitro study. J Hand Surg Am. 2006;31(7):1142–8.
2. Ritt MJ, Bishop AT, Berger RA, Linscheid RL, Berglund LJ, An KN. Lunotriquetral ligament properties: a comparison of three anatomic subregions. J Hand Surg Am. 1998;23(3):425–31. Epub 1998/06/10
3. Gupta R, Bingenheimer E, Fornalski S, McGarry MH, Osterman AL, Lee TQ. The effect of ulnar shortening on lunate and triquetrum motion—a cadaveric study. Clin Biomech (Bristol, Avon). 2005;20(8):839–45.
4. Trumble TE, Bour CJ, Smith RJ, Glisson RR. Kinematics of the ulnar carpus related to the volar intercalated segment instability pattern. J Hand Surg Am. 1990;15(3):384–92.
5. Shin AY, Deitch MA, Sachar K, Boyer MI. Ulnar-sided wrist pain: diagnosis and treatment. Instr Course Lect. 2005;54:115–28. Epub 2005/06/14
6. Palmer AK. Triangular fibrocartilage complex lesions: a classification. J Hand Surg Am. 1989;14(4):594–606. Epub 1989/07/01
7. Palmer AK, Werner FW. Biomechanics of the distal radioulnar joint. Clin Orthop Relat Res. 1984;187:26–35. Epub 1984/07/01
8. Shin AY, Weinstein LP, Berger RA, Bishop AT. Treatment of isolated injuries of the lunotriquetral ligament. A comparison of arthrodesis, ligament reconstruction and ligament repair. J Bone Joint Surg Br. 2001;83(7):1023–8. Epub 2001/10/18
9. Nelson DL, Manske PR, Pruitt DL, Gilula LA, Martin RA. Lunotriquetral arthrodesis. J Hand Surg Am. 1993;18(6):1113–20. Epub 1993/11/01
10. Sennwald GR, Fischer M, Mondi P. Lunotriquetral arthrodesis. A controversial procedure. J Hand Surg Br. 1995;20(6):755–60. Epub 1995/12/01
11. Weiss AP, Sachar K, Glowacki KA. Arthroscopic debridement alone for intercarpal ligament tears. J Hand Surg Am. 1997;22(2):344–9. Epub 1997/03/01
12. Westkaemper JG, Mitsionis G, Giannakopoulos PN, Sotereanos DG. Wrist arthroscopy for the treatment of ligament and triangular fibrocartilage complex injuries. Arthroscopy. 1998;14(5):479–83. Epub 1998/07/29
13. Omokawa S, Fujitani R, Inada Y. Dorsal radiocarpal ligament capsulodesis for chronic dynamic lunotriquetral instability. J Hand Surg Am. 2009;34(2):237–43. Epub 2009/02/03
14. Shahane SA, Trail IA, Takwale VJ, Stilwell JH, Stanley JK. Tenodesis of the extensor carpi ulnaris for chronic, post-traumatic lunotriquetral instability. J Bone Joint Surg Br. 2005;87(11):1512–5.
15. Mirza A, Mirza JB, Shin AY, Lorenzana DJ, Lee BK, Izzo B. Isolated lunotriquetral ligament tears treated with ulnar shortening osteotomy. J Hand Surg Am. 2013;38(8):1492–7. Epub 2013/07/16
16. Leon-Lopez MM, Salva-Coll G, Garcia-Elias M, Lluch-Bergada A, Llusa-Perez M. Role of the extensor carpi ulnaris in the stabilization of the lunotriquetral joint. An experimental study. J Hand Ther. 2013;26(4):312–7. quiz 7. Epub 2013/09/17

17. Wagner ER, Elhassan BT, Rizzo M. Diagnosis and treatment of chronic lunotriquetral ligament injuries. Hand Clin. 2015;31(3):477–86.
18. Reagan DS, Linscheid RL, Dobyns JH. Lunotriquetral sprains. J Hand Surg Am. 1984;9(4):502–14.
19. Kleinman WB. Diagnostic exams for ligamentous injuries. American Society for Surgery of the Hand, Correspondence Club Newsletter. 1985;51.
20. Isa AD, McGregor ME, Padmore CE, Langohr DG, Johnson JA, King GJW, et al. An in vitro study to determine the effect of ulnar shortening on distal forearm loading during wrist and forearm motion: implications in the treatment of ulnocarpal impaction. J Hand Surg Am. 2019;44(8):669–79. Epub 20190603
21. Nicoson MC, Moran SL. Diagnosis and treatment of acute Lunotriquetral ligament injuries. Hand Clin. 2015;31(3):467–76.
22. Haugstvedt JR, Rigo IZ. Arthroscopic assisted reconstruction of LT-ligament: a description of a new technique. J Wrist Surg. 2021;10(1):2–8. Epub 20200914
23. Hofmeister EP, Moran SL, Shin AY. Anterior and posterior interosseous neurectomy for the treatment of chronic dynamic instability of the wrist. Hand (N Y). 2006;1(2):63–70.
24. Shin AY, Bishop AT. Treatment options for lunotriquetral dissociation. Tech Hand Up Extrem Surg. 1998;2(1):2–17. Epub 2006/04/13
25. Antti-Poika I, Hyrkas J, Virkki LM, Ogino D, Konttinen YT. Correction of chronic lunotriquetral instability using extensor retinacular split: a retrospective study of 26 patients. Acta Orthop Belg. 2007;73(4):451–7. Epub 2007/10/18
26. Kirschenbaum D, Coyle MP, Leddy JP. Chronic lunotriquetral instability: diagnosis and treatment. J Hand Surg Am. 1993;18(6):1107–12.

Chapter 29
Midcarpal Instability

Kelsey L. Overman and Charles A. Goldfarb

Case Presentation

A 41-year-old right-hand-dominant laborer presented with a 7-month history of right wrist pain. He was manipulating a wrench to loosen a difficult bolt when he felt a pop in his wrist. The patient attempted to work through his discomfort for 2 months but had discomfort with most activities. He also reported decreased strength and complained of a painful clunk with activities that require ulnar deviation of the wrist, such as pouring liquids, or rotation (i.e., using the same wrench). He presented for evaluation secondary to continued symptoms despite anti-inflammatories and activity modification.

Diagnosis

Physical Examination/Relevant Maneuvers

- On examination of the left upper extremity, there was a noticeable volar sag of the ulnar carpus when viewing the hand from the side. Additionally, on radiograph, there was an increased piso-styloid distance compared to the contralateral upper extremity:

Supplementary Information The online version contains supplementary material available at https://doi.org/10.1007/978-3-031-55869-6_29.

K. L. Overman · C. A. Goldfarb (✉)
Department of Orthopaedic Surgery, Washington University, St. Louis, MO, USA
e-mail: goldfarbc@wustl.edu

J. Yao (ed.), *Carpal Instability*, https://doi.org/10.1007/978-3-031-55869-6_29

- The piso-styloid distance is the distance between the dorsal tip of the ulnar styloid and the volar margin of the pisiform [8]. If the distal radioulnar joint (DRUJ) is normal, an increase in the piso-styloid distance indicates volar sagging of the proximal carpal row and midcarpal instability.

- Tenderness to palpation over the ulnar carpus at the triquetrohamate joint.
- There was a clunk with the midcarpal shift test (Video 29.1):

  - The midcarpal shift test requires that the examiner control the distal forearm with one hand and the carpus with the other. The patient's distal carpal row is passively translated in a volar direction, and the wrist is then ulnarly deviated. When a normal wrist moves into an ulnar deviated position, the palmar midcarpal ligaments and the coordinated function of the flexor carpi ulnaris (FCU) and extensor carpi ulnaris (ECU) muscles allow the three carpal bones of the proximal carpal row to glide smoothly from a flexed to an extended position. Dysfunction of these supportive structures may result in midcarpal instability. The midcarpal shift test is positive when there is a clunk during this maneuver, which is a result of the articular surface of the hamate forcing the hyperflexed triquetrum into sudden extension, pulling the attached lunate and scaphoid into extension as well [17].

- Pain was elicited with the resisted pronation confrontation test:

  - With the patient's hand in a pronated position, the examiner attempts to supinate the hand while the patient resists. Patients with MCI often have significant pain with this. The test is positive if pain is improved, while the examiner stabilizes the ulnar column of the affected wrist and hand during the same maneuver [8].

- The ulnar column was found to be lax, but lunotriquetral (LT) ballottement was stable:

  - The examiner uses one hand to stabilize the radial side of the wrist and hand with the other hand on the pisotriquetrohamate complex. Ballottement of the ulnar column in a dorso-volar direction tests for excessive laxity. Specific testing of the LT ligament includes a dorsal volar shuck maneuver of the pisiform-triquetrum and the lunate. Excessive motion (compared to contralateral side) with pain elevates suspicion of LT instability. Stability of the LT joint with a lax ulnar column indicates midcarpal instability.

- The DRUJ was stable. He had no foveal tenderness:

  - It is important to eliminate other sources of pain in the wrist. With the elbow rested on the examination table, the examiner stabilizes the patient's radius with one hand while moving the ulna in a dorsal and volar position with the other hand. This maneuver ballots the DRUJ to test for instability. Stability is assessed with the forearm pronated, supinated, and in neutral position. Of note, patients with triangular fibrocartilage complex (TFCC) pain often have pain with pronation and supination of the forearm when the proximal forearm is stabilized by the examiner. This is distinguished from midcarpal instability where patients tend to have pain when the examiner holds the patient's hand at the metacarpal level during pronation and supination [8]. Pain directly at the fovea also suggests underlying TFCC pathology.

- Examination of the contralateral wrist:

  - The other wrist is examined in a similar fashion assessing both pain and provocative maneuvers. It is common to find painless midcarpal instability.

- This patient's grip strength was 60 pounds versus 120 pounds in his contralateral hand.

Diagnostic Studies

Plain radiographs may be normal, but they are important for excluding severe cases with a static volar intercalated segment instability (VISI). VISI deformities occur secondary to a disruption of radiocarpal ligaments on the ulnar side of the wrist (ulnar half of the volar arcuate ligament) and/or the lunotriquetral (LT) ligament. Radiographs are also important for excluding other pathologies and evaluating the joint surfaces before potential reconstructive surgery. Dynamic fluoroscopy and stress views are also helpful with diagnosis. Cineradiography or simple surgeon-performed live fluoroscan assessment can demonstrate the catch-up clunk on clinical examination. The lateral view is most helpful.

Computed tomography (CT) scanning and magnetic resonance imaging (MRI) are typically not indicated. However, when used, MRI can assess the integrity of the volar arcuate ligament, the intrinsic carpal ligaments, and the LT ligament.

Wrist arthroscopy rarely allows confirmation of the diagnosis of midcarpal instability, and the common findings of diffuse synovial hyperemia are a nonspecific observation [7]. Arthroscopy can be helpful excluding other pathologic conditions involving intrinsic carpal ligaments, TFCC, or carpal instability dissociative injuries.

Management Options

Patients with generalized laxity with a midcarpal clunk require no treatment unless they have pain or dysfunction. Individuals with symptomatic, mild dynamic midcarpal instability are most likely to benefit from conservative treatment. Hand therapy with a focus on proprioceptive awareness and neuromuscular rehabilitation is an important component of nonoperative management [2, 4, 6]. Isometric exercises and dynamic strengthening are also advantageous [7]. There is general agreement that splinting should be reserved for patients with significant pain and only for short periods, as prolonged immobilization may exacerbate instability. A splint with volar ulnar support can help reduce symptomatic volar sag of the proximal carpal row and holds the lunate in a neutral posture [1]. Surgery should only be considered following failure of conservative management after a minimum of 6 weeks. Surgical indications include ongoing pain, instability, and decreased function with work and daily activities.

Patients with mild symptomatic instability without a radiographic VISI deformity may benefit from arthroscopic capsular shrinkage, soft tissue stabilization, or a combination of the two. Arthroscopic capsular shrinkage targets the palmar midcarpal, ulnocarpal, and triquetrohamate ligaments, as well as the dorsal wrist capsule. Soft tissue reconstruction procedures include dorsal wrist plication, stabilization of the triquetrohamate joint by rerouting the ECU tendon, advancement of the ulnar arm of the volar arcuate ligament across the midcarpal joint, reefing of the dorsal radiocarpal and/or intercarpal ligaments, double-level tenodesis using a slip of the extensor carpi radialis brevis, and dorsal radiocarpal ligament reconstruction with a pisiform-based split tendon graft of the FCU [8, 16, 17]. Open discussion with the patient regarding the longevity of soft tissue reconstructions is important, as soft tissue creep over time, particularly in patients with ligament laxity or collagen-vascular disorders, is common.

For more severe cases, such as the presence of a static VISI deformity, significant arthritic changes, or recurrent instability after an arthroscopic or soft tissue procedure, limited intercarpal fusions, such as triquetrohamate fusion, capitolunate fusion, or a four-bone fusion, are options. The major drawback of these procedures is the decreased range of motion and subsequent functional limitations.

Management Chosen for This Case with Rationale

The patient was initially managed with anti-inflammatories, modification of daily activities, avoidance of provoking activities, splinting for a short period of time, and hand therapy for proprioceptive training and selective strengthening. The patient did not improve over 3 months and remained notably restricted at work and with activities of daily living. He requested surgical intervention. Taking into consideration the patient's instability, lack of radiographic deformity or arthritic changes, and desire to preserve mobility of his wrist and hand, we planned a diagnostic arthroscopy, thermal shrinkage of the volar extrinsic ligaments, and dorsal wrist plication of the dorsal radiocarpal and dorsal intercarpal ligaments.

The right upper extremity was suspended with finger traps in a wrist traction tower with 10 pounds of traction on the middle and ring fingers. Fluid irrigation was utilized under gravity. A diagnostic arthroscopy was performed, exploring both the radiocarpal and midcarpal joints. We debrided synovitic tissue along the dorsal and ulnar joint capsule of the radiocarpal and midcarpal joints. The volar radiocarpal, the intrinsic (SLIL and LTIL) ligaments, and the TFCC were intact. Synovectomy with a 3 mm shaver was performed over the volar ulnar wrist until the ulnocarpal ligaments were well visualized. The ligaments were prominent and, with relaxation of the distraction, had a lax appearance. In the radiocarpal joint, the ulnocarpal ligaments were addressed with a bipolar thermal shrinkage probe from the radial border near the sigmoid notch to the ulnar-most aspect at the prestyloid recess. Light "painting" of the ligaments with short bursts of energy was delivered to prevent excessive rise in local tissue temperature. In addition, fluid egress was maximized with an additional 18-gauge needle to allow fluid cooling. During this portion of the surgery, the wrist traction force is reduced to less than 5 pounds to minimize tension on the ligament.

The midcarpal joint was assessed, and a shaver was introduced through the ulnar midcarpal portal to access the arcuate ligament. Synovectomy and thermal shrinkage were performed in a similar fashion as described for the radiocarpal joint. The target for shrinkage was the ulnar limb of the arcuate ligament and the triquetrohamatecapitate ligament on the ulnar palmar surface of the midcarpal joint (Fig. 29.1a–d and Video 29.2).

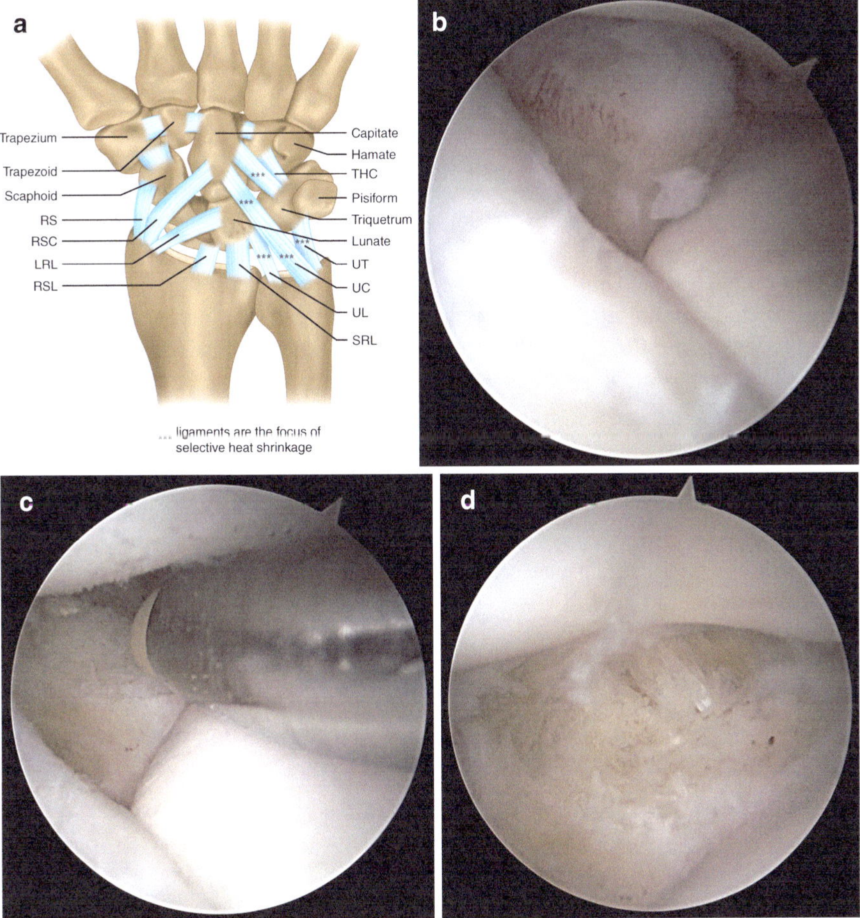

Fig. 29.1 (**a**) Line drawing of the key volar ligaments of the carpus. ** Ligaments are the focus of selective heat shrinkage. (**b**) View of the volar lunotriquetral interval at the midcarpal joint. This triangular structure should be resting between the volar lunate and triquetrum. (**c**) Heat shrinkage probe on the triangular structure and capsule beyond. (**d**) Post-heat shrinkage of the volar and ulnar midcarpal joint

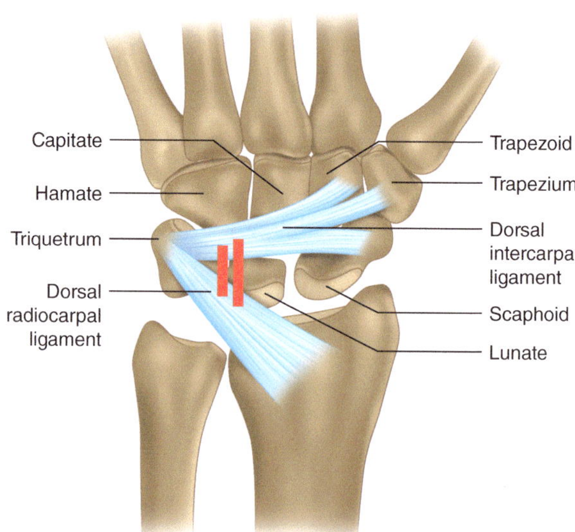

Fig. 29.2 Dorsal imbrication of the DRC and DIC ligaments. The two vertical lines indicate the position of the imbrication sutures

Attention was then turned to the dorsal wrist plication. An oblique 2.5 cm incision was made over the fifth dorsal compartment adjacent to the triquetrum. Dorsal sensory branches of the ulnar nerve were protected. The extensor digit quinti (EDQ) was protected. We mobilized the dorsal capsule, focusing on the confluence of the dorsal radiocarpal (DRC) and dorsal intercarpal (DIC) ligaments. We used multiple, 2–0 braided nonabsorbable sutures to plicate these two ligaments (Fig. 29.2).

Clinical Course and Outcome

Postoperatively, the patient was placed into a sugar-tong splint with the wrist and forearm both held in neutral. Two weeks later, sutures were removed, and he was placed in a Muenster cast. Six weeks after surgery, we began gentle range of motion with therapy. He continued to wear a short arm brace with activities until 12 weeks at which time he began weight-bearing. Five months after surgery, he returned to work full duty. One year after surgery, he had regained complete wrist motion, reported no pain, and was stable on examination.

Clinical Pearls and Pitfalls

- Diagnosis of midcarpal instability may be difficult and requires an index of suspicion and a thorough understanding of underlying anatomy and pertinent examination findings.

- The midcarpal shift test is performed by translating the distal carpal row in a volar direction and ulnarly deviating the wrist. A positive test will elicit a "clunk."
- Nonoperative management, including hand therapy, activity modification, and judicious use of bracing, is the first line of treatment.
- Arthroscopic capsular shrinkage with dorsal wrist plication can be a good option for patients with mild MCI. Given the risk of failure with an arthroscopic capsular shrinkage alone, we always perform a plication of the DRC and DIC ligaments. A salvage procedure (most commonly four-bone fusion with scaphoid excision) is performed if this procedure fails. We have limited experience with other soft tissue reconstructions.
- Patients with radiographic deformity, arthritic changes, or failed primary surgery may benefit from limited carpal fusions.

Literature Review and Discussion

Symptomatic midcarpal instability is an uncommon clinical entity characterized by a loss of synchronous motion between the proximal and distal carpal rows. Etiology can be congenital, traumatic rupture, attenuation, increased elasticity, or poor proprioception [17]. Midcarpal instability is included in the category of nondissociative carpal instability, in which there is a failure of the extrinsic wrist ligaments as opposed to the intrinsic wrist ligaments. In this condition, the midcarpal joint subluxates in a volar direction (most common), dorsal direction, or combined and then reduces with ulnar deviation. The ulnar arcuate ligament (triquetrohamate-capitate ligament) and the dorsal radiocarpal and intercarpal ligaments are important for midcarpal stability [9, 15, 16]. In mild cases, nonsurgical treatment may lead to a satisfactory outcome. In refractory cases, surgery may be warranted.

Arthroscopic thermal capsular shrinkage provides stabilization by thermal shrinkage of the extrinsic wrist ligaments and allows collagen fibrils to shorten by approximately 15–30% [11]. Mason and Hargreaves performed arthroscopic shrinkage of the volar extrinsic ligaments in 15 wrists. At 42-month follow-up, they reported improved or resolved instability in all wrists, as well as patient satisfaction in 14 of 15 patients at 3.5-year follow-up [12]. There was only a 10% loss of movement. The long-term (>10 years) follow-up of this series showed good or excellent results in 71% of patients [14]. The patients rated 12 of the 14 wrists as better than before surgery.

Von Schroeder [16] found alleviation of midcarpal instability and acceptable patient satisfaction with dorsal wrist plication for midcarpal instability in 20 out of 22 patients. The plication involved portions of the capsule as well as the DRC and DIC ligaments. Two patients with ongoing instability subsequently underwent limited intercarpal fusion.

Apart from capsulorrhaphy, soft tissue reconstructions have been less successful than limited midcarpal or four-corner fusions [3, 10, 13]. Arthrodesis eliminates ulnar sided motion between the proximal and distal rows of the carpus, thus eliminating the instability. Lichtman et al. [10] reported on six patients treated with limited midcarpal arthrodesis (three triquetrohamate arthrodesis and three 4-corner arthrodeses) for midcarpal instability. All were graded as clinically successful, and all patients returned to their former occupations. Comparatively, six of the nine patients who underwent soft tissue reconstruction failed. Goldfarb et al. [3] reported that 7 of 8 patients were satisfied with four-corner arthrodesis, and 6 of 8 of the patients had mild or no pain after the procedure. Rao and Culver reported less favorable outcomes with triquetrohamate arthrodesis, with good or excellent results in only 6 of 11 cases [13].

Although midcarpal fusions have had reasonable results for midcarpal instability, the limited carpal motion inherent in these procedures is a matter of concern with patients and may cause functional impairment. Triquetrohamate fusion and four-corner fusion correct the clunk and postural abnormality associated with midcarpal instability; however, these procedures disrupt midcarpal motion and the dart thrower's motion, leading to a marked loss of ulnar deviation, an abnormal arc of circumduction, and mixed clinical results [13]. An alternative surgical option is radiolunate fusion, which stabilizes the entire proximal row in neutral and prevents the dramatic change in lunate posture that characterizes this condition [2]. Halikis et al. reported excellent pain relief in five patients who underwent radiolunate fusion for midcarpal instability [5]. The catch-up clunk resolved in all patients. At a minimum 2.5 years of follow-up, extension was reduced by 25% compared with the contralateral side. Flexion was reduced by 32%, radial deviation was reduced by 37%, and ulnar deviation was reduced by 33% compared with the contralateral side.

Midcarpal instability is a rare condition involving dissociation between the two carpal rows. Nonsurgical management is the first line of treatment and, if unsuccessful, surgical intervention follows. Arthroscopic thermal capsulorrhaphy, soft tissue reconstruction, and a limited arthrodesis are all options. There are very few studies evaluating long-term results of the various techniques or comparing treatment options, given the infrequent occurrence of this disease process.

References

1. Chinchalkar S, Yong SA. An ulnar boost splint for midcarpal instability. J Hand Ther. 2004;17(3):377–9. https://doi.org/10.1197/j.jht.2004.04.013.
2. Garcia-Elias M. The non-dissociative clunking wrist: a personal view. J Hand Surg Eur Vol. 2008;33(6):698–711. https://doi.org/10.1177/1753193408090148.
3. Goldfarb CA, Stern PJ, Kiefhaber TR. Palmar midcarpal instability: the results of treatment with 4-corner arthrodesis. J Hand Surg. 2004;29(2):258–63. https://doi.org/10.1016/j.jhsa.2003.11.009.
4. Hagert E, Lluch A, Rein S. The role of proprioception and neuromuscular stability in carpal instabilities. J Hand Surg Eur Vol. 2016;41(1):94–101. https://doi.org/10.1177/1753193415590390.
5. Halikis MN, Colello-Abraham K, Taleisnik J. Radiolunate fusion: the forgotten partial arthrodesis. Clin Orthop Relat Res. 1997;341:30–5. https://doi.org/10.1097/00003086-199708000-00006.

6. Harwood C, Turner L. Conservative management of midcarpal instability. J Hand Surg Eur Vol. 2016;41(1):102–9. https://doi.org/10.1177/1753193415613050.

7. Higgin RPC, Hargreaves DG. Midcarpal instability: the role of wrist arthroscopy. Hand Clin. 2017;33(4):717–26. https://doi.org/10.1016/j.hcl.2017.06.003.

8. Ho PC. Palmar mid-carpal instability: my management algorithm. Chir Main. 2015;34(6):398. https://doi.org/10.1016/j.main.2015.10.193.

9. Lichtman DM, Wroten ES. Understanding midcarpal instability. J Hand Surg. 2006;31(3):491–8. https://doi.org/10.1016/j.jhsa.2005.12.014.

10. Lichtman DM, Bruckner JD, Culp RW, Alexander CE. Palmar midcarpal instability: results of surgical reconstruction. J Hand Surg. 1993;18(2):307–15. https://doi.org/10.1016/0363-5023(93)90366-B.

11. Luke TA, Rovner AD, Karas SG, Hawkins RJ, Plancher KD. Volumetric change in the shoulder capsule after open inferior capsular shift versus arthroscopic thermal capsular shrinkage: a cadaveric model. J Shoulder Elb Surg. 2004;13(2):146–9. https://doi.org/10.1016/j.jse.2003.11.008.

12. Mason WTM, Hargreaves DG. Arthroscopic thermal capsulorrhaphy for palmar midcarpal instability. J Hand Surg Eur Vol`. 2007;32(4):411–6. https://doi.org/10.1016/j.jhse.2007.03.012.

13. Rao SB, Culver JE. Triquetrohamate arthrodesis for midcarpal instability. J Hand Surg. 1995;20(4):583–9. https://doi.org/10.1016/S0363-5023(05)80273-4.

14. Ricks M, Belward P, Hargreaves D. Long-term results of arthroscopic capsular shrinkage for palmar midcarpal instability of the wrist. J Wrist Surg. 2021;10(03):224–8. https://doi.org/10.1055/s-0040-1722331.

15. Trumble TE, Bour CJ, Smith RJ, Glisson RR. Kinematics of the ulnar carpus related to the volar intercalated segment instability pattern. J Hand Surg. 1990;15(3):384–92. https://doi.org/10.1016/0363-5023(90)90048-V.

16. von Schroeder HP. Dorsal wrist plication for midcarpal instability. J Hand Surg. 2018;43(4):354–9. https://doi.org/10.1016/j.jhsa.2017.11.002.

17. Wolfe SW, Garcia-Elias M, Kitay A. Carpal instability nondissociative. J Am Acad Orthop Surg. 2012;20(9):575–85. https://doi.org/10.5435/JAAOS-20-09-575.

Further Reading

Garcia-Elias M. The non-dissociative clunking wrist: a personal view. J Hand Surg Eur Vol. 2008;33(6):698–711. https://doi.org/10.1177/1753193408090148.

Goldfarb CA, Stern PJ, Kiefhaber TR. Palmar midcarpal instability: the results of treatment with 4-corner arthrodesis. J Hand Surg. 2004;29(2):258–63. https://doi.org/10.1016/j.jhsa.2003.11.009.

Ho PC. Palmar mid-carpal instability: my management algorithm. Chir Main. 2015;34(6):398. https://doi.org/10.1016/j.main.2015.10.193.

Mason WTM, Hargreaves DG. Arthroscopic thermal capsulorrhaphy for palmar midcarpal instability. J Hand Surg Eur Vol. 2007;32(4):411–6. https://doi.org/10.1016/j.jhse.2007.03.012.

von Schroeder HP. Dorsal wrist plication for midcarpal instability. J Hand Surg. 2018;43(4):354–9. https://doi.org/10.1016/j.jhsa.2017.11.002.

Chapter 30
CIND: Radiocarpal Instability

Marc J. Richard and Nathaniel Fogel

Case Presentation

A 47-year-old male who presented with a polytrauma after a motorcycle accident who sustained a three-column thoracic spine injury, bilateral scapular body fractures, multiple facial fractures, and abdominal trauma. At the time of presentation, he complained of right wrist pain. He denied any relevant history of trauma to the right wrist. On initial exam, there was gross instability at the radiocarpal joint. Initial radiographs demonstrated ulnar translocation of the carpus as well as diastasis of the scapholunate interval (Fig. 30.1a, b). He was placed into a volar resting splint as he awaited operative intervention. After stabilization and operative management of his thoracic spine and abdominal injuries, he underwent surgical intervention for his wrist injury

M. J. Richard (✉) · N. Fogel
Department of Orthopaedic Surgery, Duke University, Durham, NC, USA
e-mail: marc.richard@duke.edu

J. Yao (ed.), *Carpal Instability*, https://doi.org/10.1007/978-3-031-55869-6_30

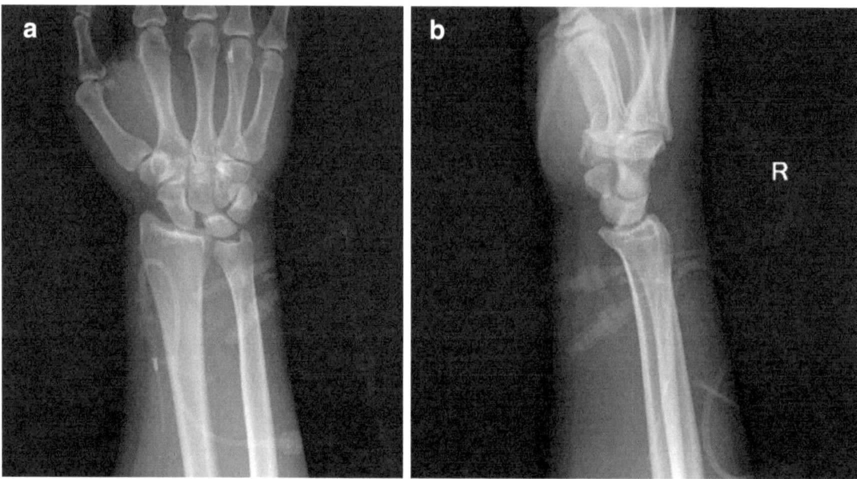

Fig. 30.1 AP (**a**) and lateral (**b**) radiographs of the right wrist demonstrating ulnar translocation of the carpus. The radiocarpal joint remains reduced on the lateral view

Diagnosis (Physical Assessment/Relevant Maneuvers: Diagnostic Studies)

Initial diagnosis of radiocarpal instability in the traumatic setting is often made on clinical examination. Gross deformity associated with persistent radiocarpal dislocation can be easily noted on physical exam and must be differentiated from deformity due to fracture. More subtle instability may only be noted upon careful inspection of radiocarpal alignment on plain radiographs, which can demonstrate static subluxation of the carpus [1]. In the traumatic setting, there is often significant instability that can be appreciated with examination of the wrist and confirmed under fluoroscopy. Diagnosis can at times be challenging as patients can have numerous other orthopedic and non-orthopedic injuries associated with what are often high-energy mechanisms. In the setting of a pure radiocarpal instability event, advanced imaging studies are not usually required. Computerized tomography (CT) imaging can be useful in the setting of injuries with associated bony pathology. MRI is rarely indicated in the acute setting but could be obtained when suspecting radiocarpal carpal instability nondissociative (CIND) seen in distal radius malunion, Madelung deformity, or malunions of the lunate or scaphoid [1]. Neurological deficits in the hand are often present, impacting the median nerve and less commonly the ulnar nerve [2]. Radiocarpal dislocations are most commonly classified radiographically with the system described by Dumontier. Type I injuries are purely ligamentous or involve only a small cortical avulsion off the radius, while type II injuries are fracture dislocation injuries with a large radial styloid fragment [3]. The Moneim classification has also been described to differentiate between radiocarpal instability events with (type II) or without (type I) intercarpal dissociation [4].

Management Options

Treatment of radiocarpal instability varies widely [5]. Initial treatment consists of closed reduction if persistent radiocarpal dislocation exists on initial presentation. Definitive treatment measures that have been described include cast immobilization, radiocarpal joint reduction and pinning, reduction and external fixator placement, open repair of ligamentous and any associated bony injuries, open ligamentous repair with application of a dorsal spanning plate, and partial/total wrist fusions [6]. Most authors advocate for at least 6 weeks of post-injury immobilization in the traumatic setting. Given the rare nature of these injuries, all series describing these treatment methods are retrospective with relatively small cohorts. Outcomes associated with these management options are further discussed later in this chapter.

Management Chosen for This Case with Rationale

The resting ulnar translocation deformity in this patient indicates significant ligamentous and capsular injury that requires reduction of the radiocarpal relationship and repair of both volar and dorsal structures. Stabilization with a dorsal spanning plate avoids the risk of potential pin-site infection seen with Kirschner (K) wires or external fixation, avoids long-term cast immobilization, and provides robust temporary stability.

The patient was positioned supine with the arm abducted on a hand table. Fluoroscopic images were obtained at the beginning of the case to better characterize the degree of radiocarpal instability. There was persistent ulnar translocation of the carpus and static scapholunate widening as had been seen on initial injury radiographs (Fig. 30.2a). There was dramatic instability to additional ulnar translation (Fig. 30.2b), and the carpus could be reduced closed with radial translation (Fig. 30.2c). On the lateral view, the carpus remained reduced in flexion and extension but could be dislocated with dorsal translation (Fig. 30.2d).

Attention was first turned to addressing the dorsal ligamentous and capsular injuries, as well as to preparing for application of a dorsal spanning plate to provide stability and maintain the radiocarpal joint reduction. Longitudinal incisions were made over the third metacarpal and the dorsal aspect of the radial shaft that were made in preparation for the dorsal plate. A cadaveric study by Azad et al. demonstrated distal fixation to the third metacarpal to be superior in restoring a more anatomic radiocarpal relationship compared to fixation to the second metacarpal [7]. A separate longitudinal incision was made just ulnar to Lister's tubercle. A majority of the extensor retinaculum had been traumatically disrupted. The extensor pollicis longus (EPL) was identified and moved out of its compartment radially and was left in this transposed position. The interval between the third and fourth extensor compartments was then utilized. The dorsal capsular and ligamentous complex was found to be avulsed off the radius. There had been a shearing injury to the dorsal cartilage of the scaphoid, and free cartilage fragments were excised. The scapholunate interosseous ligament (SLIL) was avulsed off its insertion on the lunate.

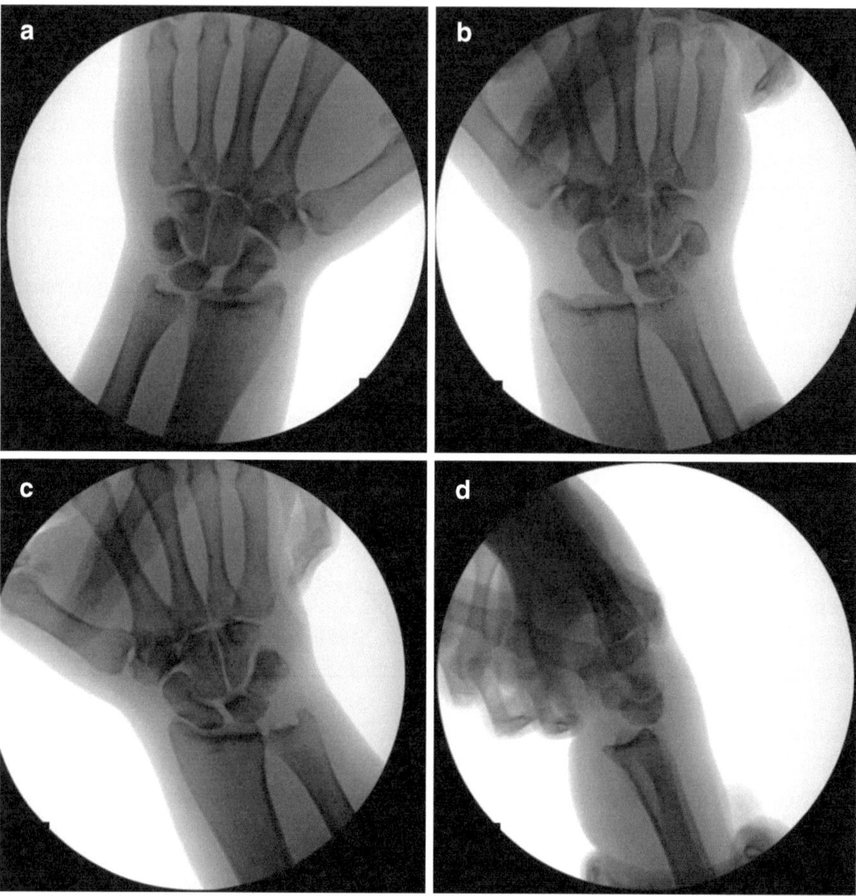

Fig. 30.2 Intraoperative fluoroscopic images demonstrating persistent ulnar translocation of the carpus and scapholunate interval widening (**a**), further instability to ulnar directed translational force (**b**), reduction of the radiocarpal relationship with radial directed translational force (**c**), and the ability to dislocate the radiocarpal joint dorsally (**d**)

The SLIL injury was addressed first. The interval was reduced with a pointed reduction clamp and held with two 0.045 inch K-wires, which were subsequently cut beneath the skin. The avulsed ligament was repaired back down to the lunate with a suture anchor (Fig. 30.3). Three additional suture anchors were placed radial to ulnar along the radius, and the entirety of the avulsed capsule and ligamentous complex including the dorsal radiocarpal ligament was repaired back down. Improved stability of the radiocarpal joint was noted at this point, but there was still pathologic mobility present. The dorsal spanning plate was then introduced and secured, holding the radiocarpal joint reduced in both AP and lateral planes. Given the persistent instability after repair of the dorsal structures and preoperative ulnar translation indicating volar ligamentous injury, attention was then turned to volar ligament repair. In the setting of ulnar translocation, we always use a combined volar and dorsal approach given the importance of repair of the radioscaphocapitate and radiolunate ligaments. Dorsal spanning plate application is our stabilization method of choice for radiocarpal instability, necessitating a dorsal

Fig. 30.3 Intraoperative fluoroscopic image demonstrating reduction and fixation of the scapholunate interval and placement of suture anchors at the lunate and dorsal distal radius for ligamentous repair

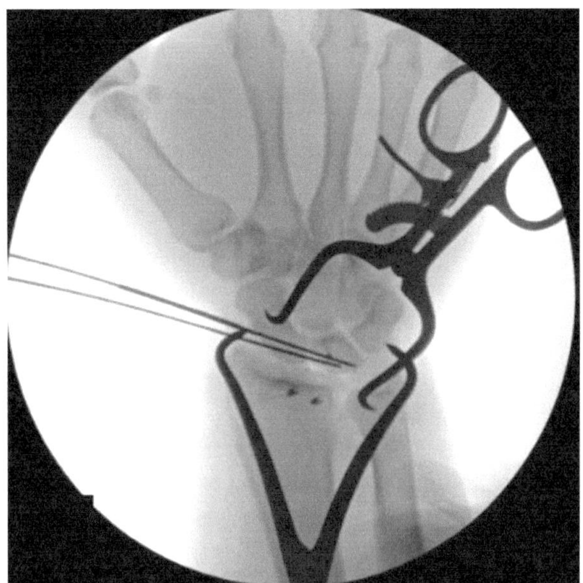

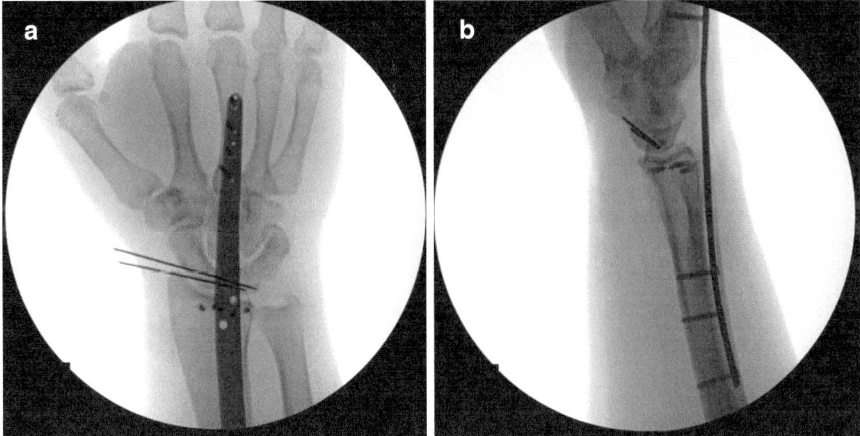

Fig. 30.4 Intraoperative AP (**a**) and lateral (**b**) fluoroscopic images demonstrating restoration of appropriate radiocarpal and intercarpal alignment after percutaneous wiring, dorsal spanning plate application, and volar and dorsal ligamentous and capsular repairs

approach as well. In the absence of ulnar translocation or any large bony fragment that needs to be addressed via a volar approach, we utilize an isolated dorsal approach. An extended carpal tunnel approach was utilized, and the complex of the insertions of the radioscaphocapitate (RSC) ligament and radiolunate ligaments was found to be avulsed off the volar lip of the radius. The ligaments were repaired back to the radius with two additional suture anchors. Final fluoroscopic images demonstrated restoration of appropriate radiocarpal and intercarpal alignment (Fig. 30.4a, b). The patient was immobilized in a volar resting splint and transitioned to a removable wrist brace at the time of suture removal, 2 weeks following the surgery.

Clinical Course and Outcome

Radiographs were obtained at 2 weeks and 2 months postoperatively, which demonstrated maintained radiocarpal alignment, no implant complication, and no interval widening of the scapholunate interval. He was indicated for removal of implants 3 months postoperatively. Fluoroscopic images obtained intraoperatively after removal of the dorsal spanning plate and K-wires demonstrated no residual radiocarpal instability to volar, dorsal, radial, or ulnar translation. At his postoperative visit 2 months after implant removal, he demonstrated wrist range of motion of 45 ° of flexion, 45 ° of extension, 70 ° of pronation, and 60 ° of supination. He reported no pain with wrist range of motion and could make a composite fist. Radiographs demonstrated mild interval ulnar translation of the carpus and widening of the scapholunate interval compared to the fluoroscopic images obtained at the time of implant removal (Fig. 30.5a, b). The patient reported no functional limitation or pain and desired to transition to home occupational therapy.

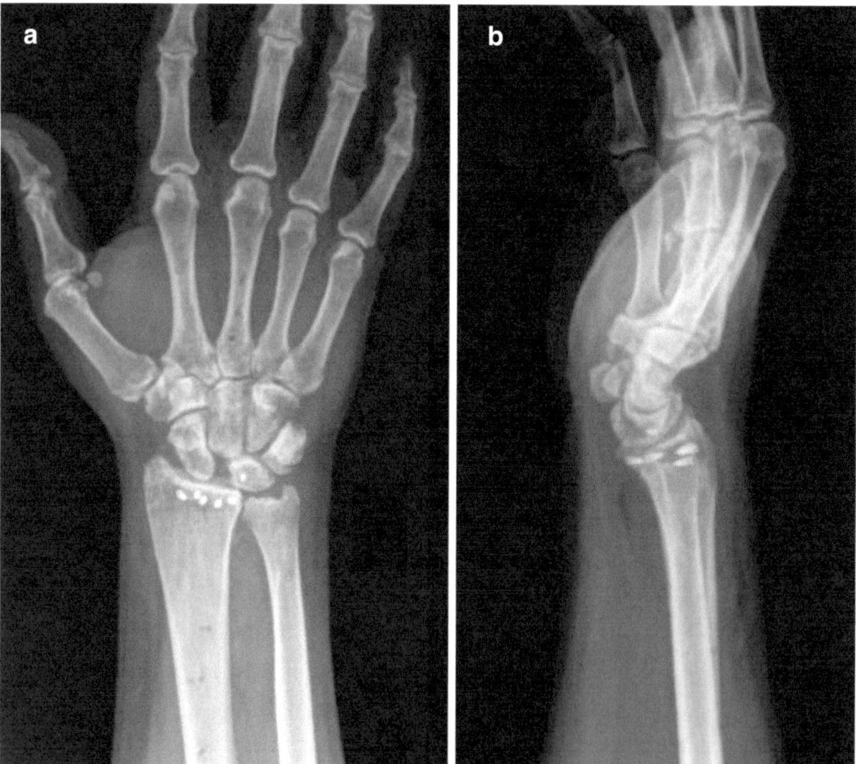

Fig. 30.5 AP (**a**) and lateral (**b**) radiographs 2 months after removal of implants show interval widening of the SLIL and mild ulnar translocation of the carpus. The patient noted no pain or functional deficits at that time

Bulleted Clinical Pearls/Pitfalls

- Repair of the volar ligaments is crucial in the setting of ulnar translation with specific attention to the attachment of the RSC and radiolunate ligaments at the volar radius.
- It is important to check for residual distal radial ulnar joint (DRUJ) instability after addressing the radiocarpal instability and treat residual DRUJ pathology as necessary.
- Consider neutralization of the ligamentous repair with a dorsal spanning plate to optimize the construct strength and radiocarpal reduction.
- Radiocarpal dislocations associated with bony avulsion injuries that can be repaired generally result in more favorable outcomes than pure ligamentous injuries.
- Radiocarpal instability related to trauma often results in loss of wrist flexion and extension motion and frequently progresses to posttraumatic arthritis regardless of the treatment method.

Literature Review and Discussion

Radiocarpal instability is a relatively rare pathology, with traumatic variants constituting 0.2% of all wrist injuries [8], and can be seen with or without separate proximal row pathology [5]. The goal of the treatment is to obtain and maintain an anatomic reduction of the radiocarpal joint while identifying and treating associated intercarpal and radiocarpal ligamentous injuries [9]. Despite a wide range of described treatment methods, decreased wrist range of motion and posttraumatic arthritis are present in nearly all patients who sustain a radiocarpal instability event [6]. Ulnar translocation of the carpus has been reported in up to 23% of patients with radiocarpal dislocation or fracture dislocation who went onto have operative management [10]. The integrity of the RSC and volar radiolunate ligaments is crucial to preventing ulnar translocation [11], and all Dumontier I injuries, which by definition are without significant bony injury to the radial styloid, should be assumed to represent avulsion of the volar ligamentous structures. While limited, there are several small series for treatment of radiocarpal instability that propose various treatment strategies. However, the heterogeneity of these injuries and common concomitant injuries makes direct comparison of studies somewhat difficult.

Wahl et al. reported a series of 13 patients with radiocarpal dislocation with ligament repair and dorsal wrist spanning fixation. Repair of dorsal capsuloligamentous structures versus dorsal and volar structures was determined on a case-by-case basis [6]. At the final follow-up, 85% of patients developed radiographic posttraumatic arthritis. Forty-five percent of patients were found to have residual DRUJ instability after ligamentous repair and stabilization. One patient with a Dumontier I injury went on to develop ulnar translocation of the carpus. Average final wrist range of motion arc was 83 °, with pronosupination arc of 163 °. As part of their study, the authors performed a comprehensive literature review and noted that only 6 studies with 8 or more patients have been published in more than 35 years, further demonstrating the limitations of the literature related to this pathology.

Dumontier et al. published a series of 27 patients and classified their injury pattern based on the presumed competence of the volar radiocarpal ligaments [4]. Various treatment methods were utilized, including closed treatment in a plaster cast, K-wire fixation, external fixation, and open reduction with ligamentous repair. All four of the patients that went onto have ulnar translocation of the carpus had type I injuries—pure ligamentous instability or with a small radial styloid fracture. They reported similar overall final range of motion arcs as Wahl et al. in both injury groups. They advocated for volar ligament repair in all type I injuries to mitigate the risk of subsequent ulnar translocation and recommended open reduction via a dorsal approach with anatomic fixation of bony injuries in type II injuries. Spiry et al. reported on 41 patients with a combination of pure radiocarpal instability events and fracture dislocation injuries [12]. For pure ligamentous injuries, they reported acceptable outcomes with a dorsal incision and radioscaphoid and radiolunate pinning alone, without any volar ligamentous repair. Their results further supported the importance of reduction and fixation of bony injuries present in Dumontier II injury patterns.

Yuan et al. reported 26 patients who underwent treatment for posttraumatic radiocarpal instability [10]. This series included long-term follow-up on 17 patients with a mean follow-up of 14.8 years. In this group, those that underwent acute open reduction internal fixation or addressed the underlying ligamentous injury acutely tended to report lower PRWE and DASH scores than those who had not. Further, those with delayed treatment required salvage procedures and tended to have worse patient-reported outcomes. The study's conclusions were tempered with the understanding that the rare nature and significant variation in the severity of concomitant bony and soft tissue injury make it difficult to make definitive statements on which treatments are superior. Despite this, the authors concluded that primary ligamentous repair trended toward overall improved long-term outcomes.

Radiocarpal instability represents a rare but challenging problem. Literature is limited and consists entirely of retrospective reviews. However, early intervention in the form of capsuloligamentous repair and bony stabilization appears to be associated with improved patient-reported outcomes compared to closed treatment and primary salvage procedures. Prospective study and further instability subtype analysis are required for better understanding of ideal treatment.

References

1. Zelenski NA, Shin AY. Management of nondissociative instability of the wrist. J Hand Surg Am. 2020;45(2):131–9.
2. Mudgal CS, Psenica J, Jupiter JB. Radiocarpal fracture-dislocation. J Hand Surg Br. 1999;24(1):92–8.

3. Dumontier C, Zu Reckendorf GM, Sautet A, et al. Radiocarpal dislocations: classification and proposal for treatment. A review of twenty-seven cases. J Bone Joint Surg Am. 2001;83(2):212–8.
4. Moneim MS, Bolger JT, Omer GE. Radiocarpal dislocation: classification and rationale for management. Clin Orthop Relat Res. 1985;192:199–209.
5. Wolfe SW, Garcia-Elias M, Kitay A. Carpal instability nondissociative. J Am Acad Orthop Surg. 2012 Sep;20(9):575–85.
6. Wahl EP, Lauder AS, Pidgeon TS, Guerrero EM, Ruch DS, Richard MJ. Dorsal wrist spanning plate fixation for treatment of radiocarpal fracture-dislocations. Hand (N Y). 2021;16(6):834–42.
7. Azad A, Choi JT, Fisch R, Gipsman A, Nicholson LT, Ghiassi A. Wrist-spanning fixation of radiocarpal dislocation: a cadaveric assessment of ulnar translation. Hand (N Y). 2021;16(4):482–90.
8. Dunn AW. Fractures and dislocations of the carpus. Surg Clin North Am. 1972;52:1513–38.
9. Ilyas AM, Mudgal CS. Radiocarpal fracture-dislocations. J Am Acad Orthop Surg. 2008;16(11):647–55.
10. Yuan BJ, Dennison DG, Elhassan BT, Kakar S. Outcomes after radiocarpal dislocation: a retrospective review. Hand (N Y). 2015;10(3):367–73.
11. Rayhack JM, Linscheid RL, Dobyns JH, Smith JH. Posttraumatic ulnar translation of the carpus. J Hand Surg Am. 1987;12:180–9.
12. Spiry C, Bacle G, Marteau E, et al. Radiocarpal dislocations and fracture-dislocations: injury types and long-term outcomes. Orthop Traumatol Surg Res. 2018;104(2):261–6.

Further Reading

Dumontier C, Zu Reckendorf GM, Sautet A, et al. Radiocarpal dislocations: classification and proposal for treatment. A review of twenty-seven cases. J Bone Joint Surg Am. 2001;83(2):212–8.
Ilyas AM, Mudgal CS. Radiocarpal fracture-dislocations. J Am Acad Orthop Surg. 2008;16(11):647–55
Spiry C, Bacle G, Marteau E, et al. Radiocarpal dislocations and fracture-dislocations: injury types and long-term outcomes. Orthop Traumatol Surg Res. 2018;104(2):261–6.
Wahl EP, Lauder AS, Pidgeon TS, Guerrero EM, Ruch DS, Richard MJ. Dorsal wrist spanning plate fixation for treatment of radiocarpal fracture-dislocations. Hand (N Y). 2021;16(6):834–42.

Chapter 31
Non-dissociative Carpal Instability in Distal Radius Fractures

Margaret Woon Man Fok and Diego L. Fernandez

Introduction

Distal radius fractures are common in adults, with a prevalence of 17.5% of all fractures [1]. It has a bimodal distribution of presentation, of which it shows correlation with fracture mechanism [2]. Distal radius fractures in male patients between 18 and 45 years old usually result from high-energy trauma, while those in patients >45 years old are usually the consequence of a lower energy mechanism (e.g., a fall on the street). Yet, irrespective of the age groups, the management of distal radius fractures has shifted from cast immobilization to surgical fixation in recent decades [3].

Anatomic reduction and rigid fixation for displaced distal radius fractures have been shown to improve the patients' outcomes [3]. Emphasis should be not only on the radial stabilization but also on the management of associated ligamentous injuries (namely, triangular fibrocartilage complex (TFCC), scapholunate (SL), and lunotriquetral (LT) ligaments). The use of wrist arthroscopy in distal radius fractures has revealed a high incidence of associated TFCC, SL, and LT injuries [4–9]. Debate arises on whether one needs to manage these injuries concomitantly [10–14]. Still no consensus has been drawn [3].

M. W. M. Fok (✉)
Department of Orthopaedics and Traumatology, Queen Mary Hospital, The University of Hong Kong, Pok Fu Lam, Hong Kong Special Adminstractive Region

D. L. Fernandez
University of Bern, Bern, Switzerland

J. Yao (ed.), *Carpal Instability*, https://doi.org/10.1007/978-3-031-55869-6_31

More recent attention has been given to the association of non-dissociative carpal instability with intra- and extra-articular fractures, radiocarpal fracture dislocations [15], and also scaphoid fractures [16]. This subgroup of CIND following acute trauma is now defined as CIND-T. Carpal malalignment is often noted in postfixation radiographs and may show a flexion (palmar) or extension (dorsal) rotational deformity of the proximal row. No identifiable intrinsic ligament tear (namely, SL and LT ligaments) is noted [15]. If this associated pathology does not receive adequate initial treatment along with reduction and fixation of the radius, the misaligned carpus evolves into a fixed irreducible deformity and subsequent wrist stiffness.

This chapter describes the association of CIND and distal radius fractures, discusses the pathomechanics, and provides treatment recommendations.

Background

Carpal instability can be a result of dissociation within a carpal row, dissociation between the carpal rows, or both. While carpal instability dissociative (CID) is characterized by instability between bones within a single carpal row, carpal instability non-dissociative (CIND) is characterized by dysfunction of the entire proximal carpal row, manifested by either the radiocarpal joint, the midcarpal joint, or both [17–19]. When both CIND and CID are present, it is termed as carpal instability combined (CIC). In addition, Wolfe et al. further subclassified CIND into CIND-palmar, CIND-dorsal, and CIND-combined. Depending on which extrinsic radiocarpal ligaments are involved, it causes the proximal row to flex (palmar) or extend (dorsal) [19]. Yet, when carpal instabilities are seen in the presence of distal radius malunion, they have been categorized as carpal instability adaptive (CIA), a term implying that the abnormalities are extrinsic to the carpus and the radiocarpal ligaments are intact. A typical example is the midcarpal malalignment following a malunited distal radius fracture [19, 20]. Due to the malunion, the volar carpal ligaments are slack and are less capable of inducing the physiologic shift of the proximal carpal row from flexion into extension as the wrist ulnarly deviates. While the carpal ligaments are not torn, the distances between their origins and insertions are decreased by the dorsal tilt of the malunited distal radius, resulting in a compensatory proximal row extension and distal row flexion. While most cases of CIA can be managed by corrective osteotomy of distal radius, there are chronic cases of which carpal malalignment cannot be corrected completely following osteotomy, i.e., CIA fixed as described by Fernandez [21].

CIND in distal radius fractures has rarely been addressed in the literature. This entity is different from CIA in that the radiocarpal ligaments are actually torn or avulsed from their insertions, instead of being intact as in CIA. As a result, carpal malalignment persists even after a satisfactory reduction of the distal radius fracture. All intrinsic ligaments including SL and LT ligaments are intact. Depending on the involved radiocarpal ligaments, CIND-T-palmar and CIND-T-dorsal might be noted [15] (Figs. 31.1 and 31.2).

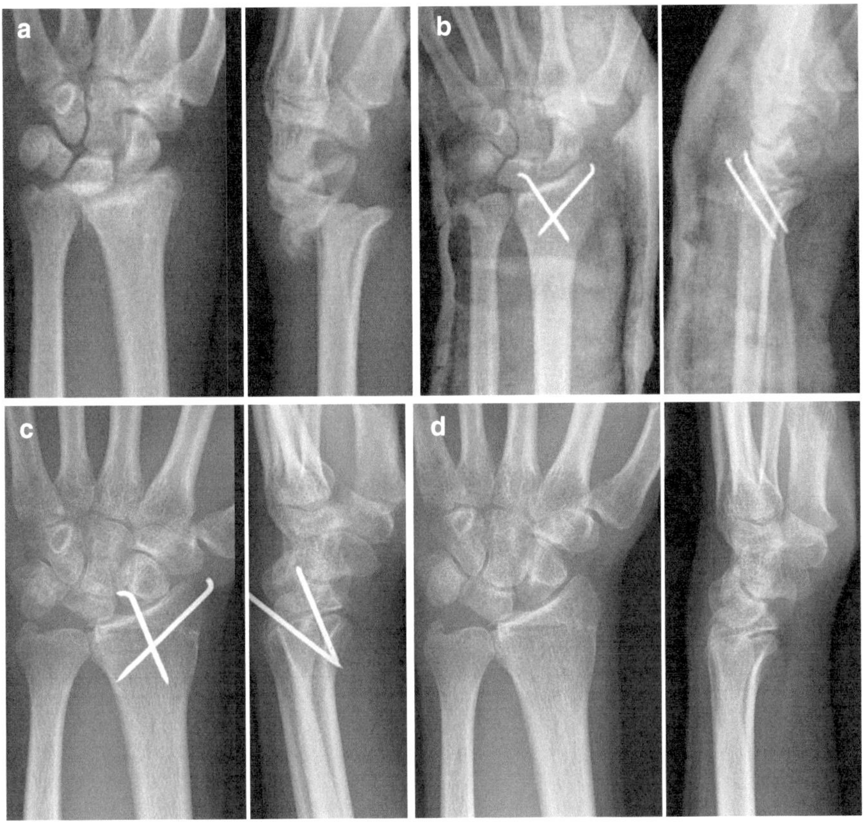

Fig. 31.1 CIND-T-palmar in a 30-year-old patient. (**a**) Fracture dislocation of left distal radius. (**b**) Close reduction and percutaneous pinning of left distal radius. (**c**) Radiographs at 6 weeks post-surgery prior to removal of K-wires. (**d**) Radiographs at 9 weeks post-surgery revealing a subacute CIND-T-palmar configuration. (*Copyright by Margaret Fok*)

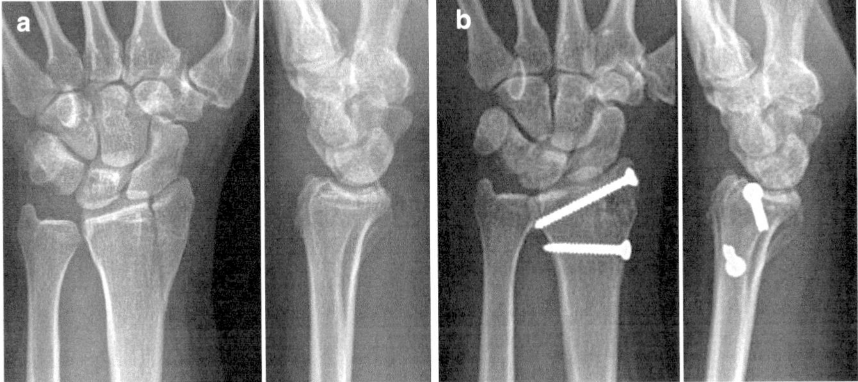

Fig. 31.2 CIND-T-dorsal in a 36-year-old patient. (**a**) Intra-articular fracture of left distal radius. (**b**) Radiographs at 4 weeks post-surgery revealing a subacute CIND-T-dorsal configuration after closed reduction and screw fixation of fracture. (*Copyright by Margaret Fok*)

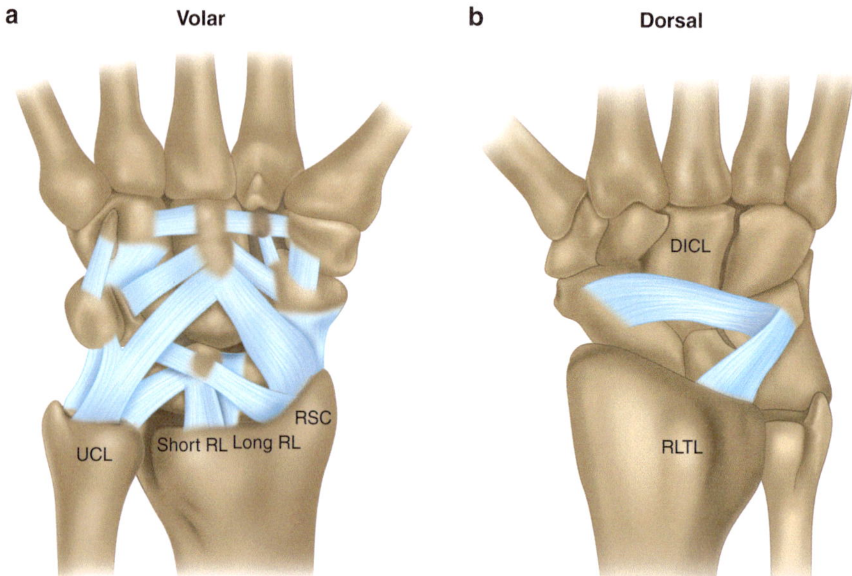

Fig. 31.3 Figures showing the radiocarpal ligaments. (**a**) Key volar radiocarpal ligaments. *UCL* ulnocarpal ligament, *RL* radiolunate ligament, *RSC* radioscaphocapitate ligament. (**b**) Key dorsal radiocarpal ligaments. *DICL* dorsal intercarpal ligament, *RLTL* radiolunotriquetral ligament. (*Copyright by Diego Fernandez*)

Biomechanics [15]

Critical to the stability of radiocarpal joint, several key ligaments are noted dorsally (dorsal intercarpal (DIC) ligament and radiolunotriquetral (RLT) ligament) and volarly (long and short radiolunate (RL) ligament, radioscaphocapitate (RSC) ligament, and ulnocarpal (UC) ligaments) (Fig. 31.3). In cadaveric lab testing, sequential sectioning of dorsal and palmar extrinsic ligaments has been performed in order to simulate the pathomechanism of CIND-T-palmar and CIND-T-dorsal in distal radius fractures.

Four cadaveric forearms were mounted on a stand (Fig. 31.4) of which axial load with 1.5 kg was applied through the wrist. An electronic sensor was then placed centrally (dorsal to palmar) in the lunate to measure the spatial displacement of the proximal row under load.

Fig. 31.4 Biomechanical
test on a cadaveric
forearm. (Copyright by
Margaret FOK)

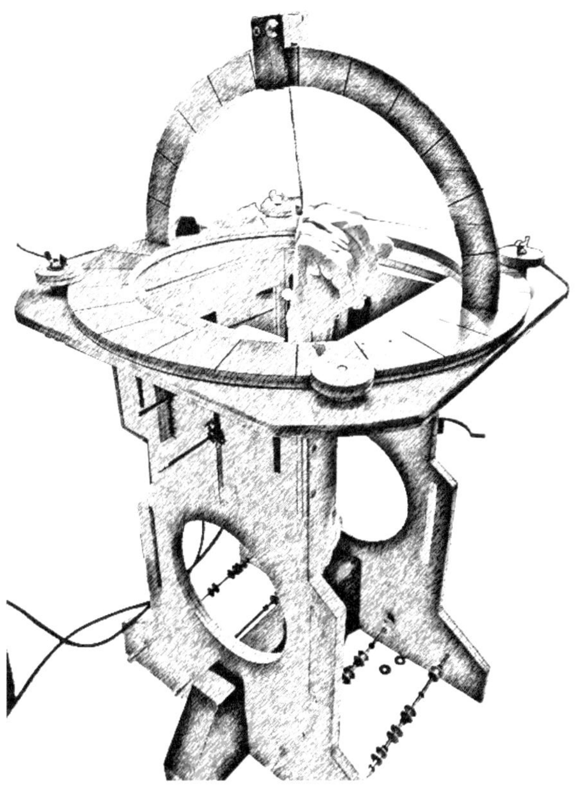

	Position of lunate via sensor (on average) during axial loading			
	Supination	Flexion	Ulnar deviation	Radial deviation
Intact wrist ligament	1.6	0.73	0.7	–
Sectioning of RT ligament	2.7	1.15	0.55	–
Sectioning of RT, long and short RL ligament	0.5	2.33	0.67	–
Sectioning of RT, long and short RL and ulnocarpal ligament	0.87	7.34	–	0.03
Sectioning of all extrinsic ligaments with wrist loaded in 30 ° flexion	0.19	4.10	–	0.14
Sectional of all extrinsic ligaments with wrist loaded in 30 ° extension	3.14	3.81	–	0.81

*SL and LT ligaments remain intact for all specimens

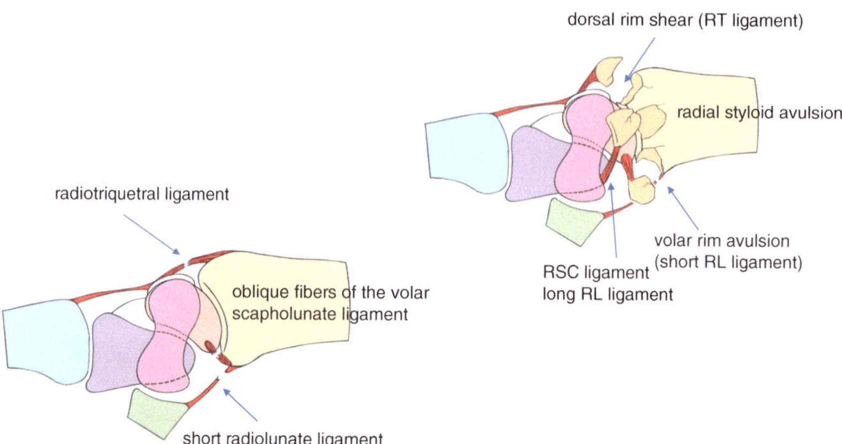

Fig. 31.5 Pathomechanism of CIND-T-palmar–avulsion fractures/ligament tear. (Copyright by *Margaret FOK)*

With sequential sectioning of dorsal and palmar extrinsic ligaments, there was an increase in flexion of the proximal carpal row. In the absence of the ulnocarpal ligament, the proximal row radially deviated instead of deviating ulnarly. Some degree of proximal carpal row supination was noted in all circumstances during axial loading.

Palmar rotation of the proximal carpal row was observed during manual axial force in three cadaveric specimens after sectioning the RT, RSC, and the long and short RL ligaments. Further flexion was noted with the sectioning of ulnocarpal ligaments. This may simulate a clinical situation of which a non-osteoporotic wrist is placed under high-energy trauma. Besides intra-articular fracture, extrinsic wrist ligament tear(s) or bony avulsions (together with the insertion/origin of the extrinsic ligaments) as in radiocarpal fracture-dislocations can result (Fig. 31.5). The volar rim of the radius contains the origin of the short RL ligament. Radial styloid fractures involve the origin of the RSL and long radiolunate ligaments. Shearing fractures of the dorsal rim of the radius imply that the origin of the RLT ligament is affected. Together, they lead to the CIND-T-palmar in distal radius fracture.

For dorsal rotation of the proximal carpal row, sequential sectioning of extrinsic ligaments did not reproduce CIND-T-dorsal. This is compatible with the findings of Wolfe et al. [19]. They postulated that in pure CIND-dorsal, deficiency of DIC and attenuation of long RL and RSC allow the capitate to subluxate dorsally when the proximal row extends during ulnar deviation. Yet, by reviewing the radiographs of patients with CIND-T-dorsal, it is noted that the malalignment was present immediately after fixation of the fracture (Fig. 31.2). Thus, it is suggested that the extension of proximal row may also depend on the displacement of intra-articular fragments at the scaphoid fossa and/or be associated to a radiocarpal extrinsic ligament injury.

Presentation

Despite the alarming radiographic findings, the clinical presentation may vary. While some patients may be asymptomatic, a symptomatic patient may present in the following manner.

A 30-year-old gentleman suffered from a fracture dislocation of left distal radius during a motorcycle accident (Fig. 31.1). Close reduction of left wrist and percutaneous pinning was performed. At 6 weeks post-surgery, the fracture was noted to be healed and K-wires were removed. Active mobilization was started. He re-presented to the clinic at 9 weeks post-surgery with wrist pain and marked stiffness. Radiographs were taken showing a subacute CIND-T-palmar configuration. Wrist arthroscopy confirmed that there were intact scapholunate and lunotriquetral ligaments. As the carpal malignment was found to be unreducible intraoperatively, radioscapholunate arthrodesis was performed (Fig. 31.6). Pain was relieved, and gentle active mobilization exercise was allowed postoperatively. Strengthening exercise was permitted once fusion was noted on radiographs. At 1-year follow-up, the clinical result was satisfactory. The carpal alignment was maintained on radiographs.

The authors have reported [15] 12 patients that presented with either CIND-T-palmar or CIND-T-dorsal after intra-articular distal radius fractures over a 5-year period. The average age was 32 years old, ranging from 18 to 36 years old, and they were involved in high-energy trauma. Ten patients presented with CIND-T-palmar at a variable time frame after the fixation of distal radius fracture, usually after active mobilization exercise was started. Two patients with CIND-T-dorsal presented at the immediate postoperative period. Yet, only 8 out of 12 patients (7 CIND-T-palmar and 1 CIND-T-dorsal) suffered from severe pain and stiffness, affecting their performance of daily activities, requiring revision surgeries.

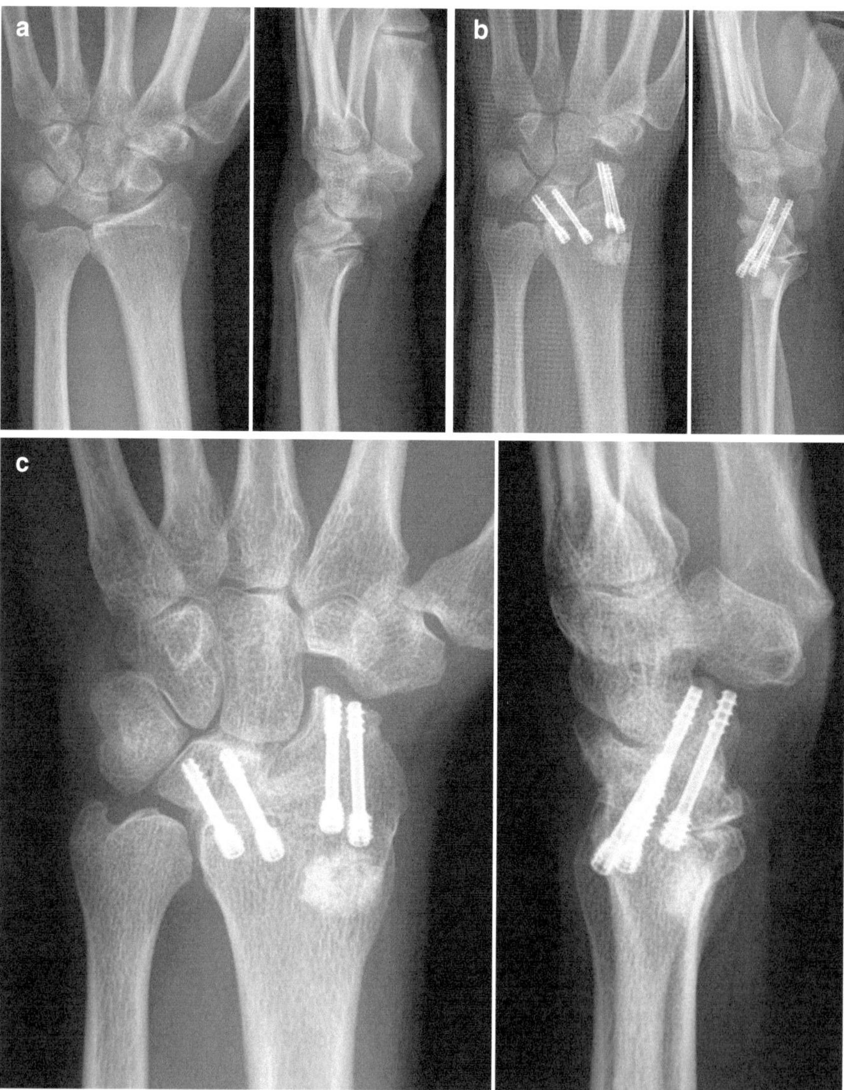

Fig. 31.6 Radioscapholunate (RSL) fusion in a patient with fixed nonreducible carpal malalignment. (**a**) Fixed CIND-T-dorsal after intra-articular distal radius fracture (patient in Fig. 31.2). (**b**) Radiographs showing RSL fusion. (**c**) Radiographs at 1 year post-RSL fusion with maintained carpal alignment. (**d–f**) Clinical result at 1 year post-RSL fusion. (*Copyright by Margaret FOK*)

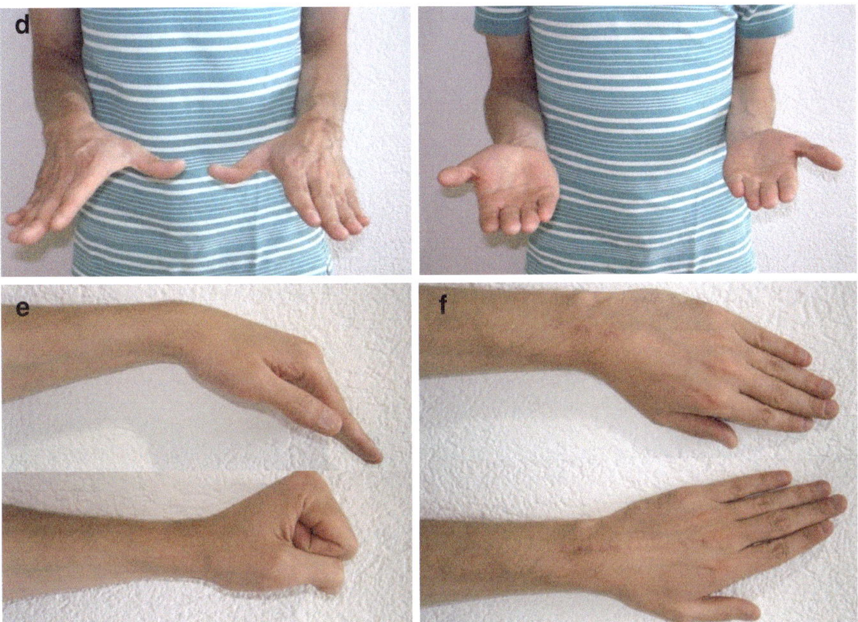

Fig. 31.6 (continued)

Diagnosis

A high index of suspicion is needed. Preoperative radiographs with volar rim avulsions, dorsal rim fractures, radial styloid fractures, as well as dorsal bony avulsions at the triquetrum may suggest the involvement of the extrinsic radiocarpal ligaments. While instability can be detected intraoperatively, it is usually picked up late by plain radiographs after distal radius fixation. An increase >30 ° (CIND-T-dorsal) or decrease <30 ° (CIND-T-palmar) in radiolunate angle with preserved SL angle is noted. Additional computer tomography (CT) of the wrist is indicated in cases where revision surgery is contemplated. One should look for articular incongruity of the distal radius and unreduced avulsion fractures at the volar and dorsal rims. MRI or diagnostic wrist arthroscopy is useful if intrinsic ligament tears are suspected.

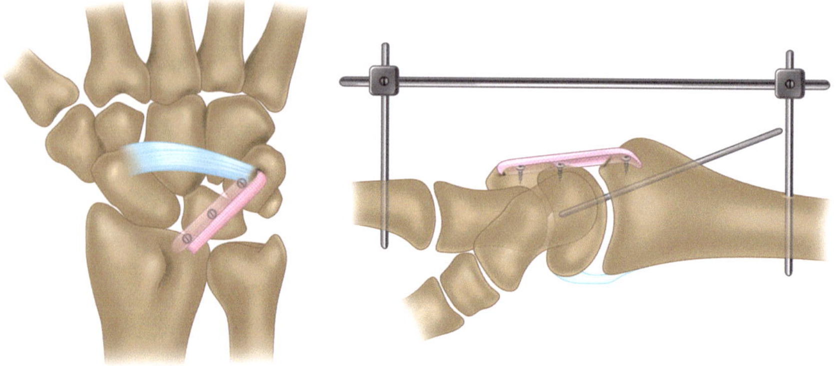

Fig. 31.7 Illustration showing capsule repair/reconstruction of radiolunotriquetral (RLT) ligament with free tendon graft (strip of extensor carpi radialis brevis (ECRB) or palmaris longus (PL)) fixed with three bone anchors). (*Copyright by Diego Fernandez*)

Management

If the patient is symptomatic and is detected early, usually within 3 months, carpal malalignment is reducible. CT is used to assess the congruity of the radiocarpal joint, as well as any unreduced avulsion fractures. Wrist arthroscopy may be used to confirm the integrity of SL and LT ligaments. Dorsal ± volar radiocarpal ligament capsular repair is then performed together with re-reduction of the distal radius if needed (Fig. 31.7). The decision of which ligament(s) to repair will depend on the surgical, CT, and arthroscopic findings. In our patient cohort, only the RTL ligament (dorsal capsule) was repaired in three instances. If the diagnosis is made in the acute stage, anatomic realignment of the carpus, trans-radial pinning of the first carpal row, and immobilization in a forearm cast or with an external fixator for 6–8 weeks allow for undisturbed healing of the ligaments without the need of suture. Wrist arthroscopy helps to confirm that ligament (capsular) alignment is anatomical. Depending on the surgeon's arthroscopic skills, a ligament suture may be added.

In patients with fixed nonreducible carpal malalignment, which may be due to the chronicity of the injury, or if intra-articular malunion with degenerative changes is present, salvage procedures such as radioscapholunate arthrodesis are indicated [15] (Fig. 31.7).

Discussion

Distal radius fractures are associated with a high incidence of ligamentous injuries. No consensus is reached on how to manage them [5–9, 22]. While some surgeons advocate to manage concomitant ligamentous injuries in all young patients with distal radius fractures [10, 11], others showed that the outcome may not be altered even without repair or reconstruction [12, 23]. Concomitant repair of these ligaments may be excessive and cause unnecessary prolonged immobilization. Based on the authors' experience (unpublished data), delayed repair in symptomatic patients can achieve satisfactory outcomes. Nevertheless, distal radius fractures associated with CIND-T require special attention because if carpal alignment is not restored, painful limited motion may ensue.

This chapter describes a group of intra-articular distal radius fractures/fracture dislocations of the wrist with concomitant extrinsic wrist ligament injuries leading to CIND-T. Unlike the Colles fractures seen in osteoporotic elderly patients, these patients tend to be young and are involved in high energy of trauma [15]. They may present with severe pain and stiffness. A high index of suspicion is needed. If they are identified earlier, the carpal malalignment may be corrected by ligament repair or reconstruction, together with an intra-articular corrective osteotomy if needed. Yet, in chronic cases where the malalignment is fixed or with post-traumatic degenerative changes, salvage procedures such as radiolunate or radioscapholunate arthrodesis may be the only option.

References

1. Court-Brown CM, Caesar B. Epidemiology of adult fractures: a review. Injury. 2006;37:691–7.
2. Candela V, Lucia PD, Carnevali C, Milanese A, Spagnoli A, Villani C, et al. Epidemiology of distal radius fractures: a detailed survey on a large sample of patients in a suburban area. J Orthop Traumatol. 2022;23:43.
3. Lichtman DM, Bindra RR, Boyer MI, Putnam MD, Ring D, Slutsky DJ, et al. Treatment of distal radius fractures. Am Acad Orthop Surg. 2010;18:180–9.
4. Mehta JA, Bain GI, Heptinstall RJ. Anatomical reduction of intra-articular fractures of the distal radius: an arthroscopically-assisted approach. J Bone Jt Surg Br Vol. 2000;82-B:79–86.
5. Geissler WB, Fernandez DL, Lamey DM. Distal radioulnar joint injuries associated with fractures of the distal radius. Clin Orthop Relat R. 1996;327:135–46.
6. Ruch DS, Vallee J, Poehling GG, Smith BP, Kuzma GR. Arthroscopic reduction versus fluoroscopic reduction in the management of intra-articular distal radius fractures. Arthrosc J Arthrosc Relat Surg. 2004;20:225–30.
7. Ruch DS, Yang CC, Smith BP. Results of acute arthroscopically repaired triangular fibrocartilage complex injuries associated with intra-articular distal radius fractures. Arthrosc J Arthrosc Relat Surg. 2003;19:511–6.
8. Lindau T, Adlercreutz C, Aspenberg P. Peripheral tears of the triangular fibrocartilage complex cause distal radioulnar joint instability after distal radial fractures. J Hand Surg. 2000;25:464–8.
9. Richards RS, Bennett JD, Roth JH, Milne K. Arthroscopic diagnosis of intra-articular soft tissue injuries associated with distal radial fractures. J Hand Surg. 1997;22:772–6.
10. Abe Y, Yoshida K, Tominaga Y. Less invasive surgery with wrist arthroscopy for distal radius fracture. J Orthop Sci. 2013;18:398–404.
11. Gong HS, Cho HE, Kim J, Kim MB, Lee YH, Baek GH. Surgical treatment of acute distal radioulnar joint instability associated with distal radius fractures. J Hand Surg Eur Vol. 2015;40:783–9.
12. Fok MWM, Fang CX, Lau TW, Fung YKE, Fung BKK, Leung FKL. The status of triangular fibrocartilage complex after the union of distal radius fractures with internal plate fixation. Int Orthop. 2018;42:1917–22.

13. Swart E, Tang P. The effect of ligament injuries on outcomes of operatively treated distal radius fractures. Am J Orthop (Belle Mead N J). 2017;46:E41–6.
14. Mrkonjic A, Lindau T, Geijer M, Tägil M. Arthroscopically diagnosed Scapholunate ligament injuries associated with distal radial fractures: a 13- to 15-year follow-up. J Hand Surg. 2015;40:1077–82.
15. Fok MWM, Fernandez DL, Maniglio M. Carpal instability nondissociative following acute wrist fractures. J Hand Surg. 2020;45:662.e1–662.e10.
16. Loisel F, Orr S, Ross M, Couzens G, Leo AJ, Wolfe S. Traumatic nondissociative carpal instability: a case series. J Hand Surg. 2022;47:285.e1–285.e11.
17. Cooney WP, Dobyns JH, Linscheid RL. Arthroscopy of the wrist: anatomy and classification of carpal instability. Arthrosc J Arthrosc Relat Surg. 1990;6:133–40.
18. Wright TW, Dobyns JH, Linscheid RL, Macksoud W, Siegert J. Carpal instability nondissociative. J Hand Surg Br Eur Vol. 1994;19:763–73.
19. Wolfe SW, Garcia-Elias M, Kitay A. Carpal instability nondissociative. J Am Acad Orthop Sur. 2012;20:575.
20. Taleisnik J, Watson HK. Midcarpal instability caused by malunited fractures of the distal radius. J Hand Surg. 1984;9:350–7.
21. Fernandez DL. Reconstructive procedures for malunion and traumatic arthritis. Orthop Clin N Am. 1993;24:341–63.
22. Mehta JA, Bain GI, Heptinstall RJ. Anatomical reduction of intra-articular fractures of the distal radius: an arthroscopically-assisted approach. J Bone J Surg Br Vol. 2000;82-B:79–86.
23. Mrkonjic A, Geijer M, Lindau T, Tägil M. The natural course of traumatic triangular fibrocartilage complex tears in distal radial fractures: a 13–15 year follow-up of arthroscopically diagnosed but untreated injuries. J Hand Surg. 2012;37:1555–60.

Chapter 32
Carpal Instability Adaptive in Distal Radius Malunions

Jerry I. Huang and Christian M. Shigley

Case Presentation

This patient is a 43-year-old female who sustained an injury to her left wrist from a fall off a horse. She initially underwent open reduction internal fixation of her left distal radius as well as open carpal tunnel release at an outside hospital. At 2 months postoperatively, she was noted to have limited forearm supination, so she was taken to the operating room for closed manipulation of her left wrist and forearm followed by immobilization in a long arm cast in maximal supination for 4 weeks. Patient presented to our clinic 4 months after her index procedure with persistent pain and limited forearm rotation and wrist flexion-extension. On examination, she had gross deformity of the left wrist with volar angulation deformity. Patient had forearm pronation to 70 °, symmetric to the contralateral wrist. She had limited forearm supination to 10 ° on the left, compared to 80 ° on the right. She had wrist flexion to 80 ° on the right and 40 ° on the left, with 80 ° wrist extension on the right, compared to 30 ° on the left. She had dorsal subluxation of the DRUJ with crepitus on DRUJ ballottement. Radiographs and CT demonstrated a volarly displaced left distal radius malunion with 25 ° of volar angulation with 3 mm ulnar positive variance and dorsal DRUJ subluxation (Figs. 32.1 and 32.2). The patient also had dorsal intersegmental instability (DISI) deformity with extension of the lunate.

J. I. Huang (✉) · C. M. Shigley
Department of Orthopaedics and Sports Medicine, University of Washington Medical Center, Seattle, WA, USA
e-mail: jihuang@uw.edu; cshig95@uw.edu

J. Yao (ed.), *Carpal Instability*, https://doi.org/10.1007/978-3-031-55869-6_32

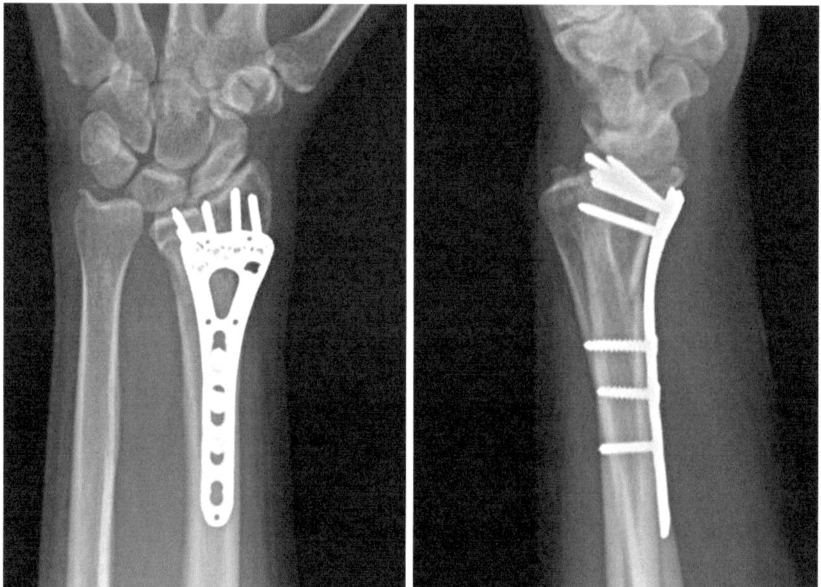

Fig. 32.1 Preoperative radiographs of the wrist with volar plate fixation of the distal radius with increased volar angulation with volar radiocarpal subluxation and shortening with 3 mm ulnar positive variance and dorsal DRUJ subluxation

Treatment options were discussed with the patient including continued therapy for range-of-motion exercises as well as use of static progression orthosis to improve forearm rotation and wrist flexion-extension. The patient had failed therapy with persistent limited forearm supination. We discussed with the patient that she had a volarly displaced distal radius malunion with significant shortening as well as dorsal DRUJ subluxation. We recommended corrective osteotomy of her left distal radius to restore the sagittal alignment of her distal radius as well as correct her carpal malalignment. We also discussed possible DRUJ stabilization with open repair of her triangular fibrocartilage complex (TFCC) and DRUJ capsulorrhaphy.

The patient was taken to the operating room, and an opening wedge osteotomy was performed volarly to correct the distal radius alignment (Figs. 32.3, 32.4, and 32.5). With correction of the volar tilt from 25 ° to approximately 10 °, the lunate position improved with improvement in radiolunate and capitolunate angles. We also restored the radial height to neutral ulnar variance. Following correction of the distal radius malunion, the distal radioulnar joint was stable with no dorsal subluxation. Postoperatively, the patient was placed in a short arm plaster splint for 2 weeks. At 2 weeks postoperatively, the patient was placed into a removable thermoplast orthosis and began gentle active range-of-motion exercises of her forearm and wrist. No strengthening of the injured extremity was seen for 3 months.

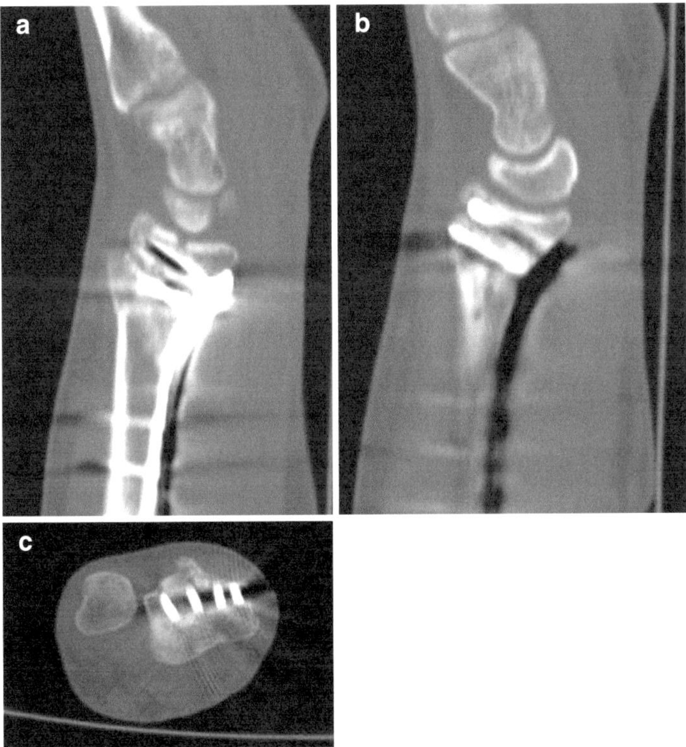

Fig. 32.2 CT scan images demonstrating increased volar angulation of the distal radius with volar radiocarpal subluxation (**a**) as well as extension of the lunate (**b**) with increased radiolunate angle. Axial cuts (**c**) demonstrated dorsal DRUJ subluxation

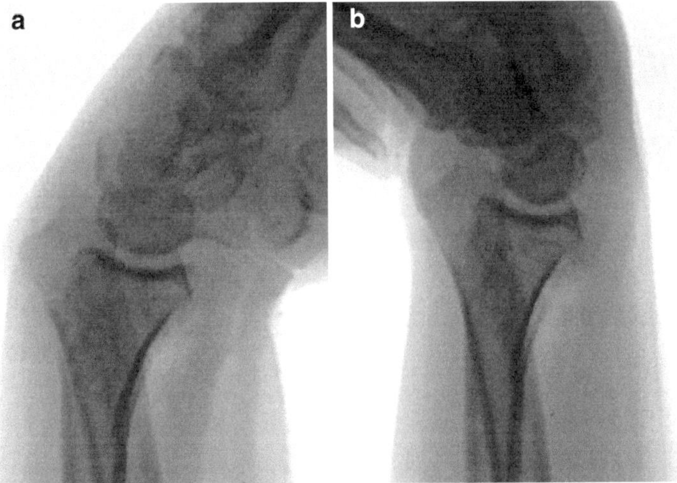

Fig. 32.3 Intraoperative fluoroscopic shots demonstrating reduction of the radiolunate angle with wrist flexion, but increased capitate flexion (**a**) compared to reduced capitolunate angle with wrist extension (**b**). An opening wedge osteotomy was performed

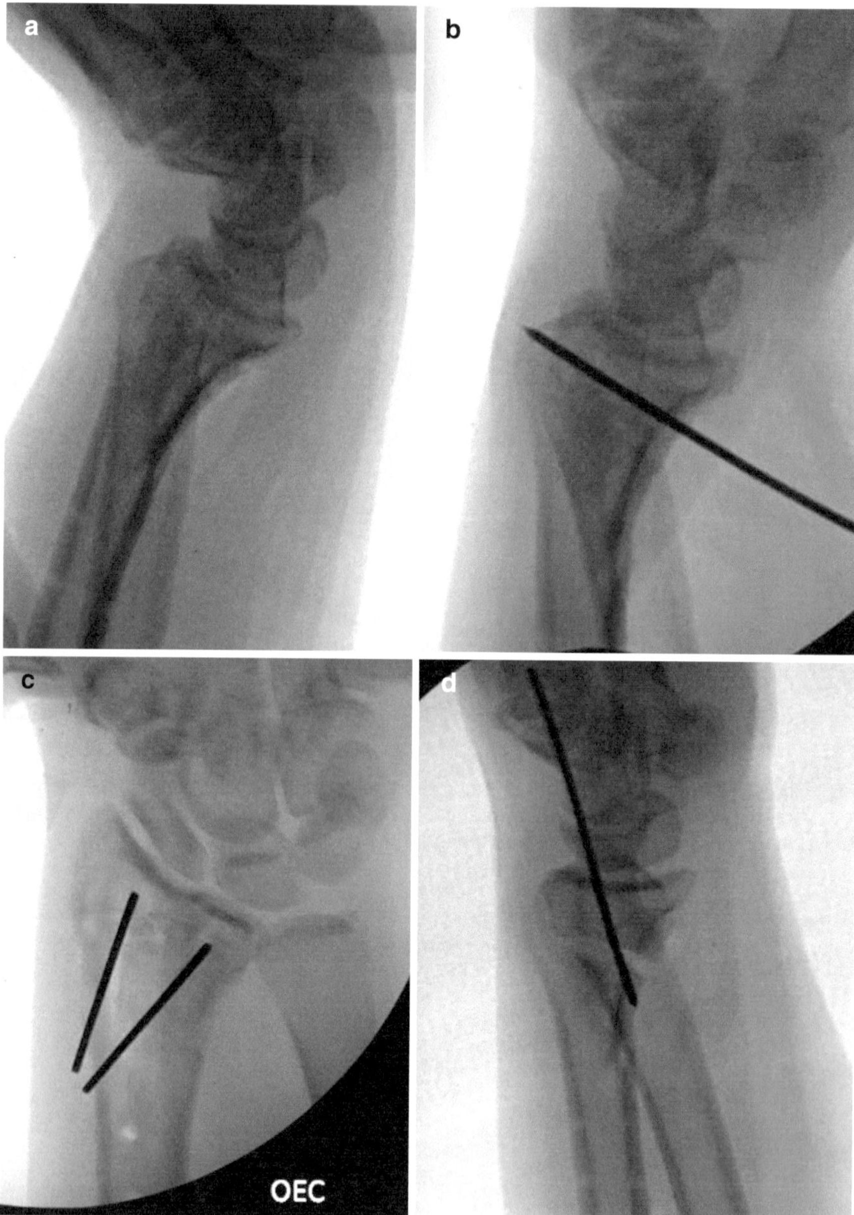

Fig. 32.4 Intraoperative fluoroscopic imaging demonstrating the amount of volar angulation of the distal radius with volar radiocarpal subluxation (**a**). A K-wire is placed at the level of the malunion parallel to the distal radial articular surface (**b**). A second K-wire is placed to mark the position of the osteotomy (**c**). An opening wedge osteotomy was performed using an oscillating saw. With elevation of the distal fragment, we restored the volar tilt back to neutral (**d**)

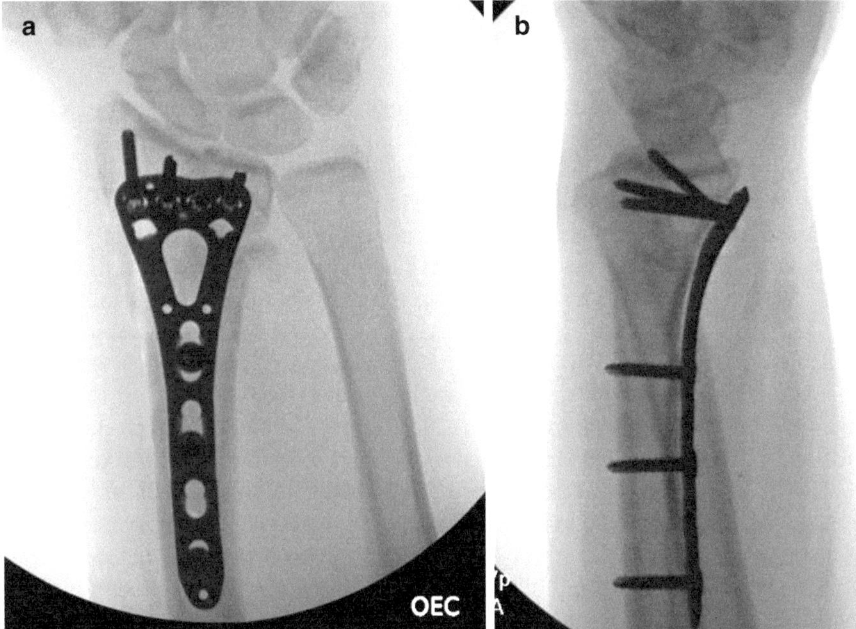

Fig. 32.5 Following opening wedge osteotomy and placement of cancellous bone chips, we were able to restore the radial height to neutral ulnar variance (**a**) as well as normal volar tilt with correction of both the radiocarpal alignment with normal capitate shift as well as normal radiolunate and capitolunate angles (**b**)

Discussion

Distal radius malunions are amongst the most common complications following treatment of distal radius fractures [1–3]. Kinematic studies have demonstrated increased strain at the distal radioulnar joint and increased torque for forearm rotation with dorsal angulation more than 30 ° and loss of forearm supination with volar angulation more than 20 ° [4, 5]. Good to excellent outcomes can be expected with distal radial corrective osteotomy (DRO) for distal radius malunions with improvement in forearm rotation and wrist range of motion, as well as patient-rated outcome scores [2, 6–8]. Relative indications for corrective osteotomy include pain with motion or activity, weakness, mechanical symptoms, decreased grip strength or range of motion, and functional limitations affecting activities of daily living [9]. For extra-articular fractures, rehabilitation should be attempted for 6 months to assess functional impact since many patients may have an acceptable clinical outcome despite abnormal radiographic parameters. Jupiter and Ring compared early vs. delayed osteotomy for distal radius malunions and found no clinical differences between intervention at 8 vs. 40 weeks [2]. However, the authors concluded that the procedure is technically easier in early reconstruction. For intra-articular fractures, early surgery is indicated to mitigate articular cartilage degeneration and development of post-traumatic arthritis.

Distal malunion can lead to changes in carpal alignment as a result of an adaptive response to changes in contact between the carpus and the distal radius with dorsal collapse being more common. McQueen et al. reported on 120 patients in a randomized trial comparing cast immobilization with open reduction internal fixation and found carpal malignment to be the most important factor predicting function in these patients [10]. Two types of patterns of carpal malalignment have been observed [11]. Type 1 is midcarpal instability where the lunate is tilted dorsally in line with the dorsally angulated distal radius, with compensatory flexion of the capitate. This pattern was first observed by Taleisnik and Watson as a dynamic form of instability as a complication of distal radius malunion [12]. The wrist adopts a zigzag shape relative to the radius, which results in reduced strength and restricted pronation and flexion [13]. Type 2 malalignment is dorsal translation of the carpus in relation to the distal radius. Uncorrected radiocarpal malalignment can result in ligament attenuation, synovitis, tendon irritation, delayed carpal tunnel syndrome, and early osteoarthritis [11]. In their series of 13 patients with adaptive carpal instability, corrective osteotomy led to relief of preoperative symptoms and correction of midcarpal instability.

Gupta et al. described the two types of adaptive carpal instability based on the effective radiolunate flexion (ERLF), which utilizes a lateral wrist X-ray to calculate the following equation [14]:

$$ERLF = (\text{Measured dorsal tilt}) + 11\,\text{degrees}\,[\text{of standard volar tilt}]$$
$$- (\text{Measured radiolunate angle})$$

Type 1 has an ERLF <25 °, representing a distal radius fragment and lunate extended together and remaining collinear. Type 2 has an ERLF >25 °, representing a dorsally subluxated lunate, relative to the distal radius fragment, so it may remain collinear with the capitate [14]. However, the ERLF has not been validated in different wrist conditions and may be influenced by wrist positioning. To overcome these limitations, recent studies have utilized capitate shift, which is the perpendicular displacement of the capitate center relative to the longitudinal radial axis [15–18]. The longitudinal radial axis should be placed along the interior aspect of the volar cortical line (proximal to the volar radial curve), compared to the central axis, because the volar cortical line is more reliable and reproducible in wrists with a distal radius fracture, without fracture and with rheumatoid arthritis [17]. In the unfractured wrist, the capitate center is normally 0.25–2.0 mm palmar relative to the volar radial cortex, and this finding is unaffected by wrist position [17, 18]. Patients with symptomatic carpal instability adaptive pattern can benefit from distal radius osteotomy to restore key radiographic parameters, such as capitate shift and volar tilt [11, 16].

De Smet et al. evaluated their clinical outcomes in 31 patients with a distal radius malunion treated with corrective osteotomy to determine the effect of improvement in radiocarpal and midcarpal alignment [11]. There was radiographic correction of volar tilt from 12 ° dorsal tilt to 6 ° volar postoperatively, and restoration of radial height from 2 mm ulnar positive variance to neutral variance. In the 20 type 1 patients, the mean ERLF was 0.8 °, while in the 11 type 2 patients, the mean ERL was 33 °. In group 1 patients, the mean radiolunate angle improved from −20 ° to −7 °, while the capitolunate angle improved from 10 ° to 0 °. The ability to correct the radiographic parameters did not correlate with age or timing of the osteotomy from the time of fracture.

Dias et al. performed a study on 250 consecutive patients with 252 distal fractures to investigate the magnitude of dorsal tilt that leads to carpal malalignment in distal radius malunions [15]. The center of the capitate normally sits slightly palmar to the longitudinal axis of the distal radius. The authors found capitate shift to have the strongest correlation to dorsal tilt and was not affected by wrist position. They found that abnormal capitate shift was observed when dorsal tilt was greater than 9 °. The same group found that correcting the dorsal tilt through an osteotomy can successfully improve carpal malalignment and capitate shift [16].

References

1. Cooney WP, Linscheid RL, Dobyns JH. External pin fixation for unstable Colles' fractures. J Bone Joint Surg Am. 1979;61:840–5.
2. Jupiter JB, Ring D. A comparison of early and late reconstruction of malunited fractures of the distal end of the radius. J Bone Joint Surg. 1996;78:739–48. https://doi org/10.2106/00004623-199605000-00014.
3. Ring D, Roberge C, Morgan T, Jupiter JB. Osteotomy for malunited fractures of the distal radius: a comparison of structural and nonstructural autogenous bone grafts. J Hand Surg Am. 2002;27:216–22. https://doi.org/10.1053/jhsu.2002.32076.
4. Hirahara H, Neale PG, Lin Y-T, Cooney WP, An K-N. Kinematic and torque-related effects of dorsally angulated distal radius fractures and the distal radial ulnar joint. J Hand Surg Am. 2003;28:614–21. https://doi.org/10.1016/S0363-5023(03)00249-1.
5. Nishiwaki M, Welsh MF, Gammon B, Ferreira LM, Johnson JA, King GJW. Effect of volarly angulated distal radius fractures on forearm rotation and distal radioulnar joint kinematics. J Hand Surg Am. 2015;40:2236–42. https://doi.org/10.1016/j.jhsa.2015.07.034.
6. Mulders MAM, d'Ailly PN, Cleffken BI, Schep NWL. Corrective osteotomy is an effective method of treating distal radius malunions with good long-term functional results. Injury. 2017;48:731–7. https://doi.org/10.1016/j.injury.2017.01.045.
7. Sato K, Nakamura T, Iwamoto T, Toyama Y, Ikegami H, Takayama S. Corrective osteotomy for volarly malunited distal radius fracture. J Hand Surg Am. 2009;34:27–33.e1. https://doi.org/10.1016/j.jhsa.2008.09.018.
8. Shea K, Fernandez DL, Jupiter JB, Martin C. Corrective osteotomy for malunited, volarly displaced fractures of the distal end of the radius. J Bone Joint Surg. 1997;79:1816–26. https://doi.org/10.2106/00004623-199712000-00007.
9. Bushnell BD, Bynum DK. Malunion of the distal radius. J Am Acad Orthop Surg. 2007;15:27–40. https://doi.org/10.5435/00124635-200701000-00004.

10. McQueen MM, Hajducka C, Court-Brown CM. Redisplaced unstable fractures of the distal radius: a prospective randomised comparison of four methods of treatment. J Bone Joint Surg Br. 1996;78:404–9.
11. De Smet L, Verhaegen F, Degreef I. Carpal malalignment in malunion of the distal radius and the effect of corrective osteotomy. J Wrist Surg. 2014;03:166–70. https://doi.org/10.1055/s-0034-1384823.
12. Taleisnik J, Watson HK. Midcarpal instability caused by malunited fractures of the distal radius. J Hand Surg Am. 1984;9:350–7. https://doi.org/10.1016/S0363-5023(84)80222-1.
13. Cognet J-M, Mares O. Distal radius malunion in adults. Orthop Traumatol Surg Res. 2021;107:102755. https://doi.org/10.1016/j.otsr.2020.102755.
14. Gupta A, Batra S, Jain P, Sharma SK. Carpal alignment in distal radial fractures. BMC Musculoskelet Disord. 2002;3:14. https://doi.org/10.1186/1471-2474-3-14.
15. Dias R, Johnson NA, Dias JJ. Prospective investigation of the relationship between dorsal tilt, carpal malalignment, and capitate shift in distal radial fractures. Bone Joint J. 2020;102-B:137–43. https://doi.org/10.1302/0301-620X.102B1.BJJ-2019-0738.R1.
16. Johnson NA, Simcock G-L, Rye D, Dias JJ. Change in capitate shift after osteotomy for distal radial fracture malunion. J Hand Surg Eur Vol. 2023;48:798–802. https://doi.org/10.1177/17531934231159786.
17. Kuhnel SP, Bigham AT, McMurtry RY, Faber KJ, King GJW, Grewal R. The capitate-to-axis-of-radius distance (CARD): a new radiographic measurement for wrist and carpal alignment in the sagittal plane. J Hand Surg Am. 2019;44:797.e1–8. https://doi.org/10.1016/j.jhsa.2018.10.024.
18. Selles C, Ras L, Walenkamp M, Maas M, Goslings J, Schep N. Carpal alignment: a new method for assessment. J Wrist Surg. 2019;08:112–7. https://doi.org/10.1055/s-0038-1673406.

Chapter 33
Arthroscopic Management of Perilunate Injuries

Bo Liu and Feiran Wu

Case Presentation

A 27-year-old, right-handed male fell from a height of 3 m onto a concrete floor with an outstretched hand. He presented to the emergency department after 16 h due to increasing pain and swelling in his right hand and wrist. Clinical examination showed diffuse swelling in the wrist compared to his contralateral side. There was tenderness over the anatomical snuffbox, lunate and triquetrum, both dorsal and palmar. Range of movement was difficult to assess due to pain both actively and passively. The patient complained of tingling in his index and middle fingers, but subjective sensation was intact according to the ten test.

Perilunate injuries are severe, highly unstable carpal dissociations characterized by a complete loss of contact between the lunate and surrounding carpus. It is comprised of a spectrum of conditions that include purely ligamentous injuries in perilunate dislocations (PLDs) and bone and ligament injuries caused by trans-scaphoid perilunate fracture-dislocations (PLFDs) [1–3]. Excessive radiocarpal hyperextension and ulnar deviation coupled with intercarpal supination have been shown to be the principal pathologic forces that disrupt the key components of the wrist [1].

The deformity in PLD-PLFDs can be variable and subtle [4]. Diagnosis can be initially missed in up to 25% of patients, even in isolated trauma [5]. Clinically, there is invariably pain and swelling, but an obvious visible abnormality may not be apparent. Signs of median nerve injury, particularly sensory, should be examined for and can be present in up to 16% of patients [6]. The most common demographic

B. Liu (✉)
Department of Hand Surgery, Beijing Ji Shui Tan Hospital, Capital Medical University and the 4th Clinical College of Peking University, Beijing, China

F. Wu
Birmingham Hand Centre, Queen Elizabeth Hospital, University Hospitals Birmingham, Birmingham, UK

J. Yao (ed.), *Carpal Instability*, https://doi.org/10.1007/978-3-031-55869-6_33

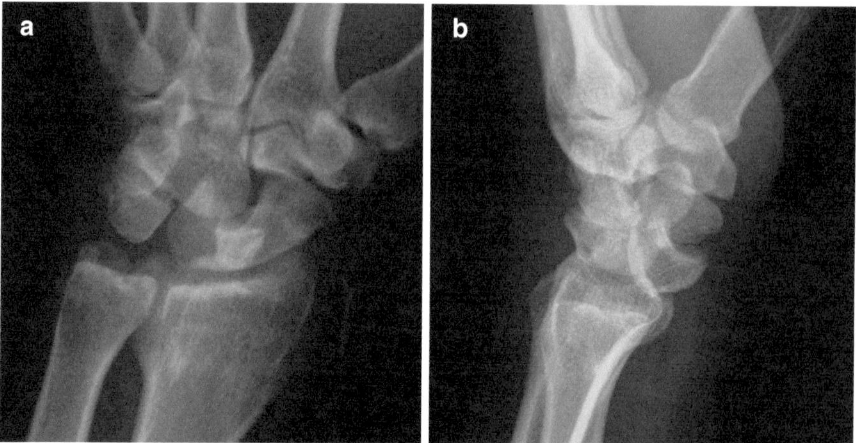

Fig. 33.1 (**a**) AP and (**b**) lateral radiographs of the patient with perilunate dislocation

is young males, with a typical mechanism being the result of a fall from two to three stories of height or road traffic accidents [6].

Diagnosis

Posterior-anterior (PA) radiographs taken of this patient's wrist showed uneven gapping between the luno-capitate and luno-triquetral joints, and disruption of Gilula's arcs. A lateral radiograph revealed that the lunate was no longer articulating with the capitate, confirming a perilunate dislocation (Fig. 33.1).

For investigation, plain PA and lateral radiographs of the wrist are almost always sufficient [7]. On PA radiographs, the space between individual carpal bones should be uniform. The articular surfaces of proximal and distal carpal rows should form smooth arcs at the radiocarpal and midcarpal articulations, i.e., Gilula's arcs. In the setting of a perilunate dislocation, these arcs are disrupted and an unusual overlap of adjacent bones is seen. On lateral radiographs, the distinctive convex shape of the distal lunate can be identified with careful inspection and should be seated in the convexity of the proximal capitate.

Management

Closed Reduction

In this case, a single attempt of a closed manual reduction was performed. The hand was elevated with finger traps, and gentle traction of 10–15 lbs was applied for 10 min. After distraction, the traction tower was released and the patient's wrist extended (maintaining longitudinal traction manually). The wrist was then gradually flexed to allow the capitate to snap back into the concavity of the lunate. To facilitate this maneuver, the operator's thumb stabilizes the lunate volarly to prevent its volar displacement by the capitate. After reduction, manual traction was released and the wrist brought back into a neutral position. Radiographs were obtained to check the success of the reduction. In this instance, the closed manual reduction was unsuccessful, and the patient was transferred to the operating room for an arthroscopic assisted reduction (AAR).

The definitive treatment of these complex injuries is always operative. Nonoperative management of perilunate injuries has unacceptably high rates of loss of reduction with poor eventual outcomes [6, 8]. We recommend a single attempt of closed manual reduction of capitolunate dislocations in the emergency department before proceeding to surgery. For acute cases, usually more than 50% of cases are successfully reduced closed after one attempt. If reduction fails, further repeated attempts are generally unsuccessful and should be avoided, particularly to avoid injury to the carpal cartilage as well as the median nerve. Repeated blind and forceful attempts can lead to further damage of the proximal capitate cartilage, an area that is already vulnerable from the index injury (Fig. 33.2). The likelihood of successful closed reductions of capitolunate dislocations significantly reduces when there is a delay of 3 days or longer following initial injury. In such scenarios, treatment should progress directly to an AAR.

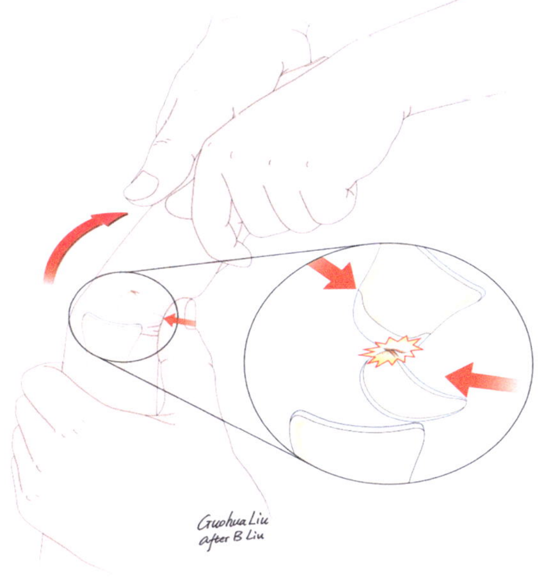

Fig. 33.2 Forceful closed manual reduction can damage the proximal capitate cartilage

Arthroscopic Reduction and Fixation

Once the patient was transferred to the operating room, under regional anesthesia, the arm was suspended in a traction tower by sterile finger traps. A dorsal 3–4 radiocarpal portal was used for initial inspection of the joint. Sufficient space for scope placement is usually not an issue as the lunate is tilted volarly and impinged against the proximal aspect of the capitate. It may also be trapped by interposed torn palmar capsular ligaments, a cause for the failure of closed reduction. Wet arthroscopy is generally required for initial joint debridement, as the initial arthroscopic view is usually obscured by traumatic synovitis, intra-articular hematoma, torn capsuloligamentous tissue, and bony or chondral debris. Joint insufflation also helps to compress small capillaries within the capsule and synovium, which aids in the control of intra-articular bleeding to achieve a clearer image.

Once a clear view was obtained, an additional 4–5 radiocarpal portal was made, and the radiocarpal joint was systematically examined. The triangular fibrocartilage complex (TFCC), volar extrinsic, and intercarpal ligaments were systematically assessed by direct inspection and manual probing. The midcarpal joint was then assessed through the radial and ulnar midcarpal portals. The SL and LT ligaments were examined by manual probing, and concomitant chondral injuries were identified and debrided. Soft tissue or bony fragments interposed between the SL and LT intervals were excised to facilitate reduction of the intercarpal joints.

Following assessment, an arthroscopic probe was introduced into the radiocarpal joint through the 4–5 portal, which allows the probe to directly face the subluxated lunate. After probe introduction, the force of wrist traction was gently increased so the tip of the probe can be hooked onto the dorsal rim of the lunate (Fig. 33.3). Two K-wires were advanced into the scaphoid and triquetrum targeting the lunate, without crossing the intercarpal intervals (Fig. 33.4). The "shoehorn maneuver" was then performed to reduce the dislocated lunate, using the probe to pull the lunate under the proximal capitate. By performing this maneuver entirely under direct arthroscopic vision, further compromise of the articular cartilage can be prevented. Once the capitolunate joint was reduced, traction was reduced and residual lunate angulation was corrected by passively flexing the wrist and transfixing the radiolunate joint with a temporary K-wire. Further correction of the rotation deformity of the scaphoid and lunate can be obtained by using a probe or depressor at the midcarpal joint if required. Once the SL and LT intervals were reduced, the K-wires in the scaphoid and triquetrum were advanced under direct vision into the lunate (Fig. 33.5).

Despite K-wire fixation, more than half of the PLDs will have grossly unstable SL joints that are easily redislocated, due to incompetence of both the primary and secondary stabilizers from the index trauma. In cases like these, we advocate augmenting the SL ligament through a dorsal mini-invasive approach and reinforcing the dorsal scapholunate complex. The dorsal scapholunate complex, including dorsal capsulo-scapholunate septum (DCSS) and the dorsal extrinsic ligaments, is a

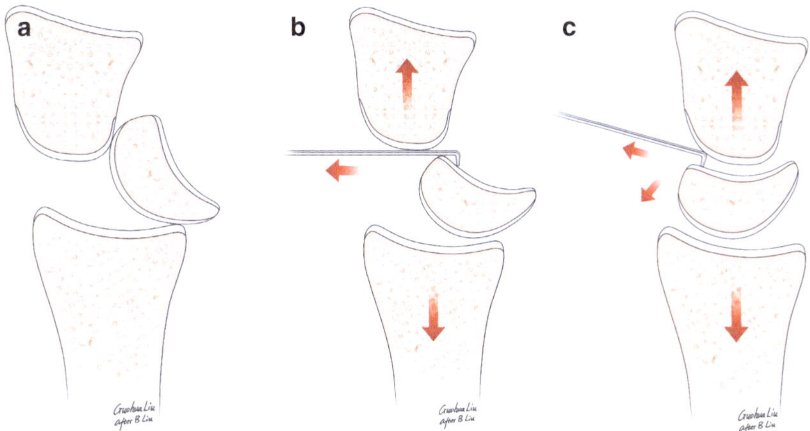

Fig. 33.3 The shoehorn maneuver to reduce the capitolunate joint (a) Before reduction; (b) Reducing the dislocation; (c) After reduction

Fig. 33.4 K-wires are advanced into the scaphoid and triquetrum prior to reducing the capitolunate joint

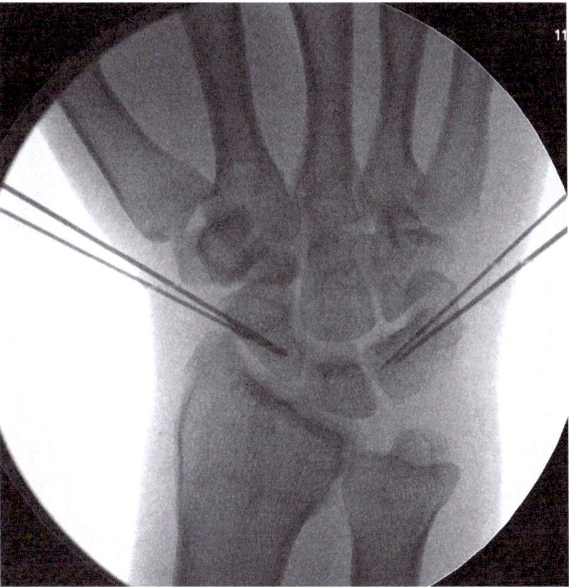

key structure for the maintenance of SL stability and subsequent long-term successful results [9, 10]. This augmentation is performed by transversely extending the 3–4 portal to a 2 cm skin opening. The extensor tendons are retracted, and a suture anchor is placed, under fluoroscopic guidance, into the scaphoid and lunate at a distance of 1 cm from the SL interval. Both sutures are delivered through the dorsal capsule and tied together to create an extra-articular reinforcement of the dorsal scapholunate complex.

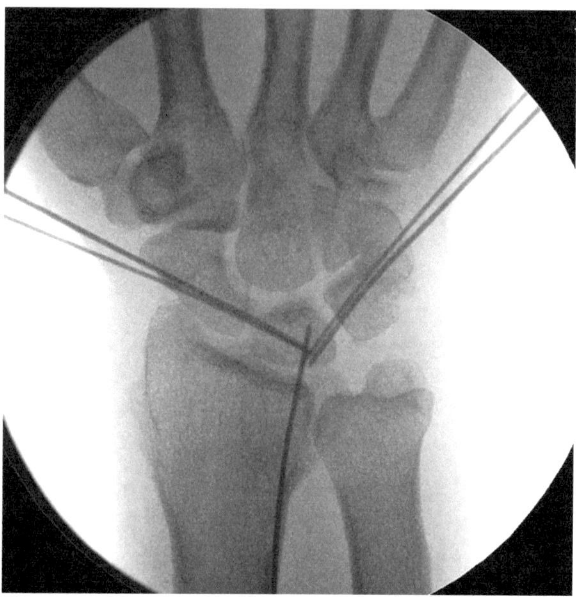

Fig. 33.5 K-wires are advanced into the lunate through the scapholunate and lunotriquetral intervals following reduction of the capitolunate joint

Arthroscopic Reduction and Fixation of PLFDs

The treatment of trans-scaphoid PLFDs is similar to the treatment of PLDs. The injuries are easily identified from orthogonal radiographs. For acute injuries under 3 days old, a single closed manual reduction is attempted in the emergency department. If this fails, or if the case presents after 3 days, patients are transferred to the operating room for AAR and fixation.

Under regional anesthesia and with the arm suspended, the radiocarpal and midcarpal joints are fully assessed using the 3–4 and 4–5 radial and ulnar midcarpal portals. When performing the "shoehorn maneuver," unlike the maneuver for PLDs, the tip of the probe is placed onto the dorsal edge of the scapholunate ligament instead of the lip of the lunate (Fig. 33.6). The wrist traction force is then gently increased up to 15 lbs, while the surgeon gently pulls and reduces the scapholunate complex under the capitate.

In PLFDs, anatomical reduction and fixation of the scaphoid fracture are the critical step in achieving a successful outcome. This fracture is generally significantly displaced in these injuries, with AAR of the scaphoid almost always necessary. To reduce the scaphoid, a guidewire is advanced along the central axis of the distal fragment from the scaphoid tubercle in a retrograde direction, without crossing the fracture line. Further K-wires can be inserted into the distal and proximal fragments to be used as fragment joysticks. Using the ulnar midcarpal portal for vision, the joysticks are manipulated to reduce the scaphoid anatomically (Fig. 33.7). The rotational and translational displacement must be checked in both the sagittal and coronal planes when checking the adequacy of reduction. Once

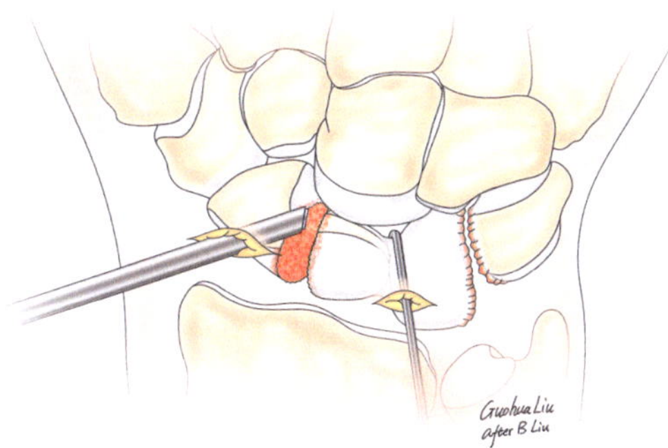

Fig. 33.6 In perilunate fracture-dislocations, the probe is hooked onto the scapholunate ligament in the shoehorn maneuver

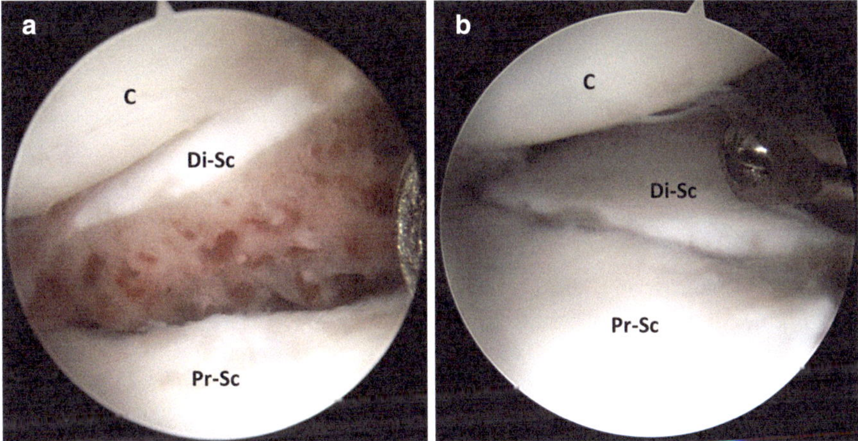

Fig. 33.7 (**a**) Pre- and (**b**) post-reduction midcarpal joint view of a scaphoid fracture. *C* capitate, *Di-Sc* distal scaphoid fragment, *Pr-Sc* proximal scaphoid fragment

reduced, the surgeon maintains the reduction while the assistant drives the central axis guidewire and a subsequent anti-rotation K-wire across the fracture site into the proximal scaphoid fragment. If a residual fracture gap persists between the scaphoid fragments, a cannulated headless compression screw can be used to compress the fracture gap and supplement the fixation. In waist fractures, the scaphoid is reamed retrograde over the central axis guidewire, and a screw is also inserted retrograde, compressing the fragments (Fig. 33.8). For proximal third or proximal pole fractures, the central guidewire is advanced proximally through the dorsal skin. A percutaneous stab incision is made in the dorsal skin where the wire exits. Reaming and screw insertion are then performed antegrade through the second incision. All K-wires are cut short and buried under the skin for both PLDs and PLFDs.

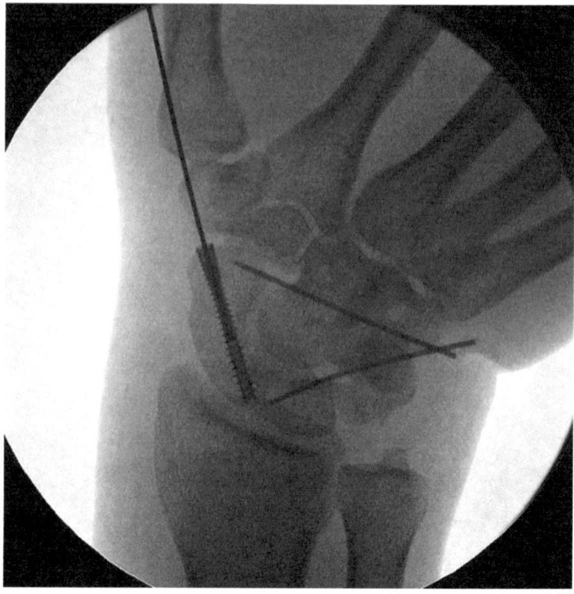

Fig. 33.8 Headless compression screw used for fixation of the scaphoid in a PLFD

Management of Associated Injuries

Frequently, arthroscopy will identify a number of concomitant injuries, many of which will need to be addressed. Traditionally, PLDs are thought of as "purely ligamentous" injuries. However, it is not uncommon to find concomitant carpal fractures in these patients, particularly following high-energy trauma. Associated displaced fractures of the triquetrum or capitate necessitate arthroscopic assisted reduction and percutaneous fixation. Other associated injuries that are typically seen include tears of the TFCC. These can be debrided or repaired as appropriate.

In PLFDs, it is common to find hemorrhage and attenuation of the scapholunate ligament. Most of these injuries are Geissler grade I or II, which are treated with immobilization only. However, only a minority will have more severe SL ligament avulsions from the lunate or gross ruptures of the SL ligament. These represent Geissler grade III or IV disruptions, and scapholunate pinning is required following an accurate reduction of the SL interval.

For patients who present with symptoms of carpal tunnel syndrome during initial presentation, we do not routinely perform carpal tunnel decompressions and the patients are managed expectantly through serial examination. The median nerve symptoms are usually due to nerve stretching and will usually resolve with reduction of the capitolunate joint.

Postoperative Care

In the current case, following fixation and burying of K-wires, the arm is immobilized in a short arm thermoplastic splint. This extends from the mid-forearm to the base of the thumb for a period of 8 weeks. At that point, the K-wires are removed under local anesthesia, and active wrist motion and gentle weight loading are initiated under the guidance of hand therapists.

For PLFDs, the proximal phalanx of the thumb is included in the splint, and weight loading and sporting activities are initiated following confirmation of scaphoid union. In patients with concurrent TFCC injuries, long arm thermoplastic splints are used with the forearm at semi-supination rotation for 6 weeks, followed by short arm splints for a further 2 weeks.

Tips and Tricks

- Surgeons attempting AAR should be proficient in the open management of PLDs and PLFDs and be ready to convert from arthroscopic to open surgery if difficulties are encountered intraoperatively.
- A poorly reduced scaphoid fracture in trans-scaphoid PLFDs will lead to unacceptably poor outcomes, and an open reduction and internal fixation should be performed if the scaphoid cannot be reduced arthroscopically.
- Arthroscopists should be proficient in the conversion of wet to dry arthroscopy techniques and may find this helpful in facilitating fracture reduction and fixation.
- Wrist traction should be used selectively, and the surgeon should clearly recognize the specific situations when wrist traction would be helpful, e.g., increasing wrist traction for AAR of the capitolunate joint and releasing traction when reducing and fixing the scaphoid fracture in trans-scaphoid PLFDs.

Conclusion

The optimal management of PLDs and PLFDs remains challenging and can be controversial. It is our philosophy to employ the method that is associated with the least surgical morbidity in order to achieve a successful outcome. Open surgery involves extensive soft tissue dissection, which could lead to capsular scarring, joint stiffness, and further impair of the already tenuous vascular supply to the scaphoid and intrinsic ligaments. The arthroscopic assisted management of such injuries offers a more precise alternative to assist with anatomical reduction and accurate percutaneous fixation.

References

1. Mayfield JK, Johnson RP, Kilcoyne RK. Carpal dislocations: pathomechanics and progressive perilunar instability. J Hand Surg. 1980;5(3):226–41. https://doi.org/10.1016/S0363-5023(80)80007-4.
2. Johnson RP. The acutely injured wrist and its residuals. Clin Orthop. 1980;149:33–44. https://doi.org/10.1097/00003086-198006000-00005.
3. Herzberg G. Perilunate and axial carpal dislocations and fracture–dislocations. J Hand Surg. 2008;33(9):1659–68. https://doi.org/10.1016/j.jhsa.2008.09.013.
4. Budoff JE. Treatment of acute lunate and perilunate dislocations. J Hand Surg. 2008;33(8):1424–32. https://doi.org/10.1016/j.jhsa.2008.07.016.
5. Herzberg G, Comtet JJ, Linscheid RL, Amadio PC, Cooney WP, Stalder J. Perilunate dislocations and fracture-dislocations: a multicenter study. J Hand Surg. 1993;18(5):768–79. https://doi.org/10.1016/0363-5023(93)90041-Z.
6. Adkison JW, Chapman MW. Treatment of acute lunate and perilunate dislocations. Clin Orthop. 1982;164:199–207.
7. Weil WM, Slade JF, Trumble TE. Open and arthroscopic treatment of perilunate injuries. Clin Orthop. 2006;445:120–32.
8. Apergis E, Maris J, Theodoratos G, Pavlakis D, Antoniou N. Perilunate dislocations and fracture-dislocations. Closed and early open reduction compared in 28 cases. Acta Orthop Scand Suppl. 1997;275:55–9.
9. Wahegaonkar A, Mathoulin C. Arthroscopic dorsal Capsulo-ligamentous repair in the treatment of chronic Scapho-lunate ligament tears. J Wrist Surg. 2013;02(02):141–8. https://doi.org/10.1055/s-0033-1341582.
10. Mathoulin C. Treatment of dynamic scapholunate instability dissociation: contribution of arthroscopy. Hand Surg Rehabil. 2016;35(6):377–92. https://doi.org/10.1016/j.hansur.2016.09.002.

Chapter 34
Perilunate Injuries: Open Management

Nicole A. Zelenski and Christine V. Schaeffer

Case Presentation

A 19-year-old right-hand-dominant male sustained a ground-level fall while playing basketball. He presented acutely to the ED with pain and deformity of his left hand with paresthesia and numbness in the median nerve distribution. He had no other injuries and was previously otherwise healthy.

Diagnosis

Radiographs

Plain radiographs demonstrated Herzberg stage I trans-scaphoid perilunate fracture-dislocation with dorsal dislocation of the capitate (Fig. 34.1a, b) [1]. The lunate is maintained within the lunate fossa. Postreduction radiographs were obtained (Fig. 34.2a, b). Surgeons should consider postreduction cross-sectional imaging to assess for occult fractures and for surgical planning. In this case, post-reduction CT confirmed a scaphoid waist fracture (Fig. 34.3).

N. A. Zelenski (✉) · C. V. Schaeffer
Division of Upper Extremity Surgery, Department of Orthopaedic Surgery, Emory University, Atlanta, GA, USA
e-mail: Nicole.ann.zelenski@emory.edu

J. Yao (ed.), *Carpal Instability*, https://doi.org/10.1007/978-3-031-55869-6_34

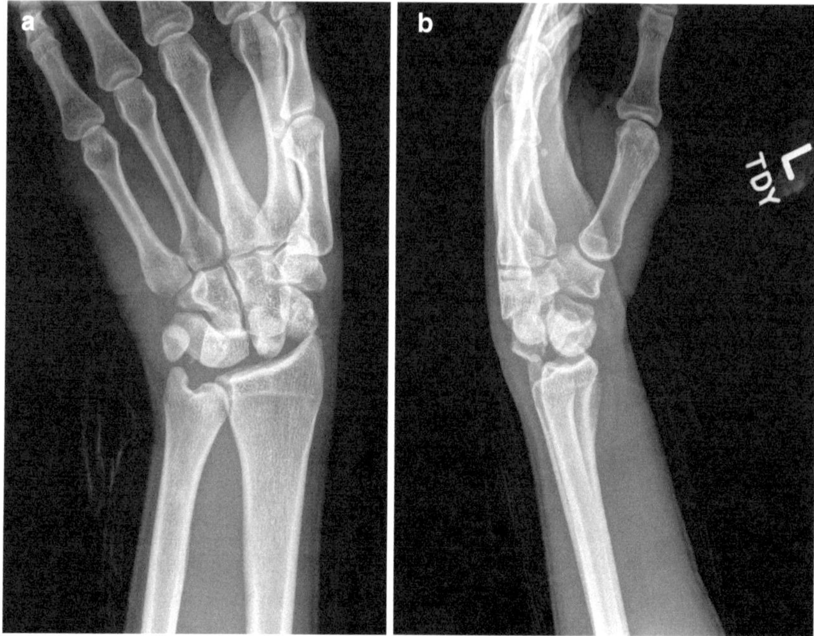

Fig. 34.1 Posterior-anterior (PA) (**a**) and lateral (**b**) plain radiographs demonstrating transscaphoid perilunate fracture-dislocation with dorsal dislocation of the capitate

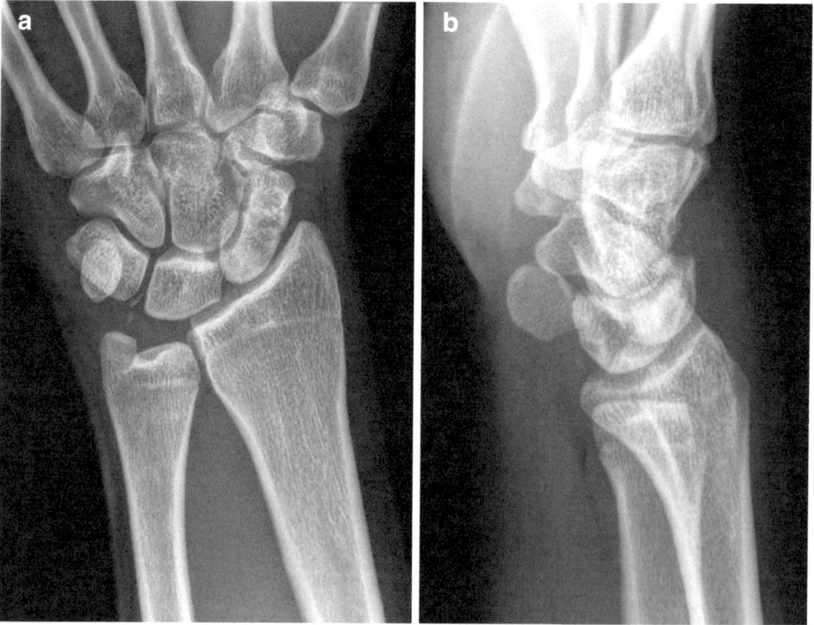

Fig. 34.2 Posterior-anterior (PA) (**a**) and lateral (**b**) plain radiographs demonstrating reduction of perilunate dislocation

Fig. 34.3 Postreduction cross-sectional imaging in the sagittal plane demonstrating associated comminuted scaphoid waist fracture

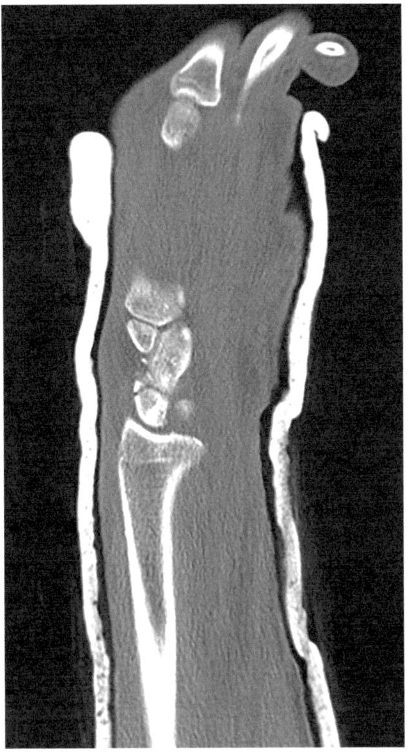

Physical Exam

Physical exam demonstrated significant wrist swelling and ecchymosis. Postreduction examination indicated 5 mm two-point discrimination in all digits with intact opposition. There were no associated upper extremity lacerations.

Management

The patient underwent closed reduction in the emergency department under conscious sedation with resolution of his nerve symptoms. Wrist immobilization is performed with dorsal or volar slab or sugar tong to keep the wrist in slight flexion with the goal of maintaining reduction until surgical fixation. In this case, a sugar tong splint was placed, and the patient was discharged. One week later, he underwent open operative fixation.

Surgical Approach

The surgical approaches described for perilunate injuries include dorsal approach, volar approach, combined dorsal/volar approach, and arthroscopic assisted. Our standard approach is a dorsal approach to the wrist. Our indications for the addition of a volar approach include the need for carpal tunnel release, a volar approach for scaphoid fixation, and residual instability or gapping of the LT after dorsal repair. In severe injuries where there is ulnar translocation of the lunate requiring repair of the long radiolunate, short radiolunate, or radioscaphocapitate, the volar approach is also added. The carpus can be stressed with ulnar directed force to detect this.

A dorsal approach is used to expose the carpus. A longitudinal incision is made on the dorsal wrist centered over the carpus, in line with the third metacarpal. Dissection is performed to the extensor retinaculum (Fig. 34.4a). Full-thickness subcutaneous flaps are raised to protect the dorsal sensory branch of the ulnar nerve (DSBUN) and the superficial branch of the radial nerve (SBRN). The extensor retinaculum is incised over the course of the extensor pollicis longus (EPL). The EPL tendon can be most easily identified distally (Fig. 34.4b), and the extensor retinaculum is incised from distal to proximal (Fig. 34.4c). The EPL is transposed radially out of the third extensor compartment. The septa between the second and third extensor compartments radially (Fig. 34.4d) and the fourth and fifth extensor compartments ulnarly (Fig. 34.4e) are incised to create retinacular flaps and expose the underlying wrist capsule. A posterior interosseous neurectomy is performed—1 cm of the nerve is excised and the ends are treated with bipolar electrocautery. Following retraction of the extensor tendons, the dorsal wrist capsule is visualized at the base of the operative field (Fig. 34.4f). The dorsal radiocarpal and dorsal intercarpal ligaments are identified, and a ligament-splitting capsulotomy is made to expose the carpus [2] (Fig. 34.4g). It is important to note that disruption or avulsion of the dorsal capsule off the radius proximally or an intrasubstance tear within the ligaments can occur in high-energy mechanisms. These deficits are used for the approach.

In the setting of an associated scaphoid fracture, scaphoid fixation can be performed via a dorsal or volar approach. Fixation is typically achieved with a headless compression screw (Fig. 34.5). In trans-scaphoid perilunate fracture dislocations, the scapholunate ligament may remain intact with the proximal pole of the scaphoid. However, concomitant injury to the scapholunate (SL) ligament is not uncommon and must be assessed and addressed if present—SL disruption was reported in 5% (5 of 104 cases) of trans-scaphoid perilunate fracture-dislocations in a multicenter study by Herzberg et al. Ninety-six percent (25 of 26 cases) of trans-scaphoid perilunate fracture-dislocations reported by Liu et al. had SL hemorrhage and some degree of attenuation on arthroscopic evaluation indicating that there is likely a spectrum of injuries [1, 3, 4]. When there is a disruption of the SL interval, the lunate position and alignment on the radius may be secured with a 0.054″ K-wire from the radius to the lunate, taking care to aim the wire into the volar lunate to allow for passage of crossing K-wires and suture anchors if necessary (Fig. 34.6). A 0.062″ K-wire can be used in the lunate as joystick to achieve neutral alignment. In very unstable perilunate injuries, the radiolunate K-wire may be left in place for

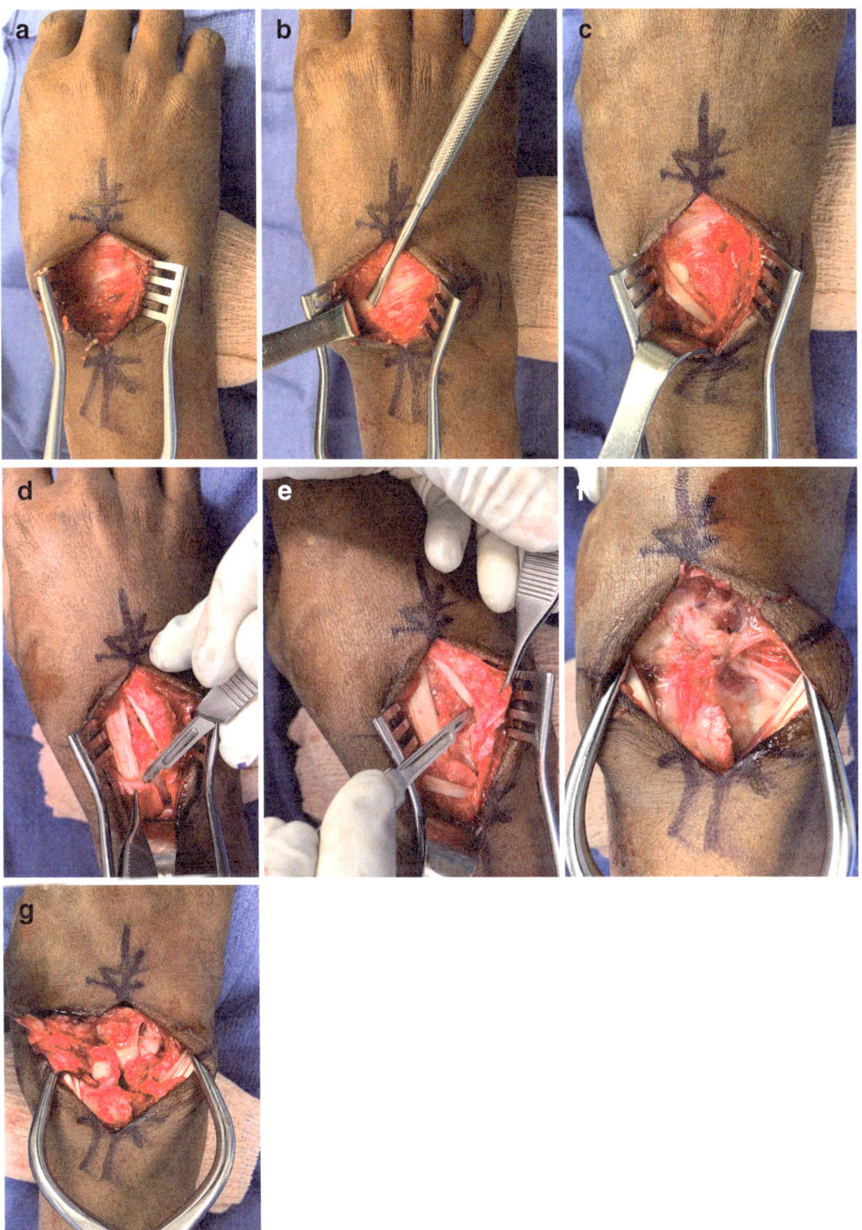

Fig. 34.4 Dorsal approach to the wrist. A longitudinal incision is made over the dorsal wrist, centered over the carpus and in line with the third metacarpal. Dissection is carried down to the extensor retinaculum (**a**). The extensor pollicis longus tendon is identified distally (**b**), and the overlying extensor retinaculum is incised from distal to proximal (**c**). The EPL tendon is transposed radially. The septa between 2–3 extensor compartments radially (**d**) and 3–4 and 4–5 compartments ulnarly (**e**) are incised to create retinacular flaps. Following retraction of the extensor tendons, the underlying wrist capsule is exposed (**f**). The carpus is exposed using the ligament-sparing approach described by Berger et al. (**g**)

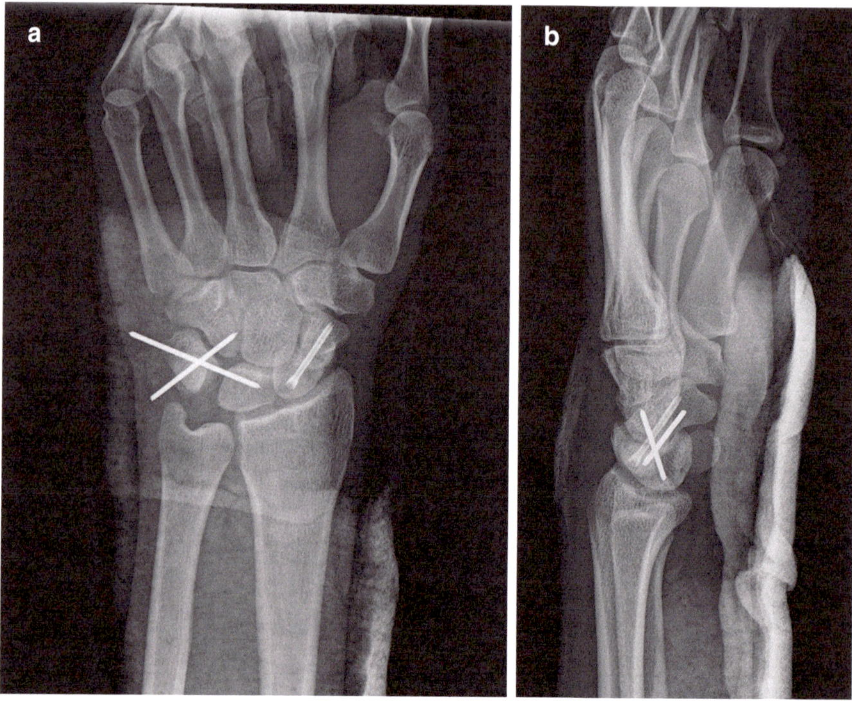

Fig. 34.5 Immediate postoperative PA (**a**) and lateral (**b**) plain radiographs demonstrating fixation of the scaphoid waist fracture with headless compression screw and K-wire fixation across the LT joint and triquetral hamate joint. Reduction of capitolunate interval is demonstrated on the lateral view (**b**)

Fig. 34.6 Lateral plain radiograph demonstrating radiolunate pin placement with 0.054 Kirshner wire to maintain neutral alignment of the lunate. The reduction of the scaphoid (yellow) and lunate (blue) is demonstrated

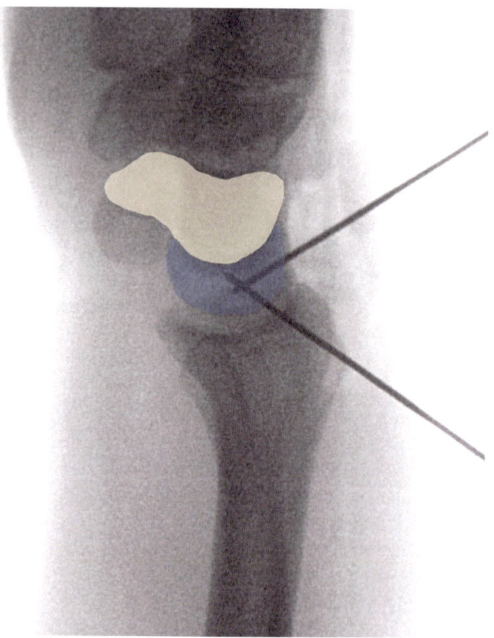

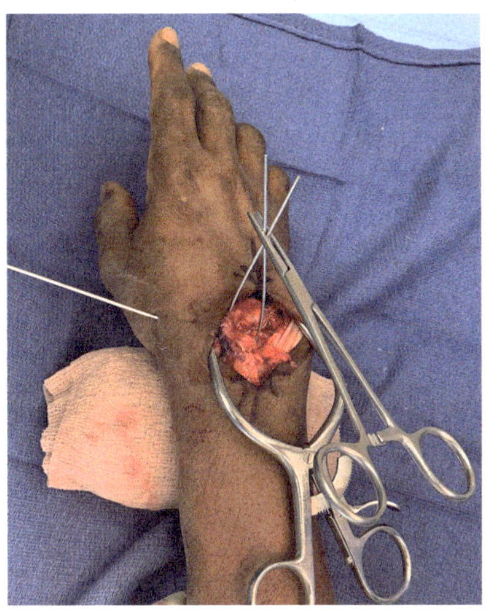

Fig. 34.7 Reduction technique for the scapholunate interval—joystick Kirschner wires are placed in the distal scaphoid and the proximal lunate. The interval is reduced through extension of the scaphoid and flexion of the lunate by clamping of the wires

added stabilization and removed at 6 weeks post-op. In cases where the radiolunate K-wire will be left in place, care must be taken to place this radial to the fourth extensor compartment to allow for smooth passage of the extensor tendons. 0.062″ K-wires can then be placed into the scaphoid to facilitate reduction. The scaphoid can be reduced to the lunate by clamping the joystick K-wires (Fig. 34.7) or using a point-to-point clamp to compress the scaphoid/lunate interval. Intraoperative fluorography should be used to confirm appropriate scapholunate angle on a lateral view (Fig. 34.6). A K-wire is placed from the scaphoid to the lunate and from the scaphoid to the capitate. The remnant scapholunate ligament is primarily repaired, when possible, with nonabsorbable suture. Suture anchors can be used in the setting of complete avulsion of the SL ligament from the dorsal scaphoid or lunate. Dorsal capsulodesis of the SL ligament repair to dorsal wrist capsular flap is performed prior to closure.

The lunotriquetral (LT) joint is then reduced in a similar fashion. A K-wire is placed across the LT joint as well as the triquetral hamate joint (Fig. 34.5). The remnant LT ligament is repaired primarily, when possible, or with the use of suture anchors. LT ligament tears are often mid-substance and can be repaired with 2–0 nonabsorbable braided suture.

In the setting of nerve symptoms, an open carpal tunnel release is performed in a standard fashion. An extended carpal tunnel approach can be utilized to repair volar ligamentous structures in the setting of persistent carpal instability following the above-described fixation or inadequate reduction via the dorsal approach. Examples of persistent instability include ulnar or volar translation of the lunate or midcarpal joint or excessive lunotriquetral mobility or volar gapping after pinning. Diagnostic wrist arthroscopy can be performed to directly assess the integrity of the volar capsule and LT interval and aid in the decision to perform an open volar approach.

Patients are placed in a volar resting splint after surgery, which is exchanged for a short arm cast at 2 weeks. The radiolunate K-wire is maintained for 4–6 weeks, and the intercarpal K-wires and cast are maintained for 8–10 weeks after which the K-wires are removed in the office and active wrist range of motion is started with guided occupational therapy. The timing for removal of K-wires is based on the natural process for ligamentous healing—tissue remodeling begins at 1–2 months post-injury with realignment of collagen fibers and increased conversion of type III to type I collagen [5]. Typically, when passive range of motion plateaus, weight-bearing can begin. A removable splint is worn for comfort, and weight-bearing is advanced at 3 months.

Outcomes

The patient's postoperative course was uneventful. The scaphoid fracture went on to union (Fig. 34.8). Wrist motion at final follow-up (14 weeks post-op) was 80 ° of flexion with 70 ° of extension (Fig. 34.9). He reported pain-free wrist motion.

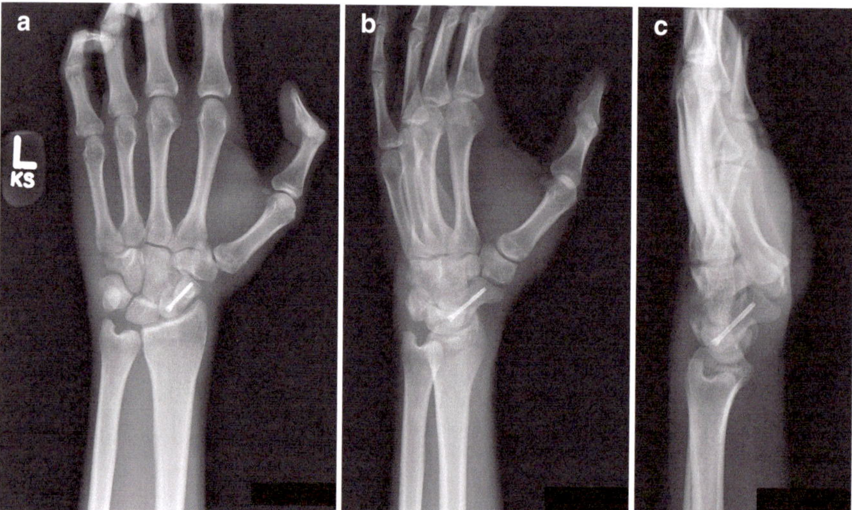

Fig. 34.8 Postoperative PA (**a**), oblique (**b**), and lateral (**c**) plain radiographs demonstrating healed scaphoid waist fracture and maintained carpal alignment

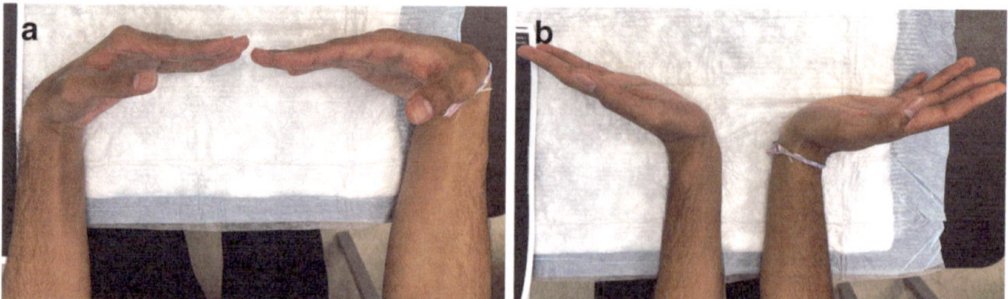

Fig. 34.9 Final postoperative range of motion following left trans-scaphoid perilunate fracture-dislocation. Wrist flexion (**a**) and extension (**b**) arcs are demonstrated, allowing for comparison of operative left wrist range of motion to the contralateral wrist

Pearls and Pitfalls

- Perilunate dislocations and fracture-dislocations present as a spectrum of injuries. This diagnosis should not be missed, and all ligamentous and bony injuries should be addressed acutely.
- Open dorsal approach to the wrist provides access for dorsal SL and LT repair and carpal fixation. Adding a volar approach allows for visualization and repair of volar capsule and LT. However, it can potentially contribute to postoperative wrist stiffness and may not be necessary for adequate treatment.
- There is an evolving role for wrist arthroscopy in the evaluation and management of perilunate injuries. The ability to evaluate the integrity of the volar capsule and intercarpal relationships with arthroscopy can aid in the identification and treatment of persistent carpal instability.
- Injury to the scapholunate ligament must be assessed and addressed, even in trans-scaphoid perilunate dislocations.
- Dorsal capsulodesis should be used to reinforce scapholunate ligament repairs.
- Radiolunate K-wire fixation can be maintained postoperatively for 4–6 weeks in unstable injury patterns. This should be placed radial to the fourth compartment to prevent injury to the extensors in the fourth dorsal compartment.

Literature Review

A recent meta-analysis reviewed 43 articles and 888 subjects [6]. The complication rate was high with the development of arthritis occurring in 30% of patients, carpal instability in 15% of patients, and avascular necrosis of the lunate in 12% of cases. Complex regional pain syndrome occurred in 11% of cases. The mean arc of motion was 118° in patients who underwent arthroscopically assisted closed reduction and percutaneous pinning and 96° in patients who underwent open reduction and internal fixation with no difference in scapholunate angle or complication rate postoperatively between the two groups. Although the authors speculated that the arthroscopically treated group may had less severe injuries, this meta-analysis indicated that arthroscopic treatment may have improved outcomes [6].

A systematic review of the literature on outcomes of acute perilunate injuries was published in 2023 [7]. Based on the 26 articles included for review, the most common surgical approach was a combined dorsal and volar (49%), followed by dorsal approach (17%) and volar approach (11%). The use of arthroscopy was described in 11.2% of articles. Higher complication rates were associated with combined dorsal/volar approach (17.4%) compared to dorsal approach alone (8.4%). The advantages of the dorsal approach include access to the carpus for bony reduction and fixation in addition to visualization of the dorsal SL ligament for repair. Meanwhile, the volar approach allows for decompression of the median nerve, facilitates reduction of the lunate, provides access to the volar capsule and volar LT ligament for repair, and can facilitate removal of volar osteochondral fragments [8]. There is some debate over the need to repair volar ligamentous structures after a perilunate dislocation. Capo found a volar carpal ligament tear present in 100% of cases [9]. It is important to note that a combined dorsal/volar approach is often implemented in the setting of a difficult reduction through an initial dorsal-only approach [10].

Higher complications rates were also reported with open fixation (17.4%) when compared to an arthroscopic approach (4.8%) to perilunate injuries in the 2023 systematic review by Liecht et al. [7]. Oh et al. performed a comparative analysis of arthroscopic assisted vs. open reduction and fixation of trans-scaphoid perilunate fracture-dislocations. In this study, there was one scaphoid nonunion (ORIF group). Wrist stability was achieved in all patients; however, the patients in the arthroscopic group had significantly better DASH scores and wrist flexion/extension arc [11]. However, given the broad-spectrum PLD injury presentations, an arthroscopic approach may not be feasible in all clinical scenarios [7].

There is also debate regarding the need to formally repair the LT ligament if the LT is reduced and K-wires are in place. Knoll et al. described LT ligament repair via a dorsal approach using bone anchors in addition to K-wire fixation, citing the established biomechanical role of the LT ligament in VISI carpal instability [12]. In 2012, Capo described a protocol of reducing and K-wiring the LT with no ligamentous repair with good results [9]. And indeed, the literature seems to suggest that primary ligamentous repair may not be necessary [6]. Despite this, dorsal ligament repair if possible and pinning are always performed in our practice.

References

1. Herzberg G, Comtet JJ, Linscheid RL, Amadio PC, Cooney WP, Stalder J. Perilunate dislocations and fracture-dislocations: a multicenter study. J Hand Surg Am. 1993;18(5):768–79. https://doi.org/10.1016/0363-5023(93)90041-Z.
2. Berger RA, Bishop AT, Bettinger PC. New dorsal capsulotomy for the surgical exposure of the wrist. Ann Plast Surg. 1995;35(1):54–9. https://doi.org/10.1097/00000637-199507000-00011.
3. Cheng CY, Hsu KY, Tseng IC, Shih HN. Concurrent scaphoid fracture with scapholunate ligament rupture. Acta Orthop Belg. 2004;70(5):485–91. https://pubmed.ncbi.nlm.nih.gov/15587040/. Accessed 25 May 2023
4. Liu B, Chen SL, Zhu J, Lei TG. Arthroscopic management of perilunate injuries. Hand Clin. 2017;33(4):709–15. https://doi.org/10.1016/J.HCL.2017.06.002.
5. Yang G, Rothrauff BB, Tuan RS. Tendon and ligament regeneration and repair: clinical relevance and developmental paradigm. Birth Defects Res C Embryo Today. 2013;99(3):203. https://doi.org/10.1002/BDRC.21041.
6. Lee CH, Lee BG, Kim JH, Yoon HS, Han KJ, Choi WS. Complications and outcomes of operative treatment for acute perilunate injuries: a systematic review. J Hand Surg Eur Vol. 2023;48:625–9. https://doi.org/10.1177/17531934221150331.
7. Liechti R, Merky DN, Grobbelaar AO, van de Wall BJM, Vögelin E, Hirsiger S. Outcomes of acute perilunate injuries-a systematic review. Eur J Trauma Emerg Surg. 2023;49:2071–84. https://doi.org/10.1007/S00068-023-02222-Y.
8. Muppavarapu RC, Capo JT. Perilunate dislocations and fracture dislocations. Hand Clin. 2015;31(3):399–408. https://doi.org/10.1016/J.HCL.2015.04.002.

9. Capo JT, Corti SJ, Shamian B, et al. Treatment of dorsal perilunate dislocations and fracture-dislocations using a standardized protocol. Hand (N Y). 2012;7(4):380–7. https://doi.org/10.1007/S11552-012-9452-Y.
10. Kremer T, Wendt M, Riedel K, Sauerbier M, Germann G, Bickert B. Open reduction for perilunate injuries—clinical outcome and patient satisfaction. J Hand Surg Am. 2010;35(10):1599–606. https://doi.org/10.1016/J.JHSA.2010.06.021.
11. Oh WT, Choi YR, Kang HJ, Koh IH, Lim KH. Comparative outcome analysis of arthroscopic-assisted versus open reduction and fixation of trans-scaphoid perilunate fracture dislocations. Arthroscopy. 2017;33(1):92–100. https://doi.org/10.1016/J.ARTHRO.2016.07.018.
12. Knoll VD, Allan C, Trumble TE. Trans-scaphoid perilunate fracture dislocations: results of screw fixation of the scaphoid and lunotriquetral repair with a dorsal approach. J Hand Surg Am. 2005;30(6):1145.e1–1145.e11. https://doi.org/10.1016/J.JHSA.2005.07.007.

Chapter 35
Perilunate Injuries Non-dislocated

G. Herzberg, M. Burnier, and C. Schaeffer

Background

High-energy trauma to the wrist can result in perilunate dislocations and fracture-dislocations (PLD-PLFD). These injuries are characterized by dorsal or volar dislocation of the capitate from the lunate including different degrees of displacements of the lunate relative to the radius [1].

Green [2] demonstrated that spontaneous reduction of PLD-PLFD may occur. There were several subsequent papers that reported cases of perilunate-like injury patterns (purely ligamentous or with associated fractures) without capitolunate dislocation [3–7]. Pin et al. described eight cases of patients with concomitant scapholunate and lunotriquetral ligamentous injuries without capitolunate dislocation in 1990 [3]. The term "floating lunate" was later quoted by Badia [4] to describe chronic cases of post-traumatic combined scapholunate and lunotriquetral dissociations. Chee [7] subsequently described their technique for reconstruction in a chronic, spontaneously reduced, pure ligamentous perilunate injury in 2013. Bony perilunate-like injuries without dislocation on initial imaging studies were described in 2013 by Bain et al. They presented 34 cases of trans-lunate injury patterns, of which 10 patients were characterized as "subluxed" without true dislocation on imaging [5]. The small number of cases described in the literature and the absence of a unifying concept to describe these perilunate-like injuries emphasized the need

G. Herzberg (✉)
Clinique Parc & Val Ouest, Lyon, France

M. Burnier
Institut Main-Membre Supérieur, Villeurbanne, France

C. Schaeffer
Emory University Hospital, Atlanta, GA, USA

J. Yao (ed.), *Carpal Instability*, https://doi.org/10.1007/978-3-031-55869-6_35

451

for a better understanding of the full spectrum of perilunate injury patterns and their classification.

The term PLIND was first proposed in 2013 [8] and defined as spontaneously reduced PLD (PLIND) or PLFD (bony PLIND). Inclusion of PLIND into the spectrum of perilunate injuries allowed for a more comprehensive understanding of these complex, high-energy injuries [9]. The modified perilunate dislocation classification including non-dislocated injury types [8] aimed to aid in the identification and appropriate management of perilunate injury variants.

The purpose of this chapter is to focus on PLIND patterns, including acute and chronic presentations.

Acute PLIND

In our case series describing 11 acute PLIND injuries [8], the patients were most commonly young male patients with high-energy injury mechanisms. Acute cases were defined as those who presented and were treated within the first week following trauma. Patients invariably presented with marked wrist swelling and pain. Plain radiographs and cross-sectional imaging demonstrated a coronal path of injury (like that seen with PLDs-PLFDs) notably without capitate dislocation (Figs. 35.1 and 35.2). Acute PLIND variants included pure ligamentous PLIND (or "floating lunate") and bony PLIND [9]. Like in PLD-PLFD, a combination of scapholunate dissociation and scaphoid waist fracture may be encountered [10]. The presence of midcarpal loose bodies as seen on initial plain radiographs and/or cross-sectional imaging was an additional indicator of PLIND diagnosis (Fig. 35.1). Diagnostic arthroscopy was a key diagnostic adjunct to confirm suspected ligamentous injuries (Fig. 35.1). Additionally, arthroscopy facilitated the removal of midcarpal loose bodies.

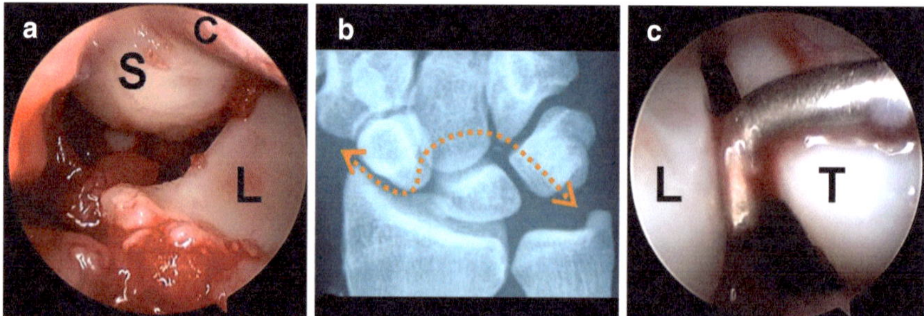

Fig. 35.1 Acute PLIND case example: (**a**) Midcarpal arthroscopy demonstrating a complete scapholunate dissociation. (**b**) PA initial radiograph of the wrist with acute ligamentous PLIND; dotted line shows the path of trauma. (**c**) Midcarpal arthroscopy demonstrating a complete lunotriquetral dissociation

The principles of surgical treatment followed those previously established for PLD-PLFD and included bony fixation and ligamentous repair vs. early salvage procedures (like proximal row carpectomy), as indicated. Surgical approaches included arthroscopic, arthroscopic assisted, or open approaches to the wrist. These approaches will be tailored to the patterns of injuries (pure ligamentous vs. bony PLIND). We currently prefer an initial diagnostic dry arthroscopy in a vertical position for acute and subacute PLIND and bony PLIND. Dry diagnostic arthroscopy is followed by a mini-open dorsal approach allowing the repair of the fibrous scapholunate junction in PLIND vs. the fixation of the scaphoid in bony PLIND. Additional K-wire carpal fixation may be performed if necessary.

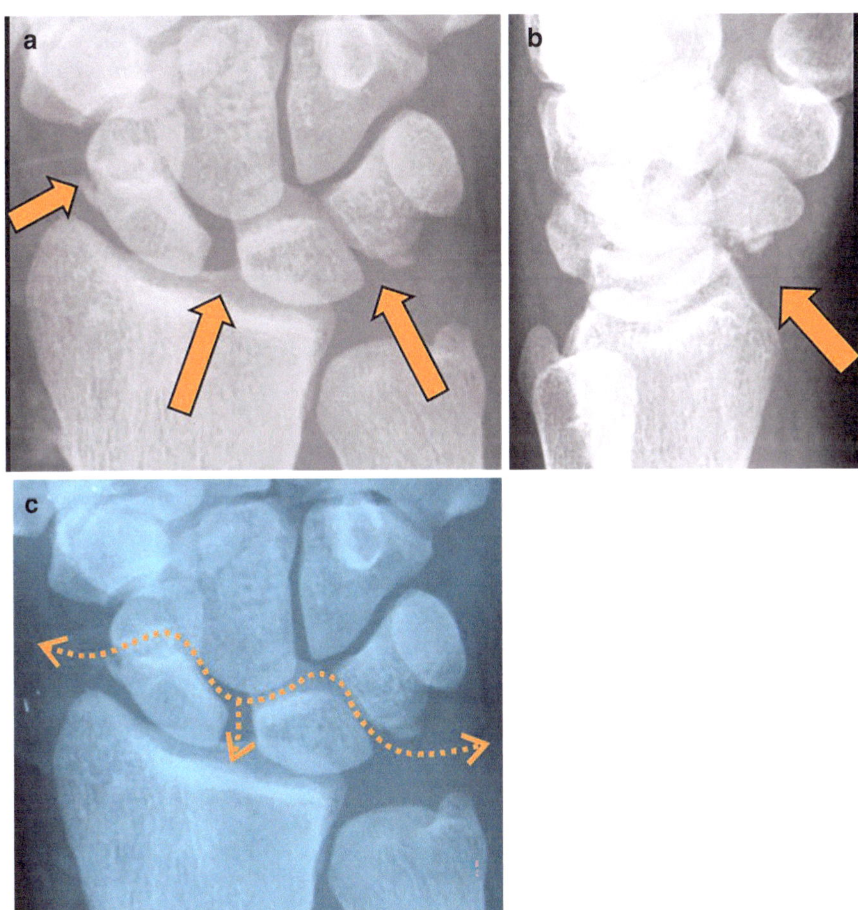

Fig. 35.2 Acute bony PLIND case example: (**a**) PA initial radiograph of the wrist showing acute, trans-scaphoid PLIND; note the widened scapholunate interval. (**b**) Significant comminution of the scaphoid fracture on plain radiograph. (**c**) Dotted line demonstrates the path of trauma

It is important to have a high index of suspicion for intracarpal osseous and ligamentous injuries to facilitate appropriate acute management. As early treatment of PLIND injuries is the same as early treatment of PLD-PLFD, one may expect similar clinical outcomes as for PLD-PLFD acutely repaired. A delay in treatment has been previously established as the main prognostic factor for PLD. Similarly, it is mandatory not to miss acute PLIND presentations.

Chronic PLIND

We defined chronic PLIND as those who presented and were treated after the 45th day of trauma, while patients who presented between 1 week and 6 weeks were considered as "late acute" or "subacute" cases. Chronic variants of PLIND (pure ligamentous vs. bony) were diagnosed in patients with delayed presentation and patients with missed, untreated acute injuries (Fig. 35.3). An extensive workup with advanced imaging in addition to a retrospective analysis of the initial imaging

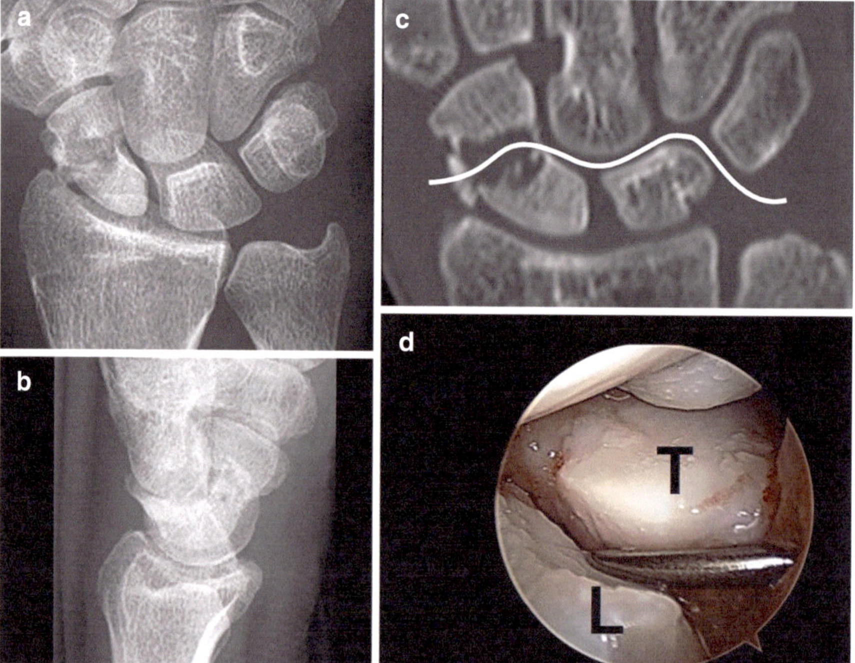

Fig. 35.3 Chronic bony PLIND case example: (**a**) PA radiograph of the wrist showing scaphoid waist nonunion with marked bone resorption. (**b**) The scapholunate angle is increased on the lateral radiograph of the wrist; no capitolunate dislocation. (**c**) Coronal view of CT scan detailing the scaphoid nonunion; white line demonstrates the path of trauma that was confirmed with arthroscopy. (**d**) Midcarpal arthroscopy demonstrating lunotriquetral dissociation

studies was required to confirm the diagnosis of PLIND. Imaging studies typically demonstrated scapholunate dissociation (SLD) or early scaphoid nonunion with additional signs of medial dissociative instability (lunotriquetral dissociation and/or triquetral fracture) and midcarpal loose bodies. Of note, the lateral carpal alignment may remain within normal limits. Diagnostic arthroscopy played a similar role as that described for the evaluation of acute PLIND [11]. Midcarpal arthroscopy allowed for characterization of the combination of lesions lateral and medial to the lunate (Fig. 35.3).

As the treatment is the same as for chronic PLD-PLFD, i.e., late reconstruction or salvage, one may expect similar clinical outcomes as for PLD-PLFD treated at a chronic stage.

Conclusions

There is now evidence that PLIND injuries are equivalent, self-reduced, PLD-PLFD (1;9).

Purely ligamentous PLIND corresponds to floating lunate as described by Badia [4] while bony PLIND was not formally described before 2013. A current modified classification (Fig. 35.4) includes PLIND injuries, both purely ligamentous and bony PLIND [8].

In any event, PLIND should not be missed since they require a treatment similar to PLD-PLFD. Unless proven otherwise, the combination of a high-energy injury, painful swollen wrist, and midcarpal chip fractures raises a high index of suspicion of an acute PLIND (Fig. 35.5).

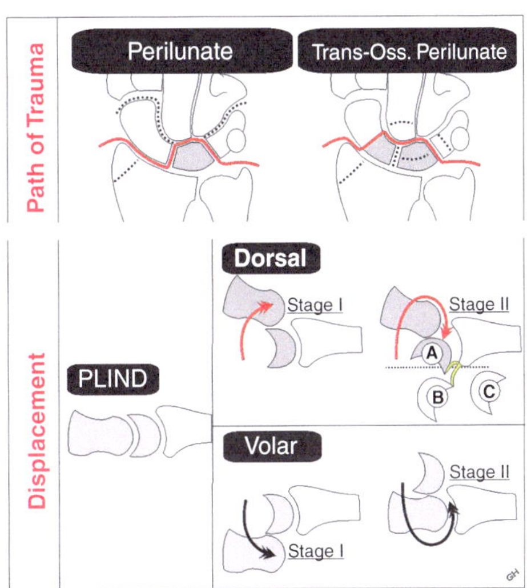

Fig. 35.4 Proposed algorithm for the diagnosis of acute PLIND. The combination of (**a**) high-energy mechanism, (**b**) marked wrist swelling/ecchymosis on physical exam, and (**c**) midcarpal loose bodies without capitolunate dislocation on PA and lateral plain radiographs is a PLIND pattern of injury until proven otherwise

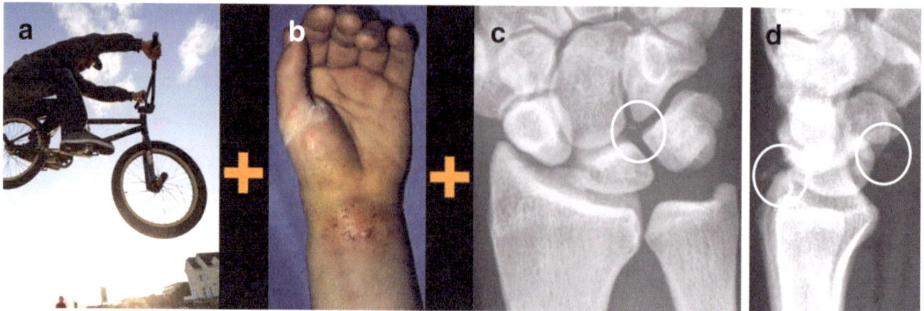

Fig. 35.5 Clinical and radiological clues to PLIND injuries

References

1. Herzberg G, Comtet JJ, Linscheid RL, Amadio PC, Cooney WP, Stalder J. Perilunate dislocations and fracture-dislocations: a multicenter study. J Hand Surg. 1993;18A(5):768–79.
2. Green DP, O'Brien ET. Open reduction of carpal dislocations: indications and operative techniques. J Hand Surg. 1978;3A(3):250–65.
3. Pin PG, Nowak M, Logan SE, Young VL, Gilula LA, Weeks PM. Coincident rupture of the scapholunate and lunotriquetral ligaments without perilunate dislocation: pathomechanics and management. J Hand Surg Am. 1990;15A:110–9.
4. Badia A, Khanchandani P. The floating lunate: arthroscopic treatment of simultaneous complete tears of the scapholunate and lunotriquetral ligaments. Hand. 2008;4(3):250–5.
5. Bain GI. Translunate fracture with associated perilunate injury: 3 case reports with introduction of the translunate arc concept. JHSA. 2008;33A(10):1770–6.
6. Briseno MR, Yao J. Lunate fractures in the face of a perilunar injury: an uncommon and easily missed pattern. J Hand Surg Am. 2011;37A(1):63–7.
7. Chee KG, Chin AYH, Chew EM, Garcia-Elias M. Antipronation spiral tenodesis: a surgical technique for the treatment of perilunate instability. J Hand Surg Am. 2012;37A:2611–8.
8. Herzberg G. Perilunate injuries, non-dislocated (PLIND). J Wrist Surg. 2013;2(4):337–45.
9. Herzberg G, Cievet Bonfils M, Burnier M. Arthroscopic treatment of translunate perilunate injury non dislocated (PLIND). J Wrist Surg. 2018;8(2):143.
10. Mayfield JK. Mechanism of carpal injuries. Clin Orthop Relat Res. 1980;149:45–54.
11. Corella F. The rocking chair sign for floating lunate. J Hand Surg Am. 2015;40A(11):2318.

Chapter 36
Partial Wrist Denervation for SLAC Wrist

Sami Tuffaha

Case Presentation

A 54-year-old right-hand-dominant female lawyer presented for an initial clinic evaluation with a history of chronic right wrist pain. Approximately 1 year prior to presentation, she fell from standing on outstretched hands and experienced the sudden onset of severe pain and swelling in her right wrist. Her primary care provider diagnosed her with a likely sprain and provisionally treated her with a wrist brace and NSAIDs. She was given a hand surgery referral but did not pursue it. After a number of weeks, her pain and swelling subsided enough to allow her to perform low-demand activities with her right hand, including typing and carrying light objects. However, she experienced moderate to severe pain with pushing and pulling heavy objects. While she regained most of her wrist range of motion 2–3 months after her initial fall, she subsequently noted progressive stiffness limiting wrist extension. She noted inability to perform yoga due to wrist stiffness and pain and also some progressive weakness in her right hand, which limited her ability to open a jar. She managed her intermittent symptoms with NSAIDs and generally avoided activities that she knew would elicit pain. Her history was notable for mild intermittent pain in her thumb bases bilaterally, which she never sought treatment for. She otherwise had no known history of osteoarthritis or inflammatory arthropathy. She was generally healthy and did not take any medications other than occasional NSAIDs to treat her wrist pain.

S. Tuffaha (✉)
Johns Hopkins University School of Medicine, Baltimore, MD, USA
e-mail: stuffah1@jhmi.edu

J. Yao (ed.), *Carpal Instability*, https://doi.org/10.1007/978-3-031-55869-6_36

Diagnosis

- Physical assessment/relevant maneuvers: On physical examination, there was mild swelling noted along the right dorsal wrist. Wrist range of motion (extension/flexion/radial/ulnar) was 40/65/10/30 on the right and 70/75/20/35 on the left; active equaled passive. Right wrist extension and radial deviation both elicited pain. Exquisite tenderness to palpation was elicited at the dorsal SL interval. Tenderness to palpation was also present along the radial radiocarpal joint. No foveal tenderness was present. Provocative testing for thumb CMC arthritis was mildly positive. A positive Watson test was elicited. Grip strength was 16 kg on the right and 24 kg on the left.
- Bilateral wrist X-rays were obtained (Fig. 36.1). A scapholunate (SL) diastasis of approximately 4 mm was observed on standard anteroposterior (AP) and clenched fist views of the right wrist, and a normal SL interval of approximately 2 mm was observed on the right side. Dorsal intercalated segment instability (DISI) was observed on the lateral view of the right wrist. Radioscaphoid joint space narrowing and sclerosis involving the entire scaphoid fossa were noted on the AP view of the right wrist. Degenerative changes were not observed at the capitolunate joint.

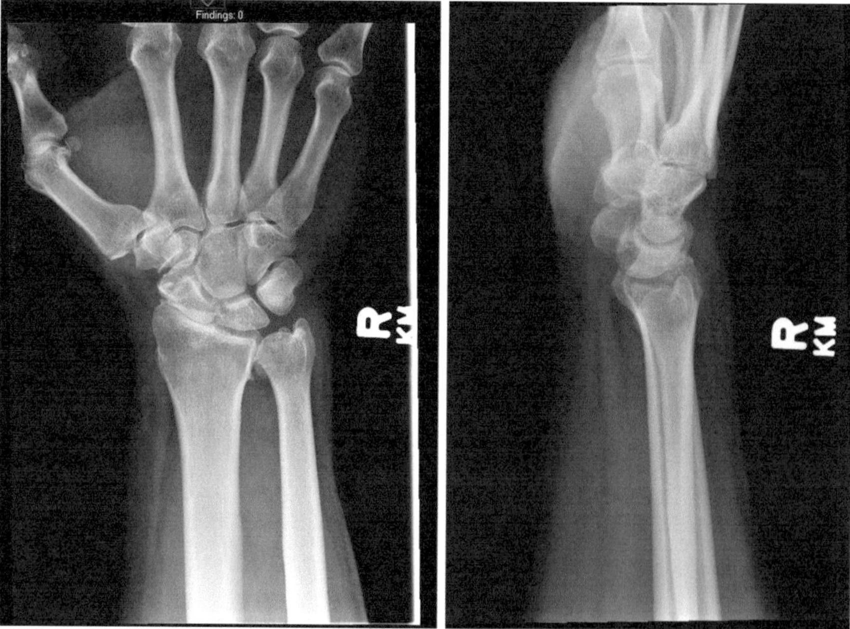

Fig. 36.1 Wrist X-ray demonstrating SLAC II with widened SL interval and radioscaphoid arthritis involving the entire scaphoid fossa on anteroposterior view (left) and DISI deformity on the lateral view (right)

Management Options

After establishing a diagnosis of stage 2 scapholunate advanced collapse (SLAC) at the patient's initial clinic evaluation, treatment options were discussed. Conservative management options included therapy, immobilization in a wrist splint or brace, and topical and systemic NSAIDs for symptomatic relief. A steroid injection was offered while discussing the likely need for repeat injections in the future. Surgical options were briefly reviewed, including partial wrist denervation with anterior interosseus nerve (AIN) and posterior interosseus nerve (PIN) neurectomies, proximal row carpectomy, and scaphoidectomy with capitolunate vs. four-corner fusion. Radial styloidectomy would not address the extent of this patient's radioscaphoid arthritis but can be considered for stage 1 SLAC. Complete wrist fusion was not necessary in this patient but can be considered for patients with more extensive arthritis or for those who fail first-line salvage procedures. Surgery for SLAC wrist is generally not offered until patients have exhausted nonsurgical options.

Management Chosen for This Patient

A steroid injection was recommended and performed at her initial clinic evaluation with approximately 6 months of significant symptomatic improvement. She requested and received a second steroid injection that again provided approximately 5–6 months of symptomatic relief. When her symptoms recurred following her second steroid injection, the patient voiced interest in considering surgical options that may provide more long-lasting benefit. She was specifically interested in partial wrist denervation as a relatively simple, low-risk surgery with rapid postoperative recovery. Diagnostic nerve blocks of the AIN and PIN were performed in clinic with 0.5% Marcaine, and the patient was instructed to monitor her symptoms for the ensuing 12 h while the block was active. She was encouraged to perform activities that are known to exacerbate her symptoms during this time and to keep a diary of symptoms. X-rays of her right wrist were found to be fairly stable from 1 year prior with only mild progression of arthritis. When she returned to clinic the following week, she reported 80–90% improvement in her symptoms following the block with return of her baseline symptoms late the next day. She was therefore deemed to be a reasonable candidate for partial wrist denervation and elected to proceed. The surgery was performed through a single 4–5 cm longitudinal incision along the distal dorsal forearm. The extensor tendons are retracted to identify the PIN coursing above the interosseus membrane (IOM) along with the deep branch of the anterior interosseus artery. PIN is divided, and approximately 2 cm of the nerve is resected to prevent spontaneous regeneration across the neurectomy site. The IOM is then longitudinally incised to expose the AIN on the deep surface of the pronator quadratus. AIN neurectomy is then performed in the same fashion as above (Fig. 36.2). Following surgery, the patient was placed in a light soft dressing with gently compressive ACE bandage.

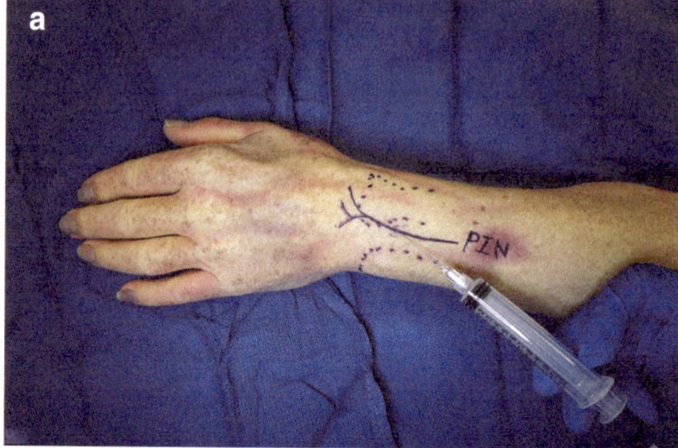

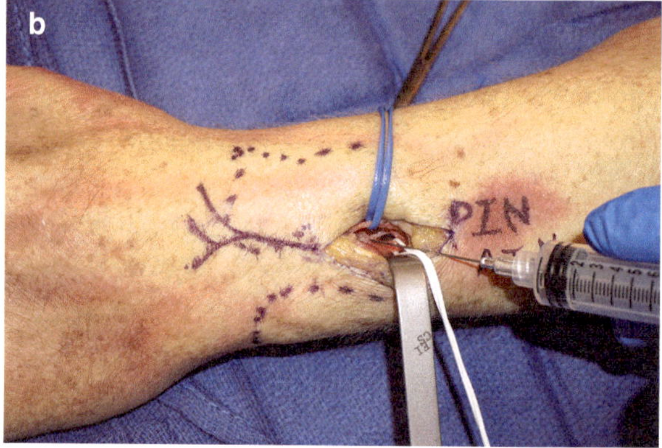

Fig. 36.2 (**a**) Photo demonstrating needle placement for diagnostic block of AINAnterior interosseus nerve (AIN) and PINPosterior interosseus nerve (PIN). (**b**) Intraoperative photo demonstrating approach for selective wrist denervation performed through a small incision on the distal dorsal wrist to expose and divide the PIN (blue vessel loop) and AIN (red vessel loop)

Clinical Course and Outcome

At her first postoperative clinic appointment, the patient noted some mild soreness at her surgical site. She was unable to ascertain whether her baseline wrist pain had improved as she was largely protecting her right hand and wrist and had not been using it much. After confirming that her surgical incision was healing appropriately, all activity restrictions were lifted at her first post-op visit. At her second postoperative visit 6 weeks following surgery, she had returned to normal use of her right hand and wrist and reported 80–90% improvement in her baseline wrist pain. She was last seen in clinic 1 year after surgery and continued to report 80–90% improvement in her symptoms. She noted continued pain and limitation in activities that involved heavy lifting and pushing with full wrist extension. She noted that the pain felt more dull than what she experienced prior to surgery. There was minimal improvement in wrist extension and radial deviation range of motion. Her right-sided grip strength improved to 19 kg. She reported being pleased with her outcome.

Clinical Pearls/Pitfalls

- Diagnostic nerve blocks are useful in determining which patients will respond well to partial wrist denervation. It is important to counsel the patient on the importance of monitoring and documenting their symptoms carefully to avoid the scenario in which the patient returns to clinic unsure of their response to the block. A favorable response to a diagnostic block does not guarantee favorable response to surgery.
- When approached through a single dorsal incision, the AIN is not always immediately located on the volar aspect of the interosseous membrane. At times, shallow blunt dissection is needed to find the AIN within the substance of the pronator quadratus muscle. Care should be taken not to injure the anterior interosseus artery to avoid bleeding that obscures the field of view, complicates identification of the nerves, and increases the risk of postoperative hematoma. The artery is typically intimate with the nerve, and careful deliberate dissection of the nerve is therefore needed to avoid this complication.
- Partial wrist denervation should not be considered a panacea. Many patients do not experience satisfactory improvement in symptoms, and recurrence of symptoms is not uncommon.

Albrecht Willem performed the first total wrist denervation in the 1960s [1], thereby introducing the concept of joint denervation more generally. Buck-Gramcko subsequently popularized Willem's technique, which involved resection of the articular branches from 10 nerves; in a series of 33 patients, two-thirds achieved complete resolution of pain or pain only with heavy manual activity, and 19 patients were reported to achieve "remarkable" improvement in function [2]. Dellon first described partial wrist denervation with division of the posterior interosseus nerve (PIN) [3] or the anterior interosseus nerve (AIN) [4]. Berger later described a technique of combining AIN and PIN neurectomies through a single dorsal incision [5, 6]. The reported experience with both complete and partial wrist denervation has been generally favorable, with satisfaction rates in most studies ranging from approximately 70% to 90% [7, 8]. One of the primary concerns with joint denervation pertains to the durability of the treatment response. Reporting on a series of 100 partial wrist denervations in 89 patients with an average follow-up of 7 years, O'Shaugnessy et al. observed that 31% of patients underwent revision surgeries in an average of 2 years following denervation. Many surgeons therefore view wrist denervation as a temporizing option to provide symptomatic relief for a limited duration of time and thereby delay the need for more invasive and morbid surgical options, particularly in young and active patients. Interestingly, a systematic review comparing partial and complete wrist denervation found a much lower rate of revision surgeries in patients who underwent complete versus partial denervation (4.7% vs. 19%) [9]. A study by Ferreres et al. also found greater durability of treatment effect with complete denervation [10]. These findings raise the possibility that incomplete denervation increases the risk of pain recurrence via collateral reinnervation. While complete wrist denervation has generally been avoided in North America as being unnecessarily invasive and morbid, perhaps this assumption should be revisited.

Wrist denervations have been shown to be safe with low reported rates of complication. There is however some ongoing debate regarding whether wrist denervation results in a loss of proprioception that may subsequently accelerate pathologic instability. Proprioceptive sensory fibers and receptors are certainly present within articular ligaments and capsular tissue [11, 12], but the clinical implications of denervating these receptors remain unclear. Rein and colleagues demonstrated reduced EMG activity from the dorsoradial ligament of the thumb CMC joint following subcutaneous and periarticular infiltration of lidocaine. Hofmeister et al. [13] and Wilhelm [14] postulated that partial wrist denervation may hasten the progression of wrist instability. However, these conclusions were anecdotal, and the worsening instability observed in some of the authors' patients may have occurred in the absence of denervation secondary to their underlying pathology. Studies that have directly evaluated this question in patients following wrist denervation and nerve blocks have not identified a measurable effect on proprioception [5, 15, 16]. Importantly, the development of Charcot joints following joint denervation has not been reported [17]. The reported experience with joint denervation does not support concern for deleterious consequences arising from loss of proprioception following joint denervation. These theoretical concerns are further diminished when considering that the standard surgical alternatives are far more destructive to the joint.

It is important to note that the quality of the reported data pertaining to wrist denervation has been called into question. A recent systematic review and meta-analysis [7] found that of the 170 studies reporting outcomes with joint denervation in the hand and wrist, only two compared treatment outcomes with another procedure [18, 19] and only one of these studies was performed prospectively [19]. Furthermore, many of the studies evaluating wrist denervation have relied on qualitative descriptors of patient-reported outcomes (i.e., "excellent," "good," "fair," "poor") or the visual analogue scale (VAS) alone. To better define treatment outcomes with wrist denervation procedures, it will be critical to perform well-controlled, prospective, comparative studies that include validated patient-reported outcomes capturing the salient features of the pertinent clinical symptoms.

References

1. Wilhelm A. Die Gelenkdenervation und ihre anatomischen Grundlagen. Ein neues Behandlungsprinzip in der Handchirurgie. Springer; 1966.
2. Buck-Gramcko D. Denervation of the wrist joint. J Hand Surg Am. 1977;2(1):54–61.
3. Dellon AL. Partial dorsal wrist denervation: resection of the distal posterior interosseous nerve. J Hand Surg Am. 1985;10(4):527–33. https://doi.org/10.1016/s0363-5023(85)80077-0.
4. Dellon AL, Mackinnon SE, Daneshvar A. Terminal branch of anterior interosseous nerve as source of wrist pain. J Hand Surg Br. 1984;9(3):316–22. https://doi.org/10.1016/0266-7681(84)90051-2.

5. Weinstein LP, Berger RA. Analgesic benefit, functional outcome, and patient satisfaction after partial wrist denervation. J Hand Surg Am. 2002;27(5):833–9. https://doi.org/10.1053/jhsu.2002.35302.

6. Berger RA. Partial denervation of the wrist: a new approach. Tech Hand Up Extrem Surg. 1998;2(1):25–35. https://doi.org/10.1097/00130911-199803000-00004.

7. Tieman TE, Duraku LS, van der Oest MJW, Hundepool CA, Selles RW, Zuidam JM. Denervation of the joints of the hand and wrist: surgical techniques and a systematic review with meta-analysis. Plast Reconstr Surg. 2021;148(6):959e–72e. https://doi.org/10.1097/PRS.0000000000008517.

8. O'Shaughnessy MA, Wagner ER, Berger RA, Kakar S. Buying time: long-term results of wrist denervation and time to repeat surgery. Hand (N Y). 2019;14(5):602–8. https://doi.org/10.1177/1558944718760031.

9. Delclaux S, Elia F, Bouvet C, Aprédoaei C, Rongières M, Mansat P. Denervation of the wrist with two surgical incisions. Is it effective? A review of 33 patients with an average of 41 months' follow-up. Hand Surg Rehabil. 2017;36(4):281–5. https://doi.org/10.1016/j.hansur.2017.04.003.

10. Ferreres A, Suso S, Foucher G, Ordi J, Llusa M, Ruano D. Wrist denervation. Surgical considerations. J Hand Surg Br. 1995;20(6):769–72. https://doi.org/10.1016/s0266-7681(95)80044-1.

11. Tomita K, Berger EJ, Berger RA, Kraisarin J, An KN. Distribution of nerve endings in the human dorsal radiocarpal ligament. J Hand Surg Am. 2007;32(4):466–73. https://doi.org/10.1016/j.jhsa.2007.01.021.

12. Hagert E, Lee J, Ladd AL. Innervation patterns of thumb trapeziometacarpal joint ligaments. J Hand Surg Am. 2012;37(4):706–714.e1. https://doi.org/10.1016/j.jhsa.2011.12.038.

13. Hofmeister EP, Moran SL, Shin AY. Anterior and posterior interosseous neurectomy for the treatment of chronic dynamic instability of the wrist. Hand (N Y). 2006;1(2):63–70. https://doi.org/10.1007/s11552-006-9003-5.

14. Wilhelm A. Denervation of the wrist. Tech Hand Up Extrem Surg. 2001;5(1):14–30. https://doi.org/10.1097/00130911-200103000-00004.

15. Gay A, Harbst K, Hansen DK, Laskowski ER, Berger RA, Kaufman KR. Effect of partial wrist denervation on wrist kinesthesia: wrist denervation does not impair proprioception. J Hand Surg Am. 2011;36(11):1774–9, https://doi.org/10.1016/j.jhsa.2011.07.027.

16. Patterson RW, Van Niel M, Shimko P, Pace C, Seitz WH. Proprioception of the wrist following posterior interosseous sensory neurectomy. J Hand Surg Am. 2010;35(1):52–6. https://doi.org/10.1016/j.jhsa.2009.10.014.

17. Milone MT, Klifto CS, Catalano LW. Partial wrist denervation: the evidence behind a small fix for big problems. J Hand Surg Am. 2018;43(3):272–7. https://doi.org/10.1016/j.jhsa.2017.12.012.

18. Riches PL, Elherik FK, Breusch SJ. Functional and patient-reported outcome of partial wrist denervation versus the Mannerfelt wrist arthrodesis in the rheumatoid wrist. Arch Orthop Trauma Surg. 2014;134(7):1037–44. https://doi.org/10.1007/s00402-014-2018-4.

19. Salibi A, Hilliam R, Burke FD, Heras-Palou C. Prospective clinical trial comparing trapezial denervation with trapeziectomy for the surgical treatment of arthritis at the base of the thumb. J Surg Res. 2019;238:144–51. https://doi.org/10.1016/j.jss.2019.01.011.

Further Reading

Berger RA. Partial denervation of the wrist: a new approach. Tech Hand Up Extrem Surg. 1998;2(1):25–35. https://doi.org/10.1097/00130911-199803000-00004.

Ferreres A, Suso S, Foucher G, Ordi J, Llusa M, Ruano D. Wrist denervation. Surgical considerations. J Hand Surg Br. 1995;20(6):769–72. https://doi.org/10.1016/s0266-7681(95)80044-1.

O'Shaughnessy MA, Wagner ER, Berger RA, Kakar S. Buying time: long-term results of wrist denervation and time to repeat surgery. Hand (N Y). 2019;14(5):602–8. https://doi.org/10.1177/1558944718760031.

Chapter 37
Case Scapholunate Ligament Partial Tear

Mark Rekant

DB who is a 43-year-old right-hand-dominant male presented with acute and continued complaints of diffuse pain about his right wrist secondary to a hyperextension injury to his right wrist while attempting to restrain an agitated patient 3 months prior to presentation to my office. He described acute pain and swelling while feeling a "popping" sensation about his wrist at the time of the injury. He also described a sense of "giving way" with acute and persistent weakness.

He had no prior wrist injuries. He was initially evaluated at a local urgent care facility when diagnosed with a wrist sprain. A splint was provided, and he was referred for an MRI study.

He presented several weeks after his injury describing ongoing right wrist pain, stiffness, and weakness despite activity modification and supportive splinting. X-rays were negative for fracture.

His exam findings about the upper extremity noted preserved elbow motion. There is diffuse tenderness about the right radiocarpal joint. There was point tenderness over the dorsal aspect of the scapholunate ligament with pain with Watson scaphoid shift testing but no gross instability. He was nontender in the anatomical snuffbox. There was no tenderness over the TFCC region. Wrist range of motion was diminished with wrist extension of $45°$, while wrist flexion was $50°$. Radial deviation was $20°$, and ulnar deviation was $40°$. He maintained full finger range of motion.

Imaging studies noted neutral ulnar variance on plain radiographs with signal changes consistent with partial tearing of the scapholunate ligament seen on MRI imaging.

M. Rekant (✉)
Philadelphia Hand to Shoulder Center, Philadelphia, PA, USA

Department of Orthopaedic Surgery, Thomas Jefferson University, Philadelphia, PA, USA

J. Yao (ed.), *Carpal Instability*, https://doi.org/10.1007/978-3-031-55869-6_37

My impression was a right wrist partial scapholunate ligament tear. My initial recommendation was supportive splinting with a forearm-based thermoplastic wrist splint. He was re-evaluated at 4 weeks and again at 8 weeks with continued complaints and similar physical examination findings. The joint decision was to proceed with arthroscopic wrist surgery. The arthroscopic findings revealed a Geissler [1] grade 2 partial tear of the scapholunate ligament involving mainly the membranous portion of the ligament with very minimal involvement of the dorsal fibers of the scapholunate ligament.

The ligament tear was treated with arthroscopic debridement and thermocapsular shrinkage of the dorsal fibers. He was then immobilized postoperatively for an additional 2 months.

Discussion

Continued wrist pain in the presence of normal plain radiographs is a common problem in the practice of hand surgeons. Pain localization in the dorsocentral aspect of the wrist is often an indication of scapholunate ligament pathology or tearing. Diagnostic studies such as wrist arthrography and magnetic resonance imaging can further aid in determining the root cause of the symptoms. When physical examination is suggestive of scapholunate ligament injury and nonoperative measures fail, wrist arthroscopy will likely provide maximal diagnostic benefit to determine the underlying cause of pain. Partial scapholunate (SL) interosseous ligament tears often are easily identified during diagnostic arthroscopy [1–9].

While complete ruptures of the SL ligament are often noted on plain radiographs with gapping of the scapholunate interval, the diagnosis of a partial tear is often not as obvious but can be a cause of continued wrist dysfunction. Watson et al. [10, 11] identified this injury as one of the main causes of dorsal wrist pain in the absence of radiographic findings (termed *dorsal wrist syndrome*). In the arthroscopic classification of wrist interosseous ligament instability by Geissler and Freeland [1] (Fig. 37.1), partial lesions are included. It should be noted that this classification quantifies the resultant

Fig. 37.1 View from midcarpal portal

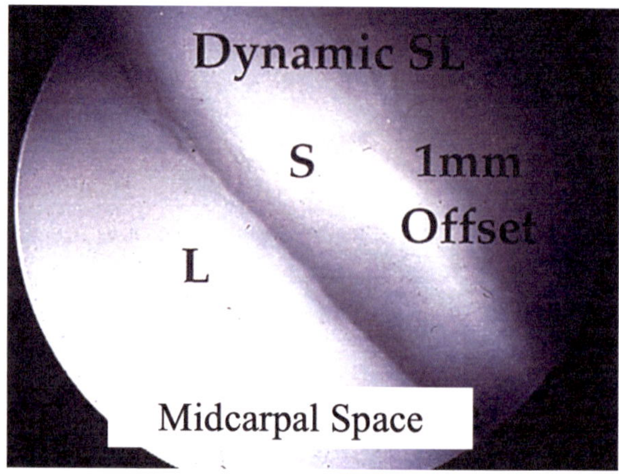

instability and not the actual size of the tear, although grade III and IV instability is thought to be the result of complete SL tears. Partial tears have been treated with arthroscopic debridement alone using synovial resectors for such lesions [3, 4]. Several studies have reported satisfactory initial results. The improved symptoms were attributed to the stabilizing effect of scar tissue formation after the debridement and to the partial denervation of the wrist [4]. However, concerns remain regarding the altered pathomechanics of a wrist with potential continued wrist instability secondary to a partial SL ligament lesion treated with debridement alone [3, 4].

The surgical technique utilized in this case consisted of a standard wrist arthroscopy performed with the patient supine and the affected extremity placed into a wrist traction apparatus. A complete diagnostic arthroscopy is performed evaluating the radiocarpal and midcarpal joints to identify any coexistent lesions. The membranous central (proximal) portion of the SLIL ligament is best visualized when the arthroscope is placed in the 3–4 radiocarpal portal. The dorsal and volar SLIL are best visualized with the arthroscope in the midcarpal ulnar (MCU) portal (Fig. 37.1), allowing a probe to be placed through the midcarpal radial (MCR) portal to assess ligament integrity. The volar SLIL is evaluated with the scope in the MCR portal. The attention is returned to the radiocarpal joint where the scapholunate ligament tear is debrided using a shaver in the 3–4 radiocarpal portal with the scope in the 6R portal. After debridement of the frayed SL ligament, the remaining portion of the SL ligament may need to be tightened using a monopolar radiofrequency probe placed through the 3–4 RC portal. The amount of heating that occurs is determined by the distance from the probe, the size of the probe, the temperature and flow rate of the arthroscopic irrigation, and the duration of application [12].

My preferred method for thermal shrinkage involves a light "painting" or touching the lax ligament with a monopolar "micro-ablator" Vulcan™ probe from Smith & Nephew™ (Washington, DC) in broad strokes along the injured ligament allowing for direct visualization of the ligamentous tightening. Overzealous RF probe application is avoided to prevent tissue and cartilage damage, which appears brown with arthroscopic visualization. After debridement and potential ligamentous tightening, the extent of the SL ligament injury is further assessed using the Geissler classification (Fig. 37.2). Geissler type II injuries can be treated with arthroscopic

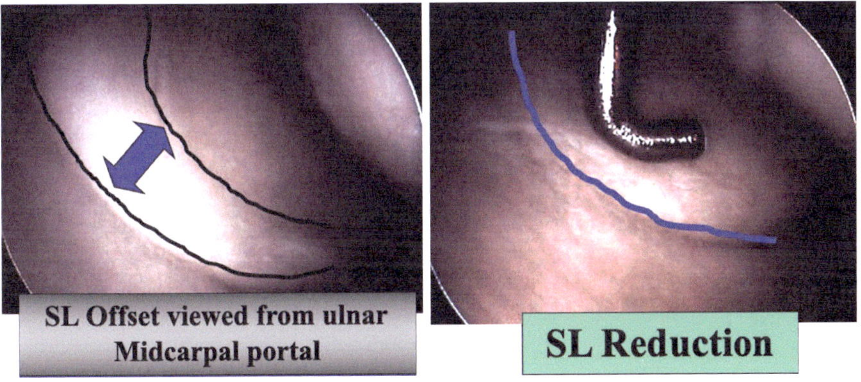

Fig. 37.2 SL offset and SL joint reduction from midcarpal vantage point

reduction of SL alignment and fixation. The lax dorsal SLIL can be tightened with thermal shrinkage.

Two 0.045 in. Kirschner wires are placed under fluoroscopic guidance into the radial aspect of the scaphoid and positioned to allow trajectory across the SL interval into the lunate (Fig. 37.3). The wires are passed into the lunate after reducing the scapholunate step-off with arthroscopic visualization and reduction (Figs. 37.4 and 37.5). The arthroscope in the MCU portal allows visualization of the reduction and alignment as the wires are passed into the lunate. The K-wires are then buried under the skin after fluoroscopic confirmation of proper placement.

An alternative technique is to secure the SL reduction with a cannulated headed or headless screw. A guidewire for a cannulated headless screw is provisionally placed across the scaphoid prior to SL joint reduction. The guidewire is then introduced into the lunate following reduction.

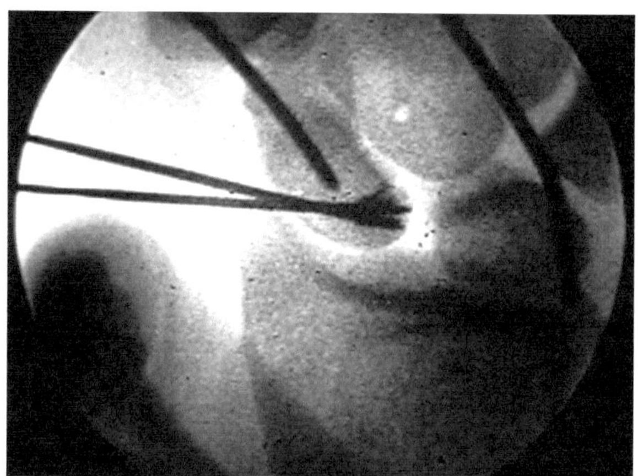

Fig. 37.3 Fluoroscopic view of Kirschner wires preset for SL joint stabilization

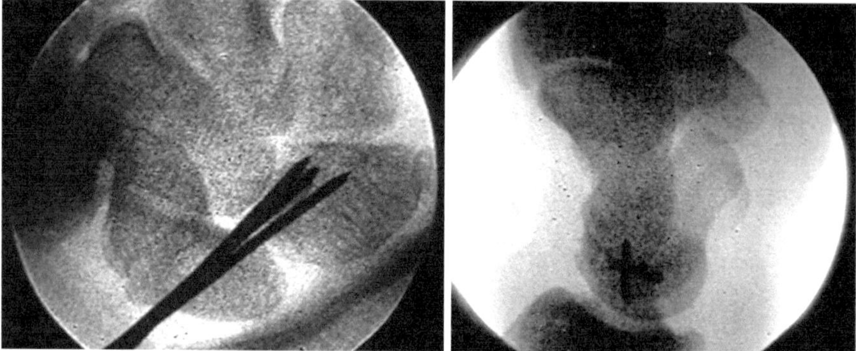

Figs. 37.4 and 37.5 AP and lateral postreduction fluoroscopy images

The screw is then passed over the guidewire after making a radial sided skin incision using blunt dissection to protect the radial sided sensory nerve branches. The scapholunate screw remains in place for a minimum of 4 months [13] although studies have indicated that the screw may remain indefinitely [14].

Further Discussion

The early diagnosis and treatment of acute scapholunate (SL) ligament injuries continue to be a challenge. Berger [15] defined the anatomy of the SL interosseous ligament (SLIL). He described the ligament having three distinct regions. The central (proximal) membranous portion is cartilaginous with a few longitudinal fibers. The dorsal portion of the interosseous ligament is histologically a true ligament. It is composed of stout transverse fibers and is the thickest portion of the SLIL. The palmar (volar) portion of the interosseous ligament is also histologically a true ligament, 1–2 mm thick, and composed of longer oblique fibers that allow rotation in the sagittal plane.

Mayfield [16] showed that the SLIL can stretch up to 225% its length before eventually tearing. An isolated injury to the SLIL initially may not cause disassociation and widening on plain or stress radiographs. A combined injury to both the intrinsic and extrinsic ligaments will cause an SL diastasis and DISI deformity. In patients with isolated SLIL injuries, plain radiograph abnormalities may not be seen initially but will occur over time as gradual attenuation of the extrinsic ligaments occurs.

This chapter presents methods to successfully manage a partial scapholunate ligament tear with arthroscopic findings of scapholunate joint instability with a "step-off." If the scapholunate joint can be easily reduced under arthroscopic guidance, the joint can be stabilized with Kirschner wires or screw fixation for a minimum of 8 weeks, which allows for collagen healing and return of stability to the scapholunate joint.

The postoperative course of treatment included 8 weeks of immobilization followed by pin removal. Hand therapy was prescribed for 1–2 months subsequent to pin removal to facilitate return to function.

References

1. Geissler WB, Freeland AE. Arthroscopically assisted reduction of intraarticular distal radial fractures. Clin Orthop. 1996;327:125–34.
2. Dautel G, Goudot B, Merle M. Arthroscopic diagnosis of scapho-lunate instability in the absence of x-ray abnormalities. J Hand Surg. 1993;18B:213–8.

3. Ruch DS, Poehling GG. Arthroscopic management of partial scapholunate and lunotriquetral injuries of the wrist. J Hand Surg. 1996;21A:412–7.
4. Weiss APC, Sachar K, Glowacki KA. Arthroscopic debridement alone for intercarpal ligament tears. J Hand Surg. 1997;22A:344–9.
5. Johnstone DJ, Thorogood S, Smith WH, Scott TD. A comparison of magnetic resonance imaging and arthroscopy in the investigation of chronic wrist pain. J Hand Surg. 1997;22B:714–8.
6. Kozin SH. The role of arthroscopy in scapholunate instability. Hand Clin. 1999;15:435–44.
7. Ruch DS, Smith BP. Arthroscopic and open management of dynamic scaphoid instability. Orthop Clin North Am. 2001;32:233–40.
8. Walsh JJ, Berger RA, Cooney WP. Current status of scapholunate interosseous ligament injuries. J Am Acad Orthop Surg. 2002;10:32–42.
9. O'Meeghan CJ, Stuart W, Mamo V, Stanley JK, Trail IA. The natural history of an untreated isolated scapholunate interosseus ligament injury. J Hand Surg. 2003;28B:307–10.
10. Watson HK, Ballet FL. The SLAC wrist: scapholunate advanced collapse pattern of degenerative arthritis. J Hand Surg. 1984;9A:358–65.
11. Watson HK, Weinzweig J, Zeppieri J. The natural progression of scaphoid instability. Hand Clin. 1997;13:39–49.
12. Owens BD, Stickles BJ, Busconi BD. Radiofrequency energy: applications and basic science. Am J Orthop. 2003;32:117–20.
13. Kuo CE, Wolfe SW. Scapholunate instability: current concepts in diagnosis and management. J Hand Surg Am. 2008;33:998–1013.
14. Rosenwasser MP, Miyasajsa KC, Strauch RJ. The RASL procedure: reduction and association of the scaphoid and lunate using the Herbert screw. Tech Hand Up Extrem Surg. 1997;1:263–72.
15. Berger RA. The gross and histologic anatomy of the scapholunate interosseous ligament. J Hand Surg Am. 1996;21(2):170–8.
16. Mayfield JK, Johnson RP, Kilcoyne RK. Carpal dislocations: pathomechanics and progressive perilunar instability. J Hand Surg Am. 1980;5(3):226–41.

Chapter 38
SLAC Wrist: Proximal Row Carpectomy

Hannah C. Langdell and Warren C. Hammert

Case Presentation

Our patient is a 58-year-old female office worker with left wrist pain. She had used a splint and had two previous steroid injections with minimal relief. Her radiographs demonstrated stage II SLAC pattern arthritis (Fig. 38.1). She was symptomatic enough to consider surgery.

H. C. Langdell
Division of Plastic, Reconstructive, Maxillofacial and Oral Surgery, Department of Surgery, Duke University Medical Center, Durham, NC, USA

W. C. Hammert (✉)
Division of Hand Surgery, Department of Orthopaedic Surgery, Duke University Medical Center, Durham, NC, USA
e-mail: warren.hammert@duke.edu

J. Yao (ed.), *Carpal Instability*, https://doi.org/10.1007/978-3-031-55869-6_38

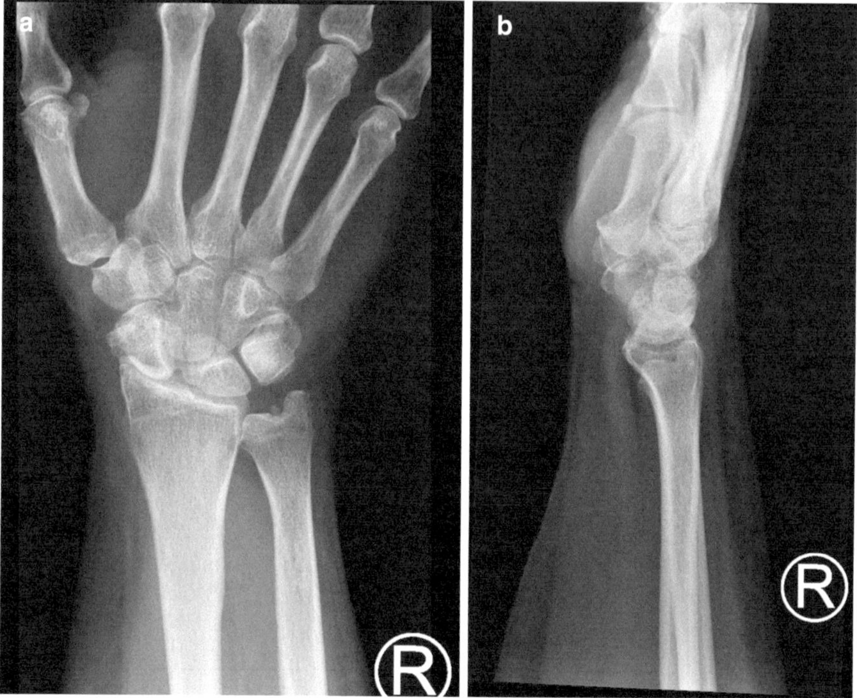

Fig. 38.1 Preoperative posteroanterior (**a**) and lateral (**b**) radiograph demonstrating stage II SLAC pattern arthritis

Diagnosis

Physical Assessment/Relevant Maneuvers

Proximal row carpectomy (PRC) is an effective surgical option in patients with symptomatic wrist arthritis who have failed conservative management. When patients present with wrist pain and arthritis, it is first important to determine the etiology. Most commonly, wrist arthritis develops as the result of trauma that over time leads to scapholunate advanced collapse (SLAC) in cases of scapholunate ligament (SLL) tears or scaphoid nonunion advanced collapse (SNAC). SLL tears, when accompanied by loss of critical stabilizers, can result in carpal malalignment with dorsal intercalated segment instability (DISI). Other causes of wrist arthritis that should be distinguished from SLAC wrist include Kienböck disease, articular chondrocalcinosis, calcium pyrophosphate deposition, and isolated scaphotrapezium-trapezoidal (STT) arthritis [1].

SLL tears or scaphoid nonunion may be asymptomatic for many years, leading to a delayed diagnosis in many patients. The natural history of SLL tears seems to be progression to SLAC arthritis, but the time frame is variable and the symptoms progress gradually over time, and scaphoid nonunion may similarly not be symptomatic, even after progression to SNAC arthritis. Upon presentation, patients often report pain, swelling, limited wrist motion, and decreased grip strength. The focal swelling and effusion at the dorso-radial wrist are the result of osteophytic growth and synovitis and result in stiffness with extension and radial deviation. Sites of pain should be localized with care to differentiate pain at the radiocarpal joint from pain at the distal radioulnar joint or ulnocarpal joint.

Diagnostic Studies

Wrist radiographs will demonstrate a predictable pattern of degenerative arthritis in patients with SLAC wrist due to scaphoid rotary subluxation and DISI. As described by Watson and Ballet, arthritis will first develop at the radial styloid (stage I), which then progresses to the radioscaphoid joint (stage II) followed by the capitolunate articulation (stage III) [2]. SNAC arthritis has the same findings in stages I and III but is slightly different in progression as stage II involves the scaphocapitate interface rather than the radioscaphoid joint. Accurately assessing which joint surfaces are involved will help determine the surgical options. Additional findings to note on radiographs are the distal radioulnar index and appearance of the thumb CMC joint and DRUJ as well as the pisotriquetral joint, as these are common locations for arthritis and treatment of the radioscaphoid joint alone may not provide complete relief if these other locations are symptomatic. Other etiologies can also be ruled out with diagnostic imaging. In pseudogout, there is a pattern of scaphoid chondrocalcinosis advanced collapse (SCAC) that can be distinguished from SLAC wrist in later stages as SCAC wrist involves scaphoid impaction onto the distal radius and scaphoid extension [3]. Despite there being differences in the diagnosis causing these patterns of arthritis, the treatments are generally the same as the radioscaphoid joint is initially involved and then progresses to the midcarpal joint.

MRI can provide additional information about the cartilage and be helpful for surgical planning but is generally not necessary. Direct inspection with wrist arthroscopy can also be helpful, but when considering PRC or limited wrist arthrodesis, direct inspection during the procedure will provide the needed information. Given some degree of uncertainty when planning the procedure, we discuss the option of converting PRC to midcarpal arthrodesis in the event that there is substantial wear on the head of the capitate. If there is just minor cartilage loss, we generally continue with the PRC with capsular interposition.

Management Options

Once patients develop symptoms due to SLAC, SCAC, or SNAC arthritis that do not resolve with nonoperative treatment, surgery can be used to address the underlying arthritic changes. We find SLAC and SNAC arthritis more common than SCAC, but the approach to treatment is the same for all, depending on the radiographic stage of arthritis. In early-stage disease (stage I), a radial styloidectomy is often sufficient to alleviate pain but may recur if the primary issue (SL instability or scaphoid nonunion) is not addressed. For most symptomatic patients with wrist arthritis that involves more than the radiostyloid articulation, a procedure to address the arthritis is often performed.

The two most common motion-sparing surgeries for SLAC wrist are limited wrist arthrodesis and PRC. The scaphoid is removed to address the radioscaphoid arthritis, and the carpus is reconstructed by either a midcarpal arthrodesis or a removal of the entire proximal carpal row. Details of the limited arthrodesis will be described in the respective chapter. PRC involves resection of the scaphoid, lunate, and triquetrum so that there is a new radiocarpal articulation between the capitate and radius [4]. Recent literature suggests lower complications and revision procedures with PRC compared to limited wrist arthrodesis [5]. It has also been suggested that patients under 35 are more likely to progress to symptomatic radiocapitate arthritis, so these younger patients are likely best treated with the limited arthrodesis [6]. Given the current evidence, our preference is for PRC in patients 35 and older when possible as outcomes are similar. We avoid the potential of nonunion, and subsequent surgeries are less likely with the PRC when compared to limited arthrodesis. Historically, it has been felt that stage III arthritis (capitolunate arthritis) is a contraindication to PRC, but with mild or early changes, this can be addressed with capsular interposition to provide a barrier between the capitate and lunate fossa of the radius.

Other surgical options are wrist denervation and wrist arthroplasty. Wrist denervation is a low-morbidity option that can be performed in elderly patients or low-demand patients who still have good range of motion to decrease the pain associated with SLAC wrist. However, the symptom relief is not completely predictable, and this procedure does not address the underlying arthritis. Earlier generation wrist arthroplasty implants have been plagued by hardware complications and poor outcomes, but there are now newer technologies that have shown improved midterm results [7, 8].

Management Chosen for This Case with Rationale

The surgical options were discussed, and through shared decision-making, she elected to proceed with PRC. Exposure was through a distally based capsular flap to be used as needed for interposition. This is our routine exposure for this operation as it maintains the option to use the flap, and we have not seen a downside to using the capsular interposition flap even when there is no cartilage loss as it theoretically provides additional soft tissue between the capitate head and lunate fossa of the radius. Upon inspection of the proximal capitate, there was a small area of cartilage loss and exposed subchondral bone. The shape of the proximal capitate was round, and it was felt that it would articulate well with the lunate facet of the radius and the capsular interposition flap would adequately cover the small area of cartilage loss.

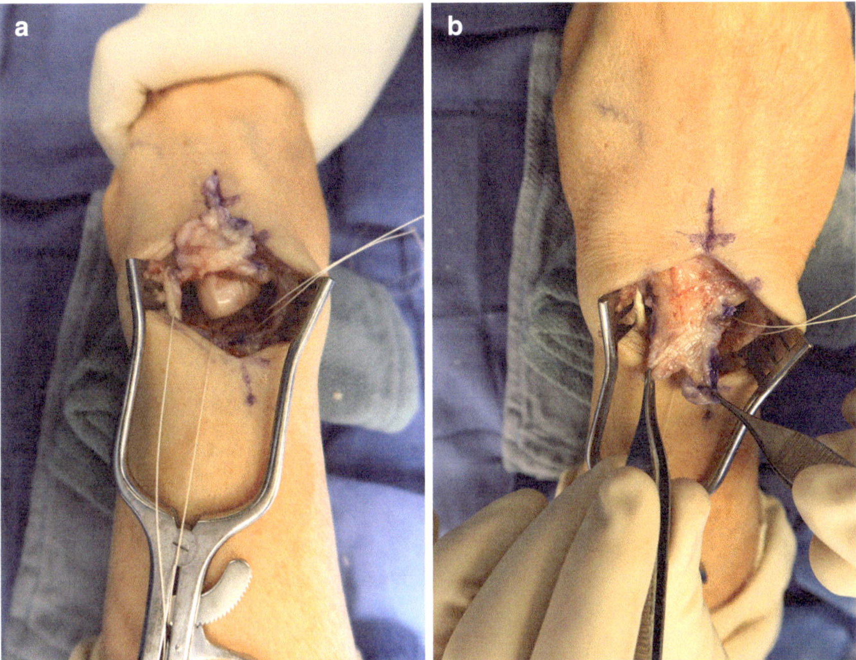

Fig. 38.2 (**a**) Intraoperative picture of capitate—note the small area of cartilage wear along dorsal ulnar aspect of capitate and (**b**) demonstration of capsular flap prior to insetting

The proximal row was removed, taking care to preserve the radioscaphocapitate (RSC) ligament (Fig. 38.2).

The distally based capsular flap was used for additional soft tissue interposition. Large absorbable sutures were placed along the volar capsule of the radioscaphoid joint and capsule at the volar ulnar aspect of the radius in a figure 8 manner to secure the capsule in the corners. We have not found the need for additional sutures as the capsule nicely drapes over the capitate head and provides the intended interposition. The capsule was loosely closed along the longitudinal incisions after ensuring that the wrist had good passive flexion and extension and the capitate was articulating in the lunate facet of the radius. The patient was placed in a volar plaster splint.

Clinical Course and Outcome

At the 1-week postoperative appointment, the patient was transitioned to a cast for an additional 2 weeks. Postoperative radiographs demonstrate the capitate articulating in the lunate fossa of the radius (Fig. 38.3). At 3 weeks following surgery, she was transitioned to a removable brace and began therapy and home exercises to regain motion and strength. Unrestricted use of the hand was allowed at 6 weeks

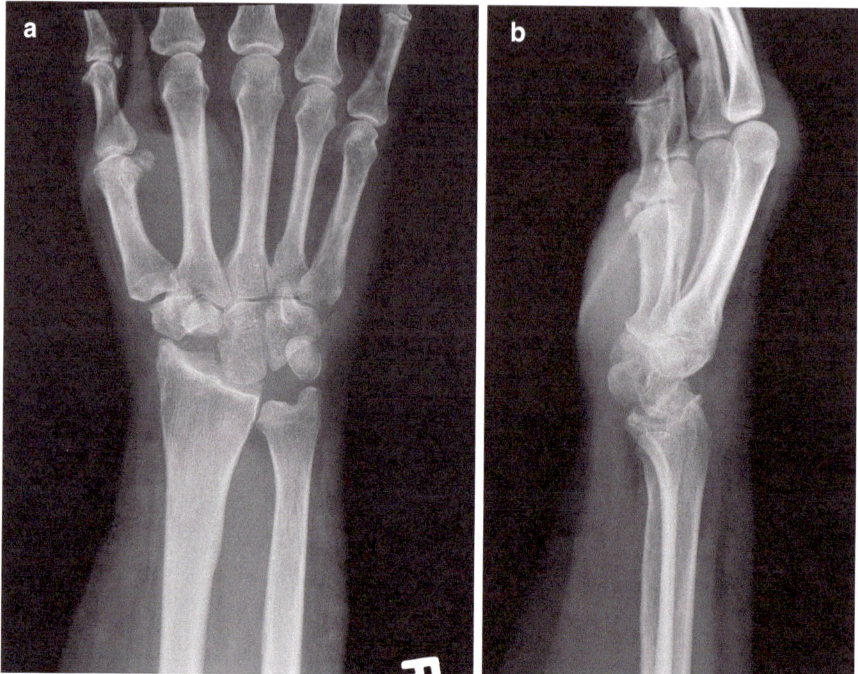

Fig. 38.3 Postoperative posteroanterior (**a**) and lateral (**b**) radiograph following PRC with capsular interposition flap demonstrated

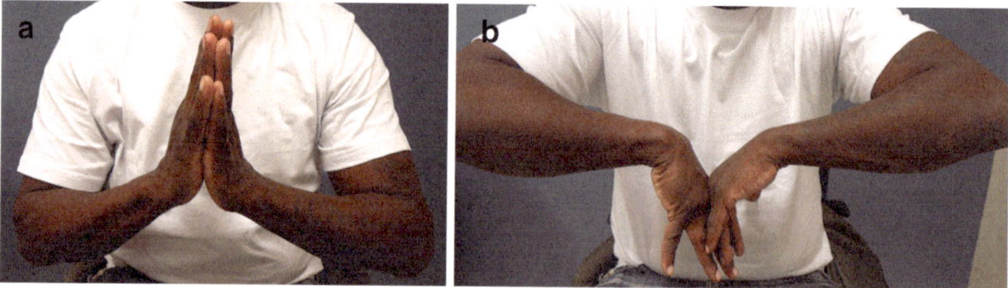

Fig. 38.4 Photographs at 6 months of a different patient who underwent left PRC depicting postoperative wrist (**a**) extension of 55° and (**b**) flexion of 30°

after surgery. Patients still typically have some discomfort with heavier activities at 6 weeks that resolves over several months. Final motion is depicted in a different patient demonstrating typical loss of flexion and extension (Fig. 38.4).

Bulleted Clinical Pearls/Pitfalls

- Anticipate about 35% loss of wrist motion and 25% loss of grip strength, but improvement in pain at rest and with activities.
- Take care to preserve the RSC ligament during removal of the scaphoid.

- Evaluate the proximal capitate prior to removal of the lunate as the option for limited arthrodesis remains if there is substantial cartilage loss on the capitate.
- Make sure that the capitate articulates in the lunate fossa of the radius. In the event that the articulation is unstable, such as injury to the radioscaphocapitate ligament or other causes, we will stabilize this with a large (0.62 in.) Kirschner wire from the capitate into the radius, maintaining the alignment and removing in 4 weeks when we begin rehabilitation.

Literature Review and Discussion

PRC results in improvement in pain and patient-reported outcomes for patients with SLAC wrist. In a cohort study of 304 patients who underwent PRC, predominantly for SLAC wrist, 82% had returned to work at 1 year, at a median time of 12 weeks postoperatively. The total Patient Rated Wrist/Hand Evaluation (PRWE) score improved from 60 preoperatively to 38 at 3 months and 26 at 12 months [9]. Similarly, Jebson et al. reported that in their series of 20 patients with wrist osteoarthritis who underwent PRC, 90% of patients had resolution of pain at an average of 13.1-year follow-up. Average wrist range of motion was 63%, and grip strength was 83% of the contralateral side [10]. Finally, Stern et al. reviewed 22 wrists that underwent PRC with an average of 14-year follow-up and found an average flexion-extension arc of 72°. Average grip strength was 91% of the contralateral hand. While radiocapitate arthrosis does develop, it does not seem to correlate with clinical outcomes [11].

PRC is often compared to four-corner fusion in the setting of SLAC wrist. Some studies show that these two operations have similar results in terms of quick Disabilities of Arm, Shoulder, and Hand (DASH) scores, pain levels, and wrist function, even in young, active patients [12, 13]. However, a meta-analysis of 1059 SLAC or SNAC wrists reported lower complication rates, lower reoperation rates, and better ROM with PRC [14]. Likewise, several large series report lower rates of secondary operations in PRC for SLAC or SNAC wrist compared to four-corner fusion and equivalent rates of conversion to total wrist arthrodesis [13, 15, 16]. Given its lower complication rate and quicker return to work, PRC is often favored for stage II SLAC wrist [15, 16]. Finally, in a systematic review of long-term outcomes of PRC including 147 patients with at least 10 years of follow-up, patients had a mean postoperative flexion-extension arc of 73.5% and grip strength of 68.4% of contralateral side. While 79% of patients had evidence of radiocapitate arthrosis, this finding was not correlated with patient-reported symptoms, any outcome measure, or time from PRC [17]. The weighted mean DASH score was 21.5 and weighted mean PRWE score was 28.7, which are comparable to the patient-reported outcome scores after four-corner fusion [18, 19]. There were 21 failures (14.3%) requiring conversion to total wrist arthrodesis or arthroplasty. Failures were evenly distributed amongst wrist pathologies, including Kienböck disease, SLAC, and SNAC wrist. Most failures were in patients younger than 35 who had an active occupation. While this review cautions against PRC in patients with active occupations due to a decrease in grip strength and a higher likelihood of reoperation, other studies have shown PRC to be successful in laborers [12, 20]. Causes of failure after PRC include unrecognized capitolunate joint arthritis, impingement of the radial styloid, and injury to the RSC ligament [20]. Conversely, factors associated with improved outcomes after PRC are age over 40, Kienböck disease as the etiology of wrist arthritis, concomitant neurectomy, and non-laborers [21]. Based on the current literature, we use the age 35 and over as a relative indication for PRC for stage II SLAC, SNAC, or SCAC arthritis. In patients under this age with risk factors for nonunion, such as smokers, we would also consider PRC.

Traditionally, PRC was contraindicated if there was existing cartilage damage to the proximal pole of the capitate or lunate fossa. However, modifications have been developed to overcome this limitation including capsular interposition with dorsal capsule or allograft, osteochondral resurfacing, resurfacing pyrocarbon implants, and partial capitate resection at the time of PRC. In a series of eight patients who underwent PRC with capsular interposition, there was improvement in visual analogue scale (VAS) pain scores postoperatively, and the mean grip strength after surgery was 66.8% of that of the contralateral hand [22]. Compared to capitate resurfacing procedures, capsular interposition was found to result in better range of motion and grip strength in a recent systematic review. While the capsular interposition group had a higher rate of conversion to arthrodesis, this was attributed to longer follow-up times in these studies [23]. The addition of capsular interposition to PRC has not been shown to affect the mean grip strength, flexion-extension arc, QuickDASH, or PRWE scores compared to performing PRC alone [24].

References

1. Weiss KE, Rodner CM. Osteoarthritis of the wrist. J Hand Surg Am. 2007;32(5):725–46. https://doi.org/10.1016/j.jhsa.2007.02.003.
2. Watson HK, Ballet FL. The SLAC wrist: scapholunate advanced collapse pattern of degenerative arthritis. J Hand Surg Am. 1984;9(3):358–65. https://doi.org/10.1016/s0363-5023(84)80223-3.
3. Romano S. Non-traumatic osteoarthritis of the wrist: chondrocalcinosis. Chir Main. 2003;22(6):285–92. https://doi.org/10.1016/j.main.2003.09.012.
4. Mulford JS, Ceulemans LJ, Nam D, Axelrod TS. Proximal row carpectomy vs four corner fusion for scapholunate (Slac) or scaphoid nonunion advanced collapse (Snac) wrists: a systematic review of outcomes. J Hand Surg Eur Vol. 2009;34(2):256–63. https://doi.org/10.1177/1753193408100954.
5. Rahgozar P, Zhong L, Chung KC. A Comparative analysis of resource utilization between proximal row carpectomy and partial wrist fusion: a population study. J Hand Surg Am. 2017;42(10):773–80. https://doi.org/10.1016/j.jhsa.2017.07.032.
6. Wall LB, Didonna ML, Kiefhaber TR, Stern PJ. Proximal row carpectomy: minimum 20-year follow-up. J Hand Surg Am. 2013;38(8):1498–504. https://doi.org/10.1016/j.jhsa.2013.04.028.
7. Giwa L, Siddiqui A, Packer G. Motec wrist arthroplasty: 4 years of promising results. J Hand Surg Asian Pac. 2018;23(3):364–8. https://doi.org/10.1142/S2424835518500388.
8. Herzberg G, Boeckstyns M, Sorensen AI, Axelsson P, Kroener K, Liverneaux P, Obert L, Merser S. "Remotion" total wrist arthroplasty: preliminary results of a prospective international multicenter study of 215 cases. J Wrist Surg. 2012;1(1):17–22. https://doi.org/10.1055/s-0032-1323642.

9. Teunissen JS, Duraku LS, Feitz R, Zuidam JM, Selles RW, Consortium BS, Wouters RM. Routinely-collected outcomes of proximal row carpectomy. J Hand Surg Am. 2022; https://doi.org/10.1016/j.jhsa.2022.09.004.

10. Jebson PJ, Hayes EP, Engber WD. Proximal row carpectomy: a minimum 10-year follow-up study. J Hand Surg Am. 2003;28(4):561–9. https://doi.org/10.1016/s0363-5023(03)00248-x.

11. Stern PJ, Agabegi SS, Kiefhaber TR, Didonna ML. Proximal row carpectomy. J Bone Joint Surg Am. 2005;87(Suppl 1, Pt 2):166–74. https://doi.org/10.2106/JBJS.E.00261.

12. Wagner ER, Werthel JD, Elhassan BT, Moran SL. Proximal row carpectomy and 4-corner arthrodesis in patients younger than age 45 years. J Hand Surg Am. 2017;42(6):428–35. https://doi.org/10.1016/j.jhsa.2017.03.015.

13. Williams JB, Weiner H, Tyser AR. Long-term outcome and secondary operations after proximal row carpectomy or four-corner arthrodesis. J Wrist Surg. 2018;7(1):51–6. https://doi.org/10.1055/s-0037-1604395.

14. Chammas PE, Hadouiri N, Chammas M, Ramos-Pascual S, Stirling P, Nover L, Klouche S. Proximal row carpectomy generates better mid- to long-term outcomes than four-corner arthrodesis for post-traumatic wrist arthritis: a meta-analysis. Orthop Traumatol Surg Res. 2022;108(7):103373. https://doi.org/10.1016/j.otsr.2022.103373.

15. Garcia BN, Lu CC, Stephens AR, Kazmers NH, Chen W, Leng J, Li L, Sauer BC, Tyser AR. Risk of total wrist arthrodesis or reoperation following 4-Corner arthrodesis or proximal row carpectomy for stage-II SLAC/SNAC arthritis: a propensity score analysis of 502 wrists. J Bone Joint Surg Am. 2020;102(12):1050–8. https://doi.org/10.2106/JBJS.19.00965.

16. Vanhove W, De Vil J, Van Seymortier P, Boone B, Verdonk R. Proximal row carpectomy versus four-corner arthrodesis as a treatment for SLAC (scapholunate advanced collapse) wrist. J Hand Surg Eur. 2008;33(2):118–25. https://doi.org/10.1177/1753193408087116.

17. Chim H, Moran SL. Long-term outcomes of proximal row carpectomy: a systematic review of the literature. J Wrist Surg. 2012;1(2):141–8. https://doi.org/10.1055/s-0032-1329547.

18. Dacho A, Grundel J, Holle G, Germann G, Sauerbier M. Long-term results of midcarpal arthrodesis in the treatment of scaphoid nonunion advanced collapse (SNAC-Wrist) and scapholunate advanced collapse (SLAC-Wrist). Ann Plast Surg. 2006;56(2):139–44. https://doi.org/10.1097/01.sap.0000194245.94684.54.

19. Merrell GA, McDermott EM, Weiss AP. Four-corner arthrodesis using a circular plate and distal radius bone grafting: a consecutive case series. J Hand Surg Am. 2008;33(5):635–42. https://doi.org/10.1016/j.jhsa.2008.02.001.

20. Green DP, Perreira AC, Longhofer LK. Proximal row carpectomy. J Hand Surg Am. 2015;40(8):1672–6. https://doi.org/10.1016/j.jhsa.2015.04.033.

21. Wagner ER, Bravo D, Elhassan B, Moran SL. Factors associated with improved outcomes following proximal row carpectomy: a long-term outcome study of 144 patients. J Hand Surg Eur Vol. 2016;41(5):484–91. https://doi.org/10.1177/1753193415597096.

22. Kwon BC, Choi SJ, Shin J, Baek GH. Proximal row carpectomy with capsular interposition arthroplasty for advanced arthritis of the wrist. J Bone Joint Surg Br. 2009;91(12):1601–6. https://doi.org/10.1302/0301-620X.91B12.22335.

23. Perry AC, Wilkes C, Curran MWT, Ball BJ, Morhart MJ. Proximal row carpectomy modifications for capitate arthritis: a systematic review. J Wrist Surg. 2023;12(1):86–94. https://doi.org/10.1055/s-0042-1751013.

24. Gaspar MP, Pham PP, Pankiw CD, Jacoby SM, Shin EK, Osterman AL, Kane PM. Mid-term outcomes of routine proximal row carpectomy compared with proximal row carpectomy with dorsal capsular interposition arthroplasty for the treatment of late-stage arthropathy of the wrist. Bone Joint J. 2018;100-B(2):197–204. https://doi.org/10.1302/0301-620X.100B2.BJJ-2017-0816.R2.

Suggested Readings

Chammas PE, Hadouiri N, Chammas M, et al. Proximal row carpectomy generates better mid- to long-term outcomes than four-corner arthrodesis for post-traumatic wrist arthritis: a meta-analysis. Orthop Traumatol Surg Res. 2022;108(7):103373. https://doi.org/10.1016/j.otsr.2022.103373.

Jebson PJ, Hayes EP, Engber WD. Proximal row carpectomy: a minimum 10-year follow-up study. J Hand Surg Am. 2003;28(4):561–9. https://doi.org/10.1016/s0363-5023(03)00248-x.

Perry AC, Wilkes C, Curran MWT, Ball BJ, Morhart MJ. Proximal row carpectomy modifications for capitate arthritis: a systematic review. J Wrist Surg. 2023;12(1):86–94. https://doi.org/10.1055/s-0042-1751013.

Chapter 39
SLAC Wrist: Midcarpal Fusion

James Tyler Frix and R. Glenn Gaston

Case Presentation

In this chapter, we present the case of a 55-year-old right-hand-dominant male who presented to our clinic with progressive left wrist pain over the last year unresponsive to NSAIDs, bracing, and cortisone injections. Pain is exacerbated by wrist flexion and extension. An avid runner and weight lifter, he has had to stop free weights and cut back on long runs due to increasing discomfort. There is a remote history of left wrist trauma from a previous military deployment, but no other issues. He is a nonsmoker and works in business management.

Physical examination revealed a well-appearing male with mild wrist swelling but without erythema or fluctuance. No other overt deformities or signs of infection were appreciated. Tenderness to palpation was noted over the dorsal radiocarpal joint and about the anatomic snuffbox. He was nontender over the ulnar fovea. He had limited wrist flexion to 50° and extension to 20° that appeared to be due to a combination of pain and mechanical block. He had full pronation and supination with excellent finger range of motion. There was pain, crepitus, and a palpable clunk with a Watson shift test that was asymmetric to the contralateral side. There was no tenderness over the PT joint, and provocative testing for CTS was negative. Grip strength was 50% that of the contralateral side, limited by pain. Baseline pain reported via the visual analog scale (VAS) was 8 out of 10.

J. T. Frix
Atrium Health Orthopedic Surgery, Charlotte, NC, USA
e-mail: James.frix@atriumhealth.org

R. G. Gaston (✉)
OrthoCarolina Hand and Upper Extremity Department, Atrium Health Department of Orthopedic Surgery, Charlotte, NC, USA
e-mail: glenn.gaston@orthocarolina.com

J. Yao (ed.), *Carpal Instability*, https://doi.org/10.1007/978-3-031-55869-6_39

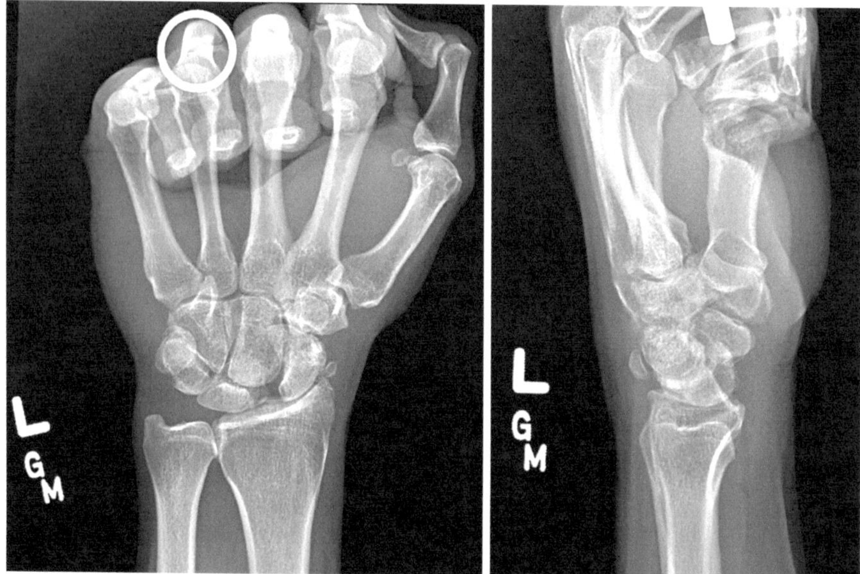

Fig. 39.1 AP and lateral view of our patient's left wrist demonstrating stage 3 scapholunate advanced collapse with scapholunate interval diastasis, radioscaphoid and capitolunate arthritis, and dorsal intercalated segment instability

Radiographic studies showed stage 3 scapholunate advanced collapse (SLAC) with significant diastasis at the scapholunate interval, narrowing at the radioscaphoid joint, and dorsal intercalated segment instability (Fig. 39.1). The patient had a type I lunate and no evidence of lunotriquetral (LT) instability. Ulnar variance was neutral.

The patient has failed conservative treatments and is amenable to surgical intervention. We discussed the risks, benefits, and expectations of surgery and obtained informed consent to proceed with scaphoid excision and midcarpal fusion with potential distal radius bone grafting. We discussed beforehand that the specific bones fused will depend on our intraoperative findings . We emphasized the importance of postoperative therapy as needed.

Diagnosis

Scapholunate advanced collapse is a predictable pattern of degenerative wrist arthritis resulting from scapholunate (SL) ligament insufficiency. This ligament is the critical link between the scaphoid and lunate maintaining proper carpal alignment and wrist kinematics. With SL disruption, the scaphoid characteristically shifts into flexion and pronation as well as frequent dorsal subluxation due to the load on the distal pole through the scaphotrapeziotrapezoid (STT) joint [2]. The lunate, in contrast, remains attached to the triquetrum through the intact LT ligaments and follows the triquetrum into an extended posture, thus increasing the scapholunate angle [2]. This pattern of carpal alignment is known as dorsal intercalated segment instability (DISI) [2, 3]. DISI alters wrist biomechanics and causes increased shear forces on the carpal joint surfaces. Cartilage thrives in compression but fails in shear, thus resulting in progressive arthritic collapse known as SLAC wrist. As the scaphoid flexes, pronates, and dorsally subluxates, its congruency with the elliptical scaphoid fossa is lost (like two overlapping spoons turned in relationship to one another), thus leading to radial styloid-scaphoid and subsequent radioscaphoid arthritis [4]. When the lunate extends, shear forces are created at the capitolunate joint, thus leading to midcarpal arthritis. The radiolunate joint, however, is typically spared from degenerative change as there are still compressive forces present between the radius and now dorsal surface of the lunate. It is this preservation of the radiolunate joint that allows for motion-sparing procedures such as midcarpal fusions.

SLAC was first described by Watson and Ballet in 1984, and since then, the understanding and management of SLAC have evolved significantly. The epidemiology of SLAC is still not well-established as the prevalence of the condition is difficult to determine, but, in their initial series, Watson and Ballet identified SLAC as the most prevalent pattern of wrist arthritis [1]. One potential reason for this difficulty is the variation of lunate morphology across populations. Two types of lunates were identified by Viegas et al. and are distinguished by the presence or absence of a medial facet for articulation with the hamate [5]. Type I lunates do not have this medial facet, while type II lunates do [5, 6]. Patients with a type II lunate have been shown to have a lower incidence of DISI deformity following SL ligament injury as compared to those with type I [6]. Rhee et al. hypothesized that the added lunohamate articulation may serve as a bony backstop which restricts lunate hyperextension after SL ligament injury, thus reducing DISI and the risk of progression to SLAC wrist [7].

Patients often report symptoms related to traumatic injury in the affected wrist for over a decade before seeking treatment and, thus, present in advanced stages [8]. Various treatment options and their associated long-term outcomes have been well-established. In this chapter, we will focus on midcarpal fusion which is typically recommended for patients with stage 2 or 3 SLAC wrist.

Diagnosis of SLAC wrist begins with a thorough history and physical examination, as patients typically present with wrist pain, crepitus, and swelling about the dorsal/radial aspect of the wrist due to underlying osteophytes and synovitis. With advanced arthritis, wrist range of motion will often be reduced with extension more affected than flexion [9]. Presentation can be acute on chronic, with patients describing a recent stressor that exacerbated years of underlying symptoms. Bilateral X-rays help establish the diagnosis, but the physical exam is crucial to rule in or out other possible associated diagnoses, such as distal radial ulna joint (DRUJ) pathology, carpal boss, CMC/STT arthritis, or ulnar impaction as associated pathology could affect treatment. Scapholunate instability can be confirmed on physical examination with the Watson test, also termed the scaphoid shift test. This is done by moving the hand into slight extension and ulnar deviation while applying pressure to the palmar aspect of the distal pole of the scaphoid and then, slowly, flexing and radially deviating the wrist. A positive test is indicated by asymmetric pain, a clunk, or sudden shift in scaphoid position as it moves over the dorsal rim of the radius [4].

Radiographic evaluation is essential for diagnosing SLAC wrist and determining the extent of joint degeneration. Imaging modalities commonly used include X-rays, computed tomography (CT) scans, and magnetic resonance imaging (MRI) [4]. Standard anteroposterior (AP) and lateral views of the wrist can help visualize arthritic changes [4]. CT scans help identify subtle changes in joint alignment and the extent of joint degeneration, thus confirming diagnostic stage, but are not typically employed in our practice for diagnosis [4]. MRI is useful in early presentations to evaluate the scapholunate ligament and surrounding soft tissue structures and can help rule in or out other potential sources of wrist pain as well as better evaluate the status of the articular cartilage [4]. As alluded to above, advanced imaging is typically unnecessary as standard AP and lateral radiographs can be supplemented with the pencil grip X-ray, also known as the clenched fist or stress view, to thoroughly evaluate the SL ligament (Fig. 39.2) [10]. An SL interval greater than 2 mm is common in the setting of an SL ligament injury and may be the only radiographic change with early presentations [4, 10]. This widening can be better appreciated with bilateral wrist radiographs for comparison to the contralateral side.

The initial radiographic classification system for scapholunate advanced collapse was proposed by Watson and Ballet in 1984 and was based on the severity of degenerative changes observed on imaging [1]. It consisted of three stages and highlighted

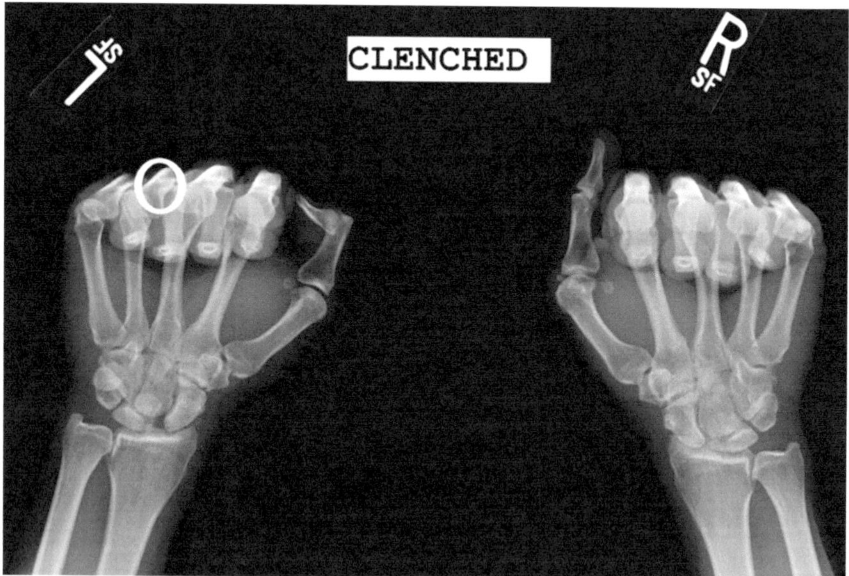

Fig. 39.2 "Pencil grip" or "clenched fist" view demonstrating significant left-sided scapholunate diastasis in our patient

progression from isolated radioscaphoid degeneration to complete capitolunate arthritis, capitate proximal advancement, and dorsal intercalated segment instability. More recently, a variation of this system which recognizes a fourth stage denoting pancarpal arthritis has gained in popularity [6]. Regardless, either system can be used to identify appropriate treatment strategies based on the extent of degenerative changes observed.

Stage 1: Radial Styloid Arthritis

In this stage, degenerative changes including joint space narrowing, osteophyte formation, and sclerosis are limited to the radial styloid process and its articulation with the scaphoid. The disease is still localized and can potentially be managed with nonsurgical interventions or targeted surgical procedures such as radial styloidectomy with or without SL reconstruction and/or denervation.

Stage 2: Scaphoid Fossa Arthritis

With stage 2, the degenerative changes progress to the entire scaphoid fossa of the distal radius. In this stage, more extensive surgical procedures like scaphoid excision with midcarpal fusion or proximal row carpectomy are typically considered given the spared midcarpal joint. Patient age and level of demand as well as risk factors for nonunion are often cited factors in deciding between these two techniques.

Stage 3: Capitolunate Arthritis

This is the final designation of the original Watson classification. It signals degenerative changes that have progressed to involve the midcarpal joint. Surgical management with scaphoid excision and midcarpal fusion becomes a primary motion-preserving option at this stage though some authors advocate for PRC with capsular interposition.

Stage 4: Pancarpal Arthritis

This is an addition to the original classification and is seen as the final stage of scapholunate advanced collapse. It highlights degenerative changes that have progressed to involve both the radiocarpal and midcarpal joints. The deep, recessed radiolunate joint is often the last area affected. Radiographic findings include diffuse joint space narrowing, sclerosis, and other associated arthritic changes throughout the wrist. At this stage, more aggressive surgical procedures, e.g., total wrist fusion or in rare cases wrist arthroplasty, may be required to alleviate pain and restore function.

Management Options

Management of SLAC wrist is dependent upon a multitude of patient and radiographic factors. Range of motion, severity of impairment, functional demands, and comorbidities that could heighten the risk of nonunion all play a role. Radiographically, the stage of disease, lunate morphology, status of LT ligament, ulnar translation of the lunate, and ulnar variance are taken into account. Treatment options are tailored based on these findings and can be broadly categorized into nonsurgical and surgical interventions.

For mild cases of SLAC, wrist conservative treatments include immobilization, avoidance of axial wrist loading, nonsteroidal anti-inflammatory drugs (NSAIDs), and corticosteroid injections [6]. These interventions aim to reduce pain and inflammation, allowing patients to maintain wrist function for as long as possible. Surgical management for SLAC wrist aims to alleviate pain and restore function to the wrist joint with selected interventions based on the patient and radiographic factors listed above.

Surgical intervention in early presentations, i.e., stage 1, may include radial styloidectomy, scaphoid stabilization procedures, and/or denervation [6]. Early surgical intervention can help thwart disease progression, but unfortunately, SLAC wrist typically presents in the later stages, leaving proximal row carpectomy (PRC), midcarpal fusion, or wrist fusion as the primary surgical option. PRC involves the removal of the proximal row of carpal bones (the scaphoid, lunate, and triquetrum) while preserving the remaining carpal bones to allow for continued wrist motion [11]. PRC or midcarpal fusion is, classically, indicated for stage 2 SLAC wrist with midcarpal fusion being the preferred treatment once progression to stage 3 is noted [6]. PRC is often favored for stage 2 SLAC wrist in older patients, lower demand patients, and patients at risk for nonunion. It is also considered in cases of ulnar translocation of the lunate or combined ulnar impaction. PRC with capsular interposition may also be an option for select patients in stage 3 [12]. Overall, favorable data exists for PRC with durable clinical outcomes in the appropriate patient population [11, 13, 14].

Midcarpal fusion is another approach with good clinical outcomes. It is a catch-all term for several differing wrist arthrodesis techniques that aim to alleviate pain from intercarpal arthritis. When referring to these individually, they are named based on the joints selected for fusion and include isolated capitolunate (CL) fusion, two-column fusion (capitolunate plus triquetrohamate), three-corner fusion (capitolunate and lunohamate), and four-corner fusion (lunate, capitate, hamate, and triquetrum) [15]. Scaphoid excision is combined with all techniques, and some clinicians also advocate for additional triquetral excision when performing CL fusion. While no one method has been proven superior, we consider isolated CL fusion as our procedure of choice due to its excellent outcomes and reproducible simplicity. One exception is in patients with a type II lunate, especially those associated with proximal hamate arthritis. In these cases, we utilize either a three-corner fusion or an isolated CL fusion paired with ostectomy of the proximal hamate depending on the size of the hamate facet of the lunate. Lastly, if LT instability is noted intraoperatively, we convert to either a two-column or a four-corner fusion.

Stage 4 SLAC wrist typically necessitates total wrist fusion or, rarely, wrist arthroplasty to alleviate pain. We also consider total fusion, regardless of stage, for patients with severely limited range of motion, or those who have already failed operative management. Any patient with a total wrist arc of motion less than $20°$, in our clinic, is a candidate for total fusion. Wrist fusion is accomplished surgically through fusing the articulations of the radiocarpal and midcarpal joints. This results in a stable, pain-free wrist joint, albeit one that lacks any motion [6]. While total wrist fusion can provide significant pain relief, the elimination of flexion-extension and radial-ulnar deviation carries the expected negative impact on hand and upper extremity function [16].

Management Chosen for This Case

Our patient presented in his fifth decade with stage 3 SLAC wrist after failed conservative management with imaging that demonstrated capitolunate arthritis, a type I lunate without ulnar translation, neutral ulnar variance, a preserved radiolunate joint, and no LT instability noted on exam or seen on radiographs. He was a non-smoker without diabetes who was healthy and active. Based on these factors and after a joint discussion with the patient, we elected to proceed with scaphoid excision and midcarpal fusion via capitolunate arthrodesis. Capitolunate fusion has gained renewed interest as an effective treatment of SLAC in recent years given improved surgical implants after initial reports suggested low union rates [17]. Early studies using K-wires demonstrated unacceptably high rates of nonunion. However, more recent studies using cannulated, headless compression screws and staples show union rates similar to four-corner fusion [15, 17–20].

We prefer isolated CL fusion, when indicated, as it provides multiple benefits when compared to four-corner fusion. It has shown to decrease OR time, implant cost, and the need for bone graft. Also, arthritis is very rarely present in the CH, TH, and LT joints, so fusion of these joints is more surgery than is needed in many patients. Lastly, CL fusion allows a more predictable restoration of triquetrohamate (TH) alignment, which impacts pisotriquetral mechanics, decreasing the subsequent risk of delayed PT arthritis [21, 22]. When doing an isolated CL fusion, the TH joint "auto-reduces" when compression across the CL is applied and thus optimizes PT mechanics. In contrast, when the TH joint is fused, we have not found any good clinical or radiographic method of ensuring proper alignment and suspect that this contributes to a high number of patients developing late PT arthritis [21]. In a multicenter prospective comparative cohort study, Duraku et al. found that capitolunate fusion had similar patient-reported outcomes and improved range of motion when compared to four-corner fusion, particularly in flexion and radial deviation [20, 23]. This is in line with other emerging literature on the technique, which has demonstrated positive clinical outcomes, improved range of motion, high union rates, and strong potential for long-term success [24, 25]. In terms of implant selection, we favor nitinol staple fixation for their simplicity, strength, high union rates, and preservation of surrounding joint surfaces [26]. In contrast, anterograde screws violate the only remaining joint surface, and both antegrade and retrograde screws have demonstrated back-out in up to 1/3 of cases [22, 27]. Plates and K-wires have had unacceptably high nonunion rates historically, and, although newer plates have reported improved fusion rates, these cannot be used for isolated CL fusions. Nitinol staples avoid these complications and allow for constant compression across the fusion site resulting in excellent outcomes. Our technique for scaphoid excision with capitolunate fusion is typically as follows.

Approach

- The patient is prepped and draped in supine position with the operative limb on a radiolucent arm board. A nonsterile tourniquet is placed at the proximal humerus.
- A 4 cm longitudinal incision is made over the dorsal aspect of wrist (Fig. 39.3). The EPL tendon is identified and protected proximally or, alternatively, if more exposure is needed, it can be transposed out of the third extensor compartment.
- The interval between the second and fourth extensor compartments is utilized distally.
- A fiber splitting T-shaped capsulotomy is made over the capitate, lunate, and scaphoid to allow for carpal exposure.

Scaphoidectomy

- The scaphoid is freed from its surrounding soft tissue attachments and excised and subsequently morselized for autograft (Fig. 39.3). This can be one of the more challenging steps of the procedure. A curved curette or McGlamry elevator placed distally into the STT interval to lever the distal pole of the scaphoid can assist with this step. Any retained, surrounding osteophytes or inflamed synovium is subsequently removed. We rarely perform a radial styloidectomy as the radial styloid is typically dorsal to the trapezium allowing the two to avoid impingement.

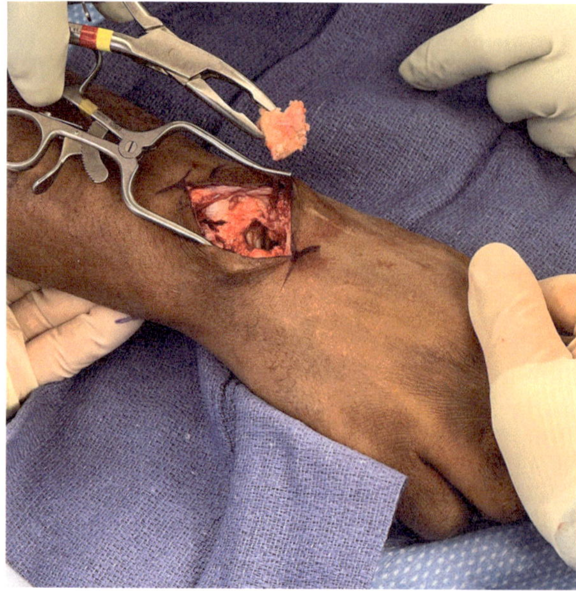

Fig. 39.3 The dorsal approach to the wrist highlighting scaphoid excision

Capitolunate Fusion

- Wrist flexion, K-wire in the lunate, and a Freer elevator in the midcarpal joint can aid in visualizing the capitolunate joint (Fig. 39.4). The joint is prepped for fusion by removing the articular cartilage of the midcarpal aspect of the capitate and lunate back to healthy/bleeding cancellous bone. We prefer a rongeur for the convex capitate head and a combination of curved osteotomes, curettes, and rongeur for the more difficult concave lunate.
- For isolated CL fusions, typically the scaphoid is a sufficient source of autograft. If additional graft is needed, Lister's tubercle is then removed allowing access to the metaphyseal distal radius for harvest of cancellous autograft.
- This cancellous graft is packed into the newly prepped space between the capitate and lunate to assist with fusion.
- The DISI deformity is reduced with palmar pressure on the head of the capitate with a bump proximal at the level of the wrist. Radial translation of the capitate helps to align the reduction in the coronal plane. If difficulty is encountered, hyperflexing the carpus and placing a K-wire longitudinally across the radiolunate joint will typically hold proper alignment of the radiolunate joint temporarily. The wrist is then extended (through the midcarpal joint), which reduces the collinear relationship of the capitate and lunate. The CL interval is then pinned (Fig. 39.5).
- Once proper capitolunate alignment has been confirmed fluoroscopically and bone graft placed, two nitinol staples are used to provide definitive fixation. Because the size of the bones is limited, proper staple placement is critical. We

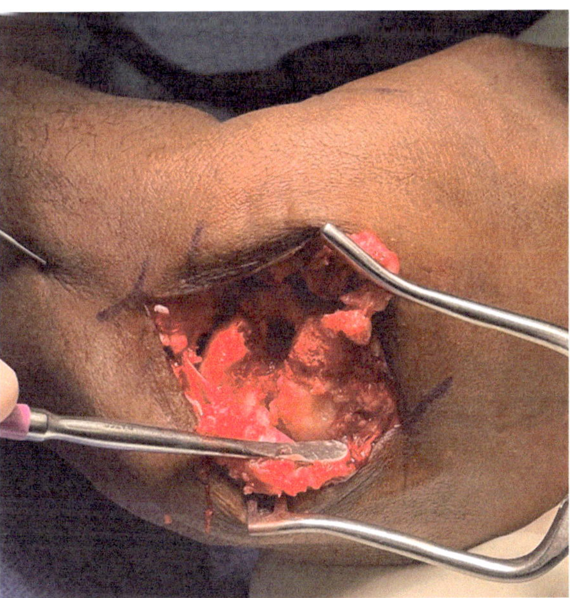

Fig. 39.4 Prepping the capitolunate joint with a K-wire placed into the lunate for fixation and assisted by a Freer elevator

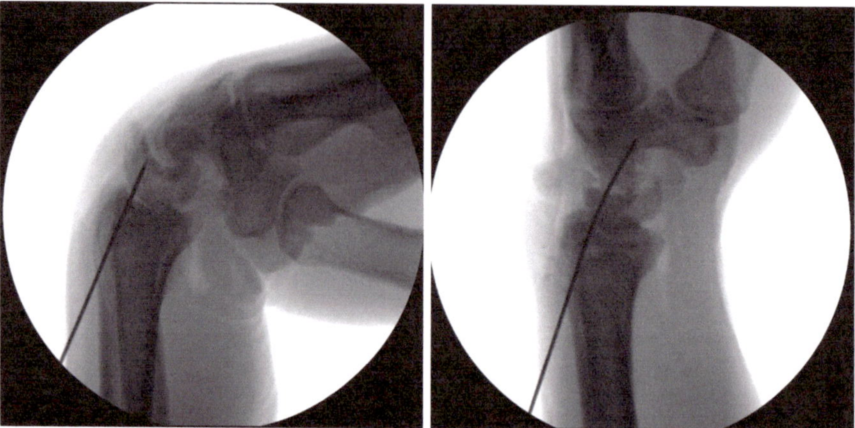

Fig. 39.5 Reducing the DISI deformity and pinning the capitolunate joint on fluoroscopic imaging

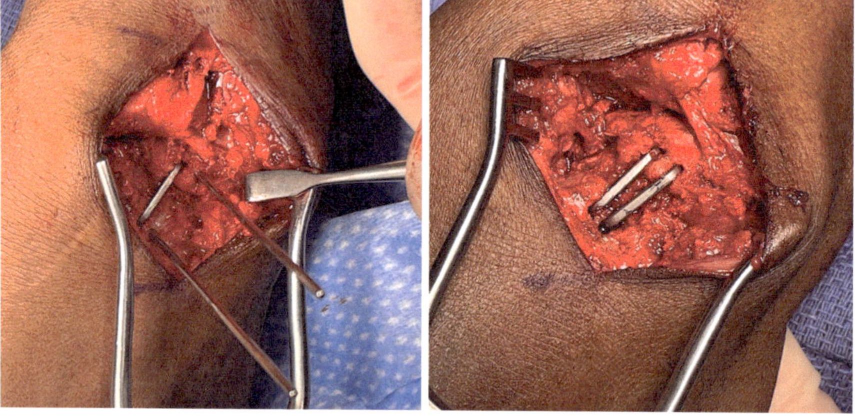

Fig. 39.6 Staple fixation following K-wire placement to ensure sufficient space and positioning

prefer to place temporary K-wires (or cannulated staple drill options with some systems) to ensure that sufficient space will exist for two staples and to enable better precision with implant placement (Fig. 39.6). Biomechanical studies show that nitinol staples can provide bicortical fixation without traversing both cortices as they provide compression 2 mm beyond the ends of the staple legs. So, our goal is to place the legs within 2 mm of the far cortices. Furthermore, all staples should be recessed or "troughed" as this prevents dorsal impingement and does not adversely affect their biomechanical performance [26].

- At this point, final fluoroscopic images are taken utilizing orthogonal views to confirm appropriate staple length and position, and a layered closure is performed (Fig. 39.7). Passive wrist extension allows direct visualization to ensure that there is no dorsal impingement of the staples on the dorsal rim of the radius.

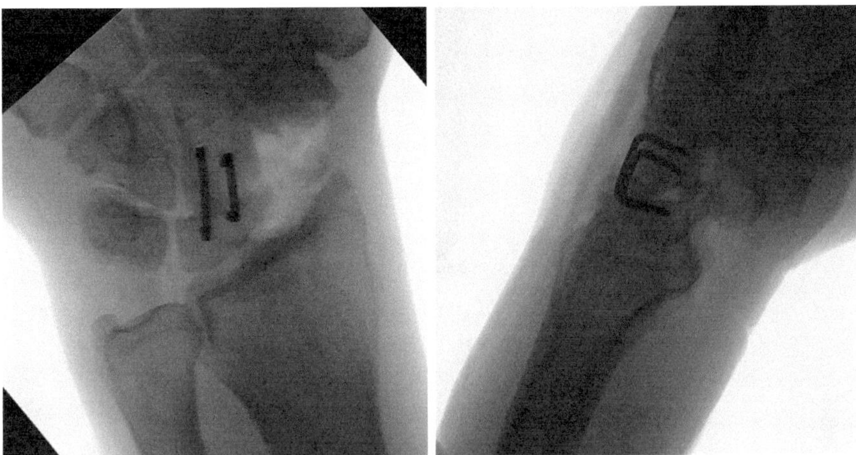

Fig. 39.7 AP and lateral fluoroscopic imaging confirming correct staple length and alignment

- The patient is then placed in a short arm splint for 2 weeks followed by an additional 2–4 weeks in a short arm cast. At 6 weeks post-op, we routinely perform a CT to ensure full osseous union before beginning full active and passive motion as well as strengthening.

Clinical Course and Outcome

Our patient returned for his first postoperative clinic visit at the 2-week mark for splint removal and wound check. At that time, he reported minimal pain and no fevers or chills. Imaging demonstrated correct hardware position (Fig. 39.8). He was placed in a short arm cast for an additional 2 weeks to protect the fusion. We discussed starting gentle digital range of motion to guard against finger stiffness at this time.

He was seen again at 4 weeks post-op for cast removal. Radiographs exhibited no signs of hardware loosening, migration, or failure (Fig. 39.9). At this point, active wrist motion was 15° extension, 25° flexion, 90° pronation, and 90° supination. He was fitted for a Velcro wrist brace to wear at all times except during showers. He was instructed to continue his daily finger motion exercises. A follow-up appointment was scheduled for 2–3 weeks with a CT scan beforehand to evaluate fusion. We released him for return to light duty at work so long as he was compliant with the wrist brace.

He returned to the office at 7 weeks post-op. At this time, CT scan showed excellent osseous union of the prior capitolunate joint (Fig. 39.10). His baseline pain was minimal, scoring a 2 on the VAS; he had returned to work, was back running again, and overall was extremely pleased with his outcome. His range of motion had

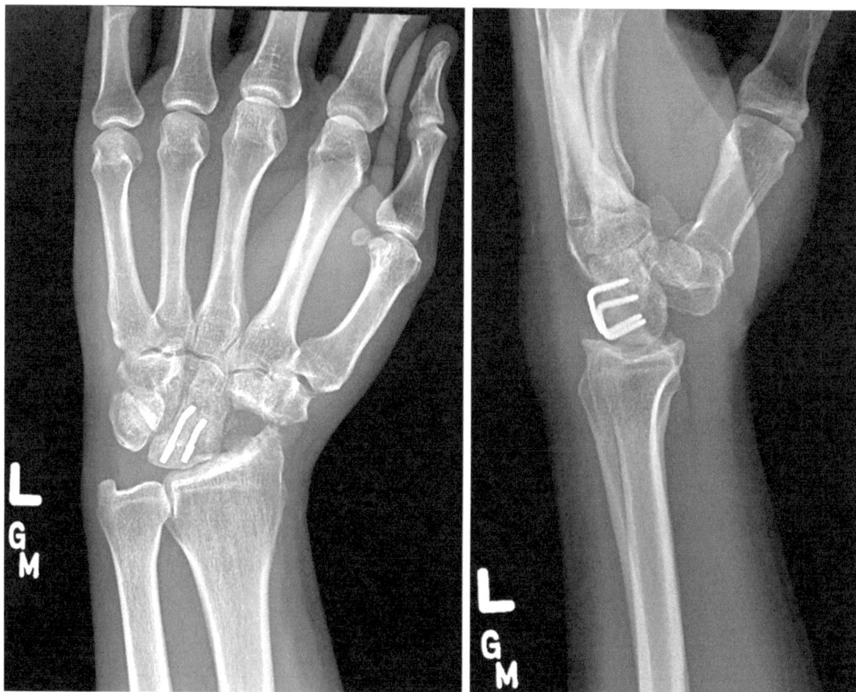

Fig. 39.8 AP and lateral radiographs at 2 weeks post-op highlighting maintained hardware position

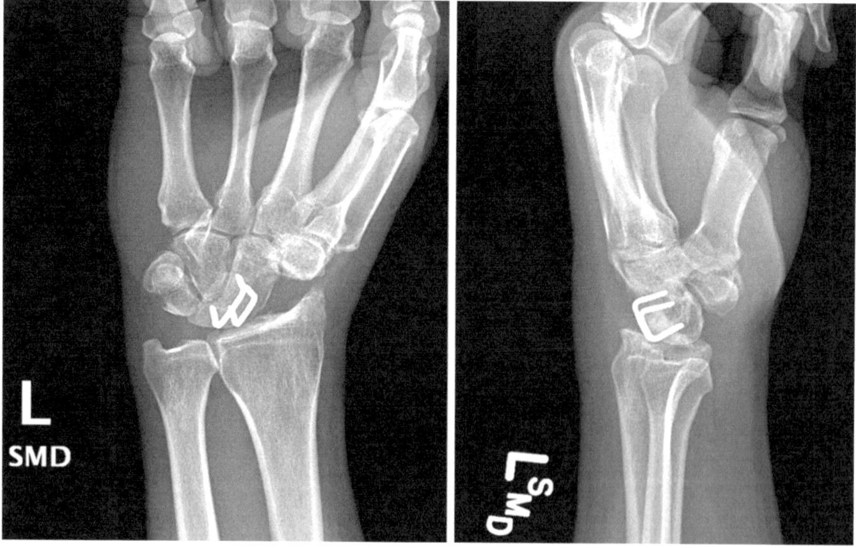

Fig. 39.9 AP and lateral radiographs at 4 weeks post-op again showing maintained alignment with no signs of hardware loosening, migration, or failure

Fig. 39.10 Selected coronal and sagittal cuts of the CT scan performed at 7 weeks post-op demonstrating full osseus union of the capitolunate joint

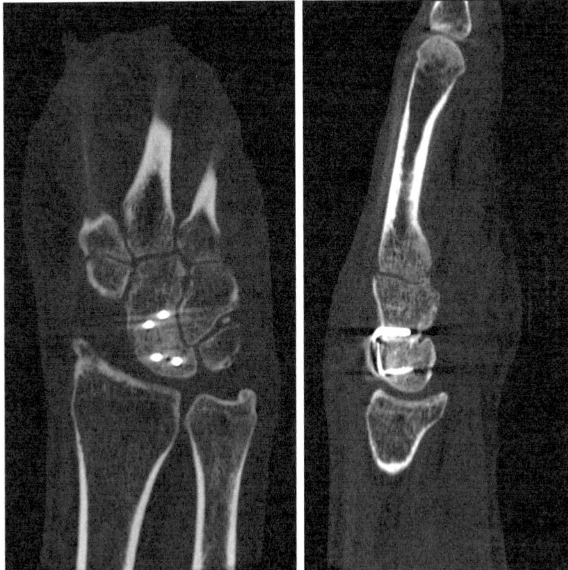

improved to a 50-degree total arc of motion in the flexion-extension plane. At this point, we allowed him to come out of the wrist brace and begin strengthening exercises while continuing his daily range-of-motion regimen. We saw him one last time at 4 months post-op and noted continued pain relief, preserved range of motion, and grip strength that had improved to 87% of the contralateral side.

Overall, this patient did well in the postoperative period and is a good example of our standard treatment protocol following capitolunate fusion. We place the vast majority of our patients in a splint for 2 weeks and cast for 2–4 weeks, and then transition to a soft wrist brace for a final 2 weeks of immobilization. We routinely get a CT scan between 6 and 8 weeks to ensure union before beginning full range-of-motion and strengthening exercises. We expect patients to achieve approximately two-thirds of their pre-op range of motion and grip strength of around 85% of the contralateral side. The goal is to preserve as much pain-free wrist motion as possible, and we follow this with the VAS. Most of our patients score between a 1 and 2 on this scale at 6–8 weeks. All in all, capitolunate fusion has proven to be a reproducible surgical technique with dependable, positive results in our patient population.

Bulleted Clinical Pearls/Pitfalls

The following are clinical pearls gathered over the years from both our successes and failures. It is our hope that these might help surgeons avoid some of our early pitfalls and, in turn, will contribute to the best possible outcomes:

- First, correct any existing carpal malalignment. Ensure that the lunate and capitate are collinear, and pay special attention to restoring the "scaphoid shadow" on AP radiographs (Fig. 39.11). In cases of SL diastasis, the capitate tends to shift relative to the lunate. By realigning the capitate to its natural position with respect to the lunate, the anatomic outline of the excised scaphoid, or its "shadow," can be restored.
- Second, recognize and address the type II lunate. Be especially mindful if performing CL fusion and dealing with proximal hamate arthritis. In these patients, we perform a proximal hamate ostectomy or, depending on the size of the hamate facet, convert to a three-corner fusion (Fig. 39.12). In patients with LT instability (either clinically or if an LT step-off is seen radiographically), consider either a four-corner or a two-column fusion as an alternative to CL fusion as this can be a source of ongoing post-op ulnar sided wrist pain.
- When using nitinol staples, take the time to trough them appropriately. This helps to avoid dorsal impingement without compromising fixation strength (Fig. 39.13).
- Lastly, consider alternative procedures such as PRC for stage 2 SLAC wrist in lower demand patients or those with a high risk of nonunion.

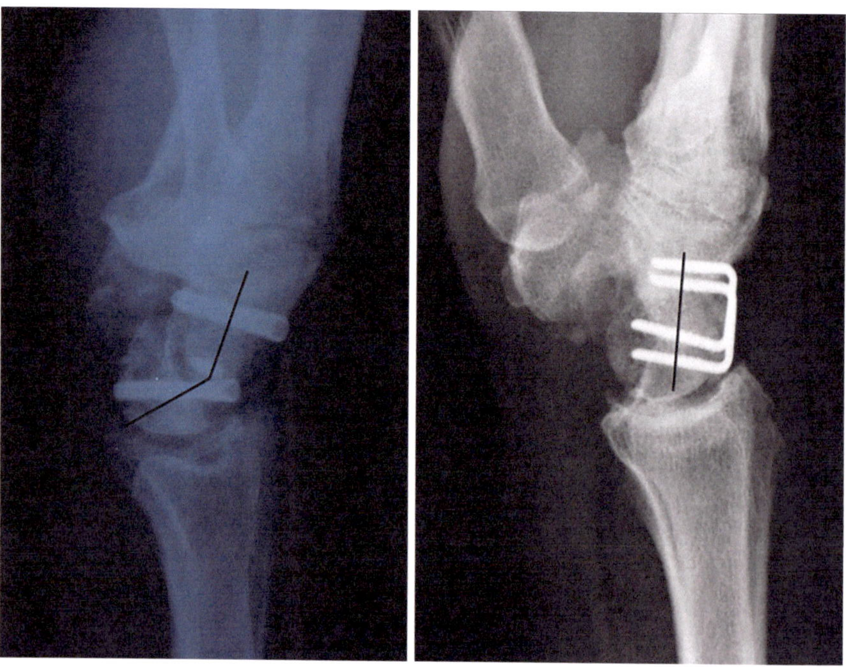

Fig. 39.11 Two laterals of the wrist demonstrating attempts at DISI correction. The left image shows suboptimal alignment using headless compression screws with the lunate off axis as compared to the capitate. In comparison, the image on the right displays an accurate anatomical DISI correction using nitinol staple fixation with the lunate collinear to the capitate

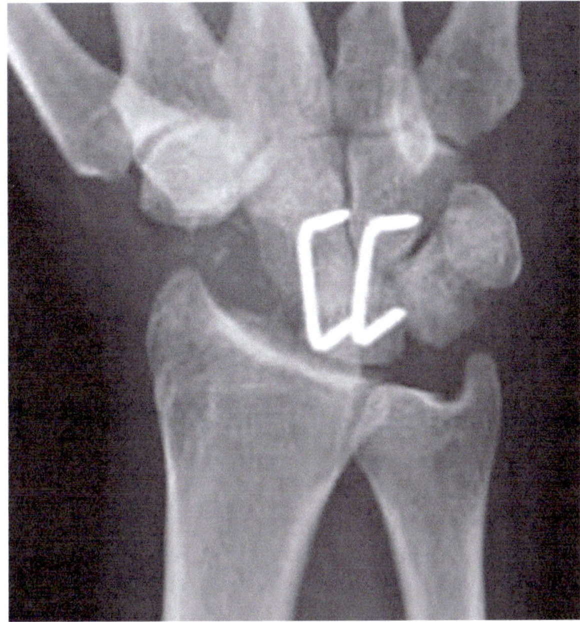

Fig. 39.12 Three-corner fusion with nitinol staples in a patient with SLAC and a type II lunate

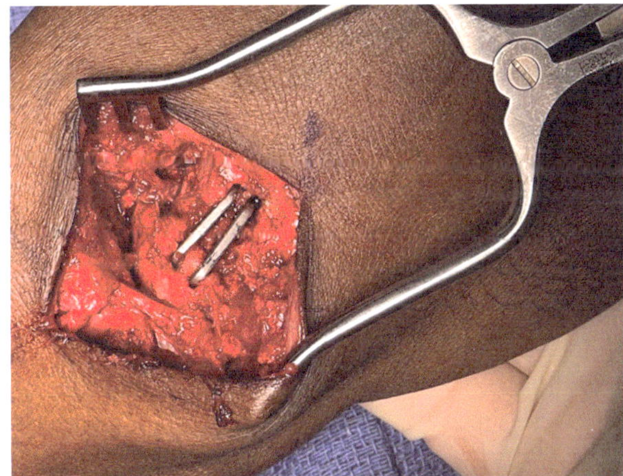

Fig. 39.13 Properly seated nitinol staples after troughing, decreasing the chance of dorsal impingement without compromising fixation strength

Literature Review and Discussion

Scapholunate advanced collapse (SLAC) is a common degenerative pattern of wrist arthritis resulting from injury to the scapholunate ligament and subsequent alterations in wrist biomechanics [1, 2, 4]. Patients often present in their fifth and sixth decades with wrist pain, decreased range of motion, and weakness or reduced grip strength [8]. Surgical intervention is the backbone of management with several different midcarpal fusion techniques being employed. The most popular of these, scaphoid excision paired with four-corner fusion, has produced good clinical results for almost three decades [28, 29]. Recently, however, capitolunate (CL) fusion has emerged as an alternative offering potential benefits over the traditional approach [22]. This literature review aims to compare the outcomes of four-corner and CL fusion in the management of SLAC wrist arthritis.

Midcarpal fusion via scaphoid excision and four-corner fusion has been widely adopted in treating wrist arthritis due to SLAC. Several studies have reported favorable outcomes, such as pain relief, functional improvement, and preserved wrist motion [30, 31]. However, as with any intervention, this technique has its limitations including potential nonunion or malunion, further surgery, and limitations in postoperative wrist range of motion, which can have a significant impact on hand and upper extremity performance [16, 30–32].

Over the years, several different techniques have arisen to achieve four-corner fusion. A systematic review by Hayes et al. analyzed many of these osteosynthesis methods including K-wires, screws, plates, and staples and concluded that the procedure resulted in significant improvement in wrist pain and function with minimal differences based on the type of the fixation used, with high union rates and low incidence of complication [32]. Dacho et al. showed that these benefits are maintained in the midterm with patients reporting significant pain relief, functional improvement, and high fusion rates upon 4-year follow-up [33].

Scaphoid excision with capitolunate fusion has emerged as a potentially faster, less invasive, and less expensive alternative to four-corner fusion. Capitolunate fusion strives to achieve the same functional outcomes of four-corner fusion with only an arthrodesis of the capitolunate joint, a less invasive strategy [20]. Early attempts to implement this technique date back to the 1990s using K-wires but were initially abandoned due to low union rates [18]. With advancements in fixation techniques, specifically using cannulated headless compression screws and nitinol staples, union rates have improved leading to a resurgence of interest in CL fusion. With this, several recent studies have shown that outcomes of CL fusion are equivalent to those of four-corner fusion [20]. The technique affords satisfactory pain relief, maintained wrist stability, and preserved range of motion [17, 20, 25]. A multicenter comparative study published last year by Duraku et al. found no significant differences in pain, function, or complications between CL and four-corner fusion techniques [20]. This study also highlighted the added benefits of increased range of motion and overall technical simplicity as compared to four-corner fusion, a hypothesis noted by Gaston et al. 10 years prior [22]. These advantages make CL fusion an attractive option especially considering the reduced need for bone graft, potential for decreased costs by utilizing fewer implants, reduced OR time, and potential for improved TH alignment, thus possibly decreasing the risk of late PT arthritis. Although capitolunate fusion has shown favorable results, further long-term studies are needed to better understand its durability and comparative effectiveness [15].

In conclusion, while midcarpal fusion with scaphoid excision and four-corner arthrodesis has been the traditional approach to treating SLAC wrist arthritis, capitolunate fusion offers a promising alternative, yet specific patient factors and radiographic factors should be considered when selecting a treatment method. With improved union rates and potential benefits such as increased ROM and decreased operative times, CL fusion may see increased adoption in the future, particularly for patients with type I lunates and stable LT joints. Despite the favorable outcomes of both techniques, careful patient selection, optimal timing of surgical intervention, adherence to appropriate surgical techniques, and postoperative protocols are critical to achieving favorable outcomes.

Further Reading

1. SLAC and SNAC Wrist: The Top Five Things That General Radiologists Need to Know [4].
2. Treatment of scapholunate ligament injury: Current concepts [2].
3. Decision making for partial carpal fusions [6].
4. Intercarpal arthrodesis: A systematic review [15].
5. Capitolunate Arthrodesis: A Systematic Review [25].
6. Two-Corner Fusion or Four-Corner Fusion of the Wrist for Midcarpal Osteoarthritis? A Multicenter Prospective Comparative Cohort Study [20].
7. Biomechanical Properties of Nitinol Staples: Effects of Troughing, Effective Leg Length, and 2-Staple Constructs [26].

This reading list offers a comprehensive guide to understanding SLAC wrist and its surgical treatment via midcarpal fusion. The first few papers cover key imaging features, decision-making processes, and management strategies behind the various midcarpal fusion techniques. The next few focus on capitolunate arthrodesis, its performance in different clinical scenarios, and its comparison to other popular fusion methods. The list concludes with a focus on the biomechanical properties of nitinol staples and our preferred fixation device for capitolunate fusion and outlines the proper technique for their use.

References

1. Watson HK, Ballet FL. The SLAC wrist: scapholunate advanced collapse pattern of degenerative arthritis. J Hand Surg Am. 1984;9(3):358–65. https://doi.org/10.1016/s0363-5023(84)80223-3.
2. Andersson JK. Treatment of scapholunate ligament injury: current concepts. EFORT Open Rev. 2017;2(9):382–93. https://doi.org/10.1302/2058-5241.2.170016.
3. Ahmadi AR, Duraku LS, van der Oest MJW, Hundepool CA, Selles RW, Zuidam JM. The never-ending battle between proximal row carpectomy and four corner arthrodesis: a systematic review and meta-analysis for the final verdict. J Plast Reconstr Aesthet Surg. 2022;75(2):711–21. https://doi.org/10.1016/j.bjps.2021.09.076.
4. Kompoliti E, Prodromou M, Karantanas AH. SLAC and SNAC wrist: the top five things that general radiologists need to know. Tomography. 2021;7(4):488–503. https://doi.org/10.3390/tomography7040042.
5. Viegas SF, Wagner K, Patterson R, Peterson P. Medial (hamate) facet of the lunate. J Hand Surg Am. 1990;15(4):564–71. https://doi.org/10.1016/s0363-5023(09)90016-8.
6. Bain GI, McGuire DT. Decision making for partial carpal fusions. J Wrist Surg. 2012;1(2):103–14. https://doi.org/10.1055/s-0032-1329548.

7. Rhee PC, Moran SL, Shin AY. Association between lunate morphology and carpal collapse in cases of scapholunate dissociation. J Hand Surg Am. 2009;34(9):1633–9. https://doi.org/10.1016/j.jhsa.2009.06.017.

8. Murphy BD, Nagarajan M, Novak CB, Roy M, McCabe SJ. The epidemiology of scapholunate advanced collapse. Hand (N Y). 2020;15(1):23–6. https://doi.org/10.1177/1558944718788672.

9. Laulan J, Marteau E, Bacle G. Wrist osteoarthritis. Orthop Traumatol Surg Res. 2015;101(Suppl. 1):S1–9. https://doi.org/10.1016/j.otsr.2014.06.025.

10. Lawand A, Foulkes GD. The "clenched pencil" view: a modified clenched fist scapholunate stress view. J Hand Surg Am. 2003;28(3):414–8.; discussion 9–20. https://doi.org/10.1053/jhsu.2003.50046.

11. Imbriglia JE, Broudy AS, Hagberg WC, McKernan D. Proximal row carpectomy: clinical evaluation. J Hand Surg Am. 1990;15(3):426–30. https://doi.org/10.1016/0363-5023(90)90054-u.

12. Gaspar MP, Pham PP, Pankiw CD, Jacoby SM, Shin EK, Osterman AL, et al. Mid-term outcomes of routine proximal row carpectomy compared with proximal row carpectomy with dorsal capsular interposition arthroplasty for the treatment of late-stage arthropathy of the wrist. Bone Joint J. 2018;100-B(2):197–204. https://doi.org/10.1302/0301-620X.100B2.BJJ-2017-0816.R2.

13. Jebson PJ, Hayes EP, Engber WD. Proximal row carpectomy: a minimum 10-year follow-up study. J Hand Surg Am. 2003;28(4):561–9. https://doi.org/10.1016/s0363-5023(03)00248-x.

14. Wall LB, Didonna ML, Kiefhaber TR, Stern PJ. Proximal row carpectomy: minimum 20-year follow-up. J Hand Surg Am. 2013;38(8):1498–504. https://doi.org/10.1016/j.jhsa.2013.04.028.

15. Athlani L, Cholley-Roulleau M, Blum A, Teixeira PAG, Dap F. Intercarpal arthrodesis: a systematic review. Hand Surg Rehabil. 2023;42(2):93–102. https://doi.org/10.1016/j.hansur.2022.12.006.

16. Adams BD, Grosland NM, Murphy DM, McCullough M. Impact of impaired wrist motion on hand and upper-extremity performance (1). J Hand Surg Am. 2003;28(6):898–903. https://doi.org/10.1016/s0363-5023(03)00424-6.

17. Hegazy G. Capitolunate arthrodesis for treatment of Scaphoid nonunion advanced collapse (SNAC) wrist arthritis. J Hand Microsurg. 2015;7(1):79–86. https://doi.org/10.1007/s12593-015-0182-6.

18. Kirschenbaum D, Schneider LH, Kirkpatrick WH, Adams DC, Cody RP. Scaphoid excision and capitolunate arthrodesis for radioscaphoid arthritis. J Hand Surg Am. 1993;18(5):780–5. https://doi.org/10.1016/0363-5023(93)90042-2.

19. Goubier JN, Teboul F. Capitolunate arthrodesis with compression screws. Tech Hand Up Extrem Surg. 2007;11(1):24–8. https://doi.org/10.1097/bth.0b013e31802caa87.

20. Duraku LS, Hundepool CA, Hoogendam L, Selles RW, van der Heijden B, Colaris JW, et al. Two-corner fusion or four-corner fusion of the wrist for midcarpal osteoarthritis? A multicenter prospective comparative cohort study. Plast Reconstr Surg. 2022;149(6):1130e–9e. https://doi.org/10.1097/PRS.0000000000009116.

21. Gaston RG, Lourie GM, Floyd WE 3rd, Swick M. Pisotriquetral dysfunction following limited and total wrist arthrodesis. J Hand Surg Am. 2007;32(9):1348–55. https://doi.org/10.1016/j.jhsa.2007.07.014.

22. Gaston RG, Greenberg JA, Baltera RM, Mih A, Hastings H. Clinical outcomes of scaphoid and triquetral excision with capitolunate arthrodesis versus scaphoid excision and four-corner arthrodesis. J Hand Surg Am. 2009;34(8):1407–12. https://doi.org/10.1016/j.jhsa.2009.05.018.

23. Got C, Vopat BG, Mansuripur PK, Kane PM, Weiss AP, Crisco JJ. The effects of partial carpal fusions on wrist range of motion. J Hand Surg Eur Vol. 2016;41(5):479–83. https://doi.org/10.1177/1753193415607827.

24. Delclaux S, Rongieres M, Apredoaei C, Bonnevialle N, Bonnevialle P, Mansat P. Capitolunate arthrodesis: 12 patients followed-up an average of 10 years. Chir Main. 2013;32(5):310–6. https://doi.org/10.1016/j.main.2013.07.002.

25. Dunn JC, Polmear MM, Scanaliato JP, Orr JD, Nesti LJ. Capitolunate arthrodesis: a systematic review. J Hand Surg Am. 2020;45(4):365:e1–e10. https://doi.org/10.1016/j.jhsa.2019.10.007.

26. McKnight RR, Lee SK, Gaston RG. Biomechanical properties of nitinol staples: effects of troughing, effective leg length, and 2-staple constructs. J Hand Surg Am. 2019;44(6):520:e1–9. https://doi.org/10.1016/j.jhsa.2018.08.017.
27. Shifflett GD, Athanasian EA, Lee SK, Weiland AJ, Wolfe SW. Proximal migration of hardware in patients undergoing midcarpal fusion with headless compression screws. J Wrist Surg. 2014;3(4):250–61. https://doi.org/10.1055/s-0034-1384750.
28. Krakauer JD, Bishop AT, Cooney WP. Surgical treatment of scapholunate advanced collapse. J Hand Surg Am. 1994;19(5):751–9. https://doi.org/10.1016/0363-5023(94)90178-3.
29. Wyrick JD, Stern PJ, Kiefhaber TR. Motion-preserving procedures in the treatment of scapholunate advanced collapse wrist: proximal row carpectomy versus four-corner arthrodesis. J Hand Surg Am. 1995;20(6):965–70. https://doi.org/10.1016/S0363-5023(05)80144-3.
30. Trail IA, Murali R, Stanley JK, Hayton MJ, Talwalkar S, Sreekumar R, et al. The long-term outcome of four-corner fusion. J Wrist Surg. 2015;4(2):128–33. https://doi.org/10.1055/s-0035-1549277.
31. Mavrogenis AF, Flevas DA, Raptis K, Megaloikonomos PD, Igoumenou VG, Antoniadou T, et al. Four-corner fusion of the wrist: clinical and radiographic outcome of 31 patients. Eur J Orthop Surg Traumatol. 2016;26(8):859–66. https://doi.org/10.1007/s00590-016-1824-5.
32. Hayes E, Cheng Y, Sauder D, Sims L. Four-corner arthrodesis with differing methods of osteosynthesis: a systematic review. J Hand Surg Am. 2022;47(5):477. e1-e9. https://doi.org/10.1016/j.jhsa.2021.06.002.
33. Dacho A, Grundel J, Holle G, Germann G, Sauerbier M. Long-term results of midcarpal arthrodesis in the treatment of scaphoid nonunion advanced collapse (SNAC-Wrist) and scapholunate advanced collapse (SLAC-Wrist). Ann Plast Surg. 2006;56(2):139–44. https://doi.org/10.1097/01.sap.0000194245.94684.54.

Chapter 40
Midcarpal Total Wrist Arthroplasty

William Runge, Parker Johnsen, and Scott Wolfe

Case Presentation

This patient is a 76-year-old right-hand-dominant male who is a former high-level tennis player and until recently played tennis almost every day. He has a history of a right proximal row carpectomy about 20 years ago, performed for SLAC arthritis at an outside center. That procedure gave him several years of excellent pain relief, but he has been sidelined over the last few years with escalating right wrist pain due to radiocapitate erosive arthritis. His priorities are eliminating his resting pain and, if possible, to play tennis and golf again.

Diagnosis

Physical Assessment/Relevant Maneuvers

There is no appreciable wrist deformity, and his forearm rotation is painless through a stable and well-aligned distal radioulnar joint (DRUJ). There is no effusion or synovitis of the wrist or DRUJ. Range of motion and grip and pinch strength are documented in Table 40.1.

W. Runge (✉) · S. Wolfe
Hospital for Special Surgery, New York, NY, USA
e-mail: wolfes@hss.edu

P. Johnsen
Cooper University, Camden, NJ, USA

J. Yao (ed.), *Carpal Instability*, https://doi.org/10.1007/978-3-031-55869-6_40

Table 40.1 Preoperative range of motion

	Flexion	Extension	RD	UD	Pronation	Supination	Fist	Grip (lb)	Pinch (lb)
Right	30	20	0	25	80	80	0	30	14
Left	70	70	10	50	80	80	0	65	14

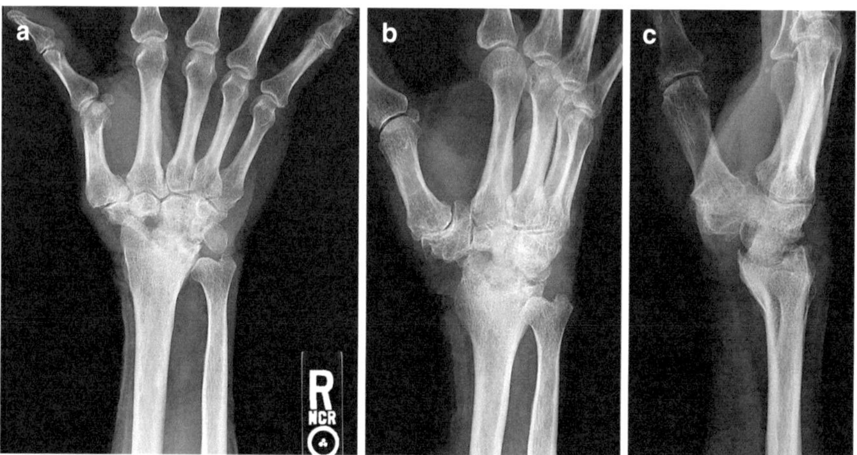

Fig. 40.1 (a–c) Preoperative radiographs of the operative wrist

Diagnostic Studies

Preoperative radiographs, shown in Figs. 40.1, 40.2 and 40.3, show the sequelae of proximal row carpectomy but also demonstrate bone-on-bone arthritis between the distal carpal row and the lunate facet of the distal radius. He also has mild-moderate basal joint arthritis, which is currently asymptomatic.

A preoperative CT of the wrist was performed to assess bone stock and for preoperative templating of the implants to be used. This revealed the expected sequelae of proximal row carpectomy with subsequent end-stage degenerative changes between the distal carpal row and radius. The CT scan also revealed deep erosion of the capitate into the radial articular surface. There were several degenerative subchondral cysts (<6 mm in diameter) on opposing sides of the radiocarpal joint, 4 mm of ulnar-negative variance, and adequate bone stock in the radius and carpus for implant arthroplasty. Representative images are shown in Fig. 40.2a–c.

The patient was sent for preoperative labs, as well as a metabolic bone workup (including CMP, PTH, vitamin D, alkaline phosphatase, procollagen I, and osteocalcin). His PTH was elevated to 74 pg/mL (normal: 14–64 pg/mL) with an elevated osteocalcin at 50 and normal procollagen I, so he was sent to a metabolic bone specialist. He was subsequently referred for a DXA test that demonstrated osteopenia, but his FRAX score met the threshold for the diagnosis of osteoporosis. He was prescribed teriparatide, in addition to calcium and vitamin D supplementation, which he started 4 months prior to surgery.

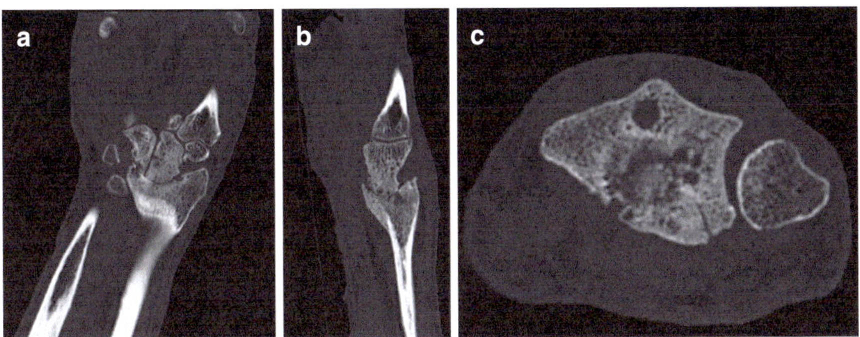

Fig. 40.2 (**a–c**) Representative (**a**) coronal, (**b**) sagittal, and (**c**) axial images from the preoperative CT scan

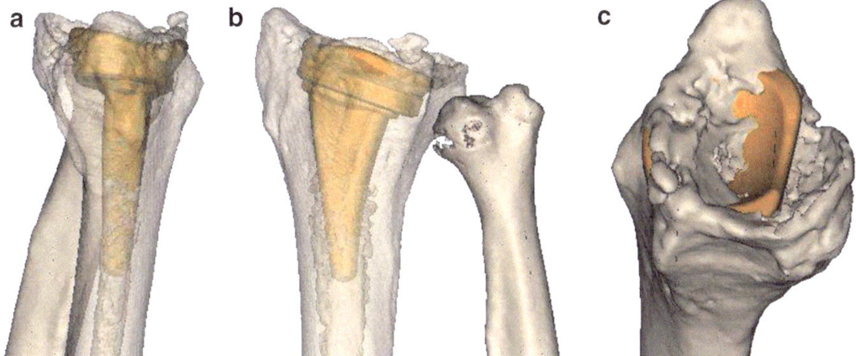

Fig. 40.3 (**a–c**) Insetting of the radial component

Management Options

Cortisone Injections

Steroid injections are always an option but are likely to be less effective in bone-on-bone disease with late-stage erosive changes. At best, a steroid injection would be expected to provide short-term relief.

Arthroscopic Debridement

Arthroscopic debridement, if even technically possible with the deep erosion of the capitate into the radius, is likely to offer little to no benefit

Denervation

Partial wrist denervation, by removal of the terminal branches of the posterior and anterior interosseous nerves, is a relatively low-risk surgery but was likely to provide minimal benefit, especially with regard to this patient's goals of more complete pain relief. A trial injection of these nerves with lidocaine would provide an estimate of the degree of pain relief.

Capsular or Allograft Interposition

Allograft interposition in the setting of proximal row carpectomy has been suggested as an intervention for patients with radiocapitellar arthritis after proximal row carpectomy, but the data for this is limited and it is likely not as durable a solution as a prosthetic implant.

Capitate Resurfacing

Capitate resurfacing could address the incongruity of the capitate and the lunate fossa following proximal row carpectomy and restore carpal height but would not address the radial sided degenerative changes such as this patient's eburnated lunate facet.

Arthrodesis

Arthrodesis is a reliable and definitive treatment option with predictable pain relief, but at the expense of motion and some functionality. This patient adamantly desired to maintain wrist motion in his dominant limb.

Total Wrist Arthroplasty

Total wrist arthroplasty has the potential to maintain or restore motion with predictable pain relief and would address the complete loss of joint surface on both sides of the joint.

Management Chosen for This Case with Rationale

After discussing the risks and benefits of total joint arthroplasty vs. total wrist arthrodesis, and the possibility of component loosening or revision, the patient elected to proceed with total wrist arthroplasty, given his desire to preserve wrist motion. He was informed that tennis or golf would place high stresses on the implant-bone interface and increase the likelihood of component loosening or revision. The senior author recommended the KinematX™ midcarpal total wrist arthroplasty (Extremity Medical, LLC, Parsippany, NJ).

Contraindications to this implant system include infection; physiologic or psychologic compromise; active wrist synovitis or severe carpal bone erosion; metal allergy; insufficient extensor tendons; inadequate skin, bone, or vascular status; severe carpal bone malalignment; displacement or absorption; metabolic or endocrinologic bone disorders; and rapid joint destruction.

Long-term patients may return to most of their normal activities including sports such as pickleball, ping-pong, swimming, and road cycling. They can swing a golf club lightly but are advised to avoid full-power swing and ground impacts. We advise that they refrain high-impact activities such as mountain biking or heavy lifting.

Preoperative 3D analysis identified the expected soft tissue tension given the prior proximal row carpectomy, and the radial component was templated to be recessed 4 mm into the radial metaphysis. Every effort would be made to preserve the ulnar head, sigmoid notch, and DRUJ. The remaining soft tissue deficit was calculated, and it was determined that a circumferential release of the soft tissue sleeve from the radius would be required to accommodate the prosthetic components. Recession of the radial component and preservation of the sigmoid notch are represented in Fig. 40.3a–c from the preoperative template. The entry point and trajectory of the radial component guide wire were carefully planned to center the stem precisely in the radial diaphysis and to reproduce anatomic volar tilt of the articulating surface. A prior study of patient outcomes following total wrist arthroplasty demonstrated that restoration of volar tilt of the radial component improved range of motion in the flexion-extension plane [1].

Figures 40.3 and 40.4 show the planned positioning of the radial and carpal components, respectively. The carpal component will require osteotomy of the midcarpal joint for the baseplate to have good bony coverage and appropriate screw trajectories.

The carpal component was aligned to be parallel to the middle metacarpal axis in both coronal and sagittal planes. Position of the carpal plate was planned to have maximum support from the osteotomized proximal capitate and hamate and to ensure that the ulnar screw would have optimal purchase in the hamate. Sizing of each component, amount of carpal bone resection, and screw lengths were all determined preoperatively.

Fig. 40.4 Planned positioning of the carpal component

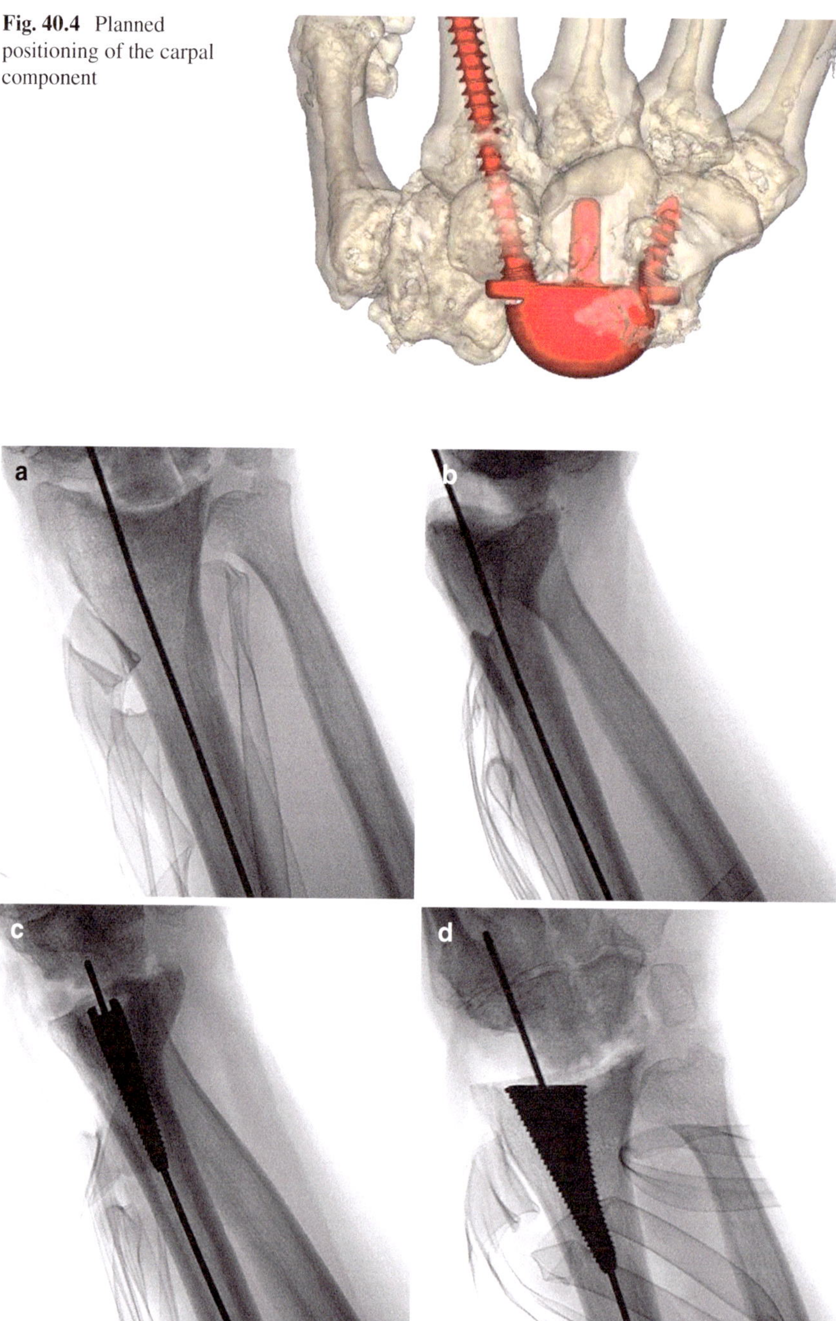

Fig. 40.5 (**a–d**) Guide wire images demonstrating centering of radial component

The procedure was performed by raising a broad ulnar based flap of retinacular tissue off the extensor tendons (from the radial diaphysis to the distal metacarpal), so that a portion could be used at closure to augment the tight capsular tissues. A distally based capsular flap was performed to allow for adequate release of the soft tissue tension. Radius preparation necessitates precise placement of the guide wire in the center of the radial shaft, use of burr and a box cutter, and sequential broaching. Carpal preparation requires attention to precise alignment of the carpal guide wire, distal row osteotomy using a cutting block, followed by reaming and drilling for the capitate center post (see Pearls and Pitfalls). Operative final fluoroscopy spots are shown in Fig. 40.5a, b. Note the centering and recession of the radius component as planned, and the maximal screw length obtained into the second metacarpal.

Final intraoperative radiographs are shown in Fig. 40.6a, b demonstrating the positioning of the components. Figure 40.7a–c demonstrates the patient's intraoperative range of motion.

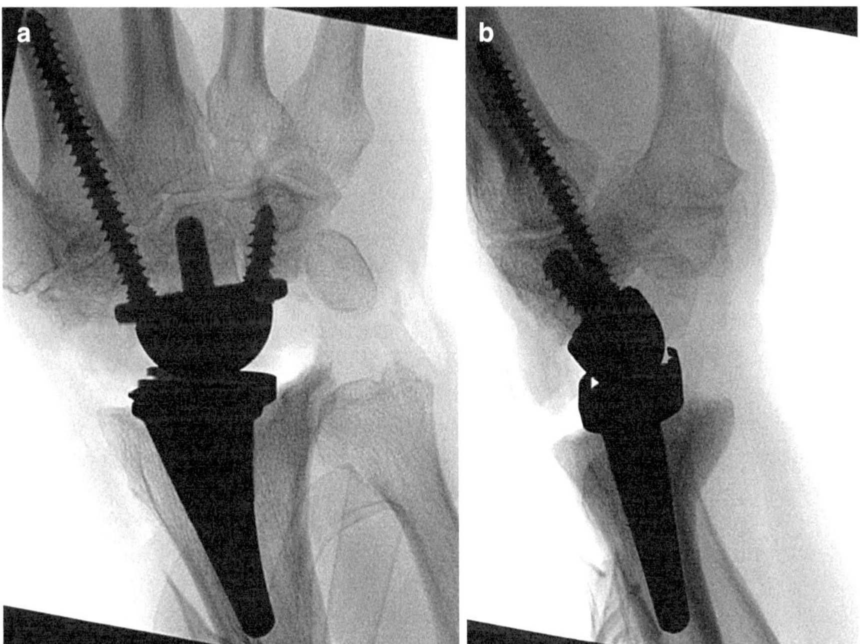

Fig. 40.6 (**a, b**) Intraoperative PA and lateral radiographs

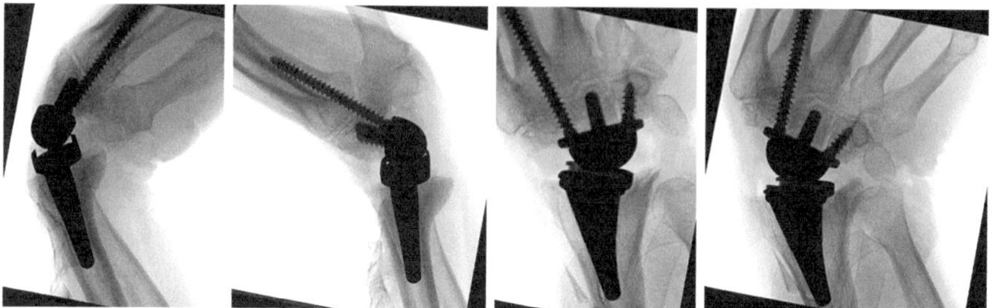

Fig. 40.7 (**a–c**) Intraoperative X-rays are also used to demonstrate the range of motion of the components

Clinical Course and Outcome

[11/3] At the first postoperative visit, on POD #8, the patient reported having been compliant with the recommendations to elevate the extremity and reported minimal pain. The plaster splint was removed, and the patient was transitioned into a removable thermoplastic wrist splint, which he would remove for active range-of-motion exercises of the wrist. Initial postoperative X-rays are shown in Fig. 40.8a–c, redemonstrating appropriate placement of components and no hardware placement changes compared to intraoperative fluoroscopic X-rays.

On the second postoperative visit, POD #13, the patient came in with clear drainage from the wound. The wound was cleaned, cultures were taken, serologies were performed, and the patient was fitted into a delta cast. This is a type of near-circumferential fiberglass cast that is cut in a clamshell fashion and has Velcro straps so that it can be removed for hygiene. For now, the patient is advised to remove it only for wound checks. He was placed on Keflex 500 mg QID empirically. His labs were normal, and the culture was negative.

On the third postoperative visit, on POD #20, the wound appearance had improved and there was no drainage. The patient was placed back into the thermoplastic wrist splint and allowed to resume OT and active range of motion of the wrist with therapy.

On the fourth postoperative visit, at 4 weeks post-op, the patient was doing well, and the wound was fully sealed with no concerning features. His range of motion was quite promising (Table 40.2). Note that his extension, radial deviation, and ulnar deviation are already improved over pre-op measurements.

The patient was followed closely for 18 months following surgery. He has returned to playing tennis and golf. X-rays at 18 months, shown in Fig. 40.9a–c after surgery, showed good evidence of bony ingrowth but some concern for radiolucency about the hamate screw. He was advised to limit his athletic activities so as not to jeopardize his fixation. At this point, he is allowed to return to casual tennis and is advised to return to golf only if he hits all balls off of a tee to avoid ground strikes. In general, patients have been counseled to permanently avoid high-impact

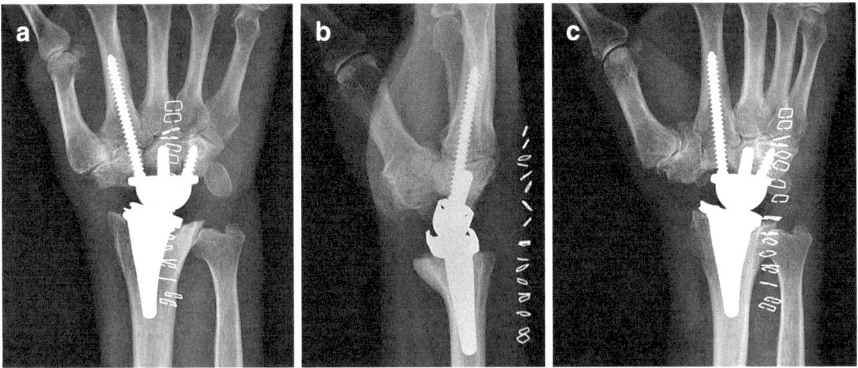

Fig. 40.8 (**a–c**) Radiographs from 11/3

Table 40.2 Range of motion at 4 weeks postoperatively

	Flexion	Extension	RD	UD	Pronation	Supination	Fist	Grip	Pinch
Right	25	25	5	30	80	55	0	n/a	n/a
Left	50	70	20	50	80	80	0	n/a	n/a

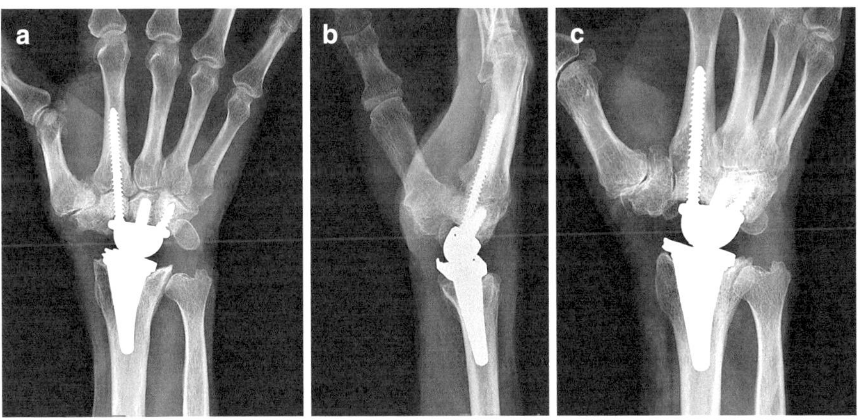

Fig. 40.9 (**a–c**) X-rays from 9/19, at 11 months after surgery

and high-load activities such as mountain biking, golf, or weight-lifting, but some patients have returned to these activities without any documented complications as of yet.

His final range of motion is shown in Fig. 40.10a–d at 17 months following surgery.

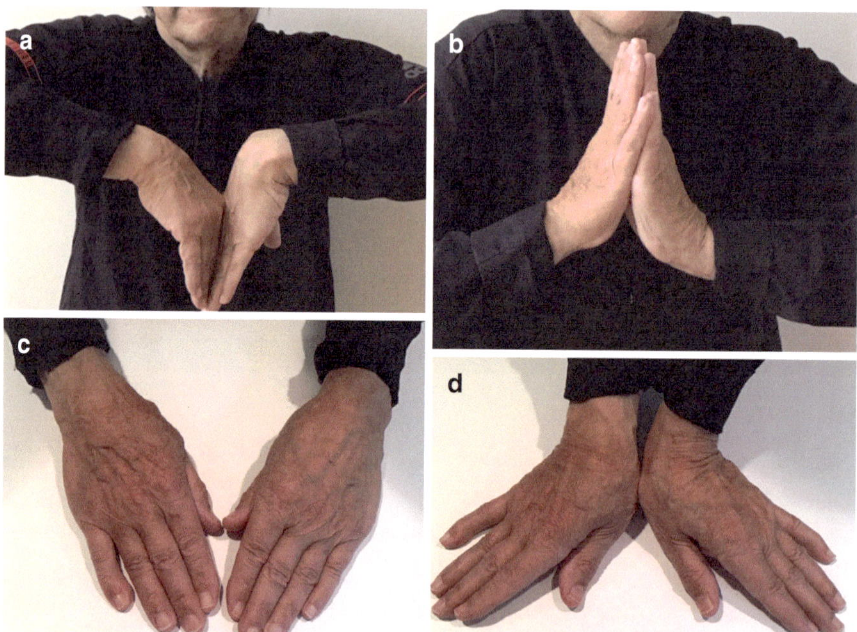

Fig. 40.10 (**a–d**) Motion at 17 months

Bulleted Clinical Pearls/Pitfalls

Use of bone cement for component fixation is performed at the surgeon's discretion. Bone graft may be used as impaction grafting to fill metaphyseal or carpal bone voids. Templating is performed preoperatively. Materialise Mimics (Leuven, Belgium) is used to reconstruct 3D models of the patient's bony anatomy from CT scans – specifically capturing the radius, capitate, and third metacarpal. We then input the KinematX 3D files to determine which size component and in what specific location it fits best (i.e., parallel to the third metacarpal for the carpal component and fit and fill with 5–10 deg. volar tilt for the radial component). The surgical team is given the plan, including precise guide wire insertion points prior to surgery. In general, components are sized sufficiently large to anticipate a good press fit for future bony ingrowth. Because the carpal cap is one size, any size radial stem can be used with any size baseplate.

Approach to the Wrist and Capsulotomy

- 7 cm Universal dorsal approach is through the third dorsal compartment with the proximal retinaculum left intact. Distal PIN is excised at the surgeon's discretion, and the second and fourth compartments are retracted.
- A distal based capsular flap is raised at the radiocarpal joint, with longitudinal limbs below the second and fifth dorsal compartment tendons. The distal based

flap allows the surgeon to adjust the tight capsular/soft tissue sleeve created from prior proximal row carpectomy. An osteotome is used to raise a thin wafer of dorsal triquetrum in continuity with the capsuloligamentous tissue to maintain anatomic alignment of the dorsal radiocarpal and radiotriquetral ligaments.

Radius Preparation and Implantation

- It is important to place the radial component guide wire in line with the long axis of the radius shaft in the coronal plane and with a 10-degree volar tilt in the sagittal plane.
- A custom elliptical motorized rasp is used to remove the remaining cartilage and shape the subchondral bone to match the shape of the metal-backed articular tray.
- A cannulated box cutter is placed over the guide wire and impacted to create a void for broaching.
- The radius is broached to size.
- A trial radial component is implanted, and the distal row reduced. Soft tissue tension is assessed, and additional soft tissue release or radial component recession is performed as needed.

Capitate/Midcarpal Preparation and Implantation

- A guide wire is driven into the capitate parallel to the third metacarpal axis in both the sagittal and coronal planes.
- The carpal cutting guide is placed over the guide wire and fixed to the distal row. The proximal capitate and hamate are osteotomized to create a flat surface for the carpal component.
- The guide wire is over-drilled to create a void for the carpal post, and the appropriately sized carpal plate is impacted in position.
- K-wires are advanced into the index metacarpal canal and into the hamate for screw fixation.
- The wires are over-drilled, and 4.0 mm angular-stable locking screws are driven into the index metacarpal and the hamate for carpal component fixation.
- The carpal cap is applied and impacted to seat a Morse taper fit.

Final Points

- A second trial reduction is performed against the radial component trial.
- Additional soft tissue release is performed as needed to maximize range of motion.
- The final radial stem and correct size modular articular tray are impacted into position, and the wrist is reduced.

- A strip of retinaculum can be used to augment deficiencies when large capsular/ soft tissue releases are necessary.
- The EPL tendon is primarily transposed radially outside of the retinaculum.

Literature Review and Discussion

Total wrist arthroplasty is a motion-sparing treatment option for pancarpal, inflammatory, post-traumatic, or osteoarthritis that offers both predictable pain relief and preservation of motion. Since the first total wrist replacement was performed by Themistocles Gluck in 1890, when he implanted an ivory ball-and-socket prosthesis into a 19-year-old with tuberculosis of the wrist [2], the development of modern wrist arthroplasty has been an iterative process, with each successive generation challenged by its own unique obstacles.

Swanson developed the first generation of widely used implants in 1967 [3, 4]. His design consisted of a single-piece implant with a proximal stem in the radius and a distal stem through the capitate into the third metacarpal shaft with a flexible hinged silicone central portion. Early outcomes were promising, with Swanson et al. reporting 90% of patients achieving functional range of motion and complete pain relief at an average of 4-year follow-up [4]. Subsequent longer term results demonstrated shortcomings of the implant, including high rates of implant fracture, ligament imbalance, and silicone synovitis [5–8]. While short-term outcomes demonstrated up to 77% good or excellent results, that number dropped to 26% when follow-up was extended to 5.8 years [6].

Recognizing the need for an implant that could accommodate the complex mobility of the wrist with more than a single degree of freedom, second-generation implants developed in the 1970s featured ball-and-socket joints. The Meuli prosthesis has been through several iterations, but it initially utilized a polyester ball and socket and was then eventually updated to a titanium and polyethylene ball and socket. The offsets were designed to position the prosthesis' center of rotation (COR) ulnar in the coronal plane and palmar in the sagittal plane in an attempt to recreate the natural wrist's COR [9–11]. The Volz implant consisted of a semi-constrained, cobalt-chrome on polyethylene implant with a hemispherical articulation that allowed for more flexion and extension than radial and ulnar deviation [12]. While both implants enjoyed initial reports of pain relief and maintenance of wrist motion, ultimately a ball-and-socket joint could not account for the moving center of rotation encountered in native wrist kinematics. Implant positioning, soft tissue balancing, and component loosening proved to be problematic, resulting in high complication rates [13–16].

First reported on in the 1990s, third-generation implants sought to improve on prior iterations by using unlinked partially constrained biaxial articulating shapes. The third-generation implants share similar attributes including ellipsoid or toroidal articulating surfaces, screw fixation of the carpal component, and porous coating on the carpal and radial stem surfaces. These implants were reported to maintain the preoperative arc of flexion-extension arc of motion and effectively reduce pain [17–19]; however, early iterations encountered high rates of carpal component loosening and dislocations [19–23]. Subsequent modifications featured an elliptical shaped bearing with increased articulating surface area that allowed for increased distribution of articular forces, decreased stress on the carpal component fixation, and less polyethylene wear. Another design incorporated mobile bearing design on the carpal component to allow ten degrees of axial rotation in an attempt to decrease stress on the bone-cement interface of the distal component ("ReMotion," Small Bone Innovation, Norristown, PA). Collectively, these improvements have resulted in near disappearance of dislocation and improvements in survival rates [20, 24, 25]. All current third-generation designs feature a convex polyethylene carpal component articulating with a concave metal radial component. A recent in vivo biplanar radiographic study compared the center of rotation of six patients with a third-generation radiocarpal design with ten healthy patient wrists and demonstrated that the implant's center of rotation shifted more than two times that of healthy wrists, raising concerns for increased stresses on the carpal component [26].

The latest generation of total wrist implants has placed emphasis on an attempt to restore the normal center of rotation in order to decrease loads on the implant and bone-implant interface and improve implant survivorship. The Maestro total wrist featured an articulating surface that simulates the curvature of the distal carpal row and demonstrated promising outcomes with regard to pain relief and range of motion [27]. Unlike its predecessors, it featured a metal convex carpal component articulating with a polyethylene metal-backed articular surface on the radial component. The Maestro was withdrawn from the market in 2019. Though unavailable in the USA, the Motec implant is a ball-and-socket design available with both metal-on-PEEK and metal-on-metal articulations. Ten-year survival rate in high-demand patients was reported at 86% [28], and postoperative patient-reported outcomes have been promising [29], although there have been reports of metal-on-metal wear. It remains to be seen if the ball-and-socket, fixed center of rotation design encounters similar challenges seen in earlier generations of implants.

The KinematX implant utilized in this case is the first total wrist prosthesis designed from the world's largest open-source database of wrist kinematics [30]. It restores the anatomic center of rotation of the wrist joint by replacing the midcarpal articulation of the wrist rather than the predecessor wrist implants that replaced the radiocarpal articulation. The midcarpal joint has been demonstrated to be essential for motions such as wrist circumduction and "dart-thrower's motion" [31, 32]. By mimicking normal kinematics and kinetics, it is predicted that implant loosening and wear will be reduced. The early outcomes of this implant system are promising in regard to pain, motion, and function and are continually analyzed via a prospective registry collected from five US centers.

While historical data may be interpreted to advocate for wrist arthrodesis over a total wrist arthroplasty due to the high complication rates seen in arthroplasty, third- and fourth-generation implant design has demonstrated marked decreases in complication rates and improvements in 10-year survival rates. A recent study utilizing national inpatient sample data demonstrated a total complication rate of 10% for wrist fusion and 7% for total wrist arthroplasty [33]. While wrist fusion remains a treatment mainstay, the resultant loss of motion can be associated with functional limitations including difficulty with perineal care and button fastening [34]. Incidence of total wrist arthroplasty in the USA has historically been low, with only a few dozen cases nationwide most years [35]. Reasons for this are likely multifactorial, but likely include the paucity of surgeons comfortable with this procedure, the lifetime weight-bearing restrictions with most prostheses, and the tolerable and reliable outcomes of wrist fusion procedures. A retrospective comparison of wrist arthrodesis and wrist arthroplasty for pancarpal post-traumatic arthritis demonstrated a mean PRWE score of 73 for the arthrodesis group and 31 for the arthroplasty group [36]. With a continuously improving complication profile, and promising outcomes regarding pain relief and function, there may be an increasing role for total wrist arthroplasty moving forward.

References

1. Akhbari B, Shah KN, Morton AM, et al. Total wrist arthroplasty alignment and its potential association with clinical outcomes. J Wrist Surg. 2021;10(4):308–15.
2. Ritt MJ, Stuart PR, Naggar L, Beckenbaugh RD. The early history of arthroplasty of the wrist. From amputation to total wrist implant. J Hand Surg Br. 1994;19(6):778–82.
3. Swanson AB. Flexible implant resection arthroplasty. Hand. 1972;4(2):119–34.
4. Swanson AB, de Groot SG, Maupin BK. Flexible implant arthroplasty of the radiocarpal joint. Surgical technique and long-term study. Clin Orthop Relat Res. 1984;187:94–106.
5. Fatti JF, Palmer AK, Mosher JF. The long-term results of Swanson silicone rubber interpositional wrist arthroplasty. J Hand Surg Am. 1986;11(2):166–75.
6. Fatti JF, Palmer AK, Greenky S, Mosher JF. Long-term results of Swanson interpositional wrist arthroplasty: part II. J Hand Surg Am. 1991;16(3):432–7.
7. Jolly SL, Ferlic DC, Clayton ML, Dennis DA, Stringer EA. Swanson silicone arthroplasty of the wrist in rheumatoid arthritis: a long-term follow-up. J Hand Surg Am. 1992;17(1):142–9.
8. DeHeer DH, Owens SR, Swanson AB. The host response to silicone elastomer implants for small joint arthroplasty. J Hand Surg Am. 1995;20(3 Pt 2):S101–9.
9. Kennedy CD, Huang JI. Prosthetic design in total wrist arthroplasty. Orthop Clin North Am. 2016;47(1):207–18.
10. Meuli HC. Arthroplasty of the wrist. Clin Orthop Relat Res. 1980;149:118–25.
11. Meuli HC, Fernandez DL. Uncemented total wrist arthroplasty. J Hand Surg Am. 1995;20(1):115–22.
12. McBeath R, Osterman AL. Total wrist arthroplasty. Hand Clin. 2012;28(4):595–609.
13. Vogelin E, Nagy L. Fate of failed Meuli total wrist arthroplasty. J Hand Surg Br. 2003;28(1):61–8.
14. Cooney WP 3rd, Beckenbaugh RD, Linscheid RL. Total wrist arthroplasty. Problems with implant failures. Clin Orthop Relat Res. 1984;187:121–8.
15. Volz RG. Total wrist arthroplasty. A clinical review. Clin Orthop Relat Res. 1984;187:112–20.
16. Gellman H, Hontas R, Brumfield RH Jr, Tozzi J, Conaty JP. Total wrist arthroplasty in rheumatoid arthritis. A long-term clinical review. Clin Orthop Relat Res. 1997;342:71–6.
17. Dv H, Heesterbeek PJ, de Vos J, M. High rate of complications and radiographic loosening of the Biaxial total wrist arthroplasty in rheumatoid arthritis: 32 wrists followed for 6 (5–8) years. Acta Orthop. 2011;82(6):721–6. Epub 2011 Nov 9
18. Cobb TK, Beckenbaugh RD. Biaxial total-wrist arthroplasty. J Hand Surg Am. 1996;21(6):1011–21.

19. Takwale VJ, Nuttall D, Trail IA, Stanley JK. Biaxial total wrist replacement in patients with rheumatoid arthritis. Clinical review, survivorship and radiological analysis. J Bone Joint Surg Br. 2002;84(5):692–9.
20. van Winterswijk PJ, Bakx PA. Promising clinical results of the universal total wrist prosthesis in rheumatoid arthritis. Open Orthop J. 2010;4:67–70.
21. Divelbiss BJ, Sollerman C, Adams BD. Early results of the universal total wrist arthroplasty in rheumatoid arthritis. J Hand Surg Am. 2002;27(2):195–204.
22. Ward CM, Kuhl T, Adams BD. Five to ten-year outcomes of the universal total wrist arthroplasty in patients with rheumatoid arthritis. J Bone Joint Surg Am. 2011;93(10):914–9.
23. Menon J. Universal total wrist implant: experience with a carpal component fixed with three screws. J Arthroplast. 1998;13(5):515–23.
24. Ferreres A, Lluch A, Del Valle M. Universal total wrist arthroplasty: midterm follow-up study. J Hand Surg Am. 2011;36(6):967–73.
25. Morapudi SP, Marlow WJ, Withers D, Ralte P, Gabr A, Waseem M. Total wrist arthroplasty using the Universal 2 prosthesis. J Orthop Surg (Hong Kong). 2012;20(3):365–8.
26. Akhbari B, Morton AM, Moore DC, Crisco JJ. Biplanar videoradiography to study the wrist and distal radioulnar joints. J Vis Exp. 2021;168:62102. Published 2021 Feb 4
27. Nydick JA, Greenberg SM, Stone JD, Williams B, Polikandriotis JA, Hess AV. Clinical outcomes of total wrist arthroplasty. J Hand Surg Am. 2012;37(8):1580–4.
28. Reigstad O, Holm-Glad T, Bolstad B, Grimsgaard C, Thorkildsen R, Rokkum M. Five- to 10-year prospective follow-up of wrist arthroplasty in 56 nonrheumatoid patients. J Hand Surg Am. 2017;42(10):788–96.
29. Yeoh D, Tourret L. Total wrist arthroplasty: a systematic review of the evidence from the last 5 years. J Hand Surg Eur Vol. 2015;40(5):458–68.
30. Akhbari B, Moore DC, Laidlaw DH, et al. Predicting carpal bone kinematics using an expanded digital database of wrist carpal bone anatomy and kinematics. J Orthop Res. 2019;37(12):2661–70.
31. Crisco JJ, Coburn JC, Moore DC, Akelman E, Weiss AC, Wolfe SW. In vivo radiocarpal kinematics and the dart thrower's motion. J Bone Joint Surg Am. 2005;87(12):2729–40.
32. Moritomo H, Apergis EP, Garcia-Elias M, Werner FW, Wolfe SW. International Federation of Societies for Surgery of the Hand 2013 Committee's report on wrist dart-throwing motion. J Hand Surg Am. 2014;39(7):1433–9.
33. Melamed E, Marascalchi B, Hinds RM, Rizzo M, Capo JT. Trends in the utilization of total wrist arthroplasty versus wrist fusion for treatment of advanced wrist arthritis. J Wrist Surg. 2016;5(3):211–6.
34. Murphy DM, Khoury JG, Imbriglia JE, Adams BD. Comparison of arthroplasty and arthrodesis for the rheumatoid wrist [published correction appears in J Hand Surg [Am]. 2003;28(5):875]. J Hand Surg Am. 2003;28(4):570–6.
35. Elbuluk AM, Milone MT, Capo JT, Bosco JA, Klifto CS. Trends and demographics in the utilization of total wrist arthroplasty. J Hand Surg Asian Pac. 2018;23(4):501–5.
36. Nydick JA, Watt JF, Garcia MJ, Williams BD, Hess AV. Clinical outcomes of arthrodesis and arthroplasty for the treatment of posttraumatic wrist arthritis. J Hand Surg Am. 2013;38(5):899–903.

Chapter 41
Acellular Dermal Allograft Arthroplasty for Wrist Arthritis

Steven J. Lee, Justin Luis, Devin W. Collins, and Michael J. Garcia

Case Presentation

A 51-year-old right-hand-dominant male presented with a previous history of right scapholunate ligament tear that progressed to stage 4 SLAC wrist. The patient is very active for his age, an accomplished amateur golfer and recreational tennis player, and enjoys strength training in the gym. His pain and dysfunction have progressed to the point where he is unable to play golf, and now he has pain with activities of daily living. He had been offered a wrist fusion by another surgeon to address his pain but was told that the lack of motion at the wrist would significantly hamper his ability to play golf at a high level and therefore obtained a second opinion for alternative treatment.

Physical Exam/Relevant Maneuvers

The patient's pertinent positive exam included a painful range of motion with wrist dorsi/volar flexion of $30°/20°$ and pronosupination of $85°/80°$. He was diffusely tender throughout his wrist, but most tender at his dorsal radiocarpal joint, and his grip strength measured 42% compared to his opposite, nondominant side. Watson's sign elicited pain without an obvious clunk.

S. J. Lee (✉) · J. Luis
Lenox Hill Hospital, New York, NY, USA
e-mail: JLUIS@NORTHWELL.EDU

D. W. Collins · M. J. Garcia
Florida Orthopedic Institute, Temple Terrace, FL, USA

J. Yao (ed.), *Carpal Instability*, https://doi.org/10.1007/978-3-031-55869-6_41

517

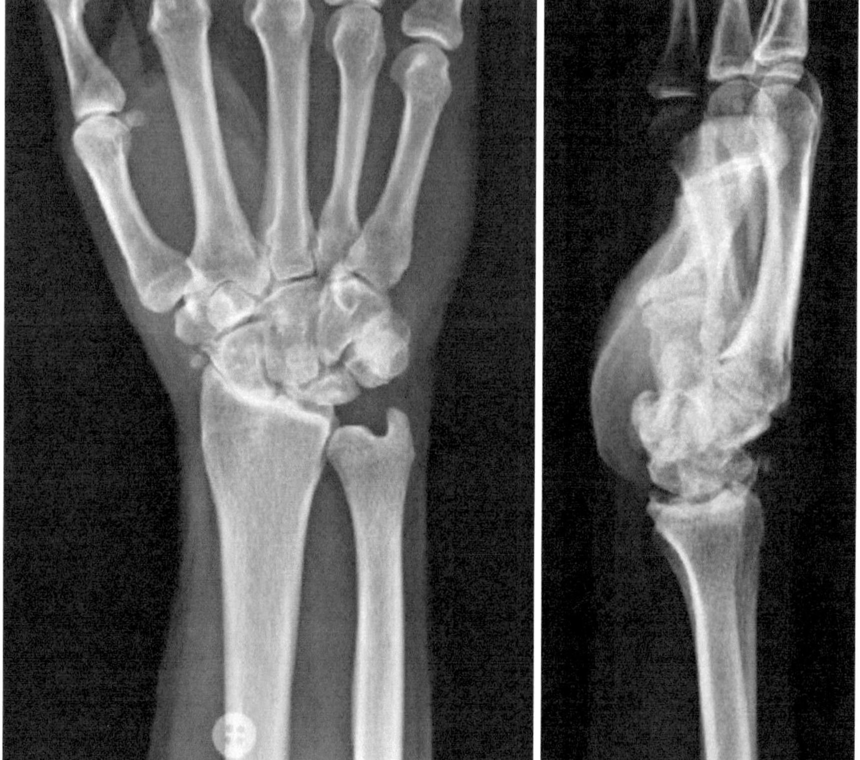

Fig. 41.1 Preoperative AP and lateral wrist X-rays showing SLAC 4

Diagnostic Studies

Radiographs and MRI ordered by the previous hand surgeon showed a complete scapholunate ligament tear with widening of 4 mm, DISI deformity with a scapholunate angle of 78°, and significant grade 4 degenerative changes at the radioscaphoid, radiolunate, and capitolunate joints in an otherwise ulnar neutral wrist (Fig. 41.1).

Management Options

The management options presented to him included nonoperative management (including pain medications, wrist splinting, platelet-rich plasma, hyaluronic acid, or cortisone injections), wrist denervation, total wrist arthroplasty, and proximal row carpectomy with acellular dermal allograft interposition arthroplasty. Partial and total wrist fusion procedures were discussed but dismissed given the patient's interest in continuing to play competitive golf. The patient already had a trial of splinting and was already taking NSAIDs but exhibited gastrointestinal complications. He had one cortisone injection but only obtained temporary relief and read that repetitive injections could promote increased arthritic changes. While understanding that pain relief might best be obtained via a wrist fusion, the patient preferred a motion-preserving operation. Preservation of motion would better allow for golf and tennis and other athletic endeavors. Total wrist arthroplasty was presented, but the combination of his very active lifestyle and reported associated complication rate was significant enough to detract him from wanting to pursue this.

Management Chosen for this Case with Rationale

The patient opted for proximal row carpectomy with acellular dermal allograft (ADA) interpositional arthroplasty, as previously described by the senior author [1]. In brief, a proximal row carpectomy was performed through a longitudinal dorsal incision, along with an anterior and posterior interosseous neurectomy. An ADA was fashioned to size and secured on to the capitate and hamate bones with suture anchors securing the radial and ulnar sides, while sutures secured the ADA via anterior to posterior drill holes in the capitate and hamate on the volar and dorsal sides. A secure capsular closure was performed, and the patient was placed into a forearm-based plaster splint for 6 weeks (Figs. 41.2, 41.3, and 41.4).

The rationale for choosing this case procedure was that even though it was presented to the patient as a relatively new procedure, the benefit of this procedure was to provide a cushion between the degenerative bones to provide pain relief while preserving functional range of motion of the wrist. It was also explained that if the ADA wore out over time, there was an option of replacing that with a new one. Finally, significant bridges would not be burned for salvage procedures in the future such as a fusion or total wrist arthroplasty. The majority of patients who have been presented with this option over a fusion or total wrist arthroplasty have opted for the ADA arthroplasty based on this reasoning.

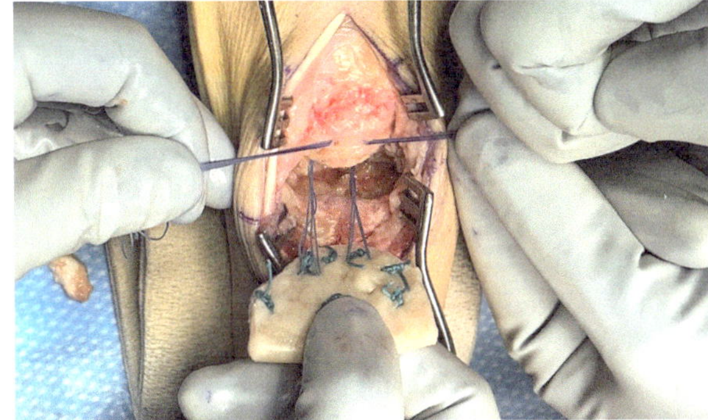

Fig. 41.2 ADA shuttled into the PRC space by pulling on sutures that are placed dorsal-volar on the capitate and hamate

Fig. 41.3 ADA secured into the PRC space

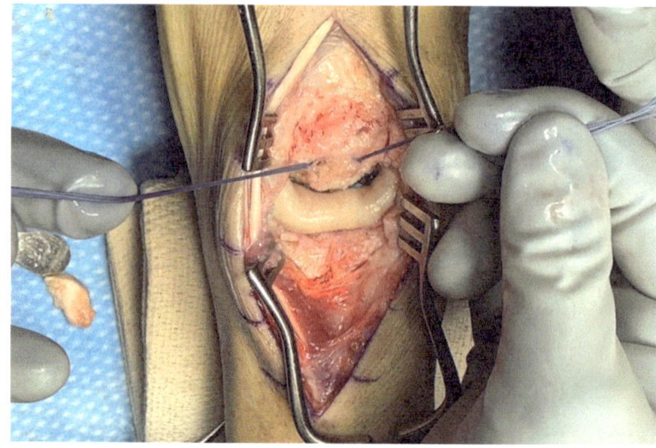

Fig. 41.4 Traction sutures are tied into the ADA to secure it into place. Separate anchors are placed on the radial side of the capitate and ulnar side of the hamate to further secure the ADA

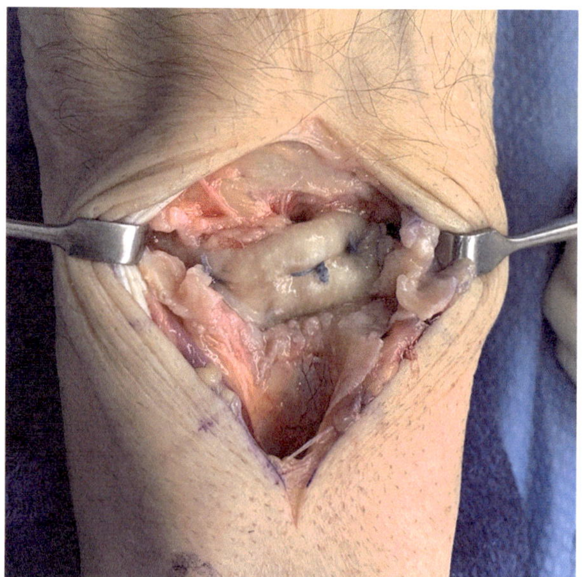

Clinical Course and Outcome

After surgery, the patient was immobilized in an orthoplast wrist splint for 6 weeks, and then started hand therapy for range of motion starting at 6 weeks. Strengthening began 8 weeks postoperatively. The patient felt better compared to before surgery at the 3-month mark and started to play golf 5 months postoperatively. His symptoms and function continued to improve for up to 1 year. At the last follow-up, the patient's wrist range of motion dorsi/volar flexion improved to within 85% and grip strength improved to 70% of the uninvolved wrist. His DASH score improved from 61 preoperatively to 8 postoperatively (Fig. 41.5).

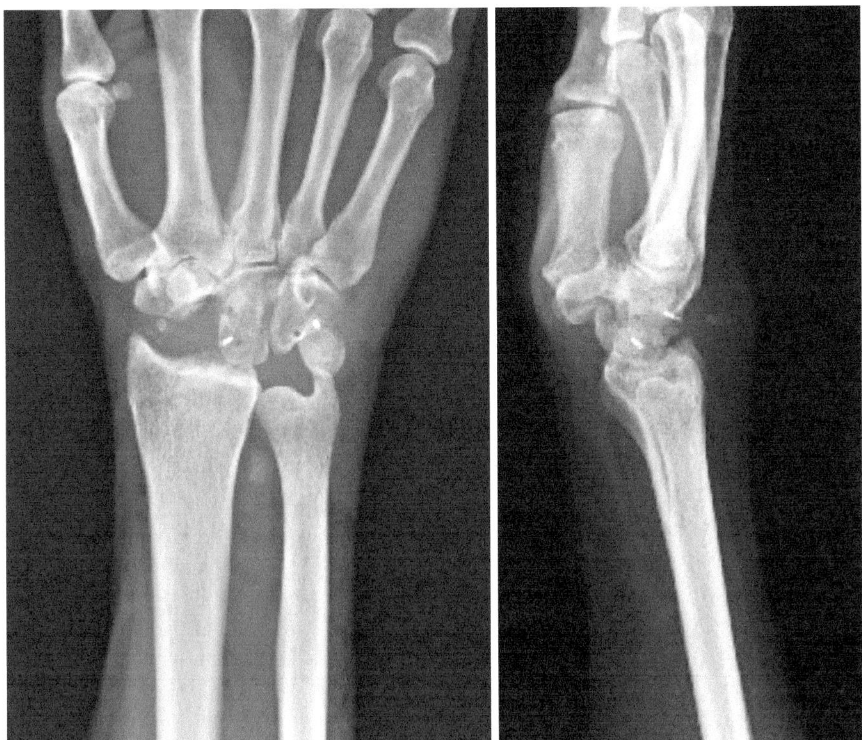

Fig. 41.5 2-Year postoperative AP and lateral wrist X-rays

Bulleted Clinical Pearls/Pitfalls ([2–4], with Figures)

- Alternative for patients who are considering total wrist fusion.
- Predictably decreases pain.
- Maintains on average 80% of the range of motion and grip strength.
- The proximal row carpectomy is performed to make space for the ADA.
- An anterior and posterior interosseous neurectomy is performed concomitantly to increase the likelihood for pain relief.
- May be repeated/revised with a new ADA if it wears down over time.
- Does not burn bridges for future salvage options, including fusion.
- May take at least 3 months for patients to feel significantly better and may improve for up to 1 year.

Literature Review and Discussion

There are many options that are available for patients with end-stage carpal instability leading to SLAC wrist. The treatment utilized depends on a number of factors including the patient's age, anticipated physical activities, previous surgeries, and especially which joint(s) are affected. For those patients in which the radiocarpal joint (stage 4) is affected despite nonoperative treatment, the traditional options are limited to radiocarpal fusions, total wrist fusions, or total joint arthroplasty. The lack of a universally accepted optimal treatment to address symptomatic carpal arthritis and/or instability has encouraged us to seek techniques that could provide predictable pain relief while preserving (or improving) range of motion and grip strength. In a prior study [1], our technique demonstrated that PRC ADA interposition arthroplasty into the radiocapitate articulation can expand the indications of PRC for more severe cases of SLAC. Moreover, we believe that this novel interposition arthroplasty technique is a valid option that can limit the morbidity of motion-sacrificing fusion for end-stage carpal arthritis, which can be performed in both an index or revision setting.

In isolated radiocarpal arthritis, limited fusions such as radioscapholunate fusions may be utilized. However, it is rare to have this be an isolated phenomenon without the scaphocapitate or capitolunate joint being affected. Therefore, end-stage carpal arthritis was often managed with total wrist arthrodesis. This treatment reliably relieves the pain associated with this problem, but the lack of motion in all wrist planes aside from pronosupination significantly reduces the patient's functional ability [2–5]. Most patients, when presented with this option, almost immediately dismiss this solution and inquire about other options and/or seek a second opinion. Furthermore, once this option is chosen, all other bridges have been burned should the patient not be satisfied with the resultant lack of motion.

Total wrist arthroplasties were frequently used with the intention of preserving motion. Several systematic reviews have shown no difference in improvement in pain and functional outcomes compared to total wrist arthrodesis, but wrist arthroplasty was shown to be associated with higher overall complication rate, especially with osteolysis, loosening, and dislocation [3–6]. With innovations in design with newer generation implants, subsequent studies argue that there has been a significant decrease in complication rate and improved range of motion and grip strength, but a recent review by Berber et al. [5] highlighted great variability in study designs. Currently, there is no consensus if wrist arthroplasty can be used as an intended motion-sparing procedure for a younger active population or in those involved in physically demanding activities or occupation. If a total wrist arthroplasty incurs one of these complications, the resultant wrist is often difficult to salvage due to the amount of bone loss that is necessary from the initial index procedure in addition to the result after implant removal.

Seeking to devise a solution to this complex nature of end-stage arthritis, others have turned their attention to soft tissue interpositional procedures. The use of interposition arthroplasty has been utilized in a wide range of areas involving different materials such as Achilles tendon, fascia lata, flexor carpi radialis, or even hematoma distraction/collagen-filling procedures with promising results [7–11]. Traditional PRC is a relatively simple way to manage those with limited arthritic changes of the capitate head with long-term studies reporting high patient satisfaction and maintenance of pain relief, range of motion, and strength [9, 10]. Despite the presence of radiographic evidence of progression of radiocapitate arthritic changes, patients were otherwise asymptomatic. There are concerns of failure of PRC when performed in younger patients that may necessitate a salvage revision [10].

We have previously described using an acellular dermal allograft for the treatment of wrist arthritis [1]. The versatility of ADA as a biological cushion and adjunctive scaffolding support have been utilized for a variety of musculoskeletal procedures in both the upper and lower extremity [1, 7, 12–16]. For thumb basal carpometacarpal arthritis (Eaton stages II and III), Adams [7] described an effective arthroscopic technique that used ADA, and in a subsequent study, Kokkalis [16] reported 100% success in pain and functional improvement with its use in LRTI. Rabinovich and Lee [1] reported significant improvement in wrist range of motion, key pinch, and grip strength, and improved VAS scores at the 6-month follow-up following interposition of ADA into the radiocapitate articulation during proximal row carpectomy (PRC) to prevent further degeneration that is commonly seen following traditional PRC techniques. Although their study lacks long-term follow-up data, their results are consistent with those of Kwon, which reported satisfactory results using a capsular interpositional flap in conjunction with PRC with an average of 41 months [8].

The reasons for using a dermal allograft in this patient are that it offers a number of benefits over other techniques that have been described. Pain relief is reliably obtained. On average, about 80% of the range of motion as well as the grip strength are preserved. Although the durability of using an ADA is not certain at this time, we currently have patients who are past 6 years without requiring a second procedure. If patients have worn out their ADA over time leading to disabling pain and dysfunction, another ADA can be inserted as a replacement and has been done successfully in those patients who have a previously failed PRC. Finally, no real bridges are burned with this technique since theoretically a wrist fusion or a total wrist arthroplasty can still be performed if the PRC ADA eventually fails to a point where a patient is requesting a different procedure.

References

1. Rabinovich RV, Lee SJ. Proximal row carpectomy using decellularized dermal allograft. J Hand Surg Am. 2018;43(4):392.e1–9. https://doi.org/10.1016/j.jhsa.2018.01.012.
2. De Smet L, Truyen J. Arthrodesis of the wrist for osteoarthritis: outcome with a minimum follow-up of 4 years. J Hand Surg Br. 2003;28(6):575–7. https://doi.org/10.1016/s0266-7681(03)00208-0.
3. Cavaliere CM, Chung KC. A systematic review of total wrist arthroplasty compared with total wrist arthrodesis for rheumatoid arthritis. Plast Reconstr Surg. 2008;122(03):813–25.
4. Nydick JA, Watt JF, Garcia MJ, Williams BD, Hess AV. Clinical outcomes of arthrodesis and arthroplasty for the treatment of posttraumatic wrist arthritis. J Hand Surg Am. 2013;38(5):899–903. https://doi.org/10.1016/j.jhsa.2013.02.013.
5. Berber O, Garagnani L, Gidwani S. Systematic review of total wrist arthroplasty and arthrodesis in wrist arthritis. J Wrist Surg. 2018;7(5):424–40. https://doi.org/10.1055/s-0038-1646956.

6. Yeoh D, Tourret L. Total wrist arthroplasty: a systematic review of the evidence from the last 5 years. J Hand Surg Eur. 2015;40(05):458–68.

7. Adams JE, Merten SM, Steinmann SP. Arthroscopic interposition arthroplasty of the first carpometacarpal joint. J Hand Surg Eur. 2007;32(3):268–74. https://doi.org/10.1016/J.JHSB.2006.12.003.

8. Kwon BC, Choi SJ, Shin J, Baek GH. Proximal row carpectomy with capsular interposition arthroplasty for advanced arthritis of the wrist. J Bone Joint Surg Br. 2009;91(12):1601–6.

9. Jebson PJ, Hayes EP, Engber WD. Proximal row carpectomy: a minimum 10-year follow-up study. J Hand Surg Am. 2003;28(4):561–9. https://doi.org/10.1016/s0363-5023(03)00248-x.

10. Wall LB, Didonna ML, Kiefhaber TR, Stern PJ. Proximal row carpectomy: minimum 20-year follow-up. J Hand Surg Am. 2013;38(8):1498–504. https://doi.org/10.1016/j.jhsa.2013.04.028.

11. Eaton RG, Akelman E, Eaton BH. Fascial implant arthroplasty for treatment of radioscaphoid degenerative disease. J Hand Surg Am. 1989;14(5):766–74. https://doi.org/10.1016/s0363-5023(89)80074-7.

12. Aynardi MC, Atwater L, Dein EJ, Zahoor T, Schon LC, Miller SD. Outcomes after interpositional arthroplasty of the first metatarsophalangeal joint. Foot Ankle Int. 2017;38(5):514–8. https://doi.org/10.1177/1071100716687366.

13. Kennedy JG, Chow FY, Dines J, Gardner M, Bohne WH. Outcomes after interposition arthroplasty for treatment of hallux rigidus. Clin Orthop Relat Res. 2006;445:210–5. https://doi.org/10.1097/01.blo.0000201166.82690.23.

14. Bailey JR, Kim C, Alentorn-Geli E, et al. Rotator cuff matrix augmentation and interposition: a systematic review and meta-analysis. Am J Sports Med. 2019;47(6):1496–506. https://doi.org/10.1177/0363546518774762.

15. Omae H, Steinmann SP, Zhao C, et al. Biomechanical effect of rotator cuff augmentation with an acellular dermal matrix graft: a cadaver study. Clin Biomech. 2012;27(8):789–92. https://doi.org/10.1016/j.clinbiomech.2012.05.001.

16. Kokkalis ZT, Zanaros G, Weiser RW, Sotereanos DG. Trapezium resection with suspension and interposition arthroplasty using acellular dermal allograft for thumb carpometacarpal arthritis. J Hand Surg Am. 2009;34(6):1029–36. https://doi.org/10.1016/j.jhsa.2009.03.001.

Chapter 42
Special Consideration for Intercarpal Ligament Injuries in the Pediatric Patient

Jason J. Yoo and Joshua M. Abzug

Case Presentation

A 16-year-old female presents with a 1-month-long history of left wrist pain after sustaining a hyperextension injury to the left wrist when her sister jumped onto her. She has had persistent wrist pain with all wrist motion made worse with wrist flexion. She has some relief with wrist bracing and use of nonsteroidal anti-inflammatory medications but continues to have substantial wrist pain.

On physical examination, the patient has mild swelling about the left wrist without deformity. She exhibits pain with active and passive range of motion of the wrist and has tenderness within the anatomical snuffbox and dorsal radial aspect of the wrist. Attempt at the Watson shift test results in significant pain preventing completion of the maneuver. There is no tenderness to palpation on the ulnar aspect of the wrist.

Radiographic examination reveals no appreciable fractures of the carpal bones nor the distal radius and ulna with concentric Gilula's lines. The scapholunate angle and the scapholunate interval are within normal limits (Fig. 42.1). There are no DISI or VISI deformities present. On pencil grip view, the left scapholunate interval appears wider than that on the right (Fig. 42.2). MRI of the wrist reveals at least a partial tear of the dorsal scapholunate ligament (Fig. 42.3).

J. J. Yoo · J. M. Abzug (✉)
Department of Orthopaedics, University of Maryland School of Medicine,
Baltimore, MD, USA
e-mail: jyoo@som.umaryland.edu; jabzug@som.umaryland.edu

J. Yao (ed.), *Carpal Instability*, https://doi.org/10.1007/978-3-031-55869-6_42

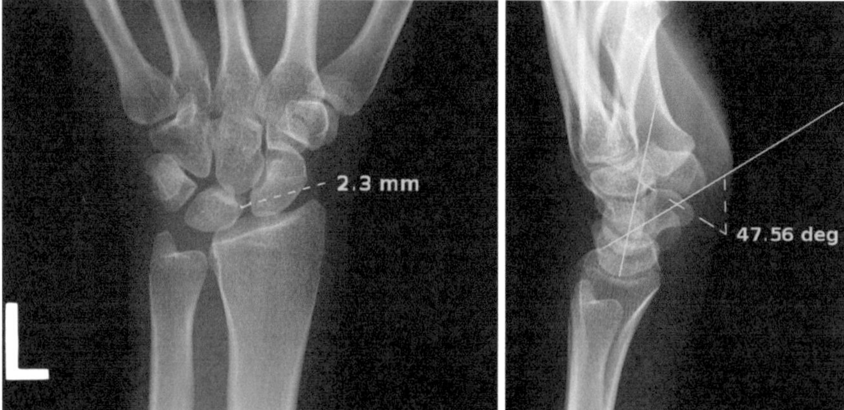

Fig. 42.1 Plain radiographs of the posteroanterior and lateral views of the left wrist showing a normal scapholunate interval of 2.3 mm and scapholunate angle of 47°

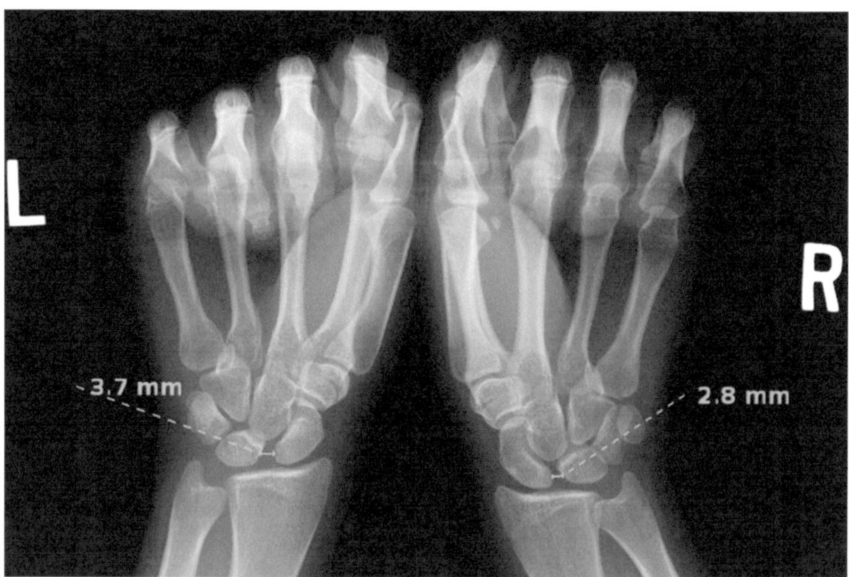

Fig. 42.2 Plain radiograph of the pencil grip view of the right and left wrists with widening of the left scapholunate interval to 3.7 mm

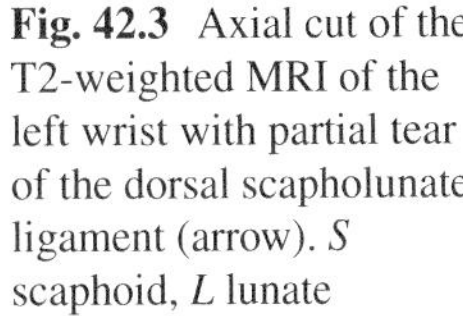

Fig. 42.3 Axial cut of the T2-weighted MRI of the left wrist with partial tear of the dorsal scapholunate ligament (arrow). *S* scaphoid, *L* lunate

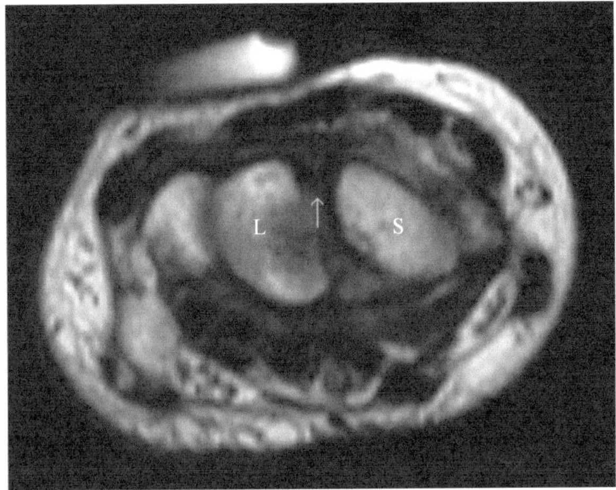

Diagnosis

Physical Assessment/Relevant Maneuvers

- Visual inspection.
- Palpation.
- Wrist range of motion.
- Maneuvers to assess intercarpal stability:

  - Scaphoid shift test.
  - Midcarpal shift test
  - Capitolunate instability pattern test.
  - Lunotriquetral ballottement test.

Diagnostic Studies

- Plain radiographs.

  - Posterior anterior, oblique, lateral, scaphoid view (PA view in ulnar deviation and slight supination).
  - Continuity of Gilula's lines.
  - Scapholunate interval.
  - Scapholunate angle.
  - Capitolunate angle.
  - Pencil grip views.

- Computed tomography.

  - The use of CT scans in the pediatric population is done judiciously due to ionizing radiation exposure.

- Magnetic resonance imaging.
- Wrist arthroscopy.

Management Options

- Observation.
- Immobilization.
- Wrist arthroscopy and debridement.
- Direct scapholunate ligament repair.
- Scapholunate ligament reconstruction.

Management Chosen for This Case

The patient exhibited signs of at least a partial scapholunate ligament injury. Physical examination revealed dorsal wrist tenderness and pain with initiation of the scaphoid shift test. On pencil grip views of the wrist, a wider scapholunate interval on the left wrist suggested the presence of some dynamic instability. Magnetic resonance imaging also localized the presence of a partial tear of the scapholunate ligament. With these physical exam and imaging findings and the patient's failure to improve after a 6-week trial of immobilization, diagnostic wrist arthroscopy was chosen for further evaluation with possible arthroscopic debridement and open ligament repair depending on the extent of injury seen on arthroscopy.

Clinical Course and Outcome

Wrist arthroscopy was performed using the standard 3-4 and 4-5 portals. Visualization of the carpus revealed intact radioscaphocapitate, long and short radiolunate ligaments. The lunotriquetral and triangular fibrocartilage complex structures were also intact. Direct visualization and probing of the scapholunate ligament demonstrated attenuation of the scapholunate ligament with a Geissler grade 2 injury (Fig. 42.4). All synovitis and loose structures were thoroughly debrided. An open ligament-sparing dorsal approach to the wrist was utilized to directly repair the dorsal intercarpal ligaments, which were also noted to be partially torn. Primary repair with nonabsorbable suture in a figure-of-eight fashion was performed. One pearl to assess the repair intraoperatively is to perform a scaphoid shift test and dart-thrower's wrist motion to directly observe the scapholunate interval to ensure that no gapping is present prior to reapproximation of the wrist capsule.

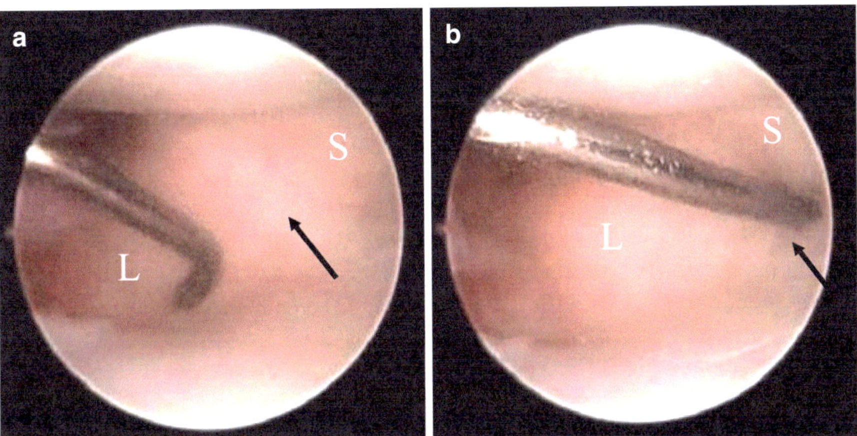

Fig. 42.4 (**a**) Arthroscopic view of the scaphoid (S), lunate (L), and scapholunate ligament (arrow). (**b**) Probing of the scapholunate ligament revealing laxity but negative drive-through sign

Postoperatively, the patient's wrist was immobilized for a total of 6 weeks. Due to social factors, the patient had a substantial delay in hand therapy resulting in wrist stiffness. Self-implemented therapy was initiated with improvement in wrist pain and motion. Wrist flexion and extension of 35° and 50°, respectively, were achieved by 4 months postoperatively with a pain-free wrist.

Clinical Pearls/Pitfalls

The normal scapholunate interval varies with age and gender in the pediatric population, as noted by a decreasing interval with increasing age until skeletal maturity is reached. Abzug et al. developed predictive equations for calculating the expected scapholunate interval based on age and gender. For males, one can use $y = -0.665(\text{age}) + 11.432$ with y as the distance in millimeters [1]. For females, $y = -0.443(\text{age}) + 7.895$.

- Contralateral wrist films can also aid in distinguishing pathologic widening of the scapholunate interval from anatomic variants.

Literature Review and Discussion

Scapholunate interosseous ligament injuries are rare in the skeletally immature patient. Due to the weak nature of the physis, wrist injuries favor physeal injury [2]. When ligamentous injuries do occur, accurate diagnosis remains a significant challenge particularly in the subgroup of patients without dynamic instability where physical examination may only reveal point tenderness.

Common radiographic parameters such as the scapholunate interval, scapholunate angle, and capitolunate angles can be used to diagnose scapholunate dissociation. However, unlike in the adult population in which the scapholunate interval of >2.5 mm is indicative of scapholunate ligament injury, radiographic parameters are less definitive in children [1, 3]. Within the pediatric population, the scapholunate interval is age dependent and can range anywhere between 1.7 and 9 mm, with higher numbers present in younger children and the normal <2 mm gapping present in children that are skeletally mature [1]. Abzug et al. described a negative linear correlation between chronological age and the radiographic scapholunate interval. It was determined that the visible radiographic distance between the scaphoid and lunate decreases with increasing age as the carpal bones ossify (Fig. 42.4). The authors developed predictive equations for calculating the expected scapholunate interval based on age and gender. For males, the following equation was predictive of the scapholunate interval with y as the distance in millimeters [1] (Fig. 42.5):

$$y = -0.665(\text{age}) + 11.432$$

For females, the following equation was predictive:

$$y = -0.443(\text{age}) + 7.895$$

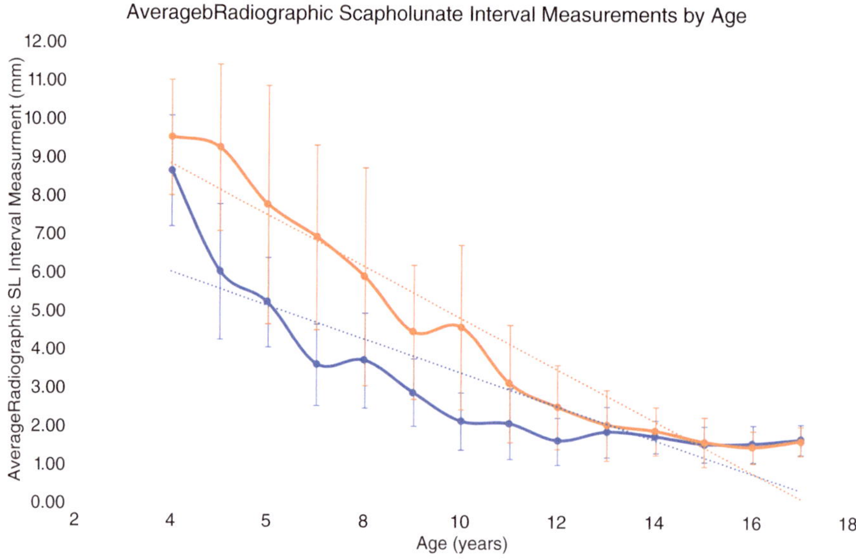

Fig. 42.5 Average radiographic scapholunate intervals based on chronological age and gender with linear regression model (dotted line). Male (orange) and female (blue). Adapted from Shaver et al. Hand 2023 [1]

Additionally, there are differences in scapholunate intervals even among gender, with females trending to have narrower scapholunate intervals at younger ages [1]. The scapholunate angle may be a more reliable indicator of scapholunate ligament injuries although younger patients may also have increased scapholunate angles [4, 5].

Comparison with contralateral radiographs and abnormal scapholunate angles may also provide an indicator of scapholunate ligament injuries [4, 5]. These factors must be considered when utilizing the scapholunate interval in the diagnosis of carpal instability.

Given the low incidence of carpal instability in the pediatric patient, treatment algorithms are largely modeled after treatment modalities used for adult carpal instability. A trial of immobilization and hand therapy without frank evidence of static instability is a reasonable first option as many patients will have resolution of pain [6]. In patients with static instability, intercarpal stability can be achieved with various methods including temporary fixation, direct ligament repair, and capsulodesis among others [7]. Kirschner wire fixation should be considered in the skeletally immature patient, and other hardware such as metal suture anchors or screws should be avoided to prevent interference with carpal growth [8]. Advanced imaging and diagnostic wrist arthroscopy may be beneficial for patients with chronic pain without definitive physical exam findings. When partial scapholunate ligamentous injuries are present (Geissler type II or III), arthroscopic debridement has been shown to be an effective therapy [7].

References

1. Shaver TB, Hogarth DA, Case AL, May CC, Abzug JM. Radiographic scapholunate interval in the pediatric population decreases in size as age increases. Hand (N Y). 2023:15589447231153166. https://doi.org/10.1177/15589447231153166.
2. Nguyen JC, Sheehan SE, Davis KW, Gill KG. Sports and the growing musculoskeletal system: sports imaging series. Radiology. 2017;284(1):25–42.
3. Megerle K, Pöhlmann S, Kloeters O, Germann G, Sauerbier M. The significance of conventional radiographic parameters in the diagnosis of scapholunate ligament lesions. Eur Radiol. 2011;21(1):176–81.
4. Joyce EA, Farrell T, McMorrow J, Mulholland D, Browne KM, Snow A. Are adult carpal angle measurements applicable to the pediatric population in the trauma setting? Skeletal Radiol. 2018;47(8):1151–6.
5. Sallam AA, Briffa N, Mahmoud SS, Imam MA. Normal wrist development in children and adolescents: a geometrical observational analysis based on plain radiographs. J Pediatr Orthop. 2020;40(9):e860–72.
6. Earp BE, Waters PM, Wyzykowski RJ. Arthroscopic treatment of partial scapholunate ligament tears in children with chronic wrist pain. J Bone Joint Surg Am. 2006;88(11):2448–55.
7. van Kampen RJ, Fox PM, Baltzer HL, Moran SL. Long-term outcomes following operative management of pediatric scapholunate ligament injuries. J Wrist Surg. 2022;12(1):56–62.
8. Zimmerman NB, Weiland AJ. Scapholunate dissociation in the skeletally immature carpus. J Hand Surg Am. 1990;15(5):701–5.

Suggested Readings

Earp BE, Waters PM, Wyzykowski RJ. Arthroscopic treatment of partial scapholunate ligament tears in children with chronic wrist pain. J Bone Joint Surg Am. 2006;88(11):2448–55.

Shaver TB, Hogarth DA, Case AL, May CC, Abzug JM. Radiographic scapholunate interval in the pediatric population decreases in size as age increases. Hand (N Y). 2023:15589447231153166. https://doi.org/10.1177/15589447231153166.

van Kampen RJ, Fox PM, Baltzer HL, Moran SL. Long-term outcomes following operative management of pediatric scapholunate ligament injuries. J Wrist Surg. 2022;12(1):56–62.

Index

Arthroscopic super-capsuloplasty
    advantage of minimal invasiveness, 155
    case report, 160
    indications, 155, 156
    innovative approach, 157
    open exposure techniques, 165
    open technique selection, 156
    postoperative care, 160
    risks and complications, 164
    skill and experience, 165
    stages of, 165
    tailored treatment approach, 156
    technique, 154, 157–159, 166
    untreated injuries, 153
    wrist anatomy and biomechanics, 153
Arthroscopic thermal capsulorrhaphy, 99
Arthroscopic thermal shrinkage
    case presentation, 95, 96
    history, 96, 97
    initial management, 98
    monopolar probes, 99
    MRI, 98
    non-surgical management, 99
    outcomes, 102
    pearls and pitfalls, 102, 103
    physical examination, 97
    plain radiographs, 98
    post-operatively patients, 101
    potential intercarpal instability, 99
    proximal portion, 101
    treatment, 99
Arthroscopic volar capsulodesis
    case presentation, 105
    diagnosis, 105, 106
    intra-operative arthroscopic images, 110
    management options, 106, 107
    open approach, 111
    outcome, 107, 111
    pearls/pitfalls, 110

B
Bilateral ulnar deviation supination stress
    test, 118
Biological circle, 225, 226
Blood vessels, 15
Bone-ligament-bone (BLB) reconstruction
    case presentation, 319
    diagnosis, 319, 320
    dorsal aspect, 325
    management, 320–322
    outcomes, 323
    palmar component, 325
    pearls/pitfalls, 324

Bone-retinaculum-bone autograft
    technique, 321

C
Calcium pyrophosphate deposition (CPPD), 38
Capitate
    carpal bones, 9
    resurfacing, 504
    shift, 426, 427
Capitolunate arthrodesis, 487
Capitolunate fusion, 487, 489
Capsular interposition, 474, 476, 478
Capsule, 154
Capsulodesis, 330
Capsulodesis with internal brace
    augmentation (CIBA)
    complication and treatment, 148, 149
    exposure, 143
    joint reduction and scapholunate ligament
        reconstruction, 143, 144
    optimal treatment strategy, 142
    outcomes, 147, 148
    pearls and pitfalls, 147
    post-operative rehabilitation, 145
    pre-operative planning, 142, 143
    techniques, 146, 147
    wound closure, 145
Carpal angles, 30
Carpal bones, 73, 155, 185
    blood vessels, 15
    capitate, 9
    dorsal radiocarpal, 12
    extrinsic carpal ligaments, 11
    hamate, 10
    intrinsic carpal ligaments, 13
    LTIL, 13
    lunate, 3
    median nerve, 14
    midcarpal ligaments, 12
    palmar radiocarpal, 11
    palmar ulnocarpal, 11
    pisiform, 5, 6
    scaphoid, 2
    SLIL, 13
    tendons, 14
    trapezium, 6, 7
    trapezoid, 8
    triangular fibrocartilage complex, 13
    triquetrum, 4
Carpal fractures, 118, 436
Carpal instability, 17, 18, 25, 410, 521, 531
    definition, 27
    dynamic and static forms, 27, 35

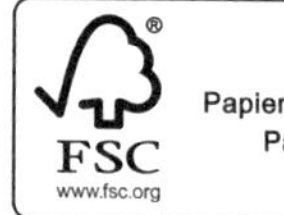

If you have any concerns about our products,
you can contact us on
ProductSafety@springernature.com

In case Publisher is established outside the EU,
the EU authorized representative is:
Springer Nature Customer Service Center GmbH
Europaplatz 3, 69115 Heidelberg, Germany

Printed by Libri Plureos GmbH
in Hamburg, Germany